Oral Pharmacology
for the Dental Hygienist

SECOND EDITION

Mea A. Weinberg, DMD, MSD, RPh
Cheryl M. Westphal Theile, RDH, EdD
New York University College of Dentistry

James Burke Fine, DDS
Columbia University College of Dental Medicine

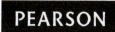

Boston   Columbus   Indianapolis   New York   San Francisco   Upper Saddle River
Amsterdam   Cape Town   Dubai   London   Madrid   Milan   Munich   Paris   Montreal   Toronto
Delhi   Mexico City   Sao Paulo   Sydney   Hong Kong   Seoul   Singapore   Taipei   Tokyo

Publisher: Julie Levin Alexander
Publisher's Assistant: Regina Bruno
Editor-in-Chief: Mark Cohen
Executive Editor: John Goucher
Assistant Editor: Nicole Ragonese
Director of Marketing: David Gesell
Executive Marketing Manager: Katrin Beacom
Marketing Coordinator: Michael Sirinides
Senior Managing Editor: Patrick Walsh
Project Manager: Christina Zingone-Luethje
Senior Operations Supervisor: Ilene Sanford
Operations Specialist: Lisa McDowell

Senior Art Director: Jayne Conte
Cover Designer: Bruce Kenselaar
Cover Art: Vitaly Korovin/shutterstock
Media Editor: Amy Peltier
Lead Media Project Manager: Lorena Cerisano
Full-Service Project Management: Bruce Hobart, Laserwords, Maine
Composition: Laserwords
Printer/Binder: LSC Communications
Cover Printer: LSC Communications
Text Font: Times Roman 10/12

Credits and acknowledgments for content borrowed from other sources and reproduced, with permission, in this textbook appear on appropriate page within text.

Library of Congress Cataloging-in-Publication Data

Weinberg, Mea A.
    Oral pharmacology for the dental hygienist / Mea A. Weinberg, Cheryl M. Westphal Theile, James Burke Fine.—2nd ed.
        p. ; cm.
    Includes bibliographical references and index.
    ISBN-13: 978-0-13-255992-8
    ISBN-10: 0-13-255992-7
    I. Theile, Cheryl M. Westphal. II. Fine, James Burke. III. Title.
    [DNLM: 1. Dentistry. 2. Pharmaceutical Preparations. 3. Dental Hygienists. 4. Drug Therapy—adverse effects. 5. Pharmacology. QV 50]
    LC Classification not assigned
    615'.10246176—dc23

2011040529

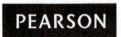

ISBN 10:   0-13-255992-7
ISBN 13:   978-0-13-255992-8

24 2022

Contents

Preface   *xiv*

Contributors   *xv*

Reviewers   *xvi*

Chapter 1 Introduction to Clinical Pharmacology   1

Introduction   2

Terminology   2

Pharmacology: The Dental Hygiene Process of Care   2

Sources of Drug Information   2

  Printed Resources   2

  Computer Resources   4

  Online Resources   4

Regulation and Classification of Drugs   4

  Development of New Drugs and Drug Safety   4

  Labeling Requirements for Over-the-Counter Drugs   5

Stages of Approval for Therapeutic and Biologic Drugs   6

  Phases of Clinical Human Studies   7

Drug Names and Properties   8

  Chemical/Generic/Trade Drug Names   8

Dental Hygiene Applications   8

Introduction   9

  Goals of Prescription Writing   9

Parts of the Prescription   9

  Units of Measurement   9

  Latin Abbreviations   10

Prescription and Nonprescription Drugs   11

Scheduled Drugs   11

Drug Container and Package Insert   12

Black Box Warning   13

Labeled and Off-Label Uses of Drugs   13

Bioequivalence and Bioavailability: Generic Drug Substitution   14

Other Factors Associated with Prescription Writing   15

  Safety of Prescription Pads   15

  Patient Adherence   15

  How to Reduce Medication Errors   15

Guidance in Prescribing   15

  Prescribing for Children   15

  Safety in Pregnancy   15

Dental Hygiene Applications   16

Key Points   16
Board Review Questions   16
Selected References   17
Web Sites   17

Chapter 2   Fundamentals of Drug Action   18
Routes of Drug Administration   19
　Enteral Administration   19
　Parenteral Administration   19
　Topical Administration   21
Pharmacokinetics   21
　Absorption   21
　Distribution   28
　Drug Elimination   29
　Drug Administration   31
Pharmacodynamics   33
　Drug–Receptor Interaction   33
　Drug Classifications in the Drug–Receptor Complex   34
　Dose–Response Relationships   34
　Potency, Efficacy, and the Ceiling Effect   35
　Toxicity   35
Drug Effects   35
Drug Interactions   37
　Factors That Modify the Effects of Drugs   37
　Placebo Response   38
Dental Hygiene Applications   38
Key Points   39
Board Review Questions   39
Selected References   40
Web Sites   40

Chapter 3   Autonomic Nervous System Drugs   41
Introduction   42
The Nervous System   42
　Nerve Cell Anatomy   42
Functions of the Autonomic Nervous System: Neurotransmitters
　and Receptors   44
　Sympathetic Nervous System (Adrenergic): Neurotransmitters   44
　Sympathetic Nervous System: Adrenergic Receptors   44
　Parasympathetic Neurotransmitters and Receptors   48
　Other Types of Neurotransmitters and Receptors   48
Autonomic Drugs   48
Sympathomimetic Drugs: Drugs Affecting Sympathetic
　Transmission   48
Adrenergic (Sympathetic) Agonists   48
　Direct-Acting Adrenergic Receptor Agonists   50
　Indirect-Acting Agonists   51
　Mixed-Acting Adrenergic Receptor Agonists   51
　Therapeutic Uses of Sympathetic Agonists   51
　Adverse Effects   51
　Drug Interactions   51

Adrenergic Receptor Antagonists   51
α_1-Adrenergic Receptor Antagonists (Blockers)   52
β-Adrenergic Receptor Antagonists   53
Indirect-Acting Adrenergic Antagonists   53
Adverse Effects of Adrenergic Blockers   53
Drug Interactions   53
Drugs Affecting Cholinergic Transmission   53
Parasympathomimetic Drugs   53
Anticholinergic Drugs   55
Dental Hygiene Applications   56
Key Points   57
Board Review Questions   58
Selected References   58
Web Sites   59
Quick Drug Guide   60

Chapter 4   **Local Anesthetics   62**
Introduction   63
History   63
Properties of Local Anesthetics   63
Chemical Properties   63
Mechanism of Action   63
Effects of pH   63
Metabolism and Excretion   64
Local Anesthetic Agents   64
Lidocaine   64
Mepivacaine   65
Prilocaine   66
Articaine   67
Bupivacaine   67
Etidocaine   67
Topical Anesthetics   67
Vasoconstrictors in Local Anesthetics   67
Epinephrine   68
Levonordefrin   68
Clinical Calculations   68
Special Patient Populations   68
Children   68
Pregnant and Nursing Women   68
Older Adults   68
Adverse Effects of Local Anesthetics   68
Allergic Reactions   68
Central Nervous System   69
Blood Disorders   69
Liver Disease   70
Treatment of Toxicity   70
Selection of the Local Anesthetic   70
Dental Management of Medically Compromised Patients   70
Diseases and Disorders   70
Drugs   71
Dental Hygiene Applications   71
Key Points   72

Board Review Questions 72
Selected References 72
Web Sites 73
Quick Drug Guide 74

Chapter 5 Sedation and General Anesthestics 75
Introduction 76
Terminology 76
Routes of Administration 76
Types of Anesthesia 76
Therapeutic Uses 76
Patient Physical Status Classification 77
Moderate Sedation in the Dental Office 77
IV/Oral/Inhalational Agents for Moderate Sedation 77
    Anti-Anxiety Agents: Benzodiazepines 78
    Sedative/Hypnotics: Barbiturates 78
    Sedative/Hypnotics: Nonbarbiturates 78
    Others 79
Monitoring 79
Nitrous Oxide 79
    Properties and Indications: Nitrous Oxide 79
    Pharmacokinetics 79
    Method of Administration 80
    Adverse Effects 80
    Contraindications 80
    Occupational Exposure 80
    Abuse of Nitrous Oxide 80
General Anesthesia 81
    History 81
    Indications 81
    Stages 81
    Classification and Chemistry 82
    Inhalational Anesthetics 82
    Injectable Anesthetics for General Anesthesia 83
    Postoperative Problems: General Anesthesia 83
Dental Hygiene Applications 84
Key Points 84
Board Review Questions 84
Selected References 85
Web Sites 85
Quick Drug Guide 86

Chapter 6 Drugs for Pain Control 87
Introduction 88
Neurophysiology of Pain 88
    Pain Components 88
    Types of Pain 88
Drug Therapy for Dental Pain 88
    Nonnarcotic Analgesics 88
Nonnarcotic Analgesics 91
    Salicylates 91
    Other Salicylate-Like Drugs 94

Nonsteroidal Anti-Inflammatory Drugs   94
    Ibuprofen and Ibuprofen-Like Drugs   94
    Selective COX-2 Inhibitors   96
    Acetaminophen   96
Opioid Analgesics   97
    Introduction   97
    Mechanism of Action   97
    Pharmacokinetics   98
    Classification   98
    Opioid Agonists: Strong Potency   98
    Opioid Agonists: Moderate Potency   100
    Other Agonists   100
    Mixed Agonist/Antagonists   100
    Antagonists   100
    Combination Narcotic Analgesic and Nonnarcotic Analgesic   101
Substance Abuse and Dependency   101
    Recognizing Drug Abuse Patients   101
Dental Hygiene Applications   102
Key Points   104
Board Review Questions   105
Selected References   106
Web Sites   106
Quick Drug Guide   107

Chapter 7   **Antibacterial Agents   110**
Antimicrobial Agents   111
    Antimicrobial Activity   111
    Adverse Effects   111
Bactericidal Antibiotics: Inhibitors of Bacterial Cell Wall
    Synthesis   113
    Penicillins   113
    Cephalosporins   116
    Nitroimadazoles   117
    Quinolones (Fluoroquinolones)   117
Bacteriostatic Antibiotics   118
    Macrolides   118
    Lincomycins   119
    Tetracyclines   120
Miscellaneous Antibiotics   121
    Sulfonamides   121
    Vancomycin   124
    Aminoglycosides   124
Prevention of Infective Endocarditis   124
    Dental Hygiene Applications   127
Antibacterial Agents: Topical   127
    Oral Rinses   127
Controlled (Sustained)-Release Drug Delivery   131
    Resorbable Controlled (Sustained)-Release Devices   131
    Dental Hygiene Applications   132
Key Points   132
Tuberculosis   132
    Testing for Tuberculosis   132

Pharmacology: Treatment of TB Infection   133
Latent Tuberculosis Infection (Prophylaxis)   133
Treatment of Active Tuberculosis   134
Special Situations   134
Dental Hygiene Applications   134
Key Points   134
Board Review Questions   134
Selected References   136
Web Sites   136
Quick Drug Guide   137

Chapter 8   Antiviral and Antifungal Agents   139
Introduction   140
Antivirals for Herpes Simplex   140
Primary Herpes Infection and Treatment   140
Recurrent Herpes Infection and Treatment   140
Antiretroviral Agents: HIV/AIDS   142
Diagnosis   145
Antiretroviral Pharmacology   145
Antiretroviral Drugs   145
Pharmacological Treatment of Systemic Opportunistic Infections   145
Pharmacological Treatment of Oral Opportunistic Lesions/ Conditions   145
Dental Hygiene Applications   146
Key Points   148
Antifungal Agents   148
Mycosis   148
Drug Interactions   152
Subcutaneous and Systemic Mycosis   152
Dental Hygiene Applications   152
Key Points   153
Board Review Questions   153
Selected References   154
Web Sites   154
Quick Drug Guide   155

Chapter 9   Antineoplastic, Immunosuppressant, and Bisphosphonate Drugs   156
Antineoplastic Drugs   157
Actions   157
Treatment   158
Adverse Effects   158
Limitations to Dental Treatment   160
Bisphosphonates   160
Hypercalcemia of Malignancy   160
Immunosuppressant Drugs   160
Dental Hygiene Applications   161
Key Points   161
Board Review Questions   161
Selected References   162

Web Sites   162
Quick Drug Guide   163

Chapter 10   Fluorides   165
Chemical Composition   166
Pharmacokinetics   166
Sources   166
Uses   166
Deliveries   167
Systemics   167
    Community Water Fluoridation   167
    School Fluoridation   167
    Prescriptions and Supplements   168
    Naturally Fluoridated Water   168
    Fluorosis   168
Topicals   168
    Self-Applied Dentifrices   169
    Mouthrinses   170
    Brush-On Gels   170
    Professionally Applied Fluoride   170
Choosing Treatment Methods   170
Toxicology   171
Dental Hygiene Applications   171
Key Points   171
Board Review Questions   172
Selected References   172
Web Sites   172
Quick Drug Guide   173

Chapter 11   Cardiovascular Drugs   174
Introduction   175
Hypertension   175
    Pathogenesis   175
    Treatment   175
    Pharmacotherapy   181
    Dental Hygiene Applications   185
Angina Pectoris   185
    Pathogenesis   185
    Pharmacotherapy/Treatment   186
    Dental Hygiene Applications   188
Heart Failure   188
    Pharmacotherapy   188
    Dental Hygiene Applications   191
Arrhythmias   191
    Dental Hygiene Applications   192
Epinephrine in Cardiac Patients   192
Lipid-Lowering Drugs   193
HMG-CoA Reductase Inhibitors (Statin Drugs)   193
Bile Acid Sequestrants   194
Fibric Acid Drugs   194
Natural Products   194

Nicotinic Acid   194
Vitamin E   195
Coenzyme Q10   196
Other Drugs   196
Combination Drugs   197
Dental Hygiene Applications   197
Thrombolytic Drugs   197
Indications   197
Dental Management of Patients on Warfarin   197
Adverse Effects   198
Drug Interactions   198
Low-Dose Heparins   199
Hematopoeitic Drugs   199
Dental Hygiene Applications   199
Key Points   199
Board Review Questions   199
Selected References   200
Quick Drug Guide   201

Chapter 12   Gastrointestinal Drugs   204
Introduction   205
Peptic Ulcer Disorders   205
Peptic-Ulcer Disease   205
Gastroesophageal Reflux Disease (GERD)   206
Summary of Treatment Guidelines for PUD and GERD   210
Irritable Bowel Syndrome   210
Pharmacotherapy   211
Nausea and Vomiting   211
Constipation   211
Pharmacotherapy   211
Diarrhea   211
Antibiotic-Associated Diarrhea   212
Treatment of Acute Diarrhea (Other than Antibiotic-Associated Diarrhea)   212
Inflammatory Bowel Disease: Ulcerative Colitis   212
Dental Hygiene Applications   213
Key Points   213
Board Review Questions   213
Selected References   214
Web Sites   214
Quick Drug Guide   215

Chapter 13   Respiratory Drugs   216
Introduction   217
Lung Anatomy   217
Pathogenesis/Diagnosis: Asthma   217
Pharmacotherapy: Controlling Asthma   219
Classification of Medications   219
Severity and Control: Basis of Drug Therapy   219
COPD (Bronchitis/Emphysema) Treatment   224
Drugs for Cold   225
Antihistamines   226

α-Adrenoceptor Agonists (Nasal Decongestants) 226
Topical (Intranasal) Corticosteroids 227
Anticholinergic Agents 227
Drugs for Cough 227
Expectorants 227
Dental Hygiene Applications 227
Key Points 228
Board Review Questions 228
Selected References 229
Web Sites 229
Quick Drug Guide 230

Chapter 14 **Neurological Drugs** **232**
Epilepsy 233
Pathophysiology 233
Anti-epileptic Drug Therapy 233
Dental Hygiene Applications 236
Parkinson's Disease 236
Clinical Presentation 236
Pathophysiology 236
Drug-Induced Parkinsonism 237
Pharmacological Treatment 237
Dental Hygiene Applications 239
Alzheimer's Disease 239
Headache 239
Migraine 239
Medication-Overuse Headaches 240
Drug Therapy 240
Alternative Treatments 241
Dental Hygiene Applications 242
Key Points 242
Board Review Questions 242
Selected References 242
Web Sites 243
Quick Drug Guide 244

Chapter 15 **Psychiatric Drugs** **246**
Introduction 247
Basic Pharmacology 247
Antipsychotic Drugs 247
Dopamine Receptors 247
Medications 248
Adverse Effects 248
Types of Antipsychotics 249
Drug Interactions of Dental Significance 249
Drugs for Mood Disorders 250
Depression 250
Bipolar Disorders (BPD) 255
Anxiolytics (Anti-Anxiety Agents) 258
Pharmacology 258
Sedative/Hypnotic Drugs 259
Barbiturates 259

Attention-Deficit/Hyperactivity Disorder (ADHD)   260
Use of Anti-Anxiety Drugs in the Dental Office   261
 Anxious Dental Patient   261
 Bruxism   261
Dental Hygiene Applications   262
Key Points   263
Board Review Questions   263
Selected References   264
Web Sites   264
Quick Drug Guide   265

Chapter 16   Endocrine and Hormonal Drugs   267
Diabetes Mellitus   268
 Type 1   268
 Type 2   268
 Insulin Resistance: Type 2 Diabetic   268
 Diagnosis   269
 Complications   270
 Control and Management   270
 Pharmacology   271
 Insulin Pharmacology: History   272
 Insulin Secretion and Absorption   273
 Goal of Insulin Therapy   273
 Insulin Regimen   273
Formulations   273
 Recombinant Human Insulin Preparations   273
 Mixing Insulin Preparations and Premixed Insulin Preparations   274
 Insulin Delivery Devices   274
 Newest Insulin Formulation   274
 Adverse Effects   274
Dental Hygiene Applications   275
Thyroid Drugs   275
 Thyroid Gland Hormones   275
 Pharmacology: Antithyroid Drugs   275
 Pharmacology: Hypothyroidism   276
 Dental Hygiene Applications   277
Adrenal (Steroid) Hormones   277
 Adrenal Glands   277
 Systemic Adrenocortical Steroids   278
 Topical Corticosteroids   280
Dental Hygiene Applications   280
Sex Hormones and Contraceptives   281
 Estrogens   282
 Nonsteroidal Estrogens   282
 Anti-Estrogens   282
 Progestins   282
 Progestin Inhibitors   284
 Estrogen/Hormonal Replacement Therapy   284
 Oral Contraceptives   284
 Drug Interactions: Sex Hormones   285
 Male Sex Hormones: Androgens and Anabolic Steroids   285
Bisphosphonates/Osteoporosis   285

Indications   285
Classification of Bisphosphonates   285
General Pharmacology: Osteoporosis   285
Risk Factors   286
Clinical Presentation   286
Management   286
Dental Hygiene Applications: Bisphosphonates   286
Dental Hygiene Applications   287
Key Points   287
Board Review Questions   287
Selected References   289
Web Sites   289
Quick Drug Guide   290

Chapter 17   Herbal and Natural Remedies   293
Homeopathy and Natural Products   294
Safety Concerns   294
Active Ingredients   294
Adverse Effects   296
Dental Implications   296
Dental Hygiene Applications   296
Key Points   297
Board Review Questions   297
Selected References   297
Web Sites   297

Glossary 299

Appendices

A Pregnancy and Breast Feeding 307

B Drug Interactions in Dentistry 309

C Adverse Effects of Common Medications Dental Patients Are Taking 316

Case Studies, Answers, and Explanations 318

Answers to Board Review Questions 322

Index 324

Preface

There is a significant amount of information about pharmacology in the medical/dental field of which it is important for the student and dental clinician to be cognizant. Pharmacology stands alone as a basic science but application of this information to dentistry must be applied to clinical settings to allow for the management of certain medical/dental conditions. This textbook studies the principles of pharmacology and their application to dental hygiene practice. With this second edition, we have maintained those attributes while adding more information on the dental management of patients taking the more commonly prescribed drugs.

This textbook was written to (1) help students understand the fundamentals of pharmacology, (2) understand about the different medications their dental patient is taking, (3) show that many medications have oral adverse effects, and (4) show there is a connection among medicine, pharmacology, and dentistry.

Oral Pharmacology for the Dental Hygienist reviews the basic concepts of pharmacology. Within most chapters are boxed-in "Patient Guidelines" sections that pertain to a specific drug that has oral adverse effects and explains how the patient can be instructed in how to maintain optimum oral health while taking that drug. "Rapid Dental Hints" remind students about key information or a task that should be performed related to the topic discussed. Additionally, there are Fun Facts found within many chapters that provide whimsical information about the disease or medications. "Quick Drug Guides" at the end of each chapter provide an easy reference to the drugs discussed within the chapter. Special sections on dental drug–drug interactions and prescriptions for common dental conditions are included. Trade names of drugs are in parentheses following the generic name. The extensive glossary should be used while reading the chapters.

The lastest information on treatment of patients on bisphosphonates and antibiotic prophylaxis of patients with total joint replacement is discussed.

We hope this book will serve as a helpful text for all dental practitioners.

Mea A. Weinberg, DMD, MSD, RPh

Cheryl M. Westphal Theile, RDH, EdD

James Burke Fine, DDS

Contributors

Elvir Dincer, DDS
Assistant Professor
Department of Dental Hygiene
Eugenio Maria de Hostos Community College of The City University New York
Bronx, New York
(Chapter 10: Fluorides)

Hana Hassan, DDS
Clinical Assistant Professor
Department of Periodontology and Implant Dentistry
New York University College of Dentistry
(Chapter 7: Antibacterial Agents)

Adrienne Lynn Ligouri, BSBE, MD, MPH
Mt. Sinai School of Medicine
New York, New York
(Chapter 10: Fluorides)

Gail Malone RDH, BS
Clinical Educator Northeast
DENTSPLY Professional
(Chapter 4: Local Anesthetics)

Robert S. Schoor, DDS
Associate Professor
Director of Postgraduate Periodontics
Department of Periodontology and Implant Dentistry
New York University College of Dentistry
New York, New York
(Chapter 5: Sedation and General Anesthetics)

Reviewers

Luis E. Arzola, DMD
Catawba Valley Community College
Hickory, North Carolina

Barbara L. Bennett, CDA, RDH
Texas State Technical College
Harlingen, Texas

Eileen Alice Derr CDA, RDH, MPA
Concorde Career College, Garden Grove
Garden Grove, California

Elvir Dincer, DDS
Hostos Community College
Bronx, New York

Marie V. Gillis, RDH, MS
Fortis Colleges
Washington, DC

Gwen Grosso, RDH
University of New Haven
West Haven, Connecticut

Stephen Holliday, DDS
Sinclair Community College
Dayton, Ohio

Barbara Lacher, BS
North Dakota State College of Science
Wahpeton, North Dakota

Elizabeth A. Riccio, DDS
Hudson Valley Community College
Troy, New York

Sandy Roe, RDH, MS
Concorde Career College
Kansas City, Missouri

Joan M. Tischler, RDH, MS
Cuyahoga Community College
Cleveland, Ohio

Angel L. Pazurek Tork, RDH, MEd
Western Technical College
Wisconsin Rapids, Wisconsin

Thomas A. Viola, RPh, CCP
Burlington County College
Burlington, New Jersey

Introduction to Clinical Pharmacology

EDUCATIONAL OBJECTIVES

After reading this chapter, the reader should be able to:

1. Describe the role of pharmacology in the dental hygiene process of care.
2. List and utilize the various online and computer drug references.
3. Discuss various federal drug laws and their impact on drug regulation.
4. Identify the various parts of a written prescription.
5. Discuss how to avoid errors in prescription writing.
6. Discuss the concept of generic substitution.

GOAL

To introduce the basic concepts of pharmacology upon which the practice of dental pharmacotherapeutics is based and to familiarize the student with various pharmacology terminologies.

KEY TERMS

Pharmacology

Pharmacology references

Drug laws

Food and Drug Administration

Prescription

Prescription drugs

Over-the-counter (OTC) drugs

Bioequivalence

Medication errors

Introduction

Although the history of pharmacology goes back only a few hundred years, medicines derived from plants, animals, and minerals have been used to treat diseases for thousands of years. Until the end of the nineteenth century, most medicines came from naturally occurring fresh plants including herbs and flowers. For example, morphine is derived from the poppy flower, and marijuana from the cannabis plant. Although these medicaments may have a therapeutic or healing effect, many substances exert a toxic effect.

Drug development has grown substantially since ancient times. Today, most drugs are no longer naturally derived but are made synthetically in laboratories; however, substances with complex structures may still be obtained from various sources. For example, cardiac glycosides used in the treatment of heart failure are derived from the *digitalis purpurea* (foxglove) plant, heparin (inhibits blood clotting; an anticoagulant) is derived from animal tissues, and insulin from gene technology. Herbal medicines such as kava, garlic, and dong quai, although not regulated by the government, are derived from plants.

> **DID YOU KNOW?**
>
> Raw opium is taken from the poppy flower and processed into codeine and morphine.

Terminology

Pharmacology is defined as the biomedical study of the interaction of chemical substances with living systems, including cells, tissues, and organisms. The term pharmacology is derived from the Greek words *pharmakos,* which means "drug," "medicine," or "poison"; and *logos,* which means "study." The subject of pharmacology is an expansive topic that ranges from how drugs enter and travel throughout the body to the responses they produce. *Drugs* are substances or chemical agents that affect biological or living systems that *do not create new physiological responses;* rather, they alter normal processes either by stimulating (increasing) or by depressing (decreasing) the function of the cell. While most drugs today are synthetic, *biologics* are agents that are naturally produced in an animal or human body. Examples of biologics are vaccines, blood and blood components, antibodies, and interferon. *Alternative drug therapy* includes herbs, vitamins, minerals, dietary supplements, and natural extracts.

There are five major subgroups of pharmacology: pharmacokinetics, pharmacodynamics, pharmacotherapeutics, pharmacogenetics, and toxicology.

Pharmacokinetics describes the way the body affects the drug including absorption, distribution, metabolism, and excretion. *Pharmacodynamics* is the action a drug has on a specific target of action in the body, including the drug's mechanism of action, receptor interactions, dose–response relationship, and therapeutic and toxic reactions. *Posology* is the study of the dosages of medicines and drugs. *Therapeutics* is the branch of medicine that deals with the treatment of disease. Drugs are used to prevent, diagnose, and treat diseases. *Pharmacotherapeutics* describes the study of how drugs may best be used in the treatment of diseases. For dental professionals, the fields of pharmacology and therapeutics are connected. *Pharmacogenetics* is the convergence of pharmacology and genetics that deals with genetic factors that influence an organism's response to a drug. For example, some individuals are termed "slow acetylators" and "fast acetylators," relating to the breakdown of an antituberculosis drug called isoniazid (INH). This is a form of genetic variation where some people cannot break down this drug as fast as others. The terms pharmacogenomics and pharmacogenetics are used interchangeably. *Toxicology* is the scientific study of poisons, chemical pollutants, and the undesirable effects of drugs on living cells, tissues, and organisms. A poison is any substance detrimental to health that may result in incapacitation, illness (e.g., cancer), or death.

Pharmacology: The Dental Hygiene Process of Care

Many new classifications of drugs have been introduced in the last decade. Over 1.5 billion prescriptions are filled annually in the United States. The majority of older adults take multiple medications, which is referred to as polypharmacy. The dental hygienist in the dental hygiene process of care begins with assessment of all medications the patient is currently taking and considers drugs that might be prescribed in the course of treatment. The names, dosages, mechanisms of action, and interactions with other drugs and herbal supplements are all critical in planning the treatment phase of dental hygiene care. The medical history must be reviewed at each visit to confirm the proper drug dosage regimen or indicate any changes in medications or drug interactions. In planned care, the prognosis and diagnosis given the drug history is taken into consideration. Certain medications' effects on oral tissue may affect the planned outcome of dental hygiene care. Risk assessment will include side effects of the medications or possible emergency situations. Implementation of educational and therapeutic services requires knowledge of the prescription and over-the-counter therapies available to the dental hygienist. Use of fluorides, analgesics, chemotherapeutics, local anesthetics, and nitrous oxide require full understanding of the pharmacological effects of these products/drugs.

Rapid Dental Hint

If a medical consultation is required from your patient's physician, be sure that the patient is getting it from the physician who is taking care of that condition.

Sources of Drug Information

Printed Resources

Many books and journals are available for **pharmacology references.** Table 1-1 lists selected sources. It should be noted that

TABLE 1-1   Selective Resources for Pharmacology

DENTAL DRUG REFERENCES	MEDICAL/PHARMACY DRUG REFERENCES	JOURNALS (NOT ALL ARE LISTED):	WEB SITES	NEWSLETTERS
ADA Guide to Dental Thera-peutics (American Dental Association)	*American Hospital Formulary Service (AHFS) Drug Information*	*U.S. Pharmacist*	www.epocrates.com	*The Medical Letter*
Dental Drug Reference with Clinical Implications (Lip-pincott Williams & Wilkins)	*Remington's Pharmaceutical Sciences*	*Drug Topics*	www.medscape.com	www.medletter.com
		Pharmacy Times	www.pdr.net	
	Physicians' Drug Reference (PDR)	*Hospital Pharmacy*	www.nursepdr.com	
Drug Information Handbook (LEXI-COMP)	*PDR® Pharmacopoeia Pocket Dosing Guide*	*Journal of the American Pharmacists Association*	www.rxlist.com	
Mosby's Dental Drug Reference	*United States Pharmacopeia Drug Information (USP DI)*	*Journal of Clinical Pharmacology*	www.uspharmacist.com	
		Journal of Clinical Pharmacy and Therapeutics	www.fda.gov/medwatch	
	Handbook of Nonprescription Drugs (American Pharmaceutical Association)	*Journal of Clinical Psychopharmacology*	www.nhlbi.nih.gov/ guidelines/index.htm	
		Journal of Pharmacokinetics and Pharmacodynamics	www.ashp.org	
	Tarascon Pocket Pharmacopoeia	*Journal of Pharmacy and Pharmacology*	www.nlm.nih.gov/ medlineplus/	
	Drug Facts and Comparison	*Journal of Pharmacy Practice and Research*	www.druginteraction. com	
	Merck Manual	*Pharmacogenetics and Genomics*	www.drugdigest.com	
		Pharmacological Reviews	www.drugs.com	
		Pharmacoepidemiology and Drug Safety		
		Therapeutic Drug Monitoring		
		World of Drug Information		

all information available online should be viewed with caution; only reputable Web sites should be used.

Many publications are updated monthly or yearly; however, many are not and may not contain the latest medications. Some popular printed text information include the *USP DI* (Thomson Publishing Corporation), *Drug Facts and Comparison* (Wolters Kluwer Health Company), and *AHFS Drug Information* (American Hospital Formulary Service). The *PDR®* (*Physicians' Desk Reference;* Thomson PDR, Montvale, NJ; www.pdr.net) is written in cooperation with participating drug manufacturers and the U.S. Food and Drug Administration (FDA), and is published annually. Other clinical information products from *PDR®* include the *PDR® Monthly Prescribing Guide™,* the mobile *PDR®,* the *PDR® Pharmacopoeia Pocket Dosing Guide,* the *PDR® for Nutritional Supplements,* the *PDR® for Herbal Medicines,* and the *PDR® Guide to Drug Interactions, Side Effects, and Indications.*

Dental drug resources, including the *ADA Guide to Dental Therapeutics,* the *Drug Information Handbook* (Lexi-Comp), and *Mosby's Dental Drug Reference,* are listed in Table 1-1.

Rapid Dental Hint

Remember to have some type of drug reference book or electronic device with you in the clinic or office for quick reference.

Computer Resources

Personal digital assistants (PDAs), which are handheld computer devices, are rapidly becoming popular for recording and storing patient information, calculating appropriate drug doses, and providing databases of medication information.

There are many software resources that are available, including MedTeach (American Society of Health System Pharmacists), Epocrates (http://www.epocrates.com), and MedFacts (http://medfacts.info.com), that can be uploaded on the computer or PDAs such as the Palm Pilot.

Additionally, over the past years many textbooks and reference books have included CD-ROMs, which can store a lot of information that complements the written material.

Online Resources

Journals provide the most recent information on medications and therapies. Over 3,000 domestic and international journals and scientific literature are available online at http://www.medline.com and http://www.pubmed.com. Medscape (www.medscape.com) is a medically and pharmaceutically based Web site that offers up to date information on medicine and pharmacology. Other Web sites are listed in Table 1-1.

Regulation and Classification of Drugs

Development of New Drugs and Drug Safety

Until the nineteenth century, there were few standards or guidelines to protect the public from drug misuse. In those days there were many medicinal concoctions that, although nontoxic, were not effective. Early drug remedies included heroin for asthma and coughs and rattlesnake oil for rheumatism. Codeine use started in the late nineteenth century and with that started the problem of addiction to these home remedies.

In 1820, the *U.S. Pharmacopoeia* (*USP*) was the first publication of drug standards in the United States. The USP listed the standards of drug purity and strength and directions for synthesis of all drugs. In 1975, the USP and the *National Formulary (NF),* published by the American Pharmaceutical Association (APhA), became one publication, the *U.S. Pharmacopoeia-National Formulary (USP-NF),* which is still published with regular updates. The USP label is found on many medication containers verifying the exact ingredients found within the container.

In the early 1900s, the United States started to develop and enforce tougher **drug laws** to protect the public from deceitful and unsafe methods practiced by medicine manufacturers. From this developed the first federal Food and Drug Act, signed into law by President Theodore Roosevelt in 1906. The act was amended in 1912, and an even stronger Food, Drug, and Cosmetic Act passed in 1938.

DID YOU KNOW?

In 1202, King John of England proclaimed the first English food law, the Assize of Bread, which prohibited adulteration of bread with such ingredients as ground peas or beans.

The United States Federal Food, Drug, and Cosmetic Act (FD&C) was a set of laws passed by Congress in 1938 that gave authority to the **Food and Drug Administration** (FDA) to regulate the safety of food, drugs, and cosmetics. These laws required drug labeling to include a list of ingredients and prohibited manufacturers from making false and misleading claims. For example, Dr. Flint's Quaker Bitters was a vegetable remedy for dyspepsia, constipation, sick headache, dizziness, and "low spirit." It was claimed that Bromoseltzer would cure all headaches (Figure 1-1). Refer to http://americanhistory.si.edu/collections/group_detail.cfm (National Museum of American History, Washington, DC).

From 1906 to 1918 manufacturers could label their products with the "guarantee" that their medicine complied with the new food and drug law (Figure 1-2). The 1906 law required manufacturers to label their products if any contained alcohol, cocaine, heroin, morphine, opium, cannabis, chloroform, or chloral hydrate (Figure 1-3). A complete listing of all ingredients was not required until 1938.

In 1968, the Electronic Product Radiation Control provisions were added to the FD&C. There are nine FD&C certified color additives used in foods in the United States and many

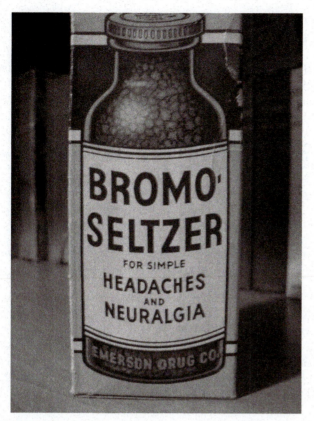

FIGURE 1-1 Early claims of relieving headaches with Bromo-Seltzer.

D&C color additives used only in drugs or cosmetics. The FD&C made the certification of food color additives mandatory (e.g., FD&C Yellow No. 5). Since 1938, there have been many amendments to the federal Food, Drug, and Cosmetic Act. Some amendments include:

Infant Formula Act, 1980

Orphan Drug Act, 1983

Drug Price Competition and Patent Term Restoration Act, 1984

Prescription Drug Marketing Act, 1987

Prescription Drug User Fee Act, 1992

Dietary Supplement Health and Education Act, 1994

Food and Drug Administration Modernization Act (FDAMA), 1997

Food Allergen Labeling and Consumer Protection Act, 2004

RDH

Rapid Dental Hint

FD&C Red No. 3 is erythrosine (tetraiodofluorescein), which is a cherry-red synthetic coal-based fluorine dye added to plaque-disclosing solutions/tablets. Question your patients regarding allergy to erythrosine.

DID YOU KNOW?

The first federal biologics law, which addressed the provision of reliable smallpox vaccine to citizens, was passed in 1813.

Labeling Requirements for Over-the-Counter Drugs

Over-the-counter (OTC) drug package labeling is required (Code of Federal Regulations) to have "drug facts" labeling appear on the outside container or wrapper of the retail package, or if there is no outside container, on all surfaces of the immediate container or wrapper. This labeling is intended to help the consumer understand how to use the product. The "drug fact" labeling (Figure 1-4)

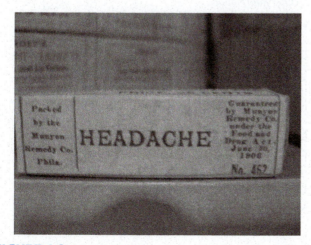

FIGURE 1-2 This headache remedy was "guaranteed" by the drug company; 1906.

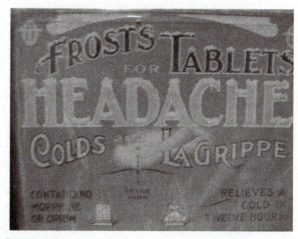

FIGURE 1-3 Tablets for headaches; it says on the label that it does not contain morphine or opium.

contains the following: active ingredient(s), purpose, use(s), warning(s), allergy alert, do not use, directions, other information, inactive ingredients, and questions or comments (with phone numbers).

Stages of Approval for Therapeutic and Biologic Drugs

All new drugs and biologics must first undergo rigid studies in animals and humans before gaining approval for use by the public. The Prescription Drug User Fee Act (PDUFA), first enacted in 1992, was designed to make the drug approval process faster and more efficient by providing the FDA with more funding through user fees from drug sponsors; however, income from the PDUFA is restricted to use for preapproval activities and not for postmarket monitoring.

Therapeutic drugs and biologics are reviewed in four different steps: preclinical investigations, clinical investigations, review of new drug applications (NDA), and postmarketing surveillance.

DID YOU KNOW?

Dental manufacturers must get FDA approval for the safety and efficacy of a therapeutic agent, such as fluoride, in their products before they can be released to the market.

DID YOU KNOW?

The Federal Trade Commission regulates the label on the juice you drink for breakfast, the cosmetics you apply, and the contact lenses you place in your eyes.

Preclinical investigations must be performed before clinical studies are done on humans. Extensive laboratory research is performed on animals and human and microbial cells cultured in the laboratory. Generally, two or more species (one rodent, one nonrodent) are tested because a drug may affect one species differently from another. Results must be submitted to the FDA before phase 1 clinical trials begin.

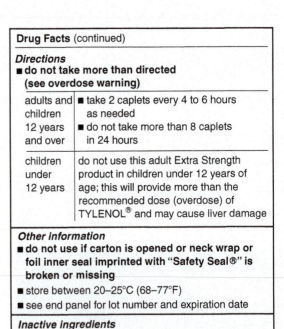

Drug Facts

Active ingredient (in each caplet)	Purpose
Acetaminophen 500 mg... Pain reliever/fever reducer	

Uses temporarily relieves minor aches and pains due to:
- headache
- muscular aches
- backache
- arthritis
- the common cold
- toothache
- menstrual cramps
- temporarily reduces fever

Warnings
Alcohol warning: If you consume 3 or more alcoholic drinks every day, ask your doctor whether you should take acetaminophen or other pain relievers/fever reducers. Acetaminophen may cause liver damage.

Do not use
- with any other product containing acetaminophen

Stop use and ask a doctor if
- new symptoms occur
- redness or swelling is present
- pain gets worse or lasts for more than 10 days
- fever gets worse or lasts for more than 3 days

If pregnant or breast-feeding, ask a health professional before use.
Keep out of reach of children.
Overdose warning: Taking more than the recommended dose (overdose) may cause liver damage. In case of overdose, get medical help or contact a Poison Control Center right away. Quick medical attention is critical for adults as well as for children even if you do not notice any signs or symptoms. ➡

Drug Facts (continued)

Directions
- **do not take more than directed (see overdose warning)**

adults and children 12 years and over	- take 2 caplets every 4 to 6 hours as needed - do not take more than 8 caplets in 24 hours
children under 12 years	do not use this adult Extra Strength product in children under 12 years of age; this will provide more than the recommended dose (overdose) of TYLENOL® and may cause liver damage

Other information
- **do not use if carton is opened or neck wrap or foil inner seal imprinted with "Safety Seal®" is broken or missing**
- store between 20–25°C (68–77°F)
- see end panel for lot number and expiration date

Inactive ingredients
cellulose, corn starch, FD&C red #40, hypromellose, magnesium stearate, polyethylene glycol, sodium starch glycolate, titanium dioxide

Questions or comments?

FIGURE 1-4 Example of "drug facts" labeling on the box of an OTC drug.

New Drug Development Time Line

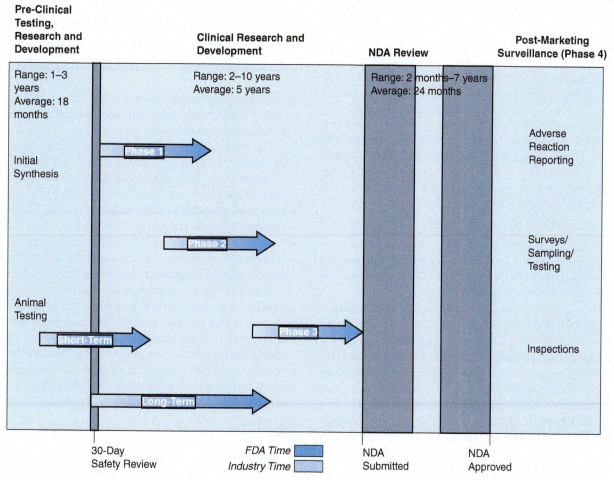

FIGURE 1-5 A new drug development time line with the four phases of drug approval.

Phases of Clinical Human Studies

Clinical human studies occur in four phases (Figure 1-5):

PHASE 1 TRIALS   This is the first time that a drug is administered in a human being. Healthy subjects receive a single dose
of a specific drug and are monitored. The primary purpose of
Phase 1 trial is to determine a proper and safe dose of the drug;
however, any toxicity should be reported.

PHASE 2 TRIALS   After safety of the drug has been documented,
another group of human subjects with the specific disease for
which the drug is intended are given the drug and monitored.
These clinical trials are often long term. This phase of studies
also determines the common short-term side effects and risks
associated with the drug. Clinical testing is an important part of
drug evaluations because of the variability of response among
people.

Approval for marketing may be accelerated if a drug is
proven to be effective and without serious side effects. The
approval process is delayed when a drug has concerns and
precautions.

Before drug testing can proceed, an NDA must be submitted.

PHASE 3 TRIALS

Review of the New Drug Application   This phase begins only
if the other phases have proven reasonably that the drug is safe
and effective. The FDA is allowed 6 months to initially review
an NDA. If it is approved, the testing goes to the final phase.
If the NDA is rejected, the approval process stops until further
notice. It takes about 17–24 months for an NDA to be reviewed.
The FDA will not approve an NDA until the new drug is proven
"safe and effective."

PHASE 4 TRIALS

Postmarketing Surveillance   This is the final stage of drug
approval that monitors the actual use of the drug in dental/
medical practice. The purpose of this phase is to monitor for
harmful or adverse drug effects in a larger population. The FDA
can withdraw a drug from the market if it is considered unsafe.
In 1997, Seldane, an antihistamine, was taken off the market
because of serious cardiac events and death.

The FDA receives comments from the public, pharmaceutical
manufacturers, and organizations pertaining to adverse drug
effects.

DRUG RECALLS Drug recalls are actions taken by the manufacturer to remove a drug or products from the market. Recalls can be initiated by the manufacturer or by the FDA. Recalls are continuously being reported; an up-to-date list is provided at www.fda.gov/opacom/7alters.html.

There are three classes of recalls: Class I, in which there is a reasonable chance that the use of or exposure to the product will cause serious adverse health problems or death; Class II, when the use or exposure to a product may cause temporary or medically reversible adverse health problems, or there is little chance of serious adverse health problems; and Class III, in which the use of or exposure to a product is not likely to cause adverse health problems.

Drug Names and Properties

Chemical/Generic/Trade Drug Names

Drugs often have several names. Every drug is given three names: a chemical name, a generic (nonproprietary) name, and a trade or brand name (proprietary name). There are more than 10,000 brand and generic varieties of drugs.

The *chemical name,* which is usually long and complicated, refers to the chemical makeup of the drug and defines its unique molecular structure. When a drug is first discovered it is given a chemical name, which is assigned using the nomenclature conventions of the International Union of Pure and Applied Chemistry (IUPAC). Several correct names may be formulated using these rules, but ordinarily the accepted chemical name will be the name listed by the Chemical Abstracts Service (CAS). The chemical name is usually too complex for general use so a shorter version or a code is used for easy reference. For example, the chemical name of acetaminophen is N-(4-hydroxyphenyl) acetamide.

> **DID YOU KNOW?**
>
> About 1,000 drugs have been designated as orphan drugs, and 200 orphan drugs have been approved by the FDA.

In the United States, the *generic name,* which is the "official" preferred name, comes from the United States Adopted Names (USAN) designations. These names are far less complicated and easier to pronounce than the chemical name. A generic drug formulation is one that contains the same therapeutically active chemical ingredients as the brand name drug marketed by the developer in the same dosage amounts and form. The Drug Price Competition and Patent Term Restoration Act of 1984 accelerated the approval of generic drugs, and were intended to reduce the cost of drugs to the consumer. There is only one generic name for each drug developed. For example, the generic name for Motrin and Advil is ibuprofen.

> **DID YOU KNOW?**
>
> The word *official* as used in the United States Pharmacopeia is synonymous with *pharmacopeial, USP,* and *compendial.*

The *trade name* or *brand name* (also referred to as proprietary name) for a drug is a registered trademark that belongs to a particular drug manufacturer and is used to designate a drug product marketed by that manufacturer. A drug can have many brand names produced by different manufacturers. For example, acetaminophen is the generic name for Tylenol, which is the trade name, and is marketed by McNeil Consumer Healthcare (Fort Washington, PA). Nuprin, Motrin, and Advil are different trade names for ibuprofen that are produced by different manufacturers.

Generic drugs are generally less expensive than brand name drugs. In the United States, a drug developer is given a patent on a drug, which includes exclusive rights to name and market that drug for 17 years after an NDA is submitted to the FDA. Unfortunately, this keeps the drug cost high because there is no competition. After 17 years, the patent expires and competing manufacturers may sell a generic version of the drug, which is a chemical equivalent, but is usually less expensive.

> **Rapid Dental Hint**
>
> Patients may not understand the differences in trade and generic names of many drugs such as analgesics. You may need to educate your patients about these products.

LOOK ALIKE–SOUND ALIKE DRUGS Many drugs have similar-looking but quite different generic names, which can cause errors in reading them on a prescription or on a patient's medical history. Most medication errors can be avoided by reviewing carefully the patient's medication history and referring to sources for drug information (Table 1-2).

Dental Hygiene Applications

Since dental hygienists play a pivotal role in clinical pharmacology in the dental practice, they should have an understanding of the fundamentals of drug therapy. Establishing a good reference

TABLE 1-2 Examples of Look Alike–Sound Alike Drugs				
LOOK ALIKE–SOUND ALIKE DRUGS 1			**LOOK ALIKE–SOUND ALIKE DRUGS 2**	
Brand Name	Ativan	Atarax	Celebrex	Celexa
Generic Name	Lorazepam	Hydroxyzine	Celecoxib	Citalopram
Indication	Anti-anxiety	Anti-anxiety	Analgesic	Antidepressant

library is important to allow the hygienist to look up and verify the medications that their patients are taking. Hygienists should be able to converse with patients about medications prescribed for them, including reviewing potential adverse effects and drug interactions, and how to take the medication. A thorough medical history should be reviewed with the patient, including any prescription and over-the-counter products and herbal supplements. The hygienist should reference any prescribed medications given to the patient to determine if there are any drug interactions with the current medications/herbal products that they are taking.

Introduction

Once a patient has been evaluated and diagnosed, the dental clinician may have the patient take certain medication(s) as part of therapy. A **prescription** is the prescriber's order to dispense a specific drug for the patient. Selection of a drug of choice depends on the characteristics of the patient and the clinical condition. The patient should be instructed on how to take the medication they are prescribed. Once a patient takes the prescribed medication, the dental clinician must monitor drug effects. For example, an antibiotic is prescribed for an endodontic infection. The patient reports the development of diarrhea. This situation must be assessed and appropriate treatment rendered. For instance, the antibiotic may need to be taken with food to prevent gastrointestinal discomfort. This information should be conveyed to the patient and the situation should still be monitored.

Goals of Prescription Writing

The goals of effective prescription writing are to:

1. Give an order for prescription medications to be dispensed to the patient.
2. Communicate with the pharmacist to minimize errors in dispensing.
3. Comply with any rules that govern prescribing and that could affect the patient's ability to obtain the drug.

Parts of the Prescription

Before the pharmacist fills a prescription, all parts of the prescription must be correctly written. The pharmacist must also determine if there is a contact number for the prescriber.

The different parts of the prescription are as follows (Figure 1-6):

1. Heading: Prescriber and patient information, including the prescriber's name, address, and telephone number and the patient's name, address, and age. The patient's age is very important and unfortunately is frequently omitted. Knowing

Rapid Dental Hint

Dental hygienists should review prescriptions for accuracy and review instructions with their patients on proper taking of the medication.

the patient's age and weight will ensure the proper dose. The date the prescription was written is important for record-keeping and because some drugs are not valid beyond a specific period or before a certain monthly date.

2. Body: Contains the symbol *Rx*, drug name (generic or brand name; see the following discussion), strength (should be written in metric units; some clinicians use apothecary—see the following discussion), and quantity to be dispensed (written as Disp: #; reflects the anticipated duration of therapy), the dosage, and complete directions for use (written as Sig: Take 2 tabs PO).

3. Closing: Contains the prescriber's signature, Drug Enforcement Administration (DEA) number (the DEA number may also be in the heading), refill information, and the check-off box to label with drug name. The expiration date for the drug must be printed on the label. Additionally, any other labeling instructions should be on the container, including warnings such as "May cause drowsiness" or "Take with food." A pharmacist cannot refill a prescription medication without authorization from the prescriber.

The prescriber is required by law only to write for drugs that pertain to his or her profession. All parts of a prescription must be written properly in order for a pharmacist to fill it. This includes the number of refills allowed, label, and the age of the patient. The name of the drug, indication for use, and duration of therapy should be written on the prescription, which will be transcribed by the pharmacist onto the label on the medication container. For example, if penicillin VK were prescribed for a dental infection, it should be written on the prescription that the antibiotic should be taken for 7 days, or take until finished, and that it is for a dental infection (see Figure 1-6).

DID YOU KNOW?

The word *prescription* stems from the Latin term that means "to write before."

Units of Measurement

There are different units of measurement that are used in the pharmacy to measure, weigh, and mix drugs: the metric system, avoirdupois system, and apothecary system.

The *metric system* of measures was formulated in France and first used in the United States in 1866. The metric system is the official system of weights and measures used by the Navy Pharmacy Department for weighing and calculating pharmaceutical preparations. Each table of the metric system contains a definitive unit. For instance, the *meter* is the unit of length, the *liter* is the unit of volume, and the *gram* is the unit of weight. Table 1-3 lists some units of measure in the metric system. Today, most prescribers and pharmacies use the metric system.

The apothecary system (Table 1-4), which is becoming obsolete, uses old measures of weights and volumes such as grains (gr). It is important not to abbreviate when using the apothecary system to prevent confusion between "grains" and "grams." Most clinicians

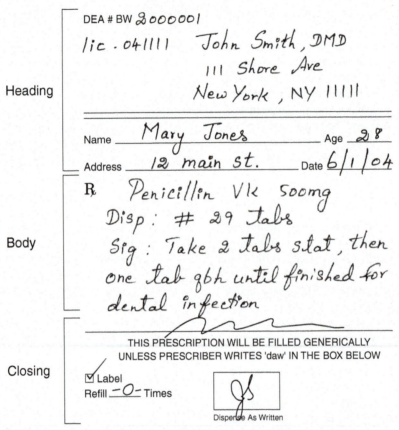

Heading

Body

Closing

DEA # BW 2000001

lic. 041111   John Smith, DMD
                    111 Shore Ave
                    New York, NY 11111

Name ___Mary Jones___   Age __28__
Address ___12 main st.___   Date __6/1/04__

R   Penicillin Vk 500mg
Disp: # 29 tabs
Sig: Take 2 tabs stat, then
one tab q6h until finished for
dental infection

THIS PRESCRIPTION WILL BE FILLED GENERICALLY
UNLESS PRESCRIBER WRITES 'daw' IN THE BOX BELOW

☑ Label
Refill __-O-__ Times

Dispense As Written

FIGURE 1-6 Part of a written prescription prescribing an antibiotic for a dental infection.

use the metric system when writing prescriptions; however, some still use the apothecary system (see Figure 1-7 on p. 11). Since 1980, the USP (United States Pharmacopoeia) and NF (National Formulary) allow the simultaneous use of both the metric and apothecary systems to report the quantity of active ingredients present in a drug product labeling. An example is quinidine sulfate 200 mg (3.086 grains).

The avoirdupois or household system of weights is used in the United States for ordinary commodities. This system defines terms such as ounce, teaspoonful, and tablespoonful.

Latin Abbreviations

Common abbreviations used in prescription writing are listed in Table 1-5 on p. 12.

> **DID YOU KNOW?**
>
> In ancient times, the symbol *Rx* was a symbol for the Roman god Jupiter, who blessed each prescription to ensure its purity.

TABLE 1-3   Metric System: Measure of Weight and Volume

Weight (the basic unit of weight is the gram)

1 kilogram (kg)	= 1,000 gram (g)
1 gram	= 1,000 *milligrams* (mg)
	= 100 centigrams (cg)
	= 10 decigrams (dg)

Volume (the basic unit of volume is the liter)

1 liter (L)	= 1,000 milliliters (mL)
	= 100 centiliters (cL)
	= 10 deciliters (dL)

TABLE 1-4   Apothecary System

Weight (the basic unit of weight is the grain)

One grain (gr)	= 0.065 grams
(g)	= rounded to 60 milligrams (mg)
20 grains	= 1 scruple
3 scruples	= 1 dram
8 drams	= 1 ounce (oz)
12 ounces	= 1 pound (lb)

Volume (the basic unit of volume is the minim)

60 minims	= 1 fluidram
8 fluidrams	= 1 fluidounce
16 fluidounces	= 1 pint (pt)
2 pints	= 1 quart (qt)
4 quarts	= 1 gallon (gal)

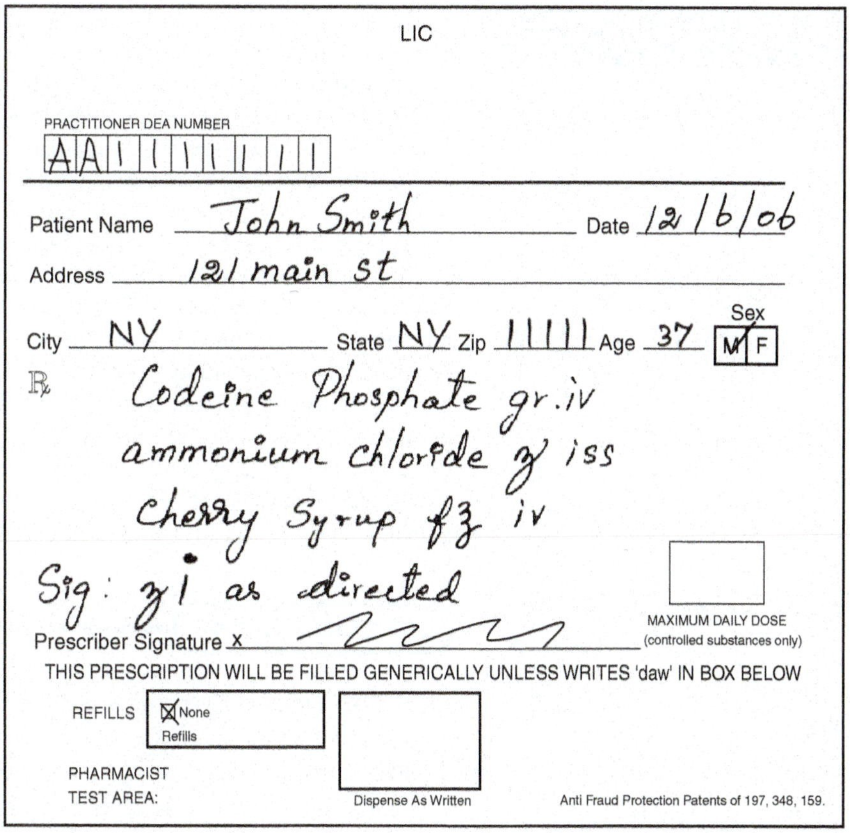
LIC

PRACTITIONER DEA NUMBER AA1111111

Patient Name John Smith Date 12/6/06

Address 121 main st

City NY State NY Zip 11111 Age 37 Sex M F

℞ Codeine Phosphate gr. iv
ammonium chloride ʒ iss
cherry Syrup fʒ iv
Sig: ʒ i as directed

Prescriber Signature X

MAXIMUM DAILY DOSE (controlled substances only)

THIS PRESCRIPTION WILL BE FILLED GENERICALLY UNLESS WRITES 'daw' IN BOX BELOW

REFILLS ☒ None Refills

PHARMACIST TEST AREA:

Dispense As Written

Anti Fraud Protection Patents of 197, 348, 159.

FIGURE 1-7 Apothecary measures of weights were often used for prescription writing, especially for compounding. This is an example of a prescription using the apothecary system for a cough syrup that the pharmacist must mix (compound).

Rapid Dental Hint

Since some over-the-counter herbs (e.g., ginger, ginkgo, ginseng) or vitamins (e.g., vitamin E) can affect blood clotting levels, the dental hygienist should ask their patients about the use of these agents.

Prescription and Nonprescription Drugs

In the United States there are two classes of drugs: **prescription** and **over-the-counter (OTC)**. Prescription drugs require a written prescription or a telephone order to the pharmacy and can only be prescribed by a dentist, physician, podiatrist, or veterinarian. In some states dental hygienists, specialized pharmacists, nurses, physician assistants, and optometrists can prescribe drugs. Prescription drugs have the federal legend statement, Rx Only. Nonprescription drugs are medications that can be obtained OTC or without a prescription. Dental hygienists should record a patient's prescription and OTC drug use.

The Food and Drug Administration regulates both prescription and OTC drugs. In 1992, the OTC Drugs Advisory Committee was created to assist the FDA in reviewing OTC drugs. An OTC drug review, which started in 1972, is a three-phase process that involves an advisory panel review, tentative final monograph publication, and a final monograph publication. A drug with OTC approval must be able to be safely self-administered.

Although nonprescription drug use has many positive aspects including cost, ease of access, and availability to the patient, there are many drawbacks such as improper use of drugs or improper indications that are potentially harmful to the individual. A consumer must be able to determine whether a drug is appropriate for his or her given condition.

In 1983, the topical prescription drug hydrocortisone was the first drug approved for OTC sales, after which many other drugs followed. Other examples include cimetadine (Tagamet) and famotidine (Pepcid) for ulcers and hyperacidity or GERD; naproxen sodium (Aleve) and ketoprofen (Actron), which are analgesics; and clotrimazole (Gyne-Lotrimin), which is an antifungal.

Scheduled Drugs

The Harrison Narcotics Act of 1914 established the first drug abuse legislation in the United States due to the high incidence of abuse of heroin, which was available over the counter. This act regulated the distribution and use of all narcotics.

Habit-forming drugs are classified according to their abuse potential for addiction and dependency and are placed in schedules by the federal Drug Enforcement Administration (DEA). Controlled substances have the potential to cause dependency, which is defined as the psychological or physiological need for

TABLE 1-5   Common Latin Abbreviations

ac	before meals
AM	morning
bid	twice a day
cap	capsule
dis	dispense
prn	as needed
q	every
qd	every day
h	hour
hs	at bedtime
qh	every hour
q8h	every 8 hours
qid	4 times a day
pc	after meals
PM	afternoon
stat	at once
sig	write on label
tid	3 times a day
po	orally (by mouth)
Rx	take thou a recipe; prescription
qs	a sufficient quantity
tab	tablet
gtts	drops
NR	no refills
mL	milliliter

a drug or substance. These drugs have restrictions and are called *controlled dangerous substances (CDS)*.

In the United States, controlled substances are drugs whose use is restricted and accounted for by the Controlled Substances Act of 1970 and later revisions. The Controlled Substances Act is also called the Comprehensive Drug Abuse Prevention and Control Act.

Hospitals and pharmacies must register with the DEA to purchase controlled drugs. Prescribers are assigned a number by the DEA in order to write prescriptions for controlled substances. This number is written on all prescriptions for controlled substances.

There are five categories of controlled substances:

- Schedule I (C-I)
- Schedule II (C-II)
- Schedule III (C-III)
- Schedule IV (C-IV)
- Schedule V (C-V)

Schedule C-I drugs have the most abuse potential and are not used clinically. Schedule C-II drugs are highly abused.

Schedule C-III drugs are less abused, and Schedule C-IV are even less abused. Schedule C-V drugs (e.g., cough syrups that contain codeine) have a very low abuse level (Figure 1-8).

Prescriptions for Schedule II drugs cannot be refilled. In some states there are special requirements that the pharmacist must fulfill with regard to dispensing Schedule II drugs, whereas prescriptions for Schedule III, IV, and V drugs can only be refilled five times within 6 months (Table 1-6).

In dentistry, controlled drugs are primarily used for dental and orofacial pain control and for sedation. For example, acetaminophen with codeine (Tylenol with codeine No. 1, 2, 3, 4) and acetaminophen with hydrocodone (Vicodin) are both C-III narcotics indicated for pain. Diazepam (Valium) and other drugs in this class that are used to calm the anxious dental patient are listed as C-IV drugs, but in many states these drugs are regulated as C-II medications. Although nitrous oxide, which is referred to as laughing gas, has a high potential for abuse, it is not scheduled.

DID YOU KNOW?

Until 1937, marijuana was legal in the United States for all purposes. In 1970, marijuana was placed in Schedule I. In the late 1990s attention was focused on making marijuana legal for medical purposes only. In 14 states (e.g., Oregon, New Jersey, Maine, Hawaii), marijuana can be prescribed for reducing nausea and vomiting in cancer patients receiving chemotherapy.

Drug Container and Package Insert

Prescription drugs are controlled by the U.S. Food and Drug Administration. The FDA Modernization Act of 1997 (FDAMA) required that before dispensing, the labels of prescription drug products (drug container) contain the symbol statement "Rx-only" instead of the "Caution: Law prohibits dispensing without prescription." The Rx only statement and the package insert (PI) are part of the packaging requirements for all prescription drugs. The package insert is literature written about the drug that accompanies all prescription drugs and is negotiated between the drug manufacturer and the FDA. The PI describes the chemical nature, indications for which the drug has been officially approved by the FDA, contraindications, warnings, adverse reactions, drug interactions, dosage and administration, and how it is supplied. All PIs are published in the *PDR®* (Thomson, Montvale, NJ).

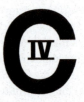

FIGURE 1-8 The capital *C* refers to a controlled substance. The roman numeral inside the *C* indicates the assigned schedule of the drug.

TABLE 1-6 Drug Schedules (Controlled Drugs)		
DRUG SCHEDULE	**ABUSE POTENTIAL**	**DRUG EXAMPLES**
C-I	Highest	No safe medical use; medical research, marijuana, hashish, PCP, LSD, heroin
C-II	High	Safe medical use; some narcotics, stimulants, and depressants. Cocaine, morphine, methadone, methamphetamine, oxycodone (Percodan/Percocet), methylphenidate (Ritalin).
C-III	Moderate	Acetaminophen with codeine (Tylenol with codeine #3, #4), acetaminophen with hydrocodone (Vicodin), anabolic steroids
C-IV	Low	Triazolam (Halcion; sedative), chloral hydrate, phenobarbital, diazepam (Valium), alprazolam (Xanax); in some states (e.g., New York, Texas) these drugs are classified as C-II
C-V	Lowest	Cough medicines that contain codeine

*Dispensing and prescription writing of controlled substances is federally regulated, but differs from state to state. Since the law is different in various states, only the federal law rules are listed in this textbook. The student is encouraged to review the laws in their state.

Beginning June 2006, the FDA required a major revision to the format of information in the PIs. Any new drug or new indication for a drug already on the market must include the newly reformatted labeling. The changes in the labeling include the addition of a section titled Highlights, which is a half-page summary at the start of the labeling that summarizes key information. In addition, the new labeling will include a table of contents following the Highlights section that will have hyperlinks to the pertinent text referenced in the table. This is an accommodation to the movement toward e-prescribing (electronic prescription writing). Information about the labeling change is posted at www.fda.gov/cder/regulatory/physLabel/default.htm. The labeling change was needed because the FDA decided that the existing labeling is too complicated, too long, and makes it too difficult to find important information.

Black Box Warning

In the United States, the FDA can require a pharmaceutical company to place a black box warning on the label of a prescription drug or in the PPI at the start of the labeling. A black box warning means that medical studies have shown that the drug causes a significant risk of serious or even life-threatening adverse effects. Black box warnings are the most serious warnings imposed by the Food and Drug Administration (FDA) for prescription medications and highlight potentially fatal, life-threatening, or disabling adverse effects for prescription drugs. A black border is placed around the text of the warning. Refer to www.fada.gov/Medwatch/safety/2006/safety06.htm.

Some examples of black box warnings include:

• January 14, 2011: Manufacturers of prescription drugs that contain acetaminophen to limit the acetaminophen dosage in each capsule or tablet to no more than 325 mg. FDA is requiring a "black box" warning label to be included on all packaging for acetaminophen products.

• March 12, 2010: Some patients cannot process or metabolize Plavix due to genetic variations, which puts them at increased risk for heart attack and stroke.

• March 2, 2006: Asthma long-acting beta$_2$-agonist including salmeterol xinafoate (Serevent Diskus) and fluticasone propionate/salmeterol xinafoate (Advair Diskus). These drugs may increase the risk of asthma-related death.

• September 28, 2006: Lamotrigine (Lamictal), a drug for seizure disorders and bipolar disorder, is not indicated for use in patients below the age of 16 years because of development of a potentially life-threatening rash.

• October 15, 2004: Antidepressants (selective serotonin reuptake inhibitors and some atypical antidepressants) may result in increased suicidal thoughts and behavior ("suicidality") in children and adolescents.

• April 11, 2005: Elderly patients with dementia-related psychosis treated with atypical antipsychotic drugs such as aripiprazole (Abilify), risperidone (Risperdal), olanzapine (Zyrexa), and quetiapine (Seroquel) are at an increased risk of death compared to a placebo.

• November 17, 2004: Depo-Provera, a contraceptive injection, carries a high risk of significant loss of bone density with long-term use.

• July 26, 2001: OxyContin is an opioid agonist and a Schedule II controlled substance with an abuse liability similar to morphine. OxyContin tablets are *not* intended for use as a prn (as needed) analgesic. OxyContin tablets are a controlled-release oral formulation of oxycodone hydrochloride indicated for the management of moderate to severe pain when a continuous, around-the-clock analgesic is needed for an extended period of time.

• June 17, 2002: Valproic acid (Depakene) has many black box warnings: (1) can cause hepatic failure resulting in fatalities, especially in children under 2 years of age; (2) can produce teratogenic effects such as neural tube defects; and (3) cases of life-threatening pancreatitis have been reported in both children and adults.

Labeled and Off-Label Uses of Drugs

The FDA approves a drug to be used for specific purposes. These approved indications or labeled uses are listed on the package insert in the drug box. Drugs may also be prescribed for a different purpose from which it is originally intended, also known as off-label use. Diphenhydramine (Benadryl) is indicated for reduction of symptoms of allergy, but may be used off label as a sleeping pill or for the relief of motion sickness.

Bioequivalence and Bioavailability: Generic Drug Substitution

Once the patent protection for an FDA-approved brand name drug expires, generic products often become available. Bioavailability and **bioequivalence** of drug products and drug product selection have emerged as critical issues in pharmacy and dentistry over the last few decades when prescribing by generic drug name. Prescribing generic drugs offers the pharmacist flexibility in selecting the drug to be dispensed and the patient possible savings.

Concern about lowering medication costs has resulted in an increase in the use of generic drug products versus brand name drugs. The extraordinary growth of the generic pharmaceutical industry and the large quantity of multisource products has provoked some questions among healthcare professionals and consumers regarding the therapeutic equivalency of these products.

The availability of different formulations of the same drug substance given at the same strength and in the same dosage form creates a challenge to healthcare professionals. Are generic drug products as good as brand name drugs? Are the generic drugs bioequivalent? The answer to both of these questions, according to the FDA, is yes. Thus, a dentist may write a prescription for tetracycline by its generic name, or may prescribe it under the brand names Sumycin, Doryx, or Vibramycin. No matter what name is used each drug must meet the same FDA standards for tetracycline.

DID YOU KNOW?

About half of all prescriptions written in the United States are for drugs that can be substituted for a generic product.

DID YOU KNOW?

Between 1492 and 1763, a colonial apothecary (pharmacist) was considered a doctor and could write prescriptions as well as dispense medications.

Bioequivalence of a drug is a pharmaceutical equivalent or alternative that contains an identical amount of the active drug as the brand name drug and does not show differences in the rate and extent of absorption. According to FDA regulations, a generic copy of a brand name drug must contain identical amounts of the same active drug ingredient in the same dosage form and route of administration and meet standards

for strength, purity, quality, and identity. *However, the inactive ingredients such as bindings, fillers, and flavorings may be different even within the same manufacturer but different batches.* These ingredients and the manufacturing process can cause clinical variability in the rate and extent of liberation of a drug from the dosing unit (e.g., tablet, capsule) and its subsequent absorption. Bioequivalence must be proved for any new form of a drug, including new dosage forms or strengths of an existing trade name drug.

The key factor when comparing brand name drugs with their generic equivalents is the bioavailability of the two drugs. Essentially, it should be determined if the two drugs get to the target tissue and act equally. Legally (FDA requirements), bioequivalence of different batches of a drug can vary by up to 20%, but such a difference does not alter the efficacy or safety of the drug. *Sometimes generic substitution is not appropriate either because standards for comparison have not been established or the actions of generic drugs may not be the same (efficacy) in everyone.*

The FDA annually publishes a book called *Approved Drug Products with Therapeutic Equivalence Evaluations* (known as the orange book) that lists the trade name drugs that are generically interchangeable.

Rapid Dental Hint

Patients may ask about the differences between generic and brand name drugs. For example, is there is a difference between ibuprofen and Advil or Motrin? Be able to explain.

A basic issue the prescriber should consider in deciding how to prescribe a drug available generically is whether there is a loss of drug efficacy or an increase in toxicity when a patient is changed from one generic formulation to another.

In most states, pharmacists are allowed to or must substitute the cheaper generic drug for a prescribed trade name drug; however, if the prescriber specifies on the prescription "Do not substitute," or signs the DAW (dispense as written) box, then the pharmacist must dispense the trade name drug. The purpose for generic drug substitution is that it is cheaper for the patient. Some states (including Florida, Kentucky, and Missouri) have a list of trade name drugs that pharmacists are not allowed to substitute generically and must be dispensed as the prescriber wrote on the prescription.

Rapid Dental Hint

The dental hygienist who is reviewing a prescription for fluoride tablets should be sure it is age-, dose-, and quantity-appropriate for the child.

> ## Rapid Dental Hint
>
> When reviewing premedication, the dental hygienist should ensure that patients take the correct number of tablets and at the right time before dental services are provided.

Other Factors Associated with Prescription Writing

Safety of Prescription Pads

Sometimes prescriptions are stolen and forged, especially for illegal prescribing of narcotics because they are cheaper and safer than street drugs. Many states require the prescriber to obtain preprinted prescription pads directly from the state that the prescriber is licensed or from approved printing manufacturers. Prescription pads should not be left unattended.

Patient Adherence

Patient adherence to the prescribed drug regimen is an important part of treatment success. Adherence implies taking a drug in the way it was prescribed or, in the case of OTC drugs, following the instructions on the label. Patient noncompliance can include not taking the medication at all, taking it at the wrong time, taking it the wrong way, or not taking it for the recommended period.

> ## Rapid Dental Hint
>
> Patient education is important for patient adherence to the drug regimen. Review with patients how and when to take drugs prescribed to them.

How to Reduce Medication Errors

The best way to avoid prescribing or **medication errors** is to write in ink and clearly (print, not script) or electronic transmission. Bad penmanship does not make for a better doctor. It is best to avoid abbreviations to avoid misinterpretations. Open-ended statements such as "Take as directed" or "As needed" should not be written. Prescriptions written for patients should be copied into the patient's chart. The number of refills should be entered on the prescription as well as the dose and dose frequency.

The FDA has started a national education campaign that focuses on eliminating the use of potentially harmful abbreviations by prescribers. The campaign addresses the use of error-prone abbreviations in all forms of communication, including written prescriptions, computer-generated labels, medication administration records, pharmacy or prescriber computer order entry screens, and commercial medication labeling, packaging, and advertising (go to www.fda.gov/cder/drug/MedErrors).

As the number of generic products continues to increase, patients, clinicians, and pharmacists must be aware of medication appearance. Patients may not question a change in the color of a generic pill that they have been taking for years only to find out that that was not the intended medication. Thus, to avoid errors patients should know what their medication looks like and be educated to always question any change in its appearance. Pharmacies should consider software that allows a description of the medication's appearance to be printed on the label (New Jersey Board of Pharmacy, April 2007).

> ## Rapid Dental Hint
>
> Review prescriptions for accuracy. Make sure the writing is legible and there are no abbreviations.

ELECTRONIC AND FAX PRESCRIBING Many states presently allow some form of electronic transmission of prescriptions, which reduces errors in reading handwritten prescriptions. In this process, the prescription is electronically transmitted via a database exchange, which is usually a computer or PDA, or email converted to fax to the patient's pharmacy. The prescription is then filled from the electronically transmitted order. The dentist is usually required to keep a written record of what is prescribed. Also, a prescription can be faxed from the dental office directly to the pharmacy.

Guidance in Prescribing

Prescribing for Children

Many drug dosage formulas have been suggested (e.g., Clark's and Young's rules) that assume incorrectly that the adult dose is correct and that the child is a small version of the adult. It is recommended that instead of using the "rules," pediatric doses should be calculated from age, weight, or body surface area (BSA).

Safety in Pregnancy

The FDA developed a system assigning all drugs a letter designation that indicates safety for use during pregnancy and lactation. The primary concern with giving certain drugs to pregnant women is that drugs are potential teratogens that may cause harm to the embryo or fetus by causing alterations in the formation of cells, tissues, and organs. Drug-induced teratogenic changes only occur during organ formation. During dental therapy, it is safest to prescribe to pregnant patients drugs that do not affect the embryo or fetus.

The categories are listed as A, B, C, D, and X. Category A is at lowest risk for harming the fetus because medical studies have not demonstrated that the drug is a risk to the fetus or pregnant women. Category D drugs (e.g., tetracycline) have been shown through medical studies to cause harm to the fetus and/or pregnant woman and should not be given. Category X drugs (e.g., estrogens) are contraindicated in women who are, or may

TABLE 1-7 Food and Drug Administration (FDA) Pregnancy Categories

SAFETY CATEGORY	DEFINITION	DRUGS
A	Studies on humans fail to show a risk to the fetus or pregnant woman. Lowest risk.	Levothyroxine (thyroid), potassium, ferrous (iron) sulfate
B	Animal studies have not shown a risk to the fetus but there are no human studies in pregnant women.	Acetaminophen, ibuprofen (becomes "C/D" in the 3rd trimester), erythromycin, chlorhexidine gluconate, azithromycin (Zithromax), penicillin, amoxicillin, metronidazole (Flagyl), clindamycin, insulin
C	Animal studies have shown a risk to the fetus but no human studies on pregnant women have been done.	Isoniazid (for tuberculosis), carbamazepine (Tegretol), fluoride, antidepressants (Zoloft, Prozac), clarithromycin (Biaxin), antihistamines (Allegra), acetaminophen with hydrocodone (Vicodin), acetaminophen with codeine (Tylenol no. 3), aspirin (D given in third trimester)
D	There is evidence that the drug may cause fetal damage, but in life-threatening situations, benefits for use in pregnant women may be acceptable despite the risk to the fetus. A "warning" will be printed on the label.	Phenytoin (Dilantin; for seizures), tetracyclines (antibiotic including doxycycoline and minocycline), anti-anxiety drugs (Valium, Xanax), warfarin (anticoagulant)
X	Studies in animals or humans have shown risk to the fetus and woman. The drug is contraindicated in women who are, or may become, pregnant.	Estrogen/progesterone

become, pregnant. Some drugs, such as cimetidine (Tagamet; for ulcers), alcohol, and tetracycline, are contraindicated in nursing women since they pass through breast milk and can cause harm to the nursing baby. Many dental drugs with A, B, and some C designations can be used safely in pregnant and lactating women. Table 1-7 lists safety categories with drug examples.

Dental Hygiene Applications

As of 2005, Oregon was the first and only state to allow dental hygienists limited prescription writing for fluoride and antimicrobial agents (e.g., gels, rinses). This change in the practice of a dental hygienist may become more prevalent and full knowledge of prescription writing may fall within the scope of practice. It is also important for the dental hygienist to be able to understand how a prescription is written because patients may ask questions about drugs that the dentist prescribed or drugs they are taking. Before a prescription is given to the patient, the dental hygienist should reference the drug and review the mechanism of action, adverse effects, how to take the medication, and if there are any drug–drug, drug–herb, or drug–food interactions.

Key Points

- Medication use impacts the dental hygiene process of care.
- Pharmacology is an integral part of dental care.

- It is important to know the medications that the dental patient is taking and how they impact the dental hygiene process of care.
- Have a few good, up-to-date resources (e.g., reference books or computerized references) for use at chairside during patient assessment.
- Every drug has three names: chemical, generic, brand.
- Prescriptions should be written clearly.
- Prescriptions should state the dose, frequency of administration, and the age of the patient.
- Do not abbreviate words.
- Communicate with the patient on how to take the medication.
- Document in the chart that the medication was reviewed with the patient and that they understood how to take the medication.
- Successful pharmacotherapy depends on patient adherence.
- Different systems of measurement have been used in pharmacy: metric, apothecary, and household.

Board Review Questions

1. Which of the following governmental agencies is responsible for approval of drugs? (p. 12)
   a. FDA
   b. EPA
   c. CIA
   d. SIA

2. Which of the following drug names refers to the structural makeup of a drug? (p. 8)
   a. Trade
   b. Proprietary
   c. Nonproprietary
   d. Chemical

3. Compared to the brand name drug, a generic name drug is usually (p. 8)
   a. cheaper.
   b. longer acting.
   c. more expensive.
   d. more effective.

4. Which of the following abbreviations stands for "twice a day"? (p. 12)
   a. bid
   b. tid
   c. qid
   d. qh

5. Which of the following is important when writing a prescription? (pp. 12–15)
   a. Avoid abbreviations when possible.
   b. Use as many abbreviations as possible.
   c. Do not write the dosage on the prescription.
   d. Always write "Take as directed."

6. The Latin abbreviation "hs" means (p. 12)
   a. at bedtime.
   b. after meals.
   c. in the right eye.
   d. as needed.

7. Which of the following schedules does acetaminophen (Tylenol) with codeine belong? (p. 13)
   a. I
   b. II
   c. III
   d. IV
   e. V

8. A patient is taking ibuprofen for arthritis. Which of the following names is given to ibuprofen? (p. 8)
   a. Generic
   b. Brand
   c. Chemical
   d. Trade

9. A pregnant woman has an endodontic abscess that requires an antibiotic. Which of the following antibiotics *should not* be prescribed? (p. 16)
   a. Penicillin
   b. Amoxicillin
   c. Tetracycline
   d. Clindamycin

10. Which of the following pregnancy categories does chlorhexidine belong? (p. 16)
    a. A
    b. B
    c. C
    d. D
    e. X

Selected References

Atkinson AJ, Lalonde RL. 2007. Introduction of quantitative methods in pharmacology and clinical pharmacology: A historical overview. *Clin Pharmacol Ther* 82:3–6.

Belgado BS. 2000. Drug information centers on the Internet. *Journal of the American Pharmaceutical Association* 41:631–632.

Gossel TA. 1998. Pharmacology back to basics. *U.S. Pharmacist* 23:70–78.

Gossel TS. 1998. Exploring pharmacology. *U.S. Pharmacist* 23:96–104.

Hansten PD, Horn, JR. 1996. Drug interactions. *Drug Interactions Newsletter* 16:893–904.

Kelly WN. 2001. Can the frequency and risks of fatal adverse drug events be determined? *Pharmacotherapy* 21(5):521–527.

Kramer JM, Cath A. 1996. Medical resources and the Internet: Making the connection. *Archives of Internal Medicine* 156:833–842.

Moeller KE, Shireman TI, Generali J, Rigler S. 2010. Pharmacy students' knowledge of black box warnings. *Am J Pharm Educ.* 74(1):1–5.

Murphy JE, Green JS, Adams LA, Squire RB, Kuo GM, McKay A. 2010. Pharmacogenomics in the curricula of colleges and schools of pharmacy in the United States. *Am J Pharm Educ.* 74(1):1–10.

Rickles NM, Noland CM, Tramontozzi A, Vinci MA. 2010. Pharmacy student knowledge and communication of medication errors. *Am J Pharm Educ.* 74(4):1–10.

Web Sites

www.pdr.net
www.drugs.com
www.rxlist.com
www.fda.gov/cder
www2.kumc.edu/instruction/prescriptStuff/format.htm
www.pslgroup.com/NEWDRUGS.HTM
http://www.elephantcare.org/abbrev.htm

PEARSON
myhealthprofessionskit™

Use this address to access the Companion Website created for this textbook. Simply select "Dental Hygiene" from the choice of disciplines. Find this book and log in using your username and password to access video clips of selected tests.

Fundamentals of Drug Action

GOAL

To provide an understanding of the basic principles of what the body does to drugs and the action of drugs on the body.

After reading this chapter, the reader should be able to:

1. Compare the differences between pharmacodynamics and pharmacokinetics.
2. Describe common routes of drug administration.
3. Describe the mechanisms of drug absorption through the various membranes in the body.
4. Describe absorption through the different routes of drug administration.
5. Describe the drug–receptor interaction.
6. Distinguish between a loading dose and a maintenance dose.
7. Describe the various factors involved in the biological variations of drug dosing.
8. List and discuss different types of drug effects.

KEY TERMS

Drug administration

Pharmacokinetics

Drug clearance

Drug dose

Pharmacodynamics

Drug receptor

Drug effects

Adverse drug event

Adverse drug reaction

Routes of Drug Administration

A drug enters the bloodstream by absorption from its site of administration. The route of administration influences the degree and rate of drug absorption. Routes of **drug administration** are broadly divided into enteral, parenteral, and topical (Table 2-1).

Enteral Administration

The enteral route of administration involves the drug being absorbed from the gastrointestinal (GI) tract and includes oral, sublingual, buccal, and rectal.

- The *oral route (PO)* is the most common, acceptable, and convenient route for the patient. When prescribed, it is often written as PO, which refers to taking the medication by mouth.

- Drugs taken by the *sublingual* (under the tongue) or *buccal* (between the cheek and tongue) routes are absorbed directly through the oral mucosa.

- *Rectal administration (PR)* of drugs in a suppository form are necessary when a drug is too irritating to the stomach; if the patient is vomiting or nauseated, or cannot swallow well; or for a local effect (e.g., lesions of the rectum or colitis). This is a very common route for infants, children and older adults.

Parenteral Administration

There are five parenteral routes of drug administration: (1) intravenous, (2) intramuscular, (3) subcutaneous, (4) intradermal, and (5) intrathecal. The first four are shown in Figure 2-1.

The parenteral route delivers drugs via a needle into the skin layers, subcutaneous tissue, muscle, CSF (cerebral spinal fluid), or veins, with the needle angled at different degrees, depending on the type of injection. This route is more invasive than enteral or topical administration and requires good aseptic technique.

- *Intravenous (IV)* injection of a drug is administered directly into the circulation via a vein; it is used for emergency situations when it is critical to get the drug into the blood as quickly as possible. Since the drug is injected directly into the blood, this route offers the fastest onset of drug action. It is easy to control the rate of drug administered, which results in predictable blood levels. This is the most common route to administer antibiotics and fluid replacement solutions to critically ill patients.

- *Intramuscular (IM)* injections are administered into the layers of skeletal muscle beneath the skin, including the deltoid muscle of the arm or gluteus muscle of the buttocks. Absorption is rapid and uniform since there are many blood vessels in muscles and the drug passes through capillary walls to enter the bloodstream. Irritating drugs can

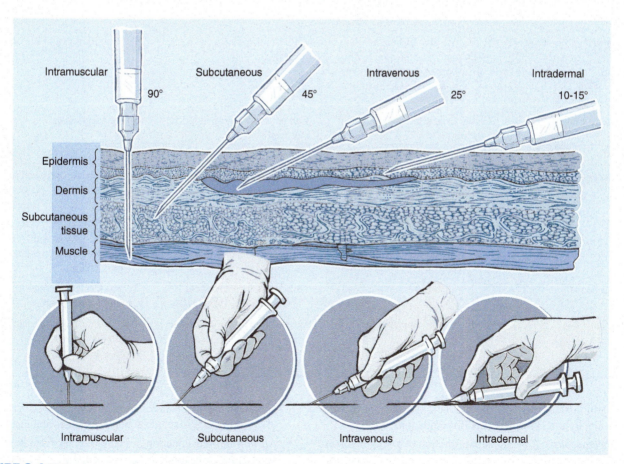

FIGURE 2-1 Different routes of parenteral drug administration.

TABLE 2-1   Routes of Drug Administration: Advantages and Disadvantages

Route	Advantages	Disadvantages	Examples
Enteral			
Oral (PO)	Most common route of administration; convenient, easy to administer	Unpredictable absorption from the gastrointestinal tract; poor adherence to schedule dosing; patient must be conscious	Antibiotics for dental infections, analgesics for dental pain, doxycycline 20 mg for chronic periodontitis
Sublingual (SL)	Provides a rapid drug response	Low doses must be given	Nitroglycerin tablets for angina
Buccal	Provides a rapid drug response	Low doses must be given	Testosterone buccal system
Rectal (PR)	Patients unable to take oral medications, older adults	Variable absorption	Analgesics, laxatives
Parenteral			
Intravenous (IV)	Drug injected directly into bloodstream; 100% of drug administered is absorbed; rapid onset	Once injected, drug cannot be retrieved	Medical emergency drugs, such as antibiotics
Intramuscular (IM)	Good absorption	Must select an appropriate injection site away from bone, large blood vessels, and nerves; soreness at site of injection. Massage injection site.	Narcotic anaglesics for severe pain, hepatitis B vaccine, flu shot
Subcutaneous (SC, SQ)	Good absorption, but slower than intramuscular; avoids enzymes in the liver that would break the drug down	Doses must be small in volume	Dental local anesthetic solutions (e.g., lidocaine), insulin
Intradermal	Easy to give to patients who cannot take the drug orally; avoids enzymes in the liver that would break the drug down	Only small volumes can be injected	Tuberculin (tuberculosis) test
Intrathecal	For local effects within spinal cord	Can get sudden drop in blood pressure	Spinal anesthesia
Topical			
Transdermal	Dosing over extended period of time; low dosage of drugs	Cannot give large volume of drug and not a rapid response	DentiPatch, nitroglycerin patch and ointment, oral contraceptive patch, nicotine patches (for smoking cessation)
Subgingival	Localized effect to oral mucous membrane, gingival crevice, skin	Only treats localized subgingival areas	Controlled-release antimicrobials (Atridox, Arestin, Perio-Chip), Oraqix
Epicutaneous	Localized effect on the skin	Only treats localized areas	Topical dental anesthetics, ointments, creams
Inhalation	Rapid drug response; local effect to the lungs or generalized effect with general anesthetics	Cannot give large volumes of drug	General anesthetics, moderate sedation drugs (nitrous), oxygen, asthma drugs

be administered by this route. One example of IM drug administration is the hepatitis B vaccination.

- *Subcutaneous (SC or SQ)* administration of a drug involves the injection of liquid into the connective tissue under the skin. This route cannot be used for irritating drugs or if a large

volume of the drug solution must be administered. Examples of drugs given SC include dental anesthetics and insulin.

- An *intradermal* injection is made directly into the dermis layer of the skin, which is below the epidermis. Intradermal injections are given to test for allergic reactions and when performing the tuberculin skin test with purified protein derivative (PPD).

- An *intrathecal* injection, which is a less common parenteral route of administration, is delivered into the spinal fluid, which bathes the spinal cord, and is used primarily for spinal anesthesia.

Topical Administration

Topical administration refers to the application of drugs to the surface of the body directly where action is desired. Examples include the skin, mucous membranes of the gingiva (local anesthetics), eyes, ears, and the gingival crevice of teeth, mouth, and throat.

- When dental drugs are applied topically into the gingival crevice, it is referred to as *subgingival* application. This route is used in dentistry to administer topical anesthetics such as Oraqix and antimicrobials such as Arestin, Atridox, and PerioChip. The intention of topically applied drugs is to produce a local effect at the site of administration; however, they may be absorbed and produce systemic effects.
- *Inhalation* administration is used for drugs that are inhaled through the mouth or nose and are used to treat asthma or rhinitis, diabetes, and for general anesthesia and moderate sedation; nitrous oxide and oxygen is most commonly delivered by this route.
- *Ophthalmic* administration of drugs is used to treat local conditions of the eye and surrounding area including infections, dryness, glaucoma, and dilation of the pupil during an eye exam. Ophthalmic drugs are available in the form of drops, irrigations, ointments, and medicated disks.
- *Otic* administration of drugs is used to treat local conditions of the ear. Otic drugs include drops and irrigations.
- *Intranasal* administration of drugs is used for both local and systemic effects. Nasal spray formulations of corticosteroids are used to treat allergic rhinitis. Nasal drops are also available.
- *Transdermal* administration is the application of a medicated adhesive patch to the skin that delivers a time-released dose of medication through the skin into the bloodstream. Examples include the nicotine patch for smoking cessation, scopolamine for motion sickness, contraceptive patches, nitroglycerin for angina, antidepressant patches (Emsam), and DentiPatch, which is a topical pre-anesthetic (lidocaine) that is applied to dry gingival tissues.

Pharmacokinetics

Pharmacokinetics describes what happens with the drug once it is in the patient. It tells how the drug is absorbed, where it goes, and how the body gets rid of it. The amount of drug in the body at any given time is determined by four processes, abbreviated ADME:

1. Absorption
2. Distribution
3. Metabolism (biotransformation)
4. Elimination or excretion

Figure 2-2a shows factors affecting the onset, duration, and intensity of a drug effect. The ultimate goal of pharmacokinetics is to have the drug reach the site of action in adequate concentrations to produce a pharmacological effect prior to elimination from the body. A *two-compartment model* describes a representation of the pharmacokinetic behavior of many drugs after oral administration. It shows the absorption of drugs into the central compartment (e.g., blood), distribution into the peripheral component (e.g., tissues), and elimination from the central component (Figure 2-2b).

Usually drugs enter the body far from the intended site of action. In order to get to the organ/tissue where it will have a pharmacological effect, the drug must be absorbed and transported through the bloodstream (systemic circulation).

Absorption

How does the drug get into the blood? A drug must be in solution to be absorbed and distributed in the body. Liquid dosage

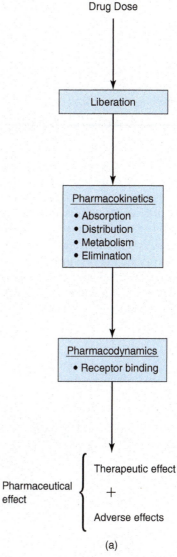

(a)

FIGURE 2-2a Generalized scheme showing the contribution of absorption, distribution, metabolism, elimination, and drug-receptor binding of drugs.

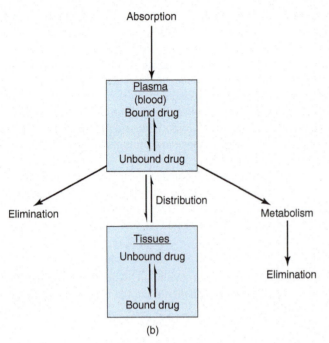

FIGURE 2-2b A two-compartment model of pharmacokinetics.

forms, such as injectables and cough syrups, are already in solution and are immediately available for absorption and transport. The drug passes through the GI tract (usually the upper part of the duodenum or small intestine), where most absorption occurs into the blood.

CELL MEMBRANES/BARRIERS Before a drug is absorbed into the blood it must pass through many *cell membranes* or tissue barriers to get to the organ/tissue where the drug will exert its pharmacological effect. Generally, a drug will be better absorbed in the small intestine than the stomach because the small intestine has a larger surface area. The final destination of a drug is referred to as the *site of drug action.*

Cell membranes form the barriers between different compartments in the body; the structure of cell membranes of the tissues in the body is illustrated in Figure 2-3. Cell membranes are composed of two layers of lipids, referred to as the biphospholipid layer with highly polar (water-soluble) heads of the molecules oriented outward and the nonpolar (fat-soluble) chains of fatty acids inside the membrane. Embedded in the membrane are proteins with small aqueous (water) holes, channels, or pores throughout. Thus, the cell membrane acts as a lipid barrier and allows lipid-soluble (*lipophilic*) drugs to penetrate cell membranes more easily by diffusion. Drugs that are water soluble (*hydrophilic*) do not diffuse easily in the lipid layer and either pass through the aqueous pores or are prevented from entering the cell and as a result are contained outside.

Optimally, a drug should have some degree of both lipid and water solubility: water solubility to go through fluids to get to the cell, and lipid solubility to get through the cell membrane. *Lipid solubility is one of the most important determinants of the pharmacokinetic characteristics of a drug.*

An orally administered drug passes down the esophagus into the gastrointestinal tract (small intestine), where it must cross the gastrointestinal mucosa (single-cell layered epithelium) into the blood before being distributed to the target tissue/organ (site of action). This is referred to as the *intestinal mucosa–blood barrier.* Intravenous drugs avoid absorption barriers by entering the bloodstream immediately upon administration.

The *placenta barrier* filters out some substances that can harm the fetus, but allows other substances, including alcohol, to cross.

Sublingually or buccally administered drugs must go through the epithelium of the oral mucosa (tongue or buccal mucosa) before entering the blood and being distributed to the site of action (Figure 2-4). This barrier is referred to as the *oral mucosa–blood barrier.*

Once the drug enters the blood, it is transported to the various tissues in the body where it will exert its pharmacological effect(s). The drug must then go through another barrier, the membrane between the blood and the tissue, called the *blood–tissue barrier.* The structure of capillary cell membranes is different in different areas in the body. If the drug is intended to go to the brain, the drug must pass through the capillaries of the brain (*blood–brain barrier*). The cell membrane of the brain is very lipid, so water-soluble substances/drugs cannot enter the brain. Only small

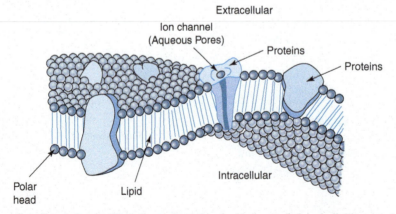

FIGURE 2-3 Diagram of a cell membrane. The cell membrane is a double layer of phospholipid molecules with highly polar heads oriented outward and the nonpolar chains of fatty acids inside the membrane. Embedded in the membrane are proteins that include ion channels for the transport of water-soluble drugs.

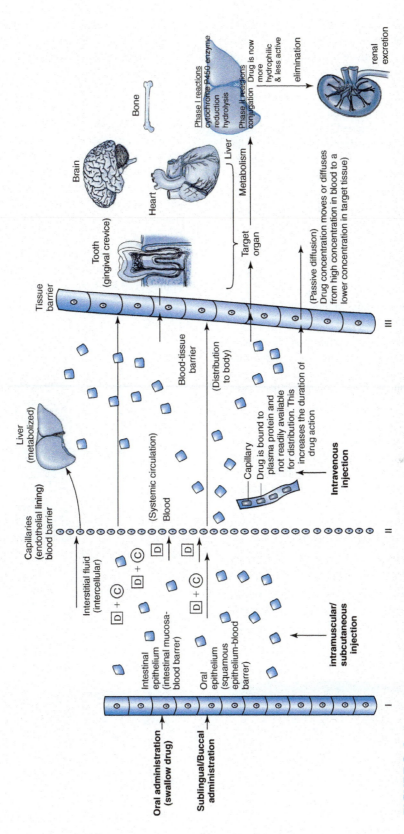

FIGURE 2-4 Absorption of a drug through cell membranes into the bloodstream (systemic circulation). The drug has to go through many tissue-blood barriers to get to the final site of action. The tissue-blood and blood-tissue barriers are: After swallowing a drug, it goes from the GI tract (gut or small intestine) into the blood (I), then from the blood through the blood-tissue barrier (II) to the site of action (organ or tissue) (III). D, drug; C, carrier.

molecular-size, lipid-soluble drugs such as general anesthetics (e.g., thiopental), alcohol, and anti-anxiety drugs get through the brain cell membrane very easily.

ABSORPTION OF DRUGS How do drugs penetrate these cell/tissue membranes? Substances move through cell membranes by passive diffusion, facilitated diffusion, active transport, or *pinocytosis.*

1. Most drugs are absorbed by *passive diffusion* across a cell barrier and into the circulation. The rate of diffusion is proportional to the concentration gradient (Figure 2-4); the rate of absorption increases as long as the concentration outside (blood) the cell is greater than the concentration inside the cell (GI fluids). As described earlier, lipid-soluble drugs go through the cell membrane while water-soluble drugs pass through the cell membrane via water channels or pores. No energy is used by the cell during passive diffusion.

2. *Facilitated diffusion* occurs when a carrier such as a protein is necessary to get a drug that is too large and/or too polar to diffuse across a lipid membrane. By definition, diffusion is a passive process that does not require energy in moving the drug across the cell membrane. Sugars, penicillin, and aspirin are transported in this way.

3. *Active transport* involves the use of carrier proteins to move drugs against the concentration gradient with expenditure of energy. This is not a common process of absorption and is limited to drugs structurally similar to endogenous substances such as vitamins (e.g., vitamin B_{12}), sugars, and amino acids.

4. *Pinocytosis* involves the engulfment of fluids or particles by a cell. The cell membrane traps the substance, forming a vesicle that will detach and move to the interior of the cell. This process involves energy expenditure and plays a minor role in drug movement.

EFFECT OF PH ON ABSORPTION OF WEAK ACIDS AND BASES

- Most drugs are either weak acids or bases (Table 2-2) and are present in solution as both ionized and nonionized forms.
  - The ionized form, which has low lipid solubility and has an electric charge, cannot easily cross a lipid membrane.
  - *The nonionized form is usually lipid soluble and readily crosses cell membranes.*

TABLE 2-2	Weak Acids and Weak Bases
WEAK ACIDS	**WEAK BASES**
Aspirin	Caffeine
Penicillin V	Codeine
Phenytoin	Erythromycin
Tetracycline	Pilocarpine (used in the treatment of dry mouth)
	Local anesthetics
	Diazepam (Valium)

- How much of the drug changes to the ionized form will depend on the pK_a of the drug and the pH of the solution. The pH refers to the concentration of the H^+ ions. The pK_a of a drug is related to the equilibrium that the drug has with its ionized form and is the pH at which the drug is 50% ionized and 50% nonionized and is a given, constant value. Generally, the pK_a of weak acids is 3–5 and weak bases is 8–10.

- Drugs that are weak acids (e.g., aspirin-pK_a 4.4, penicillin-pK_a 2.5) will be mostly nonionized (uncharged) at the acidic pH of the stomach (pH 1.4), allowing it to be absorbed readily. However, in theory, weak acids should be more readily absorbed from the stomach than weak bases. The surface area for absorption is small and the transient time of contents within the stomach is very short, so most nonionized drugs are transported farther down into the small intestine where they are absorbed (Figure 2-5).

- On the other hand, drugs that are weak bases (e.g., erythromycin, codeine, and morphine) will be more nonionized at the pH of the basic small intestine (pH 6–7) and ionized in the stomach. The nonionized portion of the drug shows

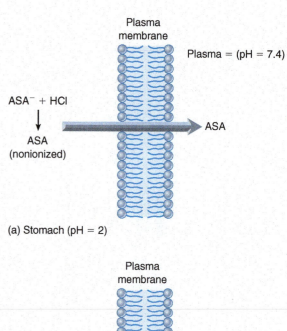

(a) Stomach (pH = 2)

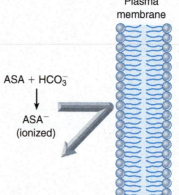

(b) Small intestine (pH = 8)

FIGURE 2-5 Effect of pH on drug absorption. (a) A weak acid such as aspirin (ASA) is in a nonionized form in an acidic environment and absorption occurs; (b) in a basic environment, aspirin is mostly in an ionized form and absorption is prevented.

great lipid solubility and therefore greater absorption in the small intestine.

- Regardless of the pH and ionization, most drug absorption, even weak acids, usually occurs in the small intestine, which has the greatest surface area.
- Enteric-coated tablets (e.g., aspirin, erythromycin) have a layer, such as wax or a cellulose acetate polymer, on the outside of the tablet that protects the stomach lining from exposure to these acidic drugs.
- Dental application:
  - Local anesthetics are weak bases. The closer the pK_a of local anesthetics are to the local tissue pH (pH 7.4), the more nonionized the drug is and the faster it will be absorbed with a quicker onset of action. The lower pK_a means that a greater fraction of the molecules exist in the nonionized form in the body, so they more easily cross nerve membranes, leading to faster onset.
  - For example, lidocaine, with a pK_a of 7.9, has a faster onset of action than bupivicaine, with a pK_a of 8.1. If the local tissue pH is more alkaline and closer to the pK_a values of the drugs, the onset of action would be faster. In the presence of inflammation, the local tissue environment becomes acidic (pH around 5–7) so there is less local anesthetic (basic) in the nonionized form than is required to cross the nerve cell membrane.

Factors Altering Absorption   Factors that can influence the *rate of drug absorption* include:

1. Blood flow to the organ (the greater the blood flow to an organ, the greater the rate of absorption). Nitroglycerin is administered under the tongue because it is rapidly absorbed because of high vascularity.
2. The small intestine has a large surface area due to microvilli present on its surface. This feature increases the rate and efficacy for absorption.
3. The salt form of the drug [e.g., hydrochloride (HCl) is the salt form of tetracycline] affects absorption and stability of the drug. Generation of a salt form of a drug is done to enhance its solubility. For example, when manufactured, local anesthetics are poorly soluble in water; however, when combined with an acid to form a salt, they can be combined with sterile water or saline.

Rapid Dental Hint

Remind patients not to eat large amounts of fatty foods at meals if taking erythromycin or codeine. This reduces the absorption of the drug.

4. The choice of the route of drug administration is influenced by drug absorption.

Absorption via Different Routes of Drug Administration

- ***ENTERAL:*** Most orally administered drugs are in the form of tablets or capsules. Once a tablet is swallowed (Figure 2-6), it travels down the esophagus into the stomach, where the active ingredient in the drug is *liberated* from its dosage form by *disintegration* into smaller particles and then dissolved; these will be in solution with the gastric fluid. This is similar to a sugar cube placed in coffee; it must disintegrate into small particles, which will then dissolve. A capsule must open before it undergoes dissolution.
  - Absorption usually occurs in the small intestine, which is ideal for absorption because of its large surface area. Oral drugs must be absorbed through two barriers—epithelial cells and blood vessel walls—in order to enter the blood.

Rapid Dental Hint

Absorption of antibiotics used in dentistry is affected by food; discuss with patients how foods affect the antibiotic being taken.

- Once absorbed into the blood, the drug is carried to the liver through the hepatic portal vein (Figure 2-7; Table 2-3); however, absorption may be slow and how much will be absorbed cannot be predicted. Generally, when mixed with certain drugs and foods, absorption may be decreased. The temperature of food also influences drug absorption; hot food slows the emptying of the stomach, while cold food enhances gastric emptying.
- Other factors affecting absorption of orally administered drugs, such as tetracycline and ciprofloxacin, include minerals (e.g., iron, calcium, magnesium) that form insoluble complexes in the intestinal tract, which slows down absorption. This limitation can be avoided by taking the drug 1 hour before or 2 hours after having dairy or minerals.

Rapid Dental Hint

Recognize that older adults and children require dose adjustments.

- Another disadvantage of the oral route is that all drugs that are taken orally must initially pass through the liver via the hepatic portal vein prior to reaching general circulation (Figure 2-7). This is called *first-pass effect*. This may inactivate the drug because it gets metabolized (broken down) in

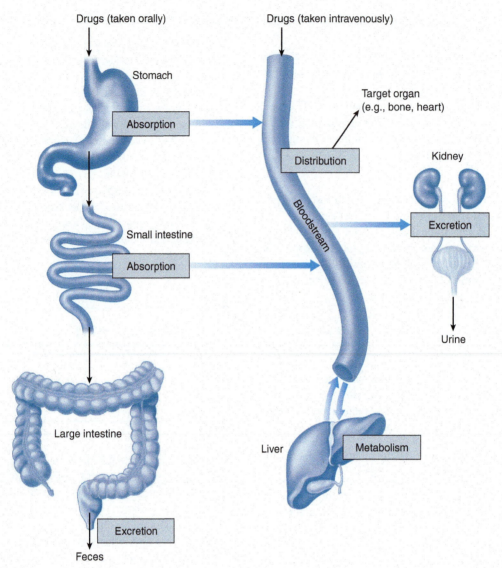

FIGURE 2-6 Movement of a drug through the body (pharmacokinetics): absorption, distribution, metabolism, and excretion.

the liver. To avoid first-pass effect, drugs are administered via IV, IM, or sublingually so the blood supply from these areas does not pass through the liver. Some drugs with a high first-pass metabolism include morphine, a narcotic analgesic, and nortriptyline, an antidepressant.

Rapid Dental Hint

Placing nitroglycerin under the tongue is effective due to the vascular nature of the floor of the mouth.

- **PARENTERAL:** Unlike enterally administered drugs, parenteral administration of drugs bypasses the gastrointestinal tract.
  - Intravenous fundministration of a drug is made directly into the circulation through a vein, bypassing absorption barriers. Most drugs used in anesthesia are given

by this route, which provides a reliable and rapid onset of action. An intravenously administered drug has 100% bioavailability because the entire drug enters the bloodstream (refer to Table 2-3).

- In subcutaneous administration, because the drug is injected into the connective tissue under the skin absorption is slow but uniform because circulation is slow. The rate of absorption depends greatly on the site of injection and on local blood flow.
- With an intramuscular injection, absorption is rapid and uniform because there are many blood vessels in muscles. Massaging or heating the area of injection increases the blood flow.
- **TOPICAL:** The major barrier to absorption from topical administration is the top layer of skin, called the *stratum corneum*, which blocks both lipid and water-soluble substances. If the skin is damaged or abraded, absorption of topical substances increases.
  - Subgingival administration: Antimicrobial agents (e.g., Atridox, Arestin, PerioChip) or Oraqix when administered

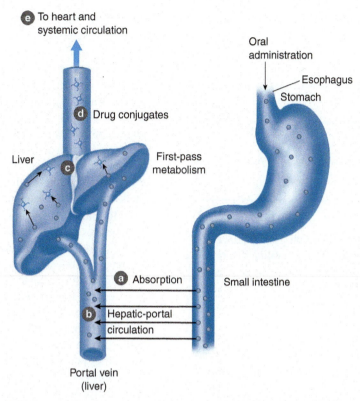

FIGURE 2-7 **First-pass metabolism (biotransformation).** Absorption of an orally administered drug.

TABLE 2-3   **Summary of Drug Action: Common Routes of Administration**

Oral

1. Tablet/capsule (e.g., tetracycline) is taken by mouth with a glass of water.

2. Tablet goes down the esophagus.

3. Drug goes into the stomach where a tablet is disintegrated (broken up) and a capsule opens up and the active ingredients in the drug are dissolved. An enteric-coated tablet is disintegrated in the duodenum (small intestine), not the stomach, because the drug is acid liable and will irritate the stomach.

4. Drug goes into the small intestine, where most drugs are absorbed.

5. The drug must cross the intestinal mucosa–blood barrier. Lipid-soluble drugs are absorbed more easily because the intestinal barrier is a lipid membrane.

6. After absorption from the small intestine, the drug goes through the portal vein into the liver.

7. As drugs go through the liver on its way to the blood, some will be metabolized extensively and inactivated before becoming available to the body (first-pass metabolism) in the liver.

8. From the liver, the transformed drug goes through capillary (blood vessel) barriers via the superior vena cava into the bloodstream for distribution in the body.

9. After the drug exerts its pharmacological action, it will either be eliminated unchanged if it is a hydrophilic drug or metabolized in the liver (by liver enzymes) to a water-soluble form that will be readily eliminated from the body (e.g., excreted via the kidneys in the urine).

10. Some drugs (large, polar drugs; estrogens, rifampicin, digitoxin, phenytoin) undergo enterohepatic recirculation, where they are excreted from the liver into the bile, then reabsorbed from the intestine, returned to the liver, and eliminated in the bile.

11. Drugs that are sufficiently lipid soluble are more readily absorbed and distributed orally. However, lipid-soluble drugs must first be converted in the liver into water-soluble metabolites that can be excreted by the kidneys.

Intravenous

1. A drug is injected directly into the blood and is rapidly distributed to the tissues.

2. In the blood, some drugs are extensively protein bound.

3. First-pass metabolism is eliminated.

4. There are no barriers to absorption; 100% bioavailablity.

5. After distribution, the drug is excreted in the urine by glomerular filtration.

6. Enterohepatic circulation: metabolism by the liver and elimination in the bile.

subgingivally into the gingival crevice are absorbed through the sulcular epithelium.

Rapid Dental Hint

Delivery of a topical anesthetic reaches the nonkeratinized sulcular epithelium, which increases its absorption. There is some absorption systemically.

- Substances can be absorbed through nasal passages or directly through the trachea. There is rapid absorption due to the presence of many capillaries in the respiratory tract. Thus, a systemic effect is achieved. It is difficult to monitor doses, and certain drugs may be irritating to the respiratory tract.
- Drugs delivered by patch therapy must be lipid soluble to pass through the layers of the skin for absorption, and are typically more concentrated than in other dosage forms. Some drugs that are administered transdermally such as nitroglycerin and smoking cessation products are intended to have systemic effects.

Distribution

Once a drug is present in the bloodstream, it is distributed throughout the body fluids to tissues and organs that it is physically able to penetrate (Figures 2-1, 2-7). After the drug leaves the blood it is distributed to the extracellular fluid [all body fluids outside of the cells; includes plasma, interstitial fluid (between cells) and lymph or enters the cells (intracellular space)]. The time it takes for this to occur is called the *distribution phase*. The volume of fluid in which a drug is able to distribute is referred to as *volume of distribution*, or V_d. This is a useful term for understanding where the drug goes and for drug calculations.

FACTORS AFFECTING DRUG DISTRIBUTION   To produce the required effect on the tissue or organ there must be an adequate dosage of the drug. A loss of drug concentration may occur during this distribution phase due to many factors:

1. Absorption across various lipid membranes and into body fat: Membrane affinity refers to the drug's attraction to cell membranes in the body. Hydrophilic drugs such as insulin do not have the capacity to penetrate lipid cell membranes; they are entirely distributed in the extracellular fluid. On the other hand, lipophilic drugs (e.g., general anesthetics, alcohol) have the capacity to cross lipid cell membranes and are more evenly distributed in all fluids.

   To be distributed to the site of action drugs must pass between cells via capillary beds. The capillary system surrounding the blood–brain barrier permits only very lipid-soluble drugs and drugs with small molecular weight

to enter the brain. In addition to being a lipid barrier, the placental barrier allows only such drugs (most drugs are smaller than 1,000 molecular weight) to pass.

2. Many drugs are bound to plasma proteins (proteins, commonly albumin, found in the plasma): While in the bloodstream, drugs may either exist in the *free form* or be bound to the many proteins, primarily albumin (Figure 2-8), which is referred to as *plasma protein binding*. The degree of protein binding depends on the concentration of the drug present in the blood and the affinity of a drug to that protein. Plasma protein binding decreases the distribution of the drug from the plasma to the intended site of action.

   Binding is generally reversible and the number of binding sites on the protein is limited, so two drugs with similar chemical structures may bind to the same site on the protein and compete. Administration of a second drug having a higher affinity for the same binding sites will displace the other drug from the site, elevating the free concentration of the displaced drug, which can result in toxic levels of the drug. Warfarin (an anticoagulant drug that prevents blood clotting) is an example of a highly plasma protein–bound drug. After being administered, 99% of the drug is bound to plasma proteins and only 2% of free warfarin molecules interact with receptors.

Rapid Dental Hint

Patients on warfarin require a medical consultation from their physician.

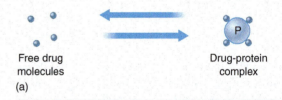

(a)

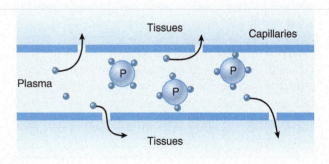

(b)

FIGURE 2-8 Plasma protein binding and drug availability.
(a) Drug exists in a free state or bound to plasma protein; (b) drug-protein complexes are too large to cross the membrane.

To summarize, *drugs that are plasma protein bound are in an inactive state; only the free drug is active.*

3. Blood flow: The greater the blood flow to an organ, the greater the rate of distribution of the drug to that organ. Thus, drugs will be distributed faster to the heart, kidneys, and brain than to the skeletal muscle, adipose tissue, and skin, which have a much lower blood flow.

Drug Elimination

Immediately after a drug is administered, the body begins to eliminate it. There are two major processes of drug elimination: *biotransformation* and *excretion* (both usually occur in combination). Renal excretion is elimination through the kidneys in the urine. Other routes of excretion include bile, feces, skin sweat, saliva, or lungs.

- *Biotransformation (metabolism)* To be eliminated readily from the body, a drug must be in a water-soluble form. Drugs are eliminated either as the original parent compound, referred to as *unchanged,* or as a drug *metabolite,* where the drug molecule must be chemically altered or biotransformed. Although some drugs are biotransformed by enzymes in the plasma, kidney, lungs, intestinal mucosa, and other tissues, *the liver is the primary site of drug biotransformation.* Generally, polar drugs that are not biotransformed are excreted unchanged in the urine. Lipophylic drugs must be biotransformed before elimination so as not to be reabsorbed from the kidneys back into the blood, prolonging the duration of drug action. Thus, a lipid-soluble drug must become less lipophilic and more water soluble to be easily eliminated by the kidneys.
  - Some drugs are *prodrugs* because when orally administered they are inactive, but become active in the body after it is metabolized. An example of a prodrug is codeine, which is metabolized to the active morphine.
- *Phases of drug biotransformation* There are two phases of biotransformation: Phase I and Phase II (Table 2-4). The purpose of *Phase I biotransformation* is to change a lipid-soluble drug to a more polar metabolite, which involves metabolic reactions including oxidation, hydrolysis, and reduction pathways. The type of biotransformation a drug undergoes depends on the chemical groups attached to the parent drug molecule.

Oxidative reactions are the most common type of Phase I metabolism. In these reactions, the liver uses enzymes to make lipid-soluble drugs more water soluble or hydrophilic. These

microsomal enzymes or *cytochrome P450 enzymes* are located primarily in the liver. When a drug is introduced into this system, it combines with oxidized P450, forming a drug–P450 complex. There are many different P450 enzymes, including:

CYP3A4: This is the most common enzyme that metabolizes many drugs used in dentistry. Some drugs that are metabolized by CYP3A4 (these are called the substrate) include lidocaine (a local anesthetic), erythromycin, and clarithromycin (Biaxin).

CYP2D6: This enzyme metabolizes codeine (a narcotic), fluoxetine (Prozac), and propranolol (heart medication).

CYP2C9: This enzyme metabolizes ibuprofen (Advil).

There are certain drugs that will either inhibit (decrease action) or induce (increase action) these CYP enzymes. For example, grapefruit juice inhibits the CYP3A4 metabolism of alprazolam (Xanax, an anti-anxiety drug), resulting in elevated serum levels of alprazolam.

Rapid Dental Hint

Be aware that there are many dental drug–drug interactions due to the CYP450 enzymes. Always look up possible drug interactions before a prescription is given to the patient.

- If a metabolic product of Phase I biotransformation is sufficiently water soluble, the kidneys may excrete it. If it is still fat soluble, enough to be reabsorbed from the kidneys back into the blood, it may be subject to *Phase II biotransformation*. In this process molecules on the drug or metabolite from Phase I are conjugated or linked with highly water-soluble compounds, such as glucoronic acid (through glucouronide formation), to make a more water-soluble product.

Factors that may influence an individual's ability to metabolize drugs include:

1. Genetics: Enzymes present in the liver are genetically determined and may either have lesser or greater amounts of enzymes, which break down the drugs.
2. Age: In the older individual, first-pass metabolism may be reduced, resulting in increased absorption of drugs. Also,

TABLE 2-4 Metabolism of Drugs: Features of Phase I and II	
Phase I: Modification of drug involving P450 enyzmes	*Phase II: Involves synthetic conjugation reactions*
Carried out in the liver	Conjugated (linked) with highly water-soluble compounds
If still fat soluble after going through Phase I, the drug will continue and may be subject to Phase II metabolism	

in the older individual there may be a reduced capacity to eliminate drugs.

3. Disease: Liver or kidney disease may reduce metabolism and elimination of drugs, resulting in increased drug levels in the body.

EXCRETION The most common route for drug excretion is through the kidney in the urine. Hydrophilic drugs are easily excreted by the kidney; patients with impaired kidney function have a reduced ability to eliminate hydrophilic drugs.

Drug clearance is the volume of plasma from which the drug is completely removed from the body per unit of time. The amount eliminated is proportional to the concentration of the drug in the blood.

Renal Excretion Plasma containing the drug and other substances is forced through the capillary blood vessels and into the glomerular capsule. Large molecules in the plasma such as proteins and cells are filtered out and remain in the blood. The resultant fluid that enters the capsule is called *glomerular filtrate.*

Some substances not removed by filtration because they are too large are eliminated by *active tubular secretion,* which requires energy, into the urine. Besides active secretion, selective

passive reabsorption of some drugs useful to the body such as water, glucose, and salts back into the blood takes place in the tubule. Additionally, a hydrophilic drug is excreted in the urine readily and will not be reabsorbed, while a lipophilic drug will be reabsorbed from the tubule back into the blood (passive diffusion) because it needs to be converted into metabolites before it is excreted.

The excretion rate is also dependent upon whether the drug is a weak acid or weak base. Weak acids are less ionized in an acidic environment. Thus, to increase the rate of excretion and reduce the chances of reabsorption of weak acids, the acid has to be ionized by increasing the pH of the urine; this can be done by administration of sodium bicarbonate. On the other hand, weak bases are less ionized as the pH of the urine increases.

Biliary Excretion In addition to renal excretion, some drugs are excreted in the bile by a process called biliary excretion. Bile, a fluid secreted by the liver, concentrates in the gallbladder and helps to break down fats and eliminates wastes and drugs in the body. These drugs undergo *enterohepatic recirculation* and are eventually metabolized by the liver and excreted into the kidneys; however, the part of the drug that is not recirculated continues in the bile and eventually is eliminated in the feces (Figure 2-9). Tetracyclines undergo enterohepatic circulation.

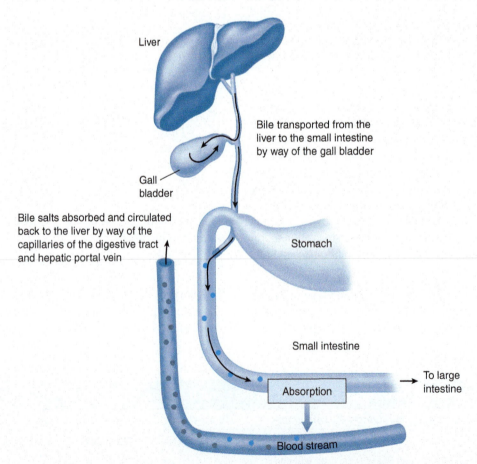

Liver

Bile transported from the liver to the small intestine by way of the gall bladder

Gall bladder

Bile salts absorbed and circulated back to the liver by way of the capillaries of the digestive tract and hepatic portal vein

Stomach

Small intestine

To large intestine

Absorption

Blood stream

FIGURE 2-9 Illustration of enterohepatic recirculation. Certain drugs are secreted into bile and eventually are eliminated in the feces (versus the urine).

CLINICAL PHARMACOKINETICS

Elimination Rate Constant and Half-life   Most drug elimination follows *first-order* kinetics: A constant percent of drug is eliminated from the body per each unit of time (Figure 2-10). That is to say, after a drug is given orally it will be absorbed by passive diffusion and the blood levels attained will be proportional to the dose administered; the greater the dose administered, the larger the blood-level concentration. As the drug is eliminated from the body, the concentration of the drug in the plasma will decrease equally over time.

There are exceptions to this rule. At high doses of some drugs (such as alcohol and aspirin), the enzyme system for biotransformation and elimination becomes saturated or overloaded and clearance is determined by how fast these pathways can work. The metabolic pathways work to their limit and cannot increase this rate even if the amount of drug delivered to them is increased. This means that the drug will be metabolized at a constant rate in spite of the amount of drug present. This is referred to as *zero-order kinetics,* in which drug elimination is at a constant rate in spite of the amount of drug present (Figure 2-11).

Half-life (*t½*) of elimination is the time it takes for the concentration of the drug in the blood to fall to half (50%) of its original value. It is an indicator of how long a drug will produce its effect in the body and defines the time interval between doses. It takes about four to five half-lives for a drug to be considered eliminated from the body.

For example, penicillin VK is given four times a day but amoxicillin is given three times a day, because amoxicillin has a longer t½ in the body (1.3 hours) versus penicillin VK (t½ 0.5 hours); therefore it does not have to be administered as frequently as penicillin (30 minutes). The larger the t½ value, the longer it takes for a drug to be eliminated from the body. Doxycycline, a tetracycline antibiotic, has a t½ of 18–22 hours, so it only has to be taken once a day after a twice-a-day loading dose on the first day. Drugs with very short half-lives, such as aspirin (t½ = 15–20 minutes) must be given every 3–4 hours. If a patient has renal or hepatic disease, the plasma half-life of a drug will increase, and the drug concentration may reach toxic levels. In these patients, drugs must be given less frequently or the dosages must be reduced.

Drug Administration

SINGLE-DOSE KINETICS

Plasma Drug Concentration Curve   After a single dose of drug is administered, the plasma concentration increases as the drug is absorbed. It reaches a peak or maximum concentration as absorption is completed and then decreases as the drug is eliminated (Figure 2-12). In most cases, except for rapid IV administration, drug distribution and absorption occur simultaneously.

Bioavailability   Bioavailability is the rate and the extent to which a drug is absorbed into the systemic circulation. The bioavailability of orally administered drugs is of special concern because it can be reduced by many factors, including the rate and extent of disintegration and dissolution, food, pH, and the effect of intestinal and liver enzymes. It is expressed as a percentage, for example, a drug delivered intravenously has 100% bioavailability because the entire amount of drug enters the bloodstream.

MULTIPLE-DOSE KINETICS

Drug Accumulation and the Steady-State Principle   If a drug that is eliminated by first-order kinetics is administered repeatedly or intermittently (e.g., amoxicillin—1 capsule every 8 hours for a dental infection), the average plasma concentration of the drug will increase or accumulate until it reaches a plateau or a steady-state plasma drug concentration (Figure 2-13). *Steady-state plasma concentration* refers to the point at which the rate of drug administration is equal to the rate of drug elimination.

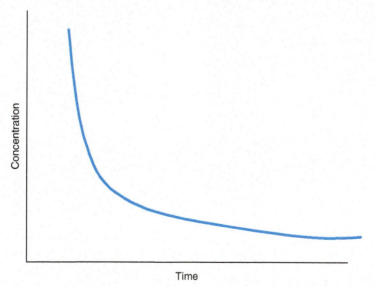

FIGURE 2-10 Most drugs exhibit first-order elimination, in which the rate of drug elimination is equivalent to the drug concentration in the blood.

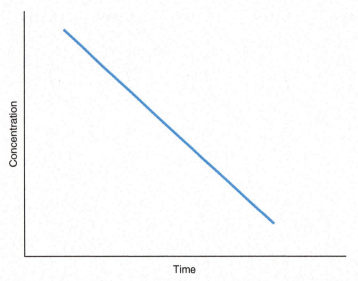

FIGURE 2-11 If drug elimination mechanisms become saturated, a drug may exhibit zero-order elimination.

The steady-state drug concentration depends on the drug dose administered and on the t½ of the drug. If the dose is doubled, the steady-state concentration is also doubled. When given at regular intervals, a drug reaches the steady-state level after approximately four to five half-lives.

DRUG DOSING Drug dose is defined as the quantity of drug administered. Dose size and dose regimen that is determined for an individual should compensate for any unusual properties of disposition that a drug may have. For example, if a drug exhibits a high rate of absorption, small doses of the drug are necessary to prevent high peak blood levels. If a drug exhibits a high rate of elimination, then more frequent doses are needed to maintain effective blood levels. Few drugs are administered as a single dose. The purpose of a *loading dose,* which is a large initial dose, is to rapidly establish a therapeutic plasma drug concentration (Figure 2-13). A large loading dose may be required initially in order to achieve a rapid response in situations that are life threatening. Subsequent doses, referred to as *maintenance doses,* are reduced. A maintenance dose maintains a desired steady-state plasma drug concentration. For example, for a dental infection penicillin VK is prescribed: 1,000 mg of penicillin VK is given immediately as a loading dose to obtain high initial blood levels, followed by 500 mg four times a day as a maintenance dose.

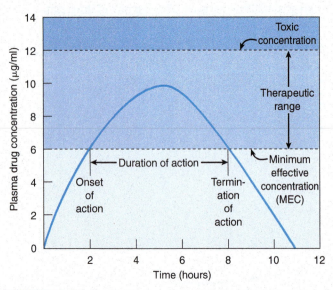

FIGURE 2-12 Graph showing oral administration of a single-dose drug. The time of onset is 2 hours and the end of drug action is 8 hours. This means that the drug has a duration of action of 6 hours. The plasma t ½ is about 4 hours (time it takes to decrease its concentration by one-half, or 50 percent).

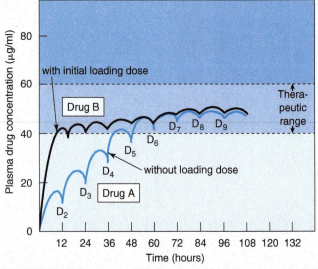

FIGURE 2-13 How repeated doses (D) of a drug cause an accumulation in the blood. Eventually, a plateau is reached where the level of drug in the blood is maintained continuously with the therapeutic range. Drug A and drug B are administered every 12 hours but drug B reaches the therapeutic range faster because a loading dose of drug B was given, but with drug A.

THERAPEUTIC DRUG RESPONSES   There are two plasma drug levels that are important in pharmacokinetics: the *minimum effective concentration* (MEC), which is the amount of drug required to produce a therapeutic effect, and the *toxic concentration,* which is the level of drug that will result in serious adverse effects (Figure 2-12). If an individual has a toothache and takes half an aspirin tablet, the plasma level will remain below the MEC and there will not be a therapeutic effect of pain relief. By taking two to three tablets, the plasma level of aspirin is increased into the therapeutic range with pain relief. If more than three tablets are taken, adverse effects will occur, resulting in toxic plasma concentration. This could be at zero-order kinetics at this point.

The *therapeutic range* or the *margin of safety* is the concentration of the drug in the plasma between the MEC and the toxic concentration. The goal to achieve a maximal response is to keep the plasma concentration in the therapeutic range. Some drugs such as warfarin and digoxin have a narrow therapeutic range, so that even a small amount above the therapeutic range can cause toxicity; penicillin has a wide margin of safety and is virtually nontoxic, even in large doses.

ADJUSTMENT OF DOSAGE   Certain conditions may reduce the clearance of drugs, which requires an adjustment of dosage.

Children and Older Adults   Children and older adults require lower drug doses than other individuals due to differences in their response to drugs. In neonates, the toxicity of drugs may be increased by delayed excretion or removal of the drug from the body because the organ systems are not yet developed. It is particularly important that the strengths of capsules or tablets be stated. Liquid preparations are especially suitable for young children; however, they may contain sucrose, which is a risk factor for caries. Older adults may have increased sensitivity to many commonly used drugs because the organs metabolize and excrete less efficiently.

Renal and Liver Impairment   Liver disease, including hepatitis and cirrhosis, may alter the response to drugs in many different ways. Drug prescribing should be kept to a minimum in all patients with severe liver disease, and sufficient information must be available to provide treatment guidelines. Certain drugs are contraindicated or require a reduced dose in patients with impaired liver function.

The use of drugs in patients with reduced kidney function (e.g., patients on dialysis) may produce toxicity because of impaired elimination from the body. The level of renal function must be determined before adjustment of doses. Either the drug dose remains the same but the dosing interval is increased or the dose is reduced while keeping the same dosing interval.

Tetracycline antibiotics are contraindicated in patients with kidney disease because the half-life is increased from about 10 hours to 57–108 hours.

Renal and liver function should be checked before prescribing any drug. Many problems can be avoided by reducing the dose or by using alternative drugs.

Pharmacodynamics

In the first section of this chapter, we reviewed how a drug gets to the site of action and what the body does to the drug. In this section, we review **pharmacodynamics,** which describes the actions a drug has on the body and involves drug–receptor interactions, mechanism of drug action, drug response, and the dose–response relationship.

Drug–Receptor Interaction

In order to initiate a physiological response, most drugs must first fit into a receptor. A **drug receptor,** usually a protein, is located on the cell membranes of every cell. A drug binds to the receptor and produces a response. The drug attaches to the receptor in a way similar to a lock and key (Figure 2-14). This type of *direct (specific) drug reaction* is the most common reaction involving drug–receptor interactions on the cell. One cell may have hundreds of receptor sites; the action of the drug is due to a change in the conformation of the receptor proteins where the drug attaches. Drugs bind to their receptor by forming Van der Waal's forces or ionic bonds (most common) with the receptor site. These bonds are reversible and weak, allowing the drug to leave the receptor easily as its tissue concentration decreases.

There are many different types of receptors. Receptors will allow binding of either a drug that is administered into the body or an endogenous substance that is synthesized and released within the body, such as a neurotransmitter (e.g.,

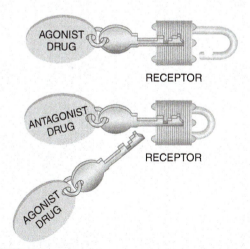

FIGURE 2-14 Illustration of a receptor on the surface of a cell with the drug. An agonist drug (key) binds to and unlocks or activates a receptor (lock). An antagonist drug (key) binds to and blocks a receptor (lock), but does not activate it. This antagonist drug prevents the agonist drug from unlocking the receptor.

acetylcholine) found in the central nervous system or a hormone such as insulin, thyroid, steroids, or histamine. A *ligand* is a molecule or drug that binds to a receptor to form a larger complex.

Some drugs (e.g., emollients, alcohol, general anesthetics, and hypnotics) do not act upon receptors, but act in an *indirect* or *nonspecific drug reaction.* Instead of relying on a receptor for drug action, these drugs saturate the water or lipid parts of the cell. The extent of drug action is proportional to the degree of drug saturation at the site of action within the cell. By reaching a certain level of saturation at a specific site on the cell, drug action occurs.

Drug Classifications in the Drug–Receptor Complex

There are three types of drug–receptor complexes (similar to a lock and key fit) (Figure 2-14): agonist, antagonist, and partial agonist. All of these types of drugs have an affinity for the receptor but they differ in what they cause the receptor to do. An *agonist* is a drug that rapidly combines with a receptor to initiate a response and rapidly dissociates or releases from the receptor; it has a high efficacy. An *antagonist* or blocker is a drug that binds to the receptor but does not dissociate and has no positive response or efficacy. It blocks the reaction of an agonist and is referred to as a blocking drug. A *partial agonist* binds to the receptor and produces a mild or submaximal therapeutic response and may inhibit the action of an agonist when given concurrently, acting like an antagonist. A *competitive antagonist* is a drug that occupies a significant proportion of the receptors and thereby prevents them from reacting maximally with an agonist. A noncompetitive antagonist may react with the receptor in such a way as not to prevent an agonist–receptor combination but to prevent the combination from initiating a response, or it may act to inhibit some subsequent event that leads to the final overt response.

Rapid Dental Hint

Naloxone (Narcan) is a narcotic antagonist drug administered to people who overdose on a narcotic drug (an agonist). Narcan competes for the same receptor site as the narcotic drug, blocking the receptor and thus reducing the narcotic's effects.

Dose–Response Relationships

New drugs must be tested in clinical trials. The outcome of treatment can be plotted as response versus log dose, where the response of the drug is measured in one of two ways: graded dose–response curve or quantal dose–response curve. The relationship between the concentration of a drug at the receptor site and the degree of the response is called the dose–response relationship.

In graded dose–response relationships, the response obtained with each dose is described in terms of a percentage of the *maximal response* and is plotted against the *log dose* of the drug (Figure 2-15). As the dose of the drug is increased, there is a gradual, progressive increase in the response until a maximum effect is seen. The drug causes a response with each dose and the maximal response is produced when all of the functional receptors are occupied and less of a response is seen when 50% of the functional receptors are occupied. Most drugs follow this *dose–response curve.* The patient's response obtained at different doses of the drug can be observed and measured. For example, after administration of a sleep-inducing drug such as a barbiturate, ataxia (unsteady muscle movement) is the first response seen, followed by sleep.

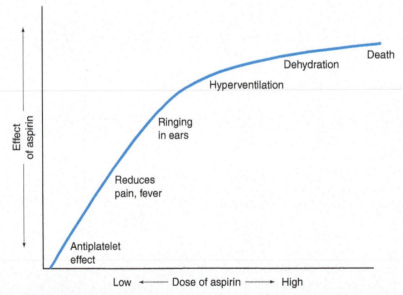

FIGURE 2-15 Dose-response relationship. As the dose of a drug increases, a maximal response or plateau is reached. Increasing the drug dose produces no additional therapeutic response.

In *quantal dose–response relationships,* the response seen with each dose of a drug exhibits an all-or-none effect.

The threshold dose is the minimum dose of a drug needed to produce a therapeutic/measurable response. It is important to maintain drug dosage concentration around the threshold level; otherwise the drug is ineffective, and in cases such as antibiotic therapy can result in bacteria that are more resistant to the drug.

Potency, Efficacy, and the Ceiling Effect

Potency refers to the measure of strength or concentration of a drug. It is usually expressed in terms of the median *effect dose* (ED_{50}), which is the dose of the drug required to produce the desired clinical effect in 50% of test animals. The potency of a drug varies inversely with a drug's ED_{50}. For example, a drug whose ED_{50} is 5 mg is 10 times more potent than a drug whose ED_{50} is 50 mg. Potency is determined by the affinity of a drug for its receptor.

Efficacy is the ability to produce a therapeutic effect regardless of the dose. Potency and efficacy often describe the success of drug therapy. For example, just knowing that 10 mg of morphine administered subcutaneously produces relief from pain tells us little about morphine's potency; it tells us only the dose required to produce a given intensity of response. However, 1.5 mg of hydromorphone or 120 mg of codeine, administered by the same route, is as effective as 10 mg of morphine in relieving the pain induced by the same stimulus, but morphine is less potent than hydromorphone and more potent than codeine. All three drugs have the same efficacy since they all produce a biological effect (Figures 2-16, 2-17).

The *ceiling effect* of a drug occurs when the therapeutic response cannot be increased with a higher dose of the drug. For example, because of its ceiling effect and poor bioavailability, increased doses of buprenorphine, a drug used in the management of opiate addiction, does not produce increased effects after a certain point, or ceiling. In fact, high doses of the drug can actually precipitate withdrawal symptoms in opiate-addicted individuals. Aspirin and NSAIDs also have a ceiling effect.

Toxicity

The ratio of a drug's toxic dose to its therapeutic dose is termed the *therapeutic index (TI).* A safe drug will have a high therapeutic index. The *median effective dose* (ED_{50}) is the drug dose that produces 50% of the maximum possible response in test animals. The dose at which 50% of test animals die is called the *lethal dose* (LD_{50}). Since a drug does not have a single toxic effect and has many therapeutic effects, it is not possible to have a list of a drug's TI; it must be calculated. The calculation is done by the following equation: $TI = LD_{50} \div ED_{50}$. A "safe" drug will have a high TI (generally at least 10). For example, the effective dose of drug A is 10 mg, and 50 mg is the average lethal dose. Thus, the TI is $50 \div 10 = 5$. This means that it would take an error in magnitude of approximately five times the average dose to be lethal to the patient.

Drug Effects

Drug effects are classified as summarized in Table 2-5.

Drugs can be extremely beneficial, lengthening life and improving its quality by reducing symptoms and improving health. Unfortunately, all drugs have adverse effects and can potentially cause injury and even death.

Responsible drug therapy requires knowing not only the efficacy of a particular drug but what combinations and conditions might aggravate a situation. In addition, the dental hygienist should be aware of unexpected reactions, such as allergies, that may occur.

Therapeutic effect is the desired and beneficial pharmaceutical effect that a drug exerts at the target site of action. For example, the primary therapeutic effect of diphenhydramine (Benadryl; an antihistamine) is to reverse allergic reactions.

An **adverse drug event** (ADE) is an undesirable experience associated with the use of a medical product. It is an unfavorable and unintended response to a drug. The FDA categorizes a serious adverse event, related to drugs or devices, as one in which the patient outcome is death, life-threatening, hospitalization,

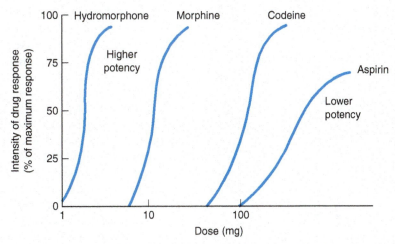

FIGURE 2-16 **Effect-log dose curve for the analgesic action of three narcotics and aspirin.** Hydromorphone is more potent than morphine and codeine, regardless of the response level at which they are compared.

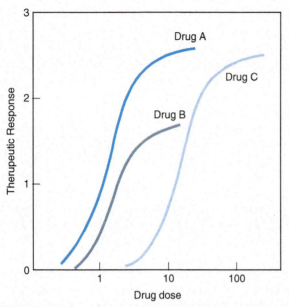

FIGURE 2-17 Drug A is more potent than Drugs B and C. Drugs A and C have equal efficacy because both drugs have reached the same maximum effect. Drug B has the least efficacy.

disability, congenital anomaly, or required intervention to prevent permanent impairment or damage. Type A adverse drug events that may lead to death are usually the result of toxicity, including prescribing too much of a correct drug (overdose) for the patient's age or weight, prescribing a drug contraindicated for the patient's condition, providing the correct drug by the wrong route or too quickly, and drug interactions. These reactions are usually predictable and preventable. Type B adverse drug events are rare and generally dose independent and are related more to the individual's response and genetic differences

---

TABLE 2-5 Drug Effects
• **Therapeutic effects**
• Intended pharmacological effect at target organ
• **Adverse drug events (ADEs)**
• Unfavorable and unintended response to a drug
• Predictable and preventable
• Medication error (e.g, miscalculations, overdose, misunderstanding of verbal orders)
• **Adverse drug reactions (ADRs)**
• Adverse effects
• Dose-related
• Predictable and affect nontarget organ sites
• **Toxic reactions**
• Dose-dependent and predictable
• Affects nontarget organ
• **Allergic reactions**
• Not dose-dependent and are unpredictable
• **Idiosyncratic reactions**
• Genetically related abnormal drug response

(e.g., some individuals are slow metabolizers of drugs degraded by certain enzymes and may be at risk for serious drug toxicity). Type B reactions are unpredictable and unpreventable.

The FDA has an Adverse Event Reporting System (AERS), which is a computerized information database designed to support the marketing safety surveillance program for all approved drug and therapeutic biological products. The FDA receives adverse drug reactions/events reports from manufacturers as required by regulation. Healthcare professionals and consumers send reports voluntarily through the MedWatch program (www.fda.gov/_medwatch). These reports become part of the database. In 2007, the FDA's Center for Drug Evaluation and Research (CDER) introduced a Web-based self-learning tutorial called FDA MedWatch and Patient Safety, which is obtained at www.connectlive.com/events/fdamedwatch. This tutorial reviews the FDA's MedWatch program.

On the other hand, an **adverse drug reaction** (ADR) has been defined by the World Health Organization (WHO) as "an effect which is noxious and unintended, and which occurs at doses used in man for prophylaxis, diagnosis, or therapy." *This term is restrictive because it only considers incidents where use of the drug is appropriate.* Medical errors are not included in this definition. Adverse drug reactions are not predictable and are unintentional because it is not known that a reaction will occur. Harm is directly caused by the drug at normal doses, during normal use. Examples of ADRs are the development of a rash after taking penicillin and bleeding from the stomach after taking corticosteroids or nonsteroidal anti-inflammatory drugs (Table 2-6). Another example of an ADR is bisphosphonate-related osteonecrosis of the jaw.

Adverse drug reactions are classified as adverse effects, toxic reactions, allergic reactions, and idiosyncratic reactions.

Side effects of a drug are additional drug actions at therapeutic levels that can be beneficial or adverse. *Side effects are dose related and predictable and are clinically evident at non-target organ sites.* For example, minoxidil (Loniten, Rogaine) was originally indicated as an antihypertensive drug, with a side effect of growing hair. Rogaine is a product for alopecia (hair loss) that is applied topically to the scalp; this is a beneficial side effect.

Adverse effects are undesirable effects that develop because drugs are not *totally* selective in their actions. Every medication has potential adverse side effects. Generally, adverse effects are dose related: the higher the dose, the greater the adverse effects. For example, adverse side effects of diphenhydramine are xerostomia, urinary retention, nausea, diarrhea, and drowsiness, which require little to no change in patient management. Categories of adverse side effects are listed by body systems, including gastrointestinal, endocrine, sense, nervous system, and hematological. Always be aware of adverse effects of a drug.

Toxicity or toxic reaction is defined as permanent damage to cell or tissue on a microscopic or macroscopic level. Acute toxicity results in an overdose when an individual dose is too large and is taken at one time. One example is the development of seizures from excessive lidocaine. Chronic toxicity occurs when the dose effects accumulate and are sometimes difficult

TABLE 2-6 Common Serious Adverse Drug Reactions

ADVERSE DRUG REACTION	DRUG CLASSIFICATION	DRUG(S)
Bleeding from the stomach	Nonsteroidal anti-inflammatory drugs (NSAIDs)	Aspirin, ibuprofen, naproxen
	Corticosteroids (anti-inflammatory)	Prednisone
Sleepiness, drowsiness, sedation	Antidepressants	Amitriptyline, fluoxetine
	Anti-anxiety drugs	Diazepam
	Antihistamines (allergies)	Diphenhydramine
Liver damage	Analgesics	Acetaminophen
	Antituberculosis drugs	Isoniazid (INH)

Source: Adapted from *Merck Manual* (18th edition).

to detect, since they may take years to develop. Toxic reactions are *predictable, dose dependent, and may be clinically evident at nontarget organ sites.* An example of drug toxicity is acetaminophen (Tylenol) overuse, which can lead to liver injury.

A drug idiosyncrasy is an unexplained, uncharacteristic response to a drug caused by hereditary factors or genetic differences. These reactions are beginning to be understood through pharmacogenetics. One example of this type of pharmacogenetic condition is seen in the X-linked genetic trait of a deficiency in the red blood cell enzyme glucose-6-phosphate dehydrogenase (G6PD). These patients can develop drug-induced hemolytic anemia after primaquine (for malaria) therapy.

The development of an allergic response requires a foreign substance called an antigen to enter the body that causes the body to produce antibodies in response to the antigen. Unlike other adverse reactions, *allergies are not dose related and are unpredictable.* The allergic response occurs when a complex is formed between the antigen and antibody, which produces an allergic reaction. Generally, the foreign substance that acts as an antigen is a macromolecule (e.g., protein). Since drugs are not proteins, in order to cause an allergic response, the drug will have to bind irreversibly with some body protein. Once the antibody forms in the body to this drug–protein complex the antibody will subsequently react with the drug alone. An allergic response can range from a mild rash to an anaphylaxis, which is life-threatening. Identifying a true drug allergy can be challenging. A true allergy versus an adverse effect of a drug must be differentiated. For example, a patient reported an upset stomach when ibuprofen was taken. This is an adverse effect, not an allergic reaction. A common drug allergy is to penicillin: 10% of the population is allergic to penicillin, including amoxicillin. Other drug allergies include pyrophosphate (anticalculus ingredient in toothpastes), cephalosporins, and sulfa drugs (sulfonamides such as Septra and Bactrim).

Drug reactions commonly manifest with dermatological symptoms. The most common skin manifestation is an erythematous, maculopapular rash that appears within 1–2 weeks after drug exposure, originates on the trunk, and eventually spreads to the limbs. Oral manifestations of allergy may be evident as erythematous, vesicular, or ulcerative mucosa.

Mutagenic effects are caused by drug-induced damage to DNA (deoxyribonucleic acid). The display of damage is evident in the children from these parents. Essentially, it is a heritable genetic defect. This is distinguished from a teratogenic defect, which refers to the drug-induced damage that develops in the fetus. Mutagenic effects depend on when the drug exposure occurred during the DNA replication cycle. It can be a minor error where the damage occurred in only one base pair, or a major error where there is an abnormal protein or no protein produced.

An example of a teratogenic drug is thalidomide, which was originally marketed as a nonaddictive sedative, but its use was discontinued due to severe teratogenic properties. Today it is being used in the treatment of oral mucosal diseases such as severe major aphthous stomatitis in HIV-infected patients and erythema nodosum.

Drug Interactions

Certain drugs given concurrently with another drug, herbal supplements, or food can cause a drug interaction that can be clinically significant and cause adverse/toxic side effects. There are many different mechanisms of drug interactions, which are further discussed in Chapter 16. For example, when tetracycline is taken with milk, it forms a complex that prevents absorption of the drug, making it ineffective as an antibiotic. Food can inhibit or delay absorption of certain antibiotics (e.g., azithromycin, metronidazole). Often a specified time interval must exist between taking certain drugs with foods or with one another.

Factors That Modify the Effects of Drugs

BIOLOGICAL VARIATION *Biological variation* explains the different responses seen among individuals within the same population, given the same dose of a drug. Certain factors are responsible for individual variation. For instance, body weight will influence drug dosing. Generally, when dealing with most adults, drug adjustment of dose to body weight is not really necessary. However, dose adjustment is necessary if the body weight is outside the normal adult range or if a potent drug with a small margin of safety is given. Smaller females may require a lower dose than males.

It is important to recognize the physiological responses that change with age. In very young children, liver enzymes are underdeveloped, resulting in a deficiency in enzyme function. The renal tubular system is not completely developed and there is a deficiency in active excretion. Also, the blood flow through the kidneys is slower. Thus, a lower drug dose may be necessary.

In older adults there is a deterioration of drug removal processes and a decrease in responsiveness of receptor sites. This makes it difficult to adjust the dose. Additionally in older adults there are decreases in renal function, body cell mass, liver enzyme activity, and metabolic activity.

There are certain enzyme deficiencies that are hereditary and may affect drug dosing. Some individuals may show slow or fast acetylation of certain drugs such as isoniazid (INH; antituberculosis drug) that is metabolized by acetylation.

The presence of disease may alter the drug response. Any disease that affects the liver or kidney will increase or extend the duration of drug action. There may also be changes in receptor site sensitivity. The most obvious example of this is aspirin. Aspirin will reduce fever in an individual with fever, but does not reduce body temperature in an individual without fever.

An *idiosyncratic response* is an unusual effect of a drug that is possible with any drug or individual.

Some individuals are unusually responsive and are called *intolerant* or *hyperresponsive*. One factor involved in this response distribution is adaptation. *Adaptation* is a homeostatic adjustment that may occur during continued or prolonged presence of a drug. The body adjusts itself and minimizes the effects of the drug.

Tolerance is the need for increasing amounts of a drug to obtain the same therapeutic effect. For instance, progressive, small increases in the amount of alcohol or a narcotic analgesic are needed to cause the same effect. Tolerance does not occur universally and is a long-term reduction in response (e.g., weeks or months). An individual may develop tolerance to a certain drug and not to others. *Tachyphlaxis,* a very rapid development of tolerance, is a rapid decreasing response (within hours or days) with repeated administration of the same dose of drug at short intervals. In dental practice, tachyphlaxis to local anesthetics may develop. For example, a local anesthetic is administered to a dental patient. Once the nerve function returns to its preinjection state and the patient requires more anesthetic because of pain, the duration and intensity of anesthesia with reinjection is greatly diminished. Thus, successive doses of the anesthetic will be less effective than those given previously.

Placebo Response

An individual given a placebo, a drug that does not have any pharmacological effect, will report experiencing effects that would have been expected when receiving the active drug. This is called the placebo effect and is a measurable, observable, or felt improvement in health not attributable to treatment. The placebo effect can also be a psychological or physiological reaction, having confidence in the drug.

Dental Hygiene Applications

In order to produce their desired pharmacological and biological effects, most drugs must interact with a receptor on/in a cell and initiate a series of physiologic events. The receptor site is the site of action of a drug.

Pharmacodynamics deals with the events of drug action; it explains what the drug does to the body. In order for the drug to produce this action, it must be absorbed through various tissue membranes, be distributed to the various tissues and organs, and be metabolized to a water-soluble form so that it can be eliminated from the body. Pharmacokinetics determines the drug concentration at the site of action.

To understand the mechanisms of drug action and the clinical use of therapeutic agents for the prevention, diagnosis, and treatment of disease, it is important to understand the basics of pharmacology that have been presented in this chapter.

Many orally administered drugs (e.g., propranolol, a cardiac drug) lose some activity due to first-pass metabolism

Rapid Dental Hint

The dental hygienist plays an integral part of the dental team. Understanding the general principles of pharmacology is important when dealing with dental patients. The medical and drug history of patients must be reviewed. Drug–drug interactions can be recognized if the clinician has an understanding of the various mechanisms of pharmacokinetics and pharmacodynamics.

through the liver. Only the nonionized form of weak acids and bases is lipid soluble and more easily absorbed from the small intestine. Morphine and lidocaine undergo extensive first-pass metabolism, which prevents them from being administered orally.

A drug will absorb through cell membranes by passive diffusion more easily if it is lipophilic. Many drugs are bound to plasma proteins to a limited extent, but some (e.g., warfarin, an anticoagulant drug) are extensively bound (more than 95%), which limits distribution to tissues and organs. Many drugs are biotransformed (metabolized) before elimination from the body. Drugs are eliminated from the body either unchanged or as water-soluble metabolites. Lipid-soluble drugs must be biotransformed to more water-soluble metabolites. A loading dose is given to establish an initial therapeutic plasma drug concentration. A lower, maintenance dose follows to maintain therapeutic plasma drug concentrations.

Key Points

- Pharmacokinetics is the study of how drugs are handled by the body.
- Pharmacodynamics is the study of how drugs work and how they interact with receptors.
- A drug exerts a pharmacological effect or response.
- Liver cytochrome P450 enzymes are involved in many drug–drug interactions
- Drugs are absorbed into the blood in a nonionized, lipid-soluble form.
- Lipid solubility is one of the most important determinants of the pharmacokinetic characteristics of a drug; rate of absorption can be predicted from knowledge of a drug's lipid solubility.
- Highly ionized drugs cannot pass lipid membranes.
- Drugs are absorbed in the nonionized, lipid-soluble form. The nonionized portion of the drug shows great lipid solubility and therefore greater absorption.
- Nonionized drugs can cross lipid membranes freely.
- Most drugs are either weak acids or weak bases.
- Acids are most highly ionized at a high pH (e.g., an alkaline environment such as the intestines).
- For weak acids, the more acidic the environment, the less ionized the drug and the more easily it crosses lipid membranes.
- Bases are most highly ionized in an acidic environment (e.g., the stomach).
- All drugs are eventually eliminated by the body by either hepatic biotransformation or renal excretion, or a combination of both.
- Water-soluble (hydrophilic) drugs are excreted through the kidney in the urine.

Board Review Questions

1. Nitroglycerin is not given orally because it (pp. 25–26)
   a. has a bad taste.
   b. dissolves slowly in the mouth.
   c. has a high first-pass metabolism.
   d. undergoes absorption in the stomach too quickly.

2. Displacement of a drug from plasma albumin binding sites would usually be expected to (p. 28)
   a. decrease the amount of distribution.
   b. increase blood levels of the drug.
   c. decrease the metabolism of the drug.
   d. increase the metabolism of the drug.

3. Which of the following routes will a drug follow after intravenous administration? (p. 27)
   a. Vein, general circulation, liver, kidney
   b. Esophagus, stomach, small intestine, liver, kidney
   c. Liver, small intestine, kidney
   d. Vein, liver, general circulation, kidney

4. An individual has overdosed on oxycodone, a narcotic analgesic, and is administered a narcotic antagonist. Which of the following features describes antagonist drugs? (pp. 33–34)
   a. Binds to the same receptor sites as agonist drugs.
   b. Binds to the receptor to reduce the actions of the agonist.
   c. Have a greater affinity to the receptor than agonists.
   d. Have a lesser affinity to the receptor than agonists.

5. A prescription for penicillin VK is given to a dental patient with an endodontic abscess. The prescription is written for an initial loading dose followed by a maintenance dose. Which of the following reasons explains the rationale for giving a loading dose for an antibiotic? (p. 32)
   a. Maintains a desired steady-state plasma level.
   b. Attains the desired blood level immediately.
   c. Decreases premature clearance of the drug.
   d. Increases the rate of drug metabolism.

6. A patient has an artificial heart valve and is taking clindamycin, an antibiotic, for prophylaxis against bacteremia. In order for the clindamycin to be absorbed into the blood, it must pass through (p. 22)
   a. three barriers: epithelial cells + blood vessels + brain
   b. two barriers: epithelial cells + blood vessel
   c. one barrier: blood
   d. no barrier: drug does directly into blood

7. All of the following statements are true about lipid-soluble drugs *except* one. Which one is the exception? (pp. 22, 24)
   a. Readily absorbed through blood vessel wall
   b. Slowly absorbed through cell membrane
   c. Goes through the blood–brain barrier
   d. Can be given by inhalation

8. Which of the following reasons explains why an intravenously administered drug such as an antibiotic achieves very high initial blood concentration levels? (pp. 19, 20, 22)
   a. Drugs made of small molecules
   b. Drugs have a high pH
   c. No barrier to absorption
   d. Expensive to give

9. Which of the following statements is true regarding absorption of local anesthetics? (pp. 24, 25)
   a. Lidocaine (pK_a 4) is not absorbed easily through lipid membranes.
   b. Lidocaine (pK_a 7.9) has a fast onset because the tissue pH is close to the pKa.
   c. Bupivicaine (pK_a 8.3) has a faster onset than lidocaine.
   d. Bupivicaine (pK_a 7.7) has a slow onset of action because it is highly unionized.

10. Which of the following terms is related to the amount of drug administered? (p. 32)
    a. Dose
    b. Response
    c. Agonist
    d. Toxicity

11. Which of the following routes of drug administration bypasses the GI tract? (pp. 19, 20)
    a. Intravenous
    b. Oral
    c. Buccal
    d. Sublingual

12. Which of the following routes of administration applies to Atridox? (pp. 20, 21)
    a. Oral
    b. Transdermal
    c. Subcutaneous
    d. Topical

13. Which of the following terms describes the development of constipation after a patient started taking acetaminophen with codeine after a tooth extraction? (pp. 35, 36)
    a. Toxicity
    b. Allergy
    c. Idiosyncrasy
    d. Adverse effect

14. A dental patient taking a bisphosphonate comes into the office for an initial visit. The patient had a tooth extracted during the week and complained of extreme pain in her jaw. Upon examination, the dentist made a diagnosis of osteonecrosis of the jaw. Which of the following terms best describes this situation? (pp. 35, 36)
    a. Adverse drug reaction
    b. Adverse drug event
    c. Allergic response
    d. Acute toxicity

15. A patient had an injection of lidocaine with epinephrine. Which of the following types of injections was given? (p. 20)
    a. Subcutaneous
    b. Intravenous
    c. Intramuscular
    d. Subgingival

Selected References

Avorn J. 1997. Putting adverse drug events into perspective. *Journal of the American Medical Association* 277:341–342.

Barker L, Bromley L. 2002. Pharmacology 2—Pharmacokinetics. *Anesthesia* 15:25–36.

Bates DW, Leape L. 2000. Adverse drug reactions. In *Melmon and Morrelli's clinical pharmacology,* 4th ed. edited by SF Carruthers, BB Hoffman, KL Melmon, DW Nierenberg. New York: McGraw-Hill, pp. 1223–1256.

Brenner GM. 2000. *Pharmacology.* Philadelphia: W.B. Saunders, pp. 9–31.

Cohen JS. 1999. Ways to minimize adverse drug reactions. Individualized doses and common sense are key. *Postgraduate Medicine* 106:163–168, 171–172.

deShazo RD, Kemp SF. 1997. Allergic reactions to drugs and biologic agents. *Journal of the American Medical Association* 278:1895–1906.

Flexner C. 1999. Pharmacokinetics for physicians—A primer. www.medscape.com/viewarticle/408238.

Gossel TA. 1998. Pharmacology: Back to basics. *U.S. Pharmacist* 23:70–78.

Gossel TS. 1998. Exploring pharmacology. *U.S. Pharmacist* 23:96–104.

Kelly WN. 2001. Can the frequency and risks of fatal adverse drug events be determined? *Pharmacotherapy* 21(5):521–527.

Lazo J, Parker K. 2005. Pharmacokinetics, Pharmacodynamics: The dynamics of drug absorption, distribution, action and elimination. In *Goodman & Gilman's the pharmacological basis of therapeutics,* 11th ed. edited by L Brunton, J Lazo, K Parker. New York: McGraw-Hill.

Levine RR. 1996. *Pharmacology: Drug actions and reactions,* 5th ed. New York: Parthenon.

Mayer MH, Dowsett SA, Brahmavar K, Hornbuckle K, Brookfield WP. 2010. Reporting adverse drug events. *US Pharm.* 35:HS-15–HS-19.

Nebeker JR, Barach P, Samore MH. 2004. Clarifying adverse drug events: A clinician's guide to terminology. *Ann Inter Med.* 140:795–801.

Pratt WB, Taylor P. 1990. *Principles of drug action: The basis of pharmacology,* 3rd ed. New York: Churchill Livingstone.

Riedl MA, Casillas, AM. 2003. Adverse drug reactions: Types and treatment options. *American Family Physician.* 68:1781–1790.

Web Sites

http://www.fda.gov/Drugs/GuidanceComplianceRegulatory Information/Guidances/ucm064982.htm

http://www.fda.gov/downloads/Drugs/GuidanceCompliance RegulatoryInformation/Guidances/ucm072123.pdf

http://www.fda.gov/downloads/Drugs/GuidanceCompliance RegulatoryInformation/Guidances/ucm072137.pdf

Autonomic Nervous System Drugs

EDUCATIONAL OBJECTIVES

After reading this chapter, the reader should be able to:

1. Understand the differences between the sympathetic and parasympathetic divisions of the autonomic nervous system.

2. Illustrate the different types of receptors and neurotransmitters in the autonomic nervous system.

3. Identify drugs affecting the autonomic nervous system (sympathetic and parasympathetic divisions).

4. Understand the differences between adrenergic and cholingeric drugs.

5. Describe the role of autonomic nervous system drugs in dentistry.

6. Explain the use of vasoconstrictors (in local anesthetics) in dental patients.

KEY TERMS

Autonomic nervous system

Neuron

Neurotransmitters

Agonists

Antagonists

Sympathomimetics

Sympatholytics

Cholinergic

Anticholinergic

GOALS

- To gain knowledge of the fundamentals of the sympathetic and para-sympathetic nervous system; this is essential for understanding the mechanism of action of many drugs used in dentistry and medicine.

- To provide knowledge about the fundamentals of the autonomic nervous system drugs used to treat various medical conditions and how these drugs affect dental treatment.

Introduction

Some medications used by dental clinicians and many drugs taken by dental patients act upon the autonomic nervous system. It is essential that the dental hygienist be familiar with these medications.

The Nervous System

Structurally, the human nervous system is divided into the central nervous system (CNS) and the peripheral nervous system (PNS). The *central nervous system* is composed of the brain and spinal cord, which receive sensory input from the peripheral nervous system. The *peripheral nervous system* is functionally divided into the **autonomic nervous system** (ANS) and the *somatic nervous system*. The somatic nervous system, also called the *voluntary* nervous system, innervates the skeletal muscles, causing contractions. The autonomic nervous system, or the *involuntary* (digestion, circulation) nervous system, is composed of motor nerve cells that transmit impulses to smooth muscles (e.g., intestinal, urinary bladder, uterus, eyes, lungs, and small arteries and veins), cardiac muscle, and glands (Figure 3-1). These impulses are involuntary and cannot be consciously controlled. The autonomic nervous system is further subdivided into *sympathetic* and *parasympathetic divisions*.

Nerve Cell Anatomy

The autonomic nervous system is a two-neuron chain. What is a neuron? A **neuron** is the unit of cellular structure of the central nervous system. In the brain there are about 10 billion neurons. Neurons are nerve cells that transmit messages throughout the body. The neurons communicate with each other and transmit information in the form of electrical influx or action potential in

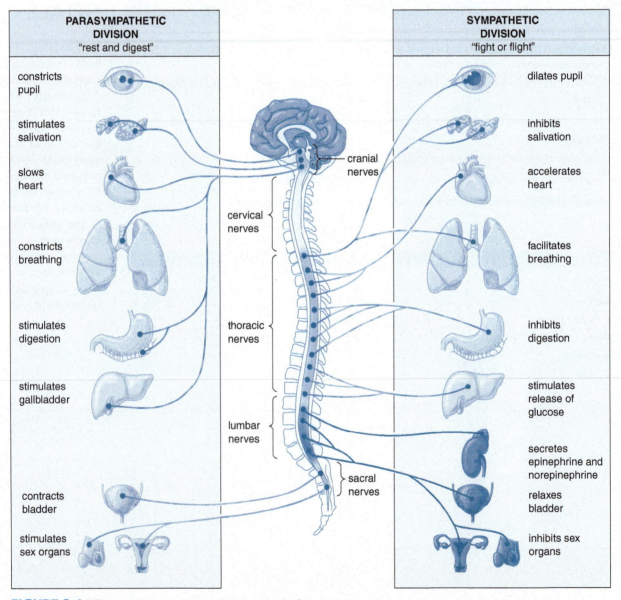

FIGURE 3-1 Effects of the sympathetic and parasympathetic nervous systems.

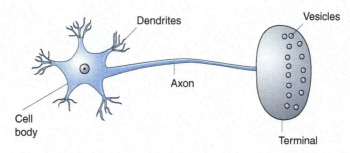

FIGURE 3-2 Diagram of a neuron.

which a stimulus of sufficient intensity is applied to a neuron. Neurons are composed of four parts (Figure 3-2):

- *Cell body* or soma, where normal cellular processes occur
- *Dendrites,* where receptors are located
- Axon, an extension or sending part
- Axon terminal, where the axon terminates; within the terminal are vesicles

Individual neurons do not directly contact one another. Instead, one neuron closely approaches another neuron, but is still separated from the other by a small space. This type of neuronal junction is called the *synapse* and the actual space is called the *synaptic cleft.* Neurons communicate with other neurons and with the target (effector) organ at these synapses. If the connection between the two neurons is outside the CNS, it is called a ganglion.

- The neurons of the *sympathetic division* originate in the thoracolumbar portion of the spinal cord as *preganglionic (or presynaptic) nerve fibers (neurons).*
- The long, *postganglionic (or postsynaptic) neurons* extend to the organs they innervate (e.g., heart, eye, lung, blood vessels, stomach and intestines, kidney, secretory glands, and urinary bladder) (Figure 3-1).

In the *parasympathetic division,* the cell bodies of the *presynaptic neurons* originate from four cranial nerves (CN III, VII, IX, and X) in the brain and from the sacral (S2–5) regions of the spinal cord. These nerves do not travel through the spinal nerves but rather the short *postganglionic neurons* synapse at or near the target organ.

NEUROTRANSMITTERS

- Because the two neurons do not actually contact each other, a nerve impulse from the brain cannot cross from one neuron to the next. Instead, in the synapse region the electrical signal that has been transmitted the length of the

preganglionic neuron located in the brain is transformed into a chemical signal through the release of a substance called a neurotransmitter (Figures 3-3, 3-4).

- **Neurotransmitters** are synthesized in the neuron and stored in vesicles or boutons located in the axon terminal of one neuron. In response to a nerve action potential (nerve impulse), the neurotransmitter is released from the vesicles into the synaptic space and binds to receptors on the postsynaptic or postganglionic neuron.
- This interaction of a neurotransmitter with a postsynaptic receptor results in the creation of a new action potential with the release of more neurotransmitters, which cross the synapse and bind to receptors on the target organ.
- This results in either an inhibitory or excitatory action of the organ (e.g., increased heart rate or decreased intestinal movement).
- *The purpose of the neurotransmitter is to carry nerve impulses across the synapse.* Once the neurotransmitter has reacted with the receptor, it is rapidly removed to allow the arrival of a second signal. The neurotransmitter is removed by enzymes, which degrade it into an inactive metabolite or by a process of "reuptake" whereby the specific neurotransmitter is taken back up into the axon terminal, where it is inactivated by enzymes.
- There are many types of neurotransmitters. The primary neurotransmitters found in the ANS are acetylcholine (ACh) and norepinephrine (NE; released from adrenal glands). Other neurotransmitters include epinephrine (EPI), dopamine, serotonin, and GABA (gamma aminobutyric acid).

RECEPTORS Receptors are structures, usually proteins, that receive neurotransmitters released from the axonal terminals of the neuron. Receptors are located on the dendrites of postganglionic neurons and on/in smooth muscle, cardiac muscle, and glands (Figure 3-2).

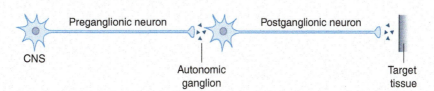

FIGURE 3-3 Basic structure of the autonomic nervous system.

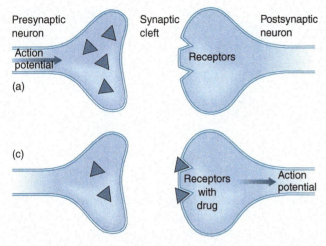

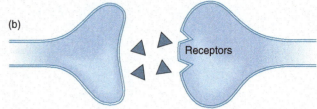

FIGURE 3-4 Synaptic transmission. (a) Action potential reaches synapse; (b) neurotransmitter released synaptic cleft; (c) neurotransmitter reaches receptors to regenerate action potential.

Functions of the Autonomic Nervous System: Neurotransmitters and Receptors

Most organs of the body are innervated by neurons of both the sympathetic and parasympathetic divisions of the ANS. The only organs not innervated by both are the sweat glands, smooth muscles of the hair follicles, the adrenal medulla, and blood vessels of the skin.

- Generally, stimulation of the sympathetic (adrenergic) and parasympathetic (cholinergic) nerves causes opposite responses (Table 3-1; Figure 3-3).

- If one division increases the activity of an organ, the other generally decreases it.

- The sympathetic nervous system is sometimes called the "fight-or-flight response."

  - Prepares the individual for emergency/stressful situations, such as those responses required during aggressive or defensive behavior. These reactions include increased heart rate, increased blood flow to the skeletal muscles, and dilation of the bronchi.

- The parasympathetic system is the "resting and digestive response."

  - Maintains the body organs at activity levels that are most efficient in maintaining normal homeostasis of the body. It slows the heart rate, lowers the blood pressure, and stimulates the gastrointestinal tract.

Sympathetic Nervous System (Adrenergic): Neurotransmitters

1. The neurotransmitter released from *every* preganglionic nerve terminal in the sympathetic division is acetylcholine, which causes excitation of the adrenergic postganglionic nerve and initiates the synthesis and release of norepinephrine (NE) from *most* postganglionic nerve terminals into the neuroeffector junction (Figure 3-5).

2. Norepinephrine then diffuses across the neuroeffector junction and exerts its effects on the effector tissue [smooth muscle (e.g., intestines, uterus, and small arteries and veins), gland, or cardiac muscle].

   a. Catecholamines, also known as adrenergic neurotransmitters, are derived from the amino acid tyrosine. The principal catecholamines are EPI, NE, and dopamine.

3. Nerve fibers that synthesize and release ACh are called *cholinergic fibers* and cause cholinergic effects.

4. Nerve fibers that secrete NE are called *adrenergic neurons* and cause adrenergic effects.

There are a few exceptions to this general rule:

1. Sweat glands are innervated only by sympathetic cholinergic pathway, which releases ACh to cause sweating. Thus, these postganglionic fibers are cholinergeric, not adrenergic.

2. The adrenal medulla is the central part of the adrenal glands located superior to the kidneys. Each adrenal medulla is innervated by a sympathetic *preganglionic* nerve, which releases ACh. The ACh then causes the release of two hormones, EPI (85%) and NE (15%). There are no postganglionic fibers innervating the adrenal medulla.

DID YOU KNOW?

Did you know that when you are scared of an insect or a snake your sympathetic nervous system gets activated to help you deal with this frightening episode?

Sympathetic Nervous System: Adrenergic Receptors

Different effector tissues (smooth muscle, cardiac muscle, and glands) contain different types of receptors with which the sympathetic neurotransmitters, NE and EPI, may interact. The two types of *adrenergic receptors* are referred to as alpha (α)- and beta (β)-receptors. Certain effector tissue contains only α-receptors, other tissues contain only β-receptors, and other tissues contain both α- and β-receptors (Figure 3-5; Tables 3-1, 3-2, 3-3, 3-4).

There are two *subtypes* of α-adrenergic receptors; α_1- and α_2-receptors:

- α_1 receptors are located on postganglionic blood vessels and smooth muscle (genitourinary system, sweat glands,

TABLE 3-1 Effects of the Autonomic Nervous System

EFFECTOR ORGAN	SYMPATHETIC (ADRENERGIC) RESPONSE (RECEPTOR)	PARASYMPATHETIC (CHOLINERGIC) RESPONSE (RECEPTOR—ALL MUSCARINIC)
Cardiac Muscle		
Heart	↑ Heart rate, contractility (β_1) ↑ BP	↓ Heart rate, contractility, blood pressure
Smooth Muscle		
Lung (bronchioles)	Dilation (relaxation) (β_2)	Constriction (contraction)
Digestive tract (stomach; small intestines) (GI)	Decreased acid secretion (α_1, β_2) Decreased motility (constipation)	Increased motility and increased acid secretion
Urinary bladder	Contraction (α_1)	Relaxation (urine flow)
Eye		
Iris	Dilation of pupil (mydriasis) (α_1)	Contraction of pupil (miosis)
Ciliary muscle	Relaxation for far vision (β_2)	Contraction for near vision
Skin		
Arrector pili muscles	Contraction ("goose bumps") (α_1)	No innervation
Liver	Breakdown of glycogen (β_2)	—
Blood Vessels		
Coronary (heart)	Constriction (α_1) Dilation (β_2)	Dilation; decreased heart rate
Mucosal linings	Constriction (α_1)	No innervation
Skin	Constriction (α_1)	No innervation
Skeletal muscles	Constriction (α_1); dilation (β_2)	No innervation
Glands		
Lacrimal (tear)	No innervation	Secretion of tears
Sweat	Sweat (muscarinic)	No innervation
Adrenal medulla	Secretion of EPI	No innervation
Salivary	Thick, mucous saliva (α_1)	Thin, watery saliva

eye, intestine). Activation of α_1-receptors influences both blood pressure and blood flow into the tissues and causes contraction of smooth muscles.

- α_2-receptors are located on postganglionic neurons and are called autoreceptors because activation of α_2-receptors causes inhibition of NE release, decreases secretion of insulin, decreases blood pressure, and decreases eye secretion.

There are three *subtypes* of β-adrenergic receptors:

- β_1-adrenergic receptors are located on cardiac tissue and when stimulated produce heart stimulation, leading to a positive chronotropic effect (increased heart rate) and a positive inotropic effect (increased contractility or strength).

- β_2-adrenergic receptors are located on the smooth muscle of the bronchioles, skeletal muscle, and blood vessels supplying the heart and kidneys. Activation of β_2-receptors causes relaxation of these smooth muscles. Whereas EPI and NE are equally potent and effective at β_1-receptors on cardiac tissue, EPI is more potent than NE on β_2-receptors.

- β_3-receptors are found on fat cells (adipocytes) and produce breakdown of lipids. Research is currently underway to develop a drug that will selectively activate this receptor because it may be useful in the treatment of obesity.

General Rules

1. Those responses due to α-*receptor* activation are primarily *excitatory* or stimulating (e.g., vasoconstriction, contraction of the uterine muscles) with the *exception* of intestinal relaxation.

2. Those responses due to β-*receptor* activation are primarily *inhibitory* or relaxing (e.g., vasodilation, relaxation of the uterine muscles and bronchial tree) with the *exception* of stimulant effects on the heart. The β-receptors of the heart are referred to as β_1-receptors. All other β-receptors (lungs, eye, uterus) are referred to as β_2-receptors.

3. *Epinephrine* released (in response to some forms of stress) by the adrenal medulla acts on both α- and β-receptors, but its effects are more potent on β_2-receptors (because it stays on these receptors longer; higher affinity). Epinephrine in the

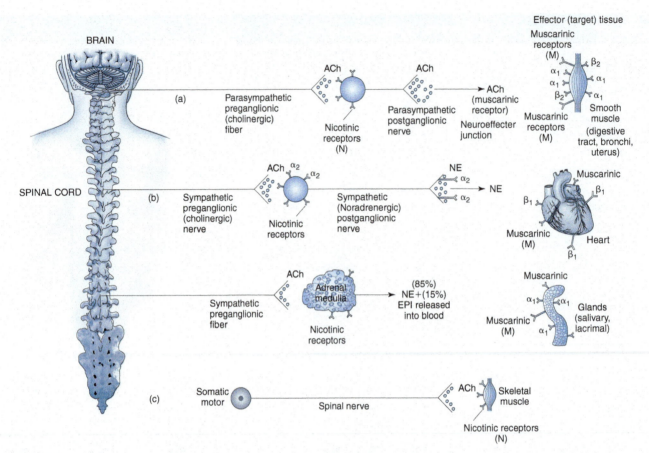

FIGURE 3-5 **(a) Parasympathetic pathway.** ACh is released from the preganglionic neuron over the synapse and stimulates cholinergic (nicotine) receptors. Then ACh is released from the postganglionic neuron, which activates the cholinergic (muscarinic) receptors on the target tissue. **(b)** Sympathetic pathway: Acetylcholine (ACh) is released from the preganglionic neuron and stimulates cholinergic (nicotine) receptors on the postganglionic neuron. Then, norepinephrine (NE) is released from the end of the postganglionic neuron, which is then transmitted to the target tissue, where it activates receptors on the surface. These adrenergic (sympathetic) receptors are either alpha (α) or beta (β). **(c)** Somatic motor pathway: nicotinic receptors on skeletal muscle.

TABLE 3-2	Neurotransmitters of the Autonomic Nervous System
PATHWAY	**NEURON/NEUROTRANSMITTER**
Sympathetic	**Smooth Muscle; Cardiac Muscle; Glands**
	Presynaptic neuron (cell body located within the CNS): Releases acetylcholine (ACh) into the synapse
	Postsynaptic neuron (cell body located outside CNS): Releases norepinephrine (NE) into the neuroeffector junction (NE will then have a pharmacological effect on the effector tissue, including smooth muscles, cardiac muscles, and glands)
	Adrenal Medulla
	Adrenal medulla (located on top of each kidney): Only presynaptic neurons, which release ACh. This stimulates the secretion of EPI (85%) and NE (15%)
	Sweat Glands
	Innervated by only sympathetic cholinergic neurons, which release ACh
Parasympathetic	**Neurons**
	Presynaptic neuron: Releases acetylcholine (ACh) into the synapse
	Postsynaptic neuron: Releases acetylcholine (ACh) into the neuroeffector junction (ACh will then have a pharmacological effect on the effector tissue)

TABLE 3-3 Classification of Autonomic Receptors

NERVOUS SYSTEM DIVISION/ NEUROTRANSMITTER	RECEPTOR	LOCATION OF RECEPTOR (FOUND ON THE SURFACE OF EFFECTOR TISSUE/ORGAN AND/ OR AXONAL TERMINAL OF NEURONS)	THERAPEUTIC OBJECTIVE
Sympathetic			
Norepinephrine (NE) (postganglionic/adrenergic receptors)	α_1	Located in smooth muscle of blood vessels and smooth muscle of most organs (e.g., heart, skin, eye, bladder, intestine, salivary glands) except the heart muscle (Note: α_1-receptors are located in blood vessels of the heart but not heart muscle, causing vasoconstriction and increased blood pressure)	Vasoconstriction (constrict blood vessels); dilates pupils (mydriasis) Urinary retention Decrease gastrointestinal motility
	α_2	Located on neurons that release NE (presynaptic); termed auto-receptors because they inhibit the amount of NE released when levels get too high; also found in eye, intestinal, hepatic, platelets, renal, and endocrine tissues	Lowers blood pressure by inhibiting release of NE at the neuroeffector junction
	β_1	Heart muscle and blood vessels of the heart Kidneys	Heart stimulation; renin secretion
	β_2	All organs except the heart muscle (e.g., smooth muscle of the bronchioles, smooth muscle of the blood vessels in skeletal muscle) Note: β_2-receptors are located in blood vessels of the heart (causing dilation and decreased blood pressure)	Relaxation of smooth muscle: bronchodilation; uterine relaxation; relaxation for distance vision
	β_3	Adipose (fat) tissue	Lipolysis (breakdown of fat)
Cholinergic/ACh (preganglionic/cholinergic receptors)	Muscarinic	Sweat glands	Increased sweating
Parasympathetic			
Acetylcholine (cholinergic) (pre- and postganglionic/ cholinergic receptors)	Nicotinic	Postsynaptic nerves and neuromuscular junction of skeletal muscle	Muscle contraction
	Muscarinic	Smooth muscle, heart, and glands	Smooth muscle contraction (bronchoconstriction), increased gastrointestinal motility (diarrhea), and secretion (mucous secretion, salivation, lacrimation—tears) Decreased heart rate
Somatic			
Acetylcholine	Nicotinic	Skeletal muscle	—

TABLE 3-4 Affinity of Neurotransmitters for Receptors

RECEPTOR/NEUROTRANSMITTER	AFFINITY TO
α_1	NE > EPI
α_2	NE > EPI
β_1 (cardiac tissue)	NE = EPI
β_2 (smooth muscle)	EPI > NE

low concentrations achieved systemically after anesthetic injections in dentistry is fairly selective for β-receptors. The β_2-receptors, when activated, cause peripheral vasodilation in skeletal muscle blood vessels, lowering peripheral resistance. At the same time, the β_1-receptors in the heart are activated to increase cardiac output. These two influences cancel each other out regarding mean blood pressure. There tends to be an increase in systolic and a decrease in diastolic blood pressure.

4. *Norepinephrine (NE)* (released from the adrenal medulla or sympathetic postganglionic nerves) acts on *all* α-receptors and *some* β-receptors and is chiefly a *vasoconstrictor.* NE does not act on the β-receptors of smooth muscles of the liver, lungs, stomach, urinary bladder, and ciliary muscle of the eye.

5. β_1-receptors predominate (95%) in the heart (coronary) blood vessels and blood vessels to skeletal muscle. EPI produces vasodilation of these blood vessels since the β-receptors outnumber the α-receptors. NE produces vasodilation of the coronary blood vessels of the heart (beta effect), but produces vasoconstriction of blood vessels to skeletal smooth muscle due to a greater effect of norepinephrine on the α-receptors.

Parasympathetic Neurotransmitters and Receptors

Parasympathetic innervation predominates over sympathetic innervation of salivary glands and lacrimal glands. Stimulation of the parasympathetic division causes secretion of saliva and tearing, bronchiole contraction, and gut relaxation.

Acetylcholine is the neurotransmitter released from the parasympathetic presynaptic and postsynaptic nerves. In each instance, the released ACh binds to and acts on cholinergic receptors contained in the postsynaptic nerve and the effector tissue. There are two types of cholinergic receptors:

- *Muscarinic cholinergic receptors* are located in tissue innervated by parasympathetic postganglionic nerves (and by sympathetic cholinergic nerves), which innervate sweat glands and smooth muscle. Activation of muscarinic receptors resembles those produced when a person ingests the poisonous mushroom *Amanita muscaria.* When activated, muscarinic receptors mediate smooth muscle contraction, and slow cardiac function and gland secretions.
- *Nicotinic cholinergic receptors* are located on skeletal muscle. Activation of nicotinic receptors on skeletal muscle causes muscle contraction. There are not many pharmacological applications of stimulating nicotinic receptors.

Acetylcholine that does not bind to the receptors is either destroyed by enzymes, taken up into the presynaptic neuron to be recycled, or diffused away from the synaptic cleft.

Other Types of Neurotransmitters and Receptors

DOPAMINE Dopamine receptors are activated by dopamine, but not by other adrenergic receptor agonists. Currently, there are five classes of dopamine receptors (D_1, D_2, D_3, D_4, and D_5), which mediate muscle relaxation in vascular smooth muscle and regulate neurotransmitter release. Dopamine plays an important role in the pathogenesis and treatment of certain brain disorders such as Parkinson's disease and schizophrenia. Antagonism of the dopamine D_2 receptor, which prevents dopamine from attaching to the receptor, is a mechanism common to antipsychotic drugs.

SEROTONIN More than 15 subtypes of serotonergic receptors have been discovered. Pharmaceutical companies have been attempting to develop compounds that will act specifically at a single receptor subtype, hoping to obtain a profound therapeutic effect that is free from adverse effects.

Serotonin, or 5-hydroxytryptamine (5-HT), is a neurotransmitter that is produced primarily by platelets, cells in the gastrointestinal tract, and neurons. Serotonin is produced locally in peripheral tissues and is also found in the brain. Its physiological effects include platelet aggregation, stimulation of gastrointestinal motility, vasoconstriction, and controlling sleep, pain, behavior, and emotions such as depression. Certain drugs can act to affect the synthesis, storage, release, or reuptake of serotonin.

Autonomic Drugs

Autonomic drugs work by acting as either agonists or antagonists at cholinergic and adrenergic receptors. Various autonomic drugs exert their effects at different steps in the neurotransmission process. Drugs that act as **agonists** bind to a receptor on the tissue and produce the maximal response, excitatory or inhibitory, obtainable in the tissue. **Antagonists** only produce a submaximal response in the tissue by blocking and reversing the effects of the neurotransmitter; an antagonist is opposite of an agonist.

Sympathomimetic Drugs: Drugs Affecting Sympathetic Transmission

Drugs that act as mediators of sympathetic transmission and cause a sympathetic response are called **sympathomimetics** or adrenergic agonists. Drugs that decrease sympathetic activity are called **sympatholytics** or *adrenergic antagonists.*

Many of the actions of sympathomimetic drugs (or the effects they produce) can be better understood in terms of specific drug–receptor interactions. The excitatory action of sympathomimetics (e.g., contraction of smooth muscle) is due to stimulation of α-receptors. This action is antagonized by an α-adrenergic blocking agent. The cardiac excitatory action of sympathomimetics is due to stimulation of the β_1-adrenergic receptors. This action is antagonized by β-blocking agents.

Adrenergic (Sympathetic) Agonists

Adrenergic agonists are divided into drugs

- that act *directly* binding to and activating the α- or β-receptors on the tissue, imitating the action of the neurotransmitter; and
- drugs that act *indirectly* (that do not themselves bind or act on the receptor, but cause the release of norepinephrine from the nerve terminals). The effects of these drugs are actually the result of the released NE interacting with the receptor sites.

Adrenergic agonists are also classified according to *receptor site specificity* (α_1, α_2, β_1, β_2) (Table 3-5). It is best to select a drug that has selectivity for the receptor intended to minimize adverse effects.

A review of the actions of adrenergic receptors:

1. *Alpha$_1$ (α_1)-receptors* are located on/in smooth muscle of the blood vessels supplying organs such as the heart, skin, and salivary glands, smooth muscle of the eye, glands, GI tract, and urinary bladder; α_2-receptors are located on the axonal terminal of neurons releasing NE. The pharmacological activation of the α_1-receptors leads to vasoconstriction, dilation of the pupils (to let more light in), and contraction of isolated smooth muscle. The exception to this rule is stimulation of α_1-receptors in the intestines, which leads to intestinal relaxation. Stimulation of α_2 receptors (autoreceptor) by released NE reduces further NE release, which is a negative feedback.

TABLE 3-5 α- and β-Adrenergic Agonists

	α-AGONISTS	CLINICAL USE	β-AGONISTS	CLINICAL USE
Direct acting	Phenylephrine (Neo-Synephrine) α_1	Nasal decongestant (vasoconstriction)	Isoproterenol (Isuprel)—nonselective β_1, β_2 (because nonselective, it is better to use a selective β_2 drug)	Asthma (bronchodilation)
	Oxymetazoline (Afrin) α_1	Nasal decongestant		
	Tetrahydrozoline (Visine) α_1	Ocular decongestant		
	Norepinephrine (Levarterenol, Levophed)	Hypotension and shock	Albuterol (Ventolin, Proventil)—selective β_2	Asthma
	Epinephrine	Prolongs action of local anesthetics, reduction in bleeding	Terbutaline (Brethine)—selective β_2	Asthma
			Metaproterenol (Alupent, Metaprel)—selective β_2	Asthma
			Epinephrine (Adrenalin)—α and nonselective β agonist	Anaphylactic shock (reverses hypotension-α_1); bronchodilator (asthma—β_2); stimulates heart in heart failure (vasoconstriction—β_1); in local anesthetics (β_2)
Central α_2 agonists	Clonidine (Catapres)—α_2 agonist	Hypertension; withdrawal from alcohol and cigarettes	Salmeterol (Serevent) β_2	Asthma
			Dobutamine (Dobutrex)—β_1, dopamine agonist	Drug of choice to stimulate heart (β_1)
	Methydopa (Aldomet)—α_2 agonist	Hypertension	Isoetharine (Bronkosol)—nonselective	Asthma (β_1, β_2)
Mixed	Ephedrine α_1/β	Nasal decongestion	Ephedrine (preferable to use a β_2 selective bronchodilator)	Bronchodilation
	Pseudoephedrine (Sudafed and others) α_1/β	Nasal decongestion	Pseudoephedrine (preferable to use a β_2 selective bronchodilator)	Bronchodilation
Indirect acting	Amphetamine, cocaine	Attention-deficit/hyperactive disorder (ADHD), narcolepsy	Topical anesthetic	

Rapid Dental Hint

In patient taking a nasal decongestant (α_1-receptor agonist), such as Afrin, epinephrine is all right to use and no special precautions are needed.

2. Beta (β_1)-receptors are located on cardiac muscle of the heart, stimulation leads to increase heart rate and force.

3. Beta (β_2)-receptors are located on smooth muscle of the bronchioles (lungs) and intestine and blood vessels supplying the heart; stimulation of these receptors causes relaxation of smooth muscle.

Direct-Acting Adrenergic Receptor Agonists

α-ADRENERGIC AGONISTS: VASOCONSTRICTION (CONSTRICTION OF BLOOD VESSELS): OCULAR AND NASAL DECONGESTANTS

- Many of the direct-acting agonists are catecholamines (e.g., epinephrine, norepinephrine, dopamine, isoproterenol, and dobutamine) and are used in the treatment of hypotension and shock by increasing blood pressure via constriction of blood vessels (vasoconstriction) (Table 3-5).
  - They bind to and activate α_1-receptors and also stimulate vasoconstriction and increase blood pressure.

- The sympathomimetic effect on nasal mucous membranes (α_1-adrenergic receptors) is constriction of the blood vessels of the nasal mucosa, which reduces vascular congestion and mucus secretions, opening the nasal passages and increasing breathing. These drugs are administered topically as nose drops or nasal sprays to produce a *decongestant effect*. Examples are phenylephrine (Neo-Synephrine) and oxymetazoline (Afrin).
  - An adverse effect of using most short-acting nasal decongestants longer than 3–5 days is rebound congestion with mucosal swelling. The topical decongestant must be slowly discontinued and replaced with normal saline (e.g., Aryl, Ocean). Additionally, local irritation including burning, sneezing, and dryness are seen.

- *Epinephrine* is unsuitable for oral administration because enzymes would destroy it and can only be given in an injectable form.
  - Epinephrine is used as a bronchodilator by stimulating β_2-receptors to counteract bronchoconstriction in anaphylactic shock, a severe, life-threatening drug reaction accompanied by hypotension.
  - Epinephrine increases glycogenolysis (β-receptor), which increases glucose production and decreases the release of insulin, resulting in hyperglycemia.
  - Being nonselective, epinephrine has adverse effects including tachycardia (increased heart rate due to β_1 stimulation), hypertension (due to α_1 stimulation), palpitations, cardiac arrhythmias (β_1), and dizziness.

- In low doses as used in dentistry, epinephrine *stimulates β_2-receptors (in blood vessels of the heart) causing vasodilation, which decreases diastolic blood pressure* but the systolic pressure increases because epinephrine increases cardiac output (β_1-*receptors*). The decrease and increase cancel each other out so there is no real change in blood pressure. On the other hand, higher doses produce more vasoconstriction and increased blood pressure by binding to α_1-receptors.

- When epinephrine has done its job, it is removed from the area via two methods:
  - Metabolized (breakdown) by monoamine oxidase (MAO) and catechol-O-methyl transferase (COMT), both enzymes present in the gastrointestinal tract
  - Reuptake back into the nerve terminal

- Levonordefrin (Neo-Cobefrin) is a vasoconstrictor found in dental local anesthetics. Levonordefrin is half as potent a vasoconstrictor as epinephrine. *It primarily stimulates α-adrenergic receptors with little to no effect on the β-adrenergic receptors.*

Rapid Dental Hint

Remember to assess your patient before choosing a local anesthetic containing epinephrine.

CENTRAL α_2-AGONISTS

- Centrally (central nervous system) active α_2-agonists stimulate α_2-receptors in the *brain* and turn off the activity of sympathetic nerves due to an inhibition of NE release from the nerve terminals; work like blockers (antagonists).
- Used to treat hypertension by decreasing heart rate.
- Adverse effects include xerostomia and orthostatic hypotension.
- The prototype drug in this class is clonidine (Catapres).

β_1/β_2-ADRENERGIC AGONISTS: ADRENERGIC BRONCHODILATION: BRONCHIAL ASTHMA

- Drugs used in the treatment of bronchial asthma affect the β_2-*adrenergic* receptors, causing dilation of the bronchial smooth muscle and vasoconstriction of the bronchial blood vessels. Drugs are administered through inhalation, orally, or injected. The prototype drug is isoproterenol (Isuprel). Since isoproterenol is nonselective and acts on both β_1- and β_2-adrenergic receptors, besides affecting the bronchioles it also affects the heart by causing an increased heart rate (β_1). Blood pressure can go up or down because there is vasodilation and increased cardiac output, which makes blood pressure increase.

- Selective β_2-adrenergic agonists (albuterol, metaproterenol, terbutaline) selectively affect only the tissues with

β_2-receptors and not cardiac muscle; as a result, there are less effects on the heart. These selective β_2-agonists, which are given via inhalation, are used in the treatment of asthma.

Indirect-Acting Agonists

- Amphetamine releases stores of NE from the sympathetic neurons, which cause vasoconstriction, cardiac excitation, and increased blood pressure. A drug called Adderall, which is indicated in narcolepsy (individual falling asleep uncontrollably) and in attention-deficit/hyperactivity disorder (ADHD), contains mixed salts of a single-entity amphetamine product (dextroamphetamine sulfate, dextroamphetamine saccharate, amphetamine aspartate monohydrate, amphetamine sulfate).

- Cocaine is a naturally occurring drug. It is the most potent vasoconstrictor and is used as a local anesthetic. Its mechanism of action is to block the reuptake of NE, increasing the concentration of NE in the synapse. The sympathomimetic effects include cardiac stimulation and elevation of blood pressure.

Mixed-Acting Adrenergic Receptor Agonists

- Ephedrine and pseudoephedrine (Sudafed) activate both α_1- and β_2-adrenergic receptors by direct and indirect methods.
  - Used as nasal decongestants due to stimulation of α_1-receptors, resulting in vasoconstriction.
  - Pseudoephedrine and ephedrine are used by drug traffickers to manufacture methamphetamine, a Schedule II controlled substance, for the illicit market. As of April 2006, federal law imposed a limit on the amount of pseudoephedrine products: Consumers can buy up to 3.6 grams a day, 9 grams for an entire month.

Therapeutic Uses of Sympathetic Agonists

- α_1-receptor agonists cause smooth muscle contraction, which leads to *vasoconstriction,* dilation of the pupils, and contraction of the bladder muscle. These drugs are used in the treatment of shock and hypotension and as a nasal/ocular decongestant.
- α_2-receptor agonists are used in the treatment of hypertension to *lower blood pressure.* These drugs will inhibit the release of NE, resulting in lower levels of NE.
- β_1-receptor agonists are used to increase the rate and force of heart contractions in patients with hypotension and shock. These drugs are given intravenously.
- β_2-receptor agonists are used to cause relaxation or dilation of smooth muscle in the lungs in patients with asthma. These long-acting drugs are given orally or inhaled. It is best to use a selective β_2 drug such as albuterol or terbutaline to keep adverse effects to a minimum.

Adverse Effects

- Taking higher doses of direct-acting catecholamines (e.g., epinephrine, isoproterenol, norepinephrine) may cause severe hypertension due to excessive cardiac stimulation; arrhythmias, tachycardia, and ventricular fibrillation may occur.
- Other adverse effects include xerostomia, nausea, vomiting, headache, dizziness, and palpitations.
- Drug abuse may occur with amphetamines and cocaine. An overdose may result in excessive cardiac stimulation. Cocaine inhibits the reuptake of NE, and amphetamine increases the release of NE into the synapse.

Rapid Dental Hint

In patients taking a tricyclic antidepressant such as amtriptyline, the amount of epinephrine must be limited to no more than two cartridges because tricyclic antidepressants inhibit the reuptake of norepinephrine so it stays in the synapse longer.

Drug Interactions

- Tricyclic antidepressants (e.g., amitriptyline, desipramine, nortriptyline, and imipramine) act by blocking the reuptake of catecholamines and thus may increase the hypertensive effects of epinephrine.
- Nonselective β_1, β_2 agonists may also cause a hypertensive crisis. Nonselective β-blockers block the β_2 vasodilatory effects of EPI. Thus, the amount of epinephrine should be limited to 0.04 mg (two cartridges of 1:100,000) in patients taking these drugs.
- A severe hypertensive reaction with death can occur when cocaine and epinephrine are taken together.

Adrenergic Receptor Antagonists

Sympatholytics are drugs that directly block the α- and β-adrenergic receptors on tissues, resulting in a decrease of sympathetic activity. These drugs are used in the treatment of cardiovascular conditions (hypertension), urinary retention, migraine headache, and glaucoma. Sympatholytics can be classified according to their effect on the receptors α-blockers and β-blockers. Essentially the symptoms produced are similar to the resting and digesting symptoms seen in the cholinergic or parasympathetic nervous system response.

DID YOU KNOW?

In literature, Sherlock Holmes injected cocaine in his arm. The author Robert Louis Stevenson wrote *Dr. Jekyll and Mr. Hyde* while under the influence of cocaine.

Most of the therapeutic effects are primarily due to the blocking of α_1- or β_1-adrenergic receptors, and any adverse effects are due to the blockade of α_2- or β_2-receptors. Because of this, drugs have been developed that selectively block either α_1- or β_1-adrenergic receptors and do not affect the other receptors, eliminating any adverse effects (Table 3-6).

α_1-Adrenergic Receptor Antagonists (Blockers)

- α_1-adrenergic blockers are used in the treatment of hypertension by blocking the vasoconstrictive actions of NE and EPI on vascular smooth muscle. This causes arteriolar vasodilation and lowers peripheral vascular resistance, which increases blood flow to the tissues so the heart does not have to work as hard.
  - Taking an initial dose of these drugs can result in orthostatic hypotension, where a sudden drop in blood pressure occurs when the individual rises quickly from a sitting or reclining position, causing dizziness or fainting. Allow the individual to remain sitting for a while before getting up.
- Alpha-blockers are classified as *nonselective α-adrenergic* blockers that bind both α_1 and α_2 receptors on smooth muscle of blood vessels. As a result, alpha-receptor sites are unable to react to norepinephrine. The *selective*

α_1-*adrenergic* blockers include prazosin (Minipress) and terazosin (Hytrin) and block only α_1-receptors.

- These drugs produce vasodilation and decrease blood pressure and they are used in the treatment of hypertension.
- Because these drugs relax the smooth muscle of the bladder and prostate, they are used in the treatment of urinary retention due to benign hypertrophy of the prostate. When the prostate becomes enlarged the flow of urine is reduced. The α_1-adrenergic blockers relax the smooth muscle, increasing urinary flow.
- Adverse effects of selective α_1-adrenergic blockers are due primarily to excessive vasodilation, which may cause hypotension, dizziness, fainting, reflex tachycardia, and palpitations.

Rapid Dental Hint

A patient that is taking an alpha-blocker has his or her blood pressure monitored. After moving the dental chair from a supine to upright position, keep the patient there for a few minutes to prevent fainting/dizziness due to orthostatic hypotension.

TABLE 3-6 Common Adrenergic Blocking Drugs (Antagonists)

DRUG CATEGORY	DRUG NAME	DRUG ACTION	CLINICAL USE
Adrenergic α_1-blockers	Prazosin (Minipress)	Selective α_1-blocker	Hypertension
	Doxazosin (Cardura)	Selective α_1-blocker	Hypertension
	Terazosin HCl (Hytrin)	Selective α_1-blocker	Hypertension, prostate hypertrophy, urinary retention
	Tamsulosin (Flomax)	Selective α_1-antagonist	Prostate hypertrophy
Selective α_2-blockers	Yohimbine (Aphrodyne)	α_2-receptor blocker	Penile erectile dysfunction (impotency)
Nonselective β-blockers (blocks both β_1 and β_2-receptors)	Naldolol (Corgard)	β_1-, β_2-blocker	Hypertension
		β_1-, β_2-blocker	
	Propranolol (Inderal)		
	Timolol (Blocadren)		Hypertension, migraine headaches, mitral valve prolapse, tremors
			Hypertension, myocardial infarction, migraine headaches, glaucoma
Selective β_1-blockers	Metoprolol (Lopressor)	Selective β_1-blocker	Hypertension
	Atenolol (Tenormin)	Selective β_1-blocker	Hypertension
	Esmolol (Brevibloc)	Selective β_1-blocker	Hypertension
	Bisoprolol fumerate (Zebeta)	Selective β_1-blocker	Hypertension
Adrenergic α- and β-blockers	Carvedilol (Coreg)	α- and β-blocker	Hypertension, atrial fibrillation,
	Labetalol (Normodyne)	α- and β-blocker	Hypertension

β-Adrenergic Receptor Antagonists (β-blockers)

Drugs classified as β-blockers are either nonselective or selective. All of the β-blockers are competitive antagonists. Therapeutic uses of β-blockers include:

- Hypertension
- Angina
- Heart arrhythmias
- Panic attacks
- Migraine headaches
- Glaucoma

NONSELECTIVE β-BLOCKERS (TREATMENT OF HYPERTENSION, ANGINA PECTORIS, GLAUCOMA)

- Nonselective β-blockers block both β_1 receptors on the heart tissue and β_2 receptors on smooth muscle, liver, lung, and other tissues—affecting all of these tissues and causing adverse effects such as a bronchospasm, bradycardia, and hypoglycemia.

- Blocking β_1-receptors located on the heart reduces sympathetic stimulation of the heart, reducing cardiac output (cardiac work is decreased) and blood pressure. Blocking β_1-receptors on the kidneys reduces the secretion of a substance called renin, involved in the formation in the bloodstream of a vasoconstrictor substance called angiotensin II that causes hypertension. Blockade of β_1-receptors in the eye reduces secretions and intraocular pressure.

- The prototype *nonselective β-blocker* is propranolol (Inderal). Its therapeutic effect is to decrease cardiac output and blood pressure and is used in the treatment of hypertension. Since it decreases oxygen demand to the heart and produces peripheral vasoconstriction, it is used in the treatment of angina and tachycardia.

  - Since it is a nonselective β_1-blocker it will also block β_2-receptors on the lungs, which may cause bronchoconstriction in asthmatics. By blocking β_2-receptors in the liver these drugs have a hypoglycemic effect, inhibiting EPI-stimulated glycogenolysis, the breakdown of glycogen into glucose. Precaution should be used in diabetics taking insulin.

  - Propranolol is also used in the prevention of migraine headache and for essential tremors, involuntary trembling of the hands.

Rapid Dental Hint

The use of local anesthetics with epinephrine for patients taking nonselective beta blockers (e.g., propranolol, nadolol, timolol) poses a significant risk of severe elevations in rblood pressure due to inability of epinephrine to bind to the β_2-receptors and consequently cause an exaggerated effect at the α_1-receptors. Therefore, limit the amount of epinephrine to two cartridges.

SELECTIVE β_1-BLOCKERS (TREATMENT OF HYPERTENSION)

- Selective β_1-blockers have a greater affinity for β_1-receptors than for β_2-receptors. These drugs are referred to as *cardioselective β-blockers* because β_1-receptors are located primarily on heart tissue. The prototype selective β-blocker is atenolol (Tenormin).

- Because these drugs are more selective toward the β_1-receptors, there are fewer adverse effects than occur with the nonselective β-blockers.

Rapid Dental Hint

There are no special precautions to follow regarding the use of epinephrine in patients taking a selective β_1-blocker; however the amount of epinephrine is limited when a patient is taking a nonselective beta-blocker such as naldolol.

Indirect-Acting Adrenergic Antagonists

These drugs do not directly block α- or β-adrenergic receptors, but they block the release of NE from nerve endings. They antagonize the effects of the sympathetic system. The two drugs in this category are reserpine and guanethidine (Ismelin), used in the treatment of hypertension.

Adverse Effects of Adrenergic Blockers

- α-blockers can cause postural hypotension and bradycardia with initial doses. Taking the drug with food may reduce the incidence of dizziness. Food may delay absorption, but does not affect the extent of absorption.

- All β-blockers can cause heart failure or heart block. Caution should be used in diabetics, as these drugs increase insulin action, resulting in hypoglycemia. Nonselective β_2-blockers may cause bronchoconstriction and are contraindicated in asthmatics.

Drug Interactions

Additive hypotensive effects occur with α_1-blockers when used concurrently with other antihypertensive drugs and diuretics.

Drugs Affecting Cholinergic Transmission

Drugs that act as mediators of cholinergic/ACh transmission are called parasympathomimetics (or **cholinergic agents**) and parasympatholytics (or **anticholinergics**) are agents that block the effects acetylcholine on parasympathetic nervous activity.

Parasympathomimetic Drugs

CHOLINERGIC AGONISTS   There are two types of cholinergic agonists: (1) directing-acting agents and (2) indirecting-acting cholinergic agonists (also referred to as cholinesterase inhibitors).

TABLE 3-7 Direct-Acting Cholinergic Agonist Agents		
DRUG NAME	**MECHANISM OF ACTION**	**CLINICAL USE**
Acetylcholine	Muscarinic and nicotinic receptor activation	Rarely used because it produces widespread effects and is rapidly broken down
Carbachol (Miostat)	Muscarinic and nicotinic receptor activation	Intraocular administration, glaucoma, miosis for eye surgery
Bethanechol (urecholine)	Muscarinic receptor stimulation	Oral administration: prevents urinary retention and increases intestinal motility after surgery
Pilocarpine (Salagen)	Greater affinity for muscarinic than for nicotinic	Intraocular administration: open-angle glaucoma Oral administration: treatment of xerostomia
Cevimeline (Evoxac)	Muscarinic receptor stimulation	Treatment of xerostomia
Methacholine	Muscarinic receptor stimulation	Diagnosis of asthma and bronchial hyperreactivity
Nicotine	Nicotine	Smoking cessation (oral, transdermal patch)

Directing-acting agents have affinity and activity at cholinergic receptors at either nicotinic or muscarinic receptors. Ideally, the drug should have a greater affinity for the muscarinic receptors because these receptors are found at the organ site. They can produce a slowing of the heart and increase smooth muscle tone of the GI and urinary tracts, which may result in nausea and evacuation of the bladder. They also may cause bronchial and pupil constriction (miosis). The nicotinic effect refers to the cholinergic action at the autonomic ganglia and at the neuromuscular junction (Table 3-7).

The prototype direct-acting cholinergic receptor agonists are acetylcholine and bethanechol (Urecholine). Acethycholine (ACh) has almost no clinical use because it is rapidly destroyed and causes a lot of adverse effects.

Natural plant alkaloids that are cholinergic agents include muscarine, nicotine, and pilocarpine. *Pilocarpine, obtained from a plant shrub, is used to treat xerostomia by binding to and stimulating cholinergic muscarinic receptors.* Muscarine, found in mushrooms, has no current medical use. Nicotine is obtained from plants and cigarettes and other tobacco products. It is contained in chewing gum and transdermal patches for smoking cessation.

One class of *indirect-acting cholinergic receptor agonists* are *cholinesterase inhibitors* (or anticholinesterase) (Table 3-8). These drugs have cholinergic action by inhibiting cholinesterase, the enzyme that breaks down acetylcholine, allowing for the accumulation of acetylcholine at the receptor site. They are divided into two classes, depending on their duration of action: reversible inhibitors, which do not bind tightly to receptors, and irreversible inhibitors, which bind irreversibly to receptors. Examples of reversible inhibitors include neostigmine and pyridostigmine, used to treat symptoms of myasthenia gravis. Physostigmine is used in the treatment of glaucoma.

TABLE 3-8 Indirect-Acting Cholinergic Agonists		
DRUG NAME	**ROUTE OF ADMINISTRATION**	**CLINICAL USES**
Reversible inhibitors		
Donepezil (Aricept)	Oral	Alzheimer's disease
Tacrine (Cognex)	Oral	Alzheimer's disease
Edrophonium	IV	Test for myasthenia gravis; antidote for curare
Neostigmine	Oral, IM, SC	Treatment for myasthenia gravis, postsurgery urine retention
Physostigmine	Topical (ocular)	Glaucoma
	IM, IV	Reverse anticholinergic overdose
Pyridostigmine	Oral, IM, IV	Myasthenia gravis
	IV	Reversal of muscle relaxants
Irreversible inhibitors		
Echothiophate	Ocular	Refractory glaucoma
Nerve gases (sarin, tabun, soman)	Absorbed through the skin, eyes	Poisoning

Rapid Dental Hint

Cevimeline (Evoxac) is a cholinergic agonist used in patients with xerostomia. There are no precautions regarding the use of epinephrine. The dose is 30 mg tid. Assess salivary flow.

Donepezil (Aricept) and tacrine (Cognex) are newer, centrally acting, reversible cholinesterase inhibitors that concentrate in the brain and are used in the treatment of Alzheimer's disease.

Rapid Dental Hint

A patient taking pilocarpine (Salagen) is taking it for xerostomia. Assess salivary flow in this patient. There are no special dental precautions in regard to using epinephrine. The initial dose is 5 mg tid, increasing to 15–30 mg a day. At least 6–12 weeks are needed.

Irreversible cholinesterase inhibitors are all organophosphates and are primarily used as pesticides. Some agents were developed as nerve gases (chemical warfare). These include tabun, sarin, and soman. Since these agents are highly lipid soluble they are absorbed through the skin and eyes. Poisoning is a problem, and can occur through these routes as well as by oral ingestion. Some agents are used medically (such as echothiophate and isofluophate in the treatment of chronic glaucoma) that are refractory to other agents.

DID YOU KNOW?

A water-nicotine mixture has been used as an insecticide since 1746. In 1828, nicotine was isolated from the leaves of the tobacco plant.

Anticholinergic Drugs

CHOLINERGIC RECEPTOR ANTAGONISTS (ANTICHOLINERGIC AGENTS)

- Cholinergic antagonists (anticholinergics) block both the muscarinic and nicotinic receptors. The muscarinic receptor antagonists compete with ACh for muscarinic receptors at the organ site, thereby inhibiting the effects of parasympathetic nerve stimulation (Tables 3-9, 3-10).

- In low doses, atropine and scopolamine cause dry mouth and inhibit sweating. In higher doses they relax smooth muscle, causing a decrease in GI and urinary tract contractions; decrease GI secretions (these drugs are used in the treatment of peptic ulcers); decrease respiratory secretions; and increase heart rate and cardiac conduction. Atropine is also used in cases of organophosphate poisoning (e.g., insecticides, nerve gas used in terrorism).

- Scopolamine is primarily used to prevent motion sickness, but has the same effects as atropine. Hyoscyamine is used primarily to treat intestinal spasms and other types of gastrointestinal disorders.

- These agents are used to dilate the pupil to allow an examination of the eye. The most popular drug used for this is topicamine (Mydriacyl).

- Nicotinic receptor antagonists include ganglionic blocking agents and neuromuscular blocking agents.

Adverse Effects   There are many adverse effects with anticholinergic agents, primarily sympathetic in nature. There is xerostomia, urinary retention, blurred vision, constipation, and tachycardia. Anticholinergic drugs are contraindicated in glaucoma and in urinary tract obstruction (e.g., benign prostatic hypertrophy [BPH]). Atropine and other muscarinic receptor antagonists are contraindicated in heart disease because they may cause tachycardia.

TABLE 3-9   Muscarinic (Cholinergic) Blocking Agents

ORGAN SYSTEM	PHARMACOLOGICAL EFFECT	DRUG NAME
CNS	Antimotion sickness	Scopolomine
	Sedation	Atropine
Eye (ocular)	Mydriasis (pupil dilation)	Atropine, homatropine
Lung (bronchi)	Bronchodilation	Ipratropium (Atrovent)
GI tract	Relaxation, slow motility (preoperative)	Dicyclomine (Bentyl), Propantheline (Pro-Banthine)
Heart	Bradycardia	Atropine
Salivary glands	Preoperative:	Methantheline (Banthine)
	Decrease salivation	Methantheline (Banthine)
Bronchial secretion	Preoperative (before surgery):	Atropine
	Decrease secretions	Atropine

TABLE 3-10 Selective Anticholinergic (Cholinergic Receptor Antagonists) Drugs

DRUG NAME	ROUTE OF ADMINSTRATION	CLINICAL USES
Muscarinic Receptor Antagonists		
Atropine sulfate	IV/IM/SC	Produces a dry field before surgery
	IV/IM	Cardiac arrythmias/bradycardia
	IV/IM	Organophosphate (nerve gas) antidote
	Inhalation	Short-term COPD
	Drops/ointment	Mydriasis before eye exam
Hyoscyamine sulfate	IV/IM/SC/PO/SL (sublingual)	Gastrointestinal (GI) spasms
Scopolamine	PO/IV/IM/SC	Adjunct to anesthesia
	PO/topical patch	Motion sickness
	Drops	Mydriasis (pupil dilation) for eye exam
Dicyclomine HCl (Bentyl)	PO	Irritable bowel syndrome
Flavoxate HCl (Uripas)	PO	Nocturia (night urination)
Ipratropium bromide (Atrovent)	Inhalation, nebulizer	Bronchodilator for chronic bronchitis and emphysema, rhinitis/common cold
Oxybutynin chloride (Ditropan)	PO	Pain/spasms in urinary incontinent patients
Tolterodine tartrate (Detrol)	PO	Urinary incontinence (less incidence of dry mouth)
Tropicamide (Mydriacyl)	Drops	Mydriasis (pupil dilation) for eye exam
Nicotinic Receptor Antagonists		
Atracurium besylate	IV	Skeletal muscle relaxation during surgery (for intubation)
Doxacurium chloride	IV	Skeletal muscle relaxation during surgery
Pancuronium bromide	IV	Skeletal muscle relaxation during surgery
Pipecuronium	IV	Skeletal muscle relaxation during surgery
Succinylcholine chloride	IV/IM	Presurgical muscle relaxation to facilitate intubation
d-tubocurarine	IV/IM	Skeletal muscle relaxation during surgery (for intubation)

DID YOU KNOW?

There is no evidence behind the popular belief that tomatoes, peppers, white potatoes, and eggplants—part of the Belladonna nightshade family—should be avoided in people with arthritis. Atropine is derived from this plant.

Drug Interactions Additive anticholinergic side effects are seen when these drugs are given concurrently with drugs that have anticholinergic effects, such as tricyclic antidepressants and antihistamines such as diphenhydramine (Benadryl).

Dental Hygiene Applications

- Many patients in the dental office will be taking one or more drugs that act on the autonomic nervous system. Drug actions of the autonomic nervous system on various organs including the heart, eye, arterioles, glands (salivary and lacrimal or tear), skin, lung, GI tract, and urinary bladder result in either stimulation or relaxation of these organs.

- A local dental anesthetic (e.g., lidocaine) containing a sympathomimetic vasoconstrictor (e.g., epinephrine) should be used with caution if the patient abuses cocaine or takes amphetamines. A severe hypertensive crisis and cardiac damage—even death—can occur due to toxic levels of EPI, which is a sympathetic agonist. Epinephrine is a vasoconstrictor, and cocaine is the most potent vasoconstrictor. Thus, epinephrine should not be used for at least 24 hours after the last dose of cocaine.

- The amount of epinephrine injected in dental anesthesia will produce primarily a β_2 response; however, if you were to push the dose beyond three or four cartridges, more α_1 effects will be seen such as increased systolic blood pressure.

- It is not a contraindication to use lidocaine with epinephrine in patients with hypertension and patients taking a tricyclic antidepressant (e.g., Elavil), but the patient should be treated similar to a cardiac patient. The administration of two to three cartridges (0.036–0.054 mg epinephrine) of 2% lidocaine with 1:100,000 epinephrine is considered safe. The patient's blood pressure should be monitored during all dental procedures.

- Levonordefrin (Neo-Cobefrin) is another type of vasoconstrictor used in the local anesthetic mepivacaine. It is half as potent a vasoconstrictor as epinephrine and it primarily stimulates α-adrenergic (sympathetic) receptors, with little to no effect on the β-adrenergic receptors. Stimulation of α_1-receptors on tissues/organs causes vasoconstriction of blood vessels, resulting in hypertension (increased systolic and diastolic blood pressure). Levonordefrin should not be used in patients taking a tricyclic antidepressant. Levonordefrin and epinephrine may be used in patients taking nonselective β-blockers, but the amount should be reduced. When evaluating a patient's medical history it is important to know every drug the patient is taking, both over the counter (OTC) and prescription. It is interesting to note that most of the adrenergic agonists (namely, α_1-adrenergeric agonists) are nasal decongestants and OTC drugs. These drugs cause a local (nasal mucosa) vasoconstiction. Patients may not realize that OTC drugs are chemical drugs and must be mentioned in the medical history.

- β_1-adrenergic receptors are found predominantly on the heart and, when stimulated, cause an increase in the rate and force of contraction. β_1-*adrenergic agonist* drugs acting selectively on β_1-receptors are used in the treatment of heart failure and are given IV. These patients will most likely not be seen in the dental office.

- β_2-receptors are found on the lungs, uterus, and arterioles and veins. β_2-*adrenergic agonist* drugs acting on β_2-receptors are used in the treatment of asthma. These drugs are selective for β_2-receptors, avoiding cardiac adverse effects. The dental clinician should be aware of which drugs are selective β_2-agonists acting only on the bronchioles.

- Patients taking α_1-blockers are being treated for hypertension. Orthostatic hypotension is an adverse effect of these drugs. To prevent syncope, allow the patient to sit in an upright position in the dental chair before getting up.

- Blood pressure should be taken at every office visit on patients taking β_1-blockers, which are used primarily in patients with hypertension to decrease blood pressure. The patient should be asked if he or she took medication that day. Use of local anesthetics containing epinephrine is not contraindicated; however, caution should be used. Two or three cartridges of 2% lidocaine with 1:100,000 epinephrine can safely be administered to a patient taking these medications.

- The primary adverse effect of anticholinergic drugs is xerostomia. The dental clinician plays an important role in teaching the patient to care for the mouth. To minimize the effects of dry mouth on the oral mucosa, the patient should be instructed to maintain good oral home care, drink plenty of water, avoid sugar candy, and avoid alcohol-containing mouthrinses. Numerous OTC salivary substitutes are available.

- Additionally, the patient may experience tachycardia, or increased heart rate, while taking anticholinergic drugs. The patient's blood pressure should be monitored at every dental visit.

Key Points

- Stimulation of the sympathetic (adrenergic) and parasympathetic (cholinergic) nerves cause opposite responses.
- Function of neurotransmitters is to carry nerve impulses (action potentials) across the synapse.
- Stimulation of the sympathetic pathway starts a "fight-or-flight" response, and activation of the parasympathetic pathway initiates a "resting and digestive" reaction.
- Sympathetic nervous division: Norepinephrine has a higher affinity and binding to all α-receptors and some β-receptors. Epinephrine has a higher affinity to β_2-receptors in blood vessels/smooth muscle.
- α_1-receptors are found in skin, coronary tissue, kidneys, mucosa, salivary glands, blood vessels, eye muscle, and sphincters of the gastrointestinal tract.
- α_1-receptor agonist drugs: nasal decongestant and treatment of hypotension.
- α_2-receptors are autoreceptors found at terminal endings of neurons that release norepinephrine. They function to inhibit release of NE and its effects.
- All α-receptor-mediated effects of sympathomimetic drugs are excitatory except in the intestines, where they cause an inhibitory type of response.
- β_1-receptors are found on heart muscle.
- All β-receptor-mediated effects of sympathomimetic drugs are inhibitory.
- β_1-receptor agonist drugs: treatment of heart conditions and shock.
- β_2-receptors are found in certain blood vessels/smooth muscle (lung, liver, intestines, bladder).
- β_2-agonist drugs: treatment of asthma.
- The cardiac excitatory effects of sympathomimetic drugs are β_1-mediated and are inhibited by a β-blocking agent.
- Sympathomimetic drugs are used primarily for their effects on the heart, bronchial tree, and nasal passages.
- Adrenergic blockers are used primarily to treat hypertension and are the most widely prescribed class of autonomic drugs.
- The primary use of β-blockers is in the treatment of hypertension.
- Cholinergic drugs are primarily used in the treatment of xerostomia (cevimeline, pilocarpine) and Alzheimer's disease (donepezil, tacrine, rivastigmine).
- Anticholinergic drugs are used to increase heart rate (atropine), urinary incontinence (oxybutynin), motion sickness (scopolamine), and irritable bowel syndrome (dicyclomine, propantheline, scopolamine).

Board Review Questions

1. Which of the following neurotransmitters is released from sympathetic postganglionic neurons? (pp. 43, 46)
   a. Dopamine
   b. Serotonin
   c. Acetylcholine
   d. Norepinephrine

2. Which of the following receptors is classified as an autoreceptor? (p. 45)
   a. Nicotinic
   b. α_1
   c. α_2
   d. β_1
   e. β_2

3. Which of the following conditions should the dental hygienist monitor if the patient is taking terazosin (Hytrin) for an enlarged prostate? (p. 52)
   a. Xerostomia
   b. Excessive sweating
   c. Excessive salivation
   d. Orthostatic hypotension
   e. Hypertension

4. In which of the following patients should the dental hygienist limit the amount of a local anesthetic containing epinephrine? (pp. 53, 57)
   a. Patient has low blood pressure
   b. Patient with xerostomia
   c. Patient taking naldolol (Corgard)
   d. Patient taking pilocarpine

5. Which of the following pathways is activated in a "fight-or-flight" situation? (p. 44)
   a. Adrenergic
   b. Cholinergic
   c. Adrenergic antagonist
   d. Somatic nervous system

6. Which of the following receptors does epinephrine in low doses primarily stimulate? (pp. 45, 57)
   a. α_1
   b. α_2
   c. β_1
   d. β_2

7. A patient is taking atenolol (Tenormin) for hypertension. Which of the following signs should be monitored? (p. 52)
   a. Kidney function
   b. Blood pressure
   c. Body temperature
   d. CNS function

8. Which of the following types of drugs is used in the treatment of nasal congestion? (pp. 47, 49, 50)
   a. β_1-agonists
   b. Selective β_2-antagonists
   c. α_1-agonists
   d. α_2-agonists

9. A patient presents to the dental office for an initial visit. There is an extensive medical history. All of the following drugs cause xerostomia as an adverse effect *except* one. Which is the exception? (pp. 54, 55)
   a. Atropine
   b. Scopolamine
   c. Pilocarpine
   d. Homatropine

10. Which of the following drugs is used in the treatment of asthma? (pp. 49, 50)
    a. Timolol
    b. Reserpine
    c. Albuterol
    d. Dobutamine

11. Which of the following drugs may cause xerostomia? (p. 55)
    a. Epinephrine
    b. Dopamine
    c. Cevimeline
    d. Atropine

12. Which of the following drugs should be limited in patients taking Elavil (a tricyclic antidepressant)? (p. 51)
    a. Epinephrine
    b. Acetylcholine
    c. Dopamine
    d. Serotonin

13. In high doses that are used in anaphylactic shock, which of the following receptors does epinephrine primarily stimulate? (p. 49)
    a. α_1
    b. α_2
    c. β_1
    d. β_2

14. Epinephrine goes through a biphasic response concerning blood pressure. After the initial increase in blood pressure, there is a decrease. This decrease in blood pressure is due to stimulation of which of the following receptors? (pp. 45, 55)
    a. α_1
    b. α_2
    c. β_1
    d. β_2

15. Which of the following receptors is stimulated when pilocarpine is taken? (pp. 54, 55)
    a. Cholinergic nicotinic
    b. Cholinergic muscarinic
    c. Adrenergic α
    d. Adrenergic β

Selected References

Bousquet P, Monassier L, Feldman J. 1998. Autonomic nervous system as a target for cardiovascular drugs. *Clin Exp Pharmacol Physiol* 25:446–448.

Bylund DB. 1995. Pharmacologic characteristics of α_2-adrenergic receptor subtypes. *Ann NY Acad Sci* 763:1–7.

Herman WW, Konzelman Jr. JL, Prisant M. 2004. New national guidelines on hypertension: A summary for dentistry. *JADA* 135:576–584.

Hieble JP, Ruffolo RR. 1996. The use of α-adrenoceptor antagonists in the pharmacological management of benign prostatic hypertrophy: An overview. *Pharmacol Res* 33:145–160.

Jaradeh SS, Prieto TE. 2003. Evaluation of the autonomic nervous system. *Phys Med Rehabil Clin N Am* 14:287–305.

Lepor H, et al. 1997. Doxazosin for benign prostatic hyperplasia: Long-term efficacy and safety in hypertensive and normotensive patients. *J Urol* 157:525–530.

Wallingford A. 2000. Beta blockers and heart disease. *Lancet* 35(4):1751–1756.

Web Sites

www.medscape.com
www.uspharmacist.com

PEARSON
myhealthprofessionskit™

Use this address to access the Companion Website created for this textbook. Simply select "Dental Hygiene" from the choice of disciplines. Find this book and log in using your username and password to access video clips of selected tests.

QUICK DRUG GUIDE

Sympathomimetics (Adrenergic Agonists)

Directing-Acting α-Agonists (vasoconstriction; ocular [eye] and nasal decongestants; treatment of hypotension and shock, antihypertensive)

- Phenylephrine (Neo-Synephrine) (nasal decongestant; increases BP) α_1
- Oxymetazoline (Afrin) (nasal and ocular decongestant) α_1
- Tetrahydrozoline (Visine) (ocular decongestant) α_1
- Norepinephrine (hypotensive shock to increased blood pressure)
- Epinephrine (shock, cardiac arrest, prolonged action of local anesthetics)
- Clonidine (Catepres) (autoreceptor; antihypertensive drug) α_2

Direct-Acting β-Agonists (anti-asthmatic/ bronchodilator; shock/heart failure)

- Isoproterenol (Isuprel) (β_1/β_2 nonselective; heart stimulation and asthma)
- Albuterol (Ventolin, Proventil) (asthma) selective β_2
- Terbutaline (Brethine) (asthma; uterus relaxation—premature labor) selective β_2
- Metaproterenol (Alupent) (asthma) selective β_2
- Epinephrine (Adrenalin) β_1/β_2 nonselective
- Dobutamine (Dobutrex) (shock/heart failure) β_1/β_2
- Isoetharine (Bronkosol) (asthma) selective β_2
- Salmeterol (Serevent) (asthma) selective β_2

Indirect-Acting Agonists

- Amphetamine (increase NE release) (ADHD)
- Cocaine (inhibits NE reuptake into nerve terminals) (topical anesthetic)

Mixed-Acting Agonists (nasal decongestants)

- Ephedrine α_1, β_2
- Pseudoephedrine (Sudafed and others) α_1, β

Centrally Acting α_2-agonists (hypertension)

- Clonidine (Catapres)
- Methyldopa (Aldomet)

Adrenergic Antagonists (Blockers)

α-Blockers

Nonselective α_1/α_2-Receptor Blockers

- Phenoxybenzamine (Dibenzyline) (hypertensive episodes in pheochromocytoma)
- Phentolamine (hypertensive episodes in pheochromocytoma)

Selective α_1-Blockers (antihypertensive drugs)

- Prazosin (Minipress)
- Doxazosin (Cardura)
- Terazosin (Hytrin) (also indicated in prostate hypertrophy)
- Tamsulosin (Flomax) (prostate hypertrophy)

Selective α_2-Blockers (impotency in men)

- Yohimbine (Aphrodyne)

β-Blockers

Selective β_1-Blockers (cardioselective; antihypertensive drugs)

- Metoprolol (Lopressor)
- Atenolol (Tenormin)
- Esmolol (Brevibloc)
- Bisoprolol (Zebeta)

Nonselective $\beta_{1,2}$-Blockers (affects both heart and other tissues with β-receptors; antihypertensive drugs; also has α-1 blocking action)

- Naldolol (Corgard) (hypertension)
- Propranolol (Inderal) (hypertension)
- Timolol (Blocadren) (glaucoma)

α- and β-Blockers (antihypertensives)

- Carvedilol (Coreg)
- Labetalol (Normodyne)

Indirect-Acting Adrenergic Antagonists (do not directly block α or β adrenergic receptors; block the release of NE from the nerve endings; treatment of hypertension)

- Reserpine
- Guanethidine

Parasympathomimetics

Direct-Acting Cholinergic Receptor Agonists (reduction in intraocular pressure, miosis; stimulate GI smooth muscle postoperative)

- Bethanechol (Urecholine)—Stimulates GI smooth muscle postoperative; prevents urine retention
- Carbachol (Miostat)—Glaucoma (open-angle)
- Cevimeline (Evoxac)—Treatment of xerostomia
- Pilocarpine (Pilocar)—Glaucoma (open-angle), xerostomia

Indirect-Acting Cholinergic Receptor Agonists

- Donepezil (Aricept)—Alzheimer's disease
- Edrophonium—Diagnosis of myasthenia gravis
- Galantamine (Razadyne)—Alzheimer's disease
- Neostigmine—Diagnosis of myasthenia gravis
- Physostigmine—Concurrently used with pilocarpine for glaucoma; diagnosis of myasthenia gravis
- Echothiophate and isoflurophate—Longer-acting drugs for glaucoma
- Rivastigmine (Exelon)—Alzheimer's disease

Parasympatholytics (Anticholinergics)

Muscarinic-Receptor Antagonists

- Atropine—Prototype; preoperative medication to dry up secretions, prevents bradycardia during spinal anesthesia; cholinergic poisoning
- Dicyclomine (Bentyl)—Irritable bowel syndrome (decreases GI motility/antispasmodic)
- Flavoxate (Uripas)—Urinary incontinence
- Ipratropium (Atrovent)—Bronchodilator
- Oxybutynin (Ditropan)—Spasm in urinary incontinence
- Propantheline—Irritable bowel syndrome (decreases GI motility/antispasmodic)
- Scopolamine—Motion sickness
- Tolterodine (Detrol)—Urinary incontinence
- Tropicamide (Mydriacyl)—Mydriasis (pupil dilation) for eye exam

Ganglionic-Blocking Drugs

- Trimethaphan—Produces controlled hypotension during surgery

Neuromuscular blocking agents

- Succinylcholine—To induce skeletal muscle relaxant during surgery to help with intubation
- d-Tubocurarinre—To induce skeletal muscle relaxant during surgery to help with intubation

Local Anesthetics

GOAL

To gain knowledge of local anesthetics used in dentistry and their use in medically compromised patients.

EDUCATIONAL OBJECTIVES

After reading this chapter, the reader should be able to:

1. Discuss the mechanism of action of local anesthetics.
2. Classify local anesthetics used in dentistry.
3. Describe adverse effects of local anesthetics.
4. Describe the signs and symptoms of anesthetic toxicity.
5. Discuss the use of vasoconstrictors in medically compromised patients.

KEY WORDS

Local anesthetics

Nerve membrane

Vasoconstrictors

Epinephrine

Introduction

Local anesthetics are drugs used to prevent pain by inhibiting the conduction of nerve impulses along a nerve fiber. The degree of local anesthesia obtained is dependent on the method of administration, for example, surface (applied directly to the surface that is to be anesthetized, such as the cornea), topical (drug is applied to the skin in the form of a cream/gel), infiltration (drug is injected below the skin), nerve block (injection close to a major nerve bundle), epidural (injection into the outer part of the spinal cord), or spinal (injection into the spinal canal).

History

The first local anesthetic agent to be used in dentistry was cocaine. In 1859, Albert Niemann discovered the intraoral anesthetic (numbing effect) of cocaine. Coca leaves were purified into coca extract and finally into cocaine. In 1884, Dr. Carl Koller, an Austrian ophthalmologist, performed the first surgery using topical cocaine on the cornea. In the same year, Dr. William Halsted used cocaine as an anesthetic agent for the first dental procedure. Due to the high incidence for addiction and a short duration of action, cocaine was no longer used for injections during dental procedures. Then, in 1905, procaine, a synthetic substitute, was developed.

> **DID YOU KNOW?**
>
> Sigmund Freud, a famous psychiatrist, used cocaine on his patients as well as experimenting on himself, and became addicted.

Properties of Local Anesthetics

Chemical Properties

The chemical structure of local anesthetics includes an aromatic segment with either an amide bond or an ester bond to a basic side chain (Figure 4-1). Benzocaine is an exception to this, possessing no basic group. A bond links the lipophilic (fat-soluble) portion of the molecule with the hydrophilic (water-soluble) component. Local anesthetics without a hydrophilic portion are used only for topical administration. Local anesthetics of intermediate potency and duration of action, such as lidocaine, mepivacaine, and prilocaine, are mainly used in dentistry.

The active ingredient in an anesthetic is called the anesthetic *base,* which is a weak base. A weak base does not ionize fully in an aqueous (body fluid) solution, resulting in a low pH level, which makes them poorly soluble in water and unstable in solution. Thus, most anesthetics are combined with an acid such as hydrochloride (HCl) to form a salt because it is more stable and soluble (dissolvable) than the base.

Mechanism of Action

The **nerve membrane** or sheath is the site of action of local anesthetics. The pH (concentration of hydrogen H+ ion) of local anesthetics is generally about 4–5. Once the anesthetic solution is injected into the tissue, it changes rapidly to the more basic pH of the tissue, close to 7.4. In an aqueous solution such as body fluids, a local anesthetic will dissociate (dissolve and break down) into a nonionized (uncharged; neutral nonelectrolyte) form and an ionized (charged; electrolyte) form. When injected, the anesthetic is not in an active form. *To be active, the nonionized or uncharged portion of the local anesthetic acts like a nonpolar (not water-soluble), lipid-soluble compound that will readily transverse the lipid nerve cell membrane.* Once inside the nerve, the ionized molecules block the sodium channels in the membrane, decreasing the permeability (passage) of the nerve membrane to sodium ions. This prevents the generation of action potentials (a stimulus applied to a nerve allowing sodium to move into the neuron) (Figure 4-2). The duration of action depends on the length of time that the drug can stay in the nerve to block the sodium channels.

Effects of pH

Local anesthetics are weak bases. The pK_a, which is a known value, has a direct effect on the onset of local anesthetics. PK_a determines the amount of base present in a solution, which also depends on the pH of the solution. When the pH is equal to the pK_a of a local anesthetic, then equal amounts of base and

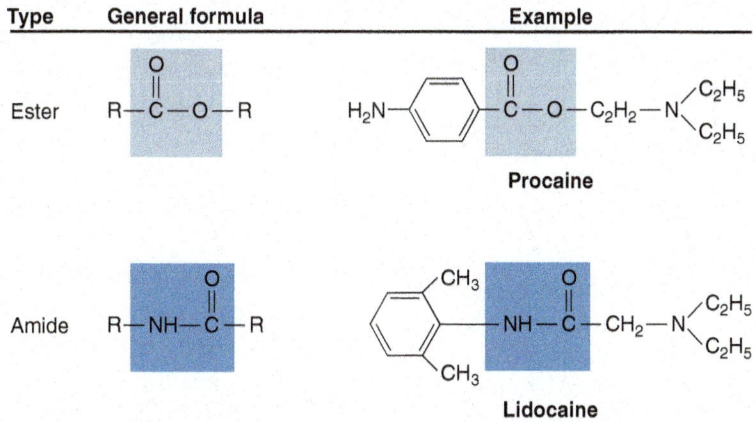

FIGURE 4-1 Chemical structures of ester and amide local anesthetics.

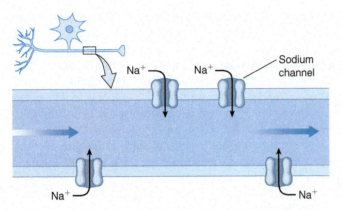

(a) Normal nerve conduction

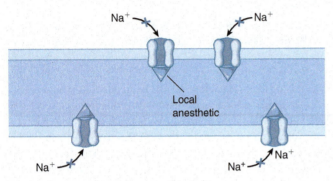

(b) Local anesthetic blocking sodium channels

FIGURE 4-2 How a local anesthetic blocks nerve conduction.

TABLE 4-1	Patient Physical Status Classification
ASA I	Normal, healthy patient
ASA II	Patient with mild systemic disease: type 2 diabetes, hypertension
ASA III	Patient with severe systemic disease: stable angina, type 1 diabetes, chronic obstructive pulmonary disease
ASA IV	Patient with severe systemic disease that is a constant threat to life: heart attack within 6 months, unstable angina, uncontrolled diabetes or uncontrolled epilepsy
ASA V	Moribund patient who is not expected to survive without the operation: patient is not expected to survive 24 hours with or without medical intervention
ASA VI	A declared brain-dead patient whose organs are being removed for donor purposes
E	Emergency operation used to modify any of the above classifications

Source: ASA, American Society of Anesthesiologists; E, emergency.

ionized species of the local anesthetic exist in solution. Thus, the lower the pK_a value of the anesthetic, the more rapid the onset of action.

For instance:

Tissue pH = 7.4; mepivacaine pK_a = 7.6;

lidocaine pK_a = 7.9

There would be more molecules of carbocaine existing in the diffusible nonionized form because its pK_a is closer to tissue pH and thus will cross the membrane more readily.

TISSUE INFLAMMATION At sites of tissue inflammation (e.g., abscesses) where the pH of the tissues is acidic (a pH of around 6 or lower), the hydrogen ion concentration is increased, which increases the ionization of the local anesthetic and decreases the penetrability through the nerve sheath and its effectiveness.

Metabolism and Excretion

Metabolism of local anesthetic depends on whether it is an ester or amide. The *ester* local anesthetics are hydrolyzed (broken down) by plasma cholinesterase into para-aminobenzoic ACID (PABA). *Amide* local anesthetics are metabolized mainly in the liver by microsomal enzymes. Prilocaine has the lowest toxicity because it is metabolized the fastest. Active metabolites are excreted by the kidneys in the urine. Patients with severe kidney disease must have the dose reduced. Cocaine is the only local anesthetic that is excreted unchanged in the urine.

Before any type of anesthesia is administered, the patient's physical status must be determined. Table 4-1 reviews the classifications made by the American Society of Anesthesiologists (ASA).

Local Anesthetic Agents

• Table 4-2 lists the various ester and amide agents and Table 4-3 lists the maximum recommended doses (MRD) of the local anesthetic agent. Each cartridge contains 1.7–1.8 ml of solution. *It should be noted that in 2005 most U.S. manufacturers of local anesthetics made a label change, which states that each cartridge contains a minimum of 1.7 ml and a maximum of 1.8 ml. Calculations in this text will be based on 1.7 ml.* Today, amide agents have replaced the use of esters because of the lower incidence of allergies. Some amide agents include lidocaine, mepivacaine, prilocaine, articaine, bupivacaine, and etidocaine.

Lidocaine

• First introduced in 1943, it is the most widely used amide anesthetic.

• It is available in an injectable form as:

  • 2% plain (without a vasoconstrictor)

  • 2% with 1:100,000 epinephrine (0.017 mg) (Note: All local anesthetic cartridges are now labeled on the cartridge as having a volume of 1.7 ml and not 1.8 ml)

  • 2% with 1:50,000 epinephrine (0.034 mg)

TABLE 4-2   Local Anesthetic Agents

DRUG	pK$_a$	VASOCONSTRICTOR	DURATION OF ACTION (WITH VC) (INFILTRATION) (PULPAL ANESTHESIA)	DURATION OF SOFT TISSUE ANESTHESIA (MIN)
Esters				
Benzocaine 20% topical	-----	None	N/A	N/A
Tetracaine (Pontocaine) topical, injectable	-----	None	N/A	N/A
Amides				
Lidocaine 2% (Xylocaine) topical, injectable	7.9	EPI 1:100,000	60–90 min	180–300 min
		EPI 1:50,000	60–90 min	180–300 min
		Plain	5–10 min	60–120 min
Mepivacaine 2% (with vasoconstrictor), 3% (without vasoconstrictor) (Carbocaine; Polocaine)	7.6	Levonordefrin 1:20,000 plain	60–90 min 20–40 min Moderate (with vasoconstrictor)	180–300 min 120–180 min
Prilocaine 4% (Citanest) (without vasoconstrictor)	7.9	EPI 1:200,000 (Citanest foret) plain	60–90 min 10–15 min	180–480 min 90–120 min
Bupivacaine 0.5% (Marcaine)	8.1	EPI 1:200,000	90–180 min	4–9 hours (up to 12 hours)
Etidocaine (Duranest)	7.7	EPI 1:200,000	40–240 min	240–540 min
Articaine 4% (Zorcaine, Septocaine, Ultracaine D-S, Ultracaine D-S Forte)	7.8	EPI 1:100,000 1:200,000 (Ultracaine D-S)	60–90 min 45–60 min	3–6 hours 2–5 hours
Topicals, others				
Oraqix Periodontal Gel (Lidocaine/prilocaine)	-----	None	N/A	Oraqix: 14–31 min
DentiPatch (Lidocaine Transoral Delivery)				

Source: Haas DA. 2002. An update on local anesthetics in dentistry. *J Can Dent Assoc* 68(9):546–551.

- As a topical anesthetic it is available as an ointment, cream, jelly, or solution (2–10%).
  - Lidocaine viscous 2% solution is indicated for a local anesthetic effect in patients with painful oral lesions such as aphthous ulcers.
- The amount of lidocaine per cartridge is 34 mg.
- Lidocaine is a potent vasodilator and has a very short duration of action. Thus, a vasoconstictor (epinephrine) is added.
- Lidocaine is used in medicine as an anti-arrhythmic to control cardiac (heart) excitability.
- Lidocaine has a rapid onset (2–3 minutes).
- It is metabolized in the liver by cytochrome P450 enzymes.
- The maximum safe dose of lidocaine with epinephrine in a healthy adult is 2.2 mg/lb or 4.4 kg/kg of body weight and should not exceed 500 mg. The maximum dose in a child should not exceed 4.4 mg/kg of body weight in a single sitting.
- Lidocaine has a pregnancy category B.

Rapid Dental Hint

Lidocaine viscous 2% is a prescription drug used for its local anesthetic effect in aphthous ulcers or in gaggers. Patient is instructed to swish with the solution and expectorate.

Mepivacaine

- First used in 1960.
- The brand names are Carbocaine and Polocaine.
- It has mild vasodilation activity and is good for short-duration procedures without a vasoconstrictor.
- Equal in potency to lidocaine
- It is available in an injectable form as:
  - 2% mepivacaine with 1:20,000 levonordefrin
  - 3% mepivacaine plain (without vasoconstrictor)

TABLE 4-3 Recommended Maximum Doses of Local Anesthetics with Vasoconstrictor

ANESTHETIC	MAXIMUM DOSE	NO. OF CARTRIDGES
Articaine	Adult: 7 mg/kg (up to 500 mg)	7
	Child: 5 mg/kg	
Bupivacaine	Adult: 1.3 mg/kg (up to 90 mg)	10
	Child: 2 mg/kg	
Lidocaine (with epinephrine)	Adult: 4.4 mg/kg (up to 500 mg)	13
	Child: 4.4 mg/kg (3.2 mg/lb)	
Mepivacaine	Adult: 4.4 mg/kg (up to 300 mg)	11 (7 if plain)
	Child: 4.4 mg/kg	
Prilocaine	Adult: 6.0 mg/kg (up to 400 mg)	8
	Child: 6.0 mg/kg	

Example of calculation:

The maximum amount (number of cartridges) of lidocaine for a 40 lb child:

1. First convert lbs into kg

   Since 2.2 lbs = 1 kg, 2.2 × 18 = 40

   Thus, 40 lbs = 18 kg

2. Since the maximum dose is presented mg/kg, it is necessary to convert kg into mg.
   It is known that the maximum dose is 7 mg/kg (see above), which equals 7 mg per 1 kg of body weight.
   Thus, 7 × 18 kg = 126 mg

3. 2% lidocaine = 20 mg/ml (lidocaine: 20 mg of lidocaine/ml of solution) and each cartridge has 1.7 ml of solution, so there is 34 mg lidocaine/cartridge (20 × 1.7).

4. 126 mg divided by 20 mg/ml = 6 ml.

5. For example, if there is 1.7 ml per cartridge, the maximum number of cartridges is 3.5 (6 divided by 1.7).

Most U.S. manufacturers of local anesthetics made a labeling change in 2005. Each cartridge contains a minimum of 1.7 ml and a maximum of 1.8 ml. Calculations in this chapter used 1.7 ml.

Source: Haas DA. 2002. An update on local anesthetics in dentistry. *J Can Dent Assoc* 68(9):546–551.

- The amount of mepivacaine per cartridge is 51 mg (3% solution) and 34 mg (2% solution).

- The vasoconstrictor used in mepivacaine is levonordefrin. It is a less potent vasoconstrictor than epinephrine but is more likely to cause an increase in blood pressure.

- It has a rapid onset of action (1½–2 minutes) and is best used for dental procedures that require no more than 30 minutes of anesthesia.

- The maximum dose is 2.0–3.0 mg/lb or 4.4–6.6 mg/kg of body weight, not to exceed a total dose at any single dental sitting of 300–400 mg in adults. In children, 2.0–3.0 mg/lb is recommended, up to a maximum of five cartridges.

- Mepivacaine has a pregnancy category C.

Rapid Dental Hint

Remember to review the medical history before deciding on the appropriate local anesthetic.

Prilocaine

- First introduced in 1960. The brand name is Citanest.

- It causes less tissue vasodilation than lidocaine. The advantage of using this agent is that it provides prolonged anesthesia with the least concentration of epinephrine.

- Prilocaine is available in an injectable form as:
  - 4% prilocaine (Citanest forte) with 1:200,000 epinephrine
  - 4% prilocaine (Citanest plain) (without a vasoconstrictor)

- There is less cardiac effect and it is especially useful in patients who are difficult to anesthetize.

- Onset of action is slower than lidocaine (2–4 minutes).

- Anesthesia is adequate for up to 90 minutes

- It is metabolized (converted) to *O*-toluidine, which is toxic and may cause methemoglobinemia if allowed to accumulate (see blood disorders). Prilocaine should not be used in infants. Prilocaine is contraindicated in patients taking acetaminophen because it can produce elevations in methemoglobin levels.

- Maximum recommended dose is 2.7 mg/lb or 6.0 mg/kg of body weight for adults and a maximum dose of 400 mg at one appointment.

- Prilocaine has a pregnancy category B.

Rapid Dental Hint

Dilution concentration of epinephrine: 1 : 50,000 (strongest) > 1 : 100,000

Articaine

- An analogue of prilocaine.
- It was first used in the United States. FDA approved in 2000.
- Brand names are Septocaine, Zorcaine, and Ultracaine.
- Articaine is available in an injectable form as:
  - 4% articaine with 1:100,000 epinephrine
  - 4% articaine with 1:200,000 epinephrine
- It has a unique structure, containing both an amide linkage and as ester side chain. Since the ester does not metabolize to PABA, individuals allergic to ester are not allergic to articaine. It has a slightly faster onset of action and better diffusion than the other agents and long and profound anesthesia.
- 1.5 times more potent than lidocaine.
- The 4% solution has a higher incidence of paresthesia on mandibular blocks.
- Onset of action: infiltration 1:200,000 is 1–2 minutes and mandibular block is 2–3 minutes. 1:100,000 infiltration is 1–2 minutes and block is 2–2½ minutes.
- Maximum recommended dose is 3.2 mg/lb or 7.0 mg/kg in adults (maximum dose 500 mg at one appointment) and children 2.27 mg/lb or 5.0 mg/kg.
- Articaine has a pregnancy category C.

Rapid Dental Hint

The amount of lidocaine 2% solution in one cartridge (1.7 ml) is 34 mg.

Bupivacaine

- First made in 1956 as an epidural agent.
- The brand name is Marcaine.
- First available in the United States in 1983.
- Available in an injectable form 0.54% solution with epinephrine 1:200,000.
- It has a slow onset (up to 30 minutes, but can last two or three times longer than lidocaine and mepivacaine, up to 7 hours).
  - Bupivacaine is usually used for lengthy dental procedures such as full mouth reconstruction and extensive and long periodontal or implant procedures.

- Bupivacaine can cause cardiotoxicity (e.g., ventricular arrhythmias).
- Maximum recommended dose is 0.6 g/lb or 1.3 mg/kg of body weight for adults with a maximum dose of 90 mg in one appointment.
- Pregnancy category of C.

Etidocaine

- A newer amide anesthetic that is similar to bupivacaine except it has a faster onset of action (3 minutes versus 6–10 minutes).
- The brand name is Duranest.
- Maximum recommended dose is 3.6 mg/lb or 8.8 mg/kg of body weight for adults, with a maximum dose of 400 mg in one appointment.
- It has a pregnancy category of B.

Topical Anesthetics

A topical anesthetic may be used before an injection of a local anesthetic to reduce discomfort associated with needle penetration. Systemic absorption of the topical anesthetic (e.g., lidocaine, benzocaine) must be considered when calculating the total amount of anesthetic administered. Benzocaine has a pregnancy category of C and tetracaine B. Both anesthetics are contraindicated in patients taking a sulfa drug. Benzocaine is not administered by injection because of its tissue-irritating properties. If the patient is allergic to ester, topical benzocaine is contraindicated. Lidocaine and tetracaine produce effective local anesthesia whether they are injected into the tissue or used topically.

Lidocaine 2.5%/prilocaine 2.5% is an anesthetic disc marketed under the name EMLA that is intended to reduce the pain of needle puncture. It is a cream that is applied 1 hour before the injection or needle procedure and lasts for 1–2 hours after removal.

Oraqix, a gel that contains lidocaine 2.5%/prilocaine 2.5%, is administered into the gingival crevice for periodontal debridement. It has a pregnancy category of B.

Vasoconstrictors in Local Anesthetics

Local anesthetics cause vasodilation, which increase the rate of absorption into the bloodstream (systemic circulation). This decreases the effectiveness of the local anesthetic and increases the anesthetic blood level, which may result in overdose. Essentially, there are two **vasoconstrictors** used in local anesthetic solutions: epinephrine and levonordefrin (Neo-Cobefrin). The addition of a vasoconstrictor counteracts the vasodilating effects of the anesthetic. Thus, the vasoconstrictor will:

- Constrict the blood vessels in the tissue, resulting in a decrease in blood flow to the site of injection.
- Slow the absorption of the agent into the bloodstream.
- Lower blood levels that would decrease the risk of an overdose.

- Decrease or prevent bleeding (hemostasis) at the site of injection.
- Allow higher concentrations of the local anesthetic remaining in the nerve for a longer time (increase the duration of anesthetic effect). For example, 2% lidocaine lasts for about 10 minutes. With the addition of epinephrine, the duration of action is prolonged to about 60 minutes.

Rapid Dental Hint

In patient taking cardioselective β_2-blockers, there are no special precautions with epinephrine.

Epinephrine

Epinephrine is a more potent vasoconstrictor than levonordefrin. Epinephrine has no cardiac effect on the healthy individual. Epinephrine stimulates both α- and β-adrenergic (sympathetic) receptors at the same time; however, β_2-stimulation predominates at low doses and α-stimulation predominates at moderate to high doses.

Subcutaneous injection of epinephrine in *low doses* as used in dentistry will stimulate predominantly β_2-receptors because these receptors have a higher affinity for epinephrine. Therefore, epinephrine can selectively stimulate β_2-receptors, resulting in vasodilation of skeletal and smooth muscle causing a decrease in diastolic blood pressure. Stimulation of β_1-receptors causes an increase in systolic blood pressure. The decrease in diastolic and increase in systolic pressure cancel each other out, so there is no increase in mean blood pressure. However, at high doses, the α_1-receptors will be occupied, resulting in an increase in blood pressure.

Epinephrine is available in many concentrations: 1:50,000, 1:100,000, and 1:200,000. *The maximum safe dose for epinephrine in healthy individuals is 0.2 mg and in cardiac patients is 0.04 mg.*

Levonordefrin

Levonordefrin (Neo-Cobefrin) is half as potent a vasoconstrictor as epinephrine. It primarily stimulates α-adrenergic (sympathetic) receptors, with little to no effect on the β-adrenergic receptors. Stimulation of α_1 receptors on tissues/organs causes vasoconstriction of blood vessels, resulting in hypertension (increased systolic and diastolic blood pressure). Epinephrine produces a greater stimulation of β_2-receptors than α_1-receptors, causing vasodilation and decreasing diastolic blood pressure. Higher doses produce more vasoconstriction and increased blood pressure. Since it is less effective/potent than epinephrine, it is used in higher concentrations (e.g., 1:20,000).

Mepivacaine 2% is available with levonordefrin as the vasoconstrictor. The onset of action is fast (30–120 minutes in the maxilla and 1–4 minutes in the mandible). The duration of action is about 1–2½ hours in the maxilla and 2½–5½ hours in the mandible.

Clinical Calculations

Calculations of the recommended doses and maximum doses of anesthetics, the amount of the drug, and vasoconstrictor should be documented (Tables 4–3, 4–4).

Special Patient Populations

Children

The primary concern in children is the ease of overdose. Before administering a local anesthetic to a child, the child's weight must be used to calculate the appropriate dose (Table 4–4). In children under 10 years of age it is rarely necessary to administer more than ½ cartridge of lidocaine 2% with epinephrine per procedure.

It is best to administer a low-concentration solution such as lidocaine 2% with epinephrine 1:100,000. Bupivacaine should not be used because it has a long duration of action.

Pregnant and Nursing Women

Local anesthetics with vasoconstrictors can be used safely in pregnant and nursing women. Because of its low concentration, lidocaine is preferred. The concentration of vasoconstrictors is low, so there is not likely to be any effect on uterine blood flow. Below are the pregnancy categories for each anesthetic.

Articaine	C
Bupivacaine	C
Lidocaine	B
Mepivacine	C
Prilocaine	B

Older Adults

There have been no documented differences in the response to local anesthetics with vasoconstrictors in older adults versus younger adults; however, it is best to administer below the maximum recommended doses because the elderly may have slower metabolism.

Rapid Dental Hint

For adults whose weight is 150 lbs and up, the maximum dose of lidocaine and articaine is about 500 mg.

For children, the dose is reduced to about ⅓ to ½ depending on the child's weight.

Adverse Effects of Local Anesthetics

Allergic Reactions

One of the most common adverse effects of local anesthetics that are reported by patients is allergy. However, in most cases it usually is not a true allergy and may be more of a reaction toward

TABLE 4-4   Calculation of the Amount of Local Anesthetic and Vasoconstrictor

Calculate the amount of lidocaine and EPI in 2 cartridges of 2% lidocaine/1:100,000 EPI:

1. Each cartridge contains 1.7 ml of drug. Lidocaine 2% is equivalent to 34 mg lidocaine.
2. Amount of epinephrine in 1:100,000 solution is 0.017 mg.
3. For example, if you use two cartridges, you have used 0.034 mg EPI and 68 mg of lidocaine.

AMOUNT (IN MG) OF ANESTHETIC (1.7-1.8 ML CARTRIDGE); CALCULATIONS ARE BASED ON 1.7 ML SOLUTIONS

PERCENTAGE CONCENTRATION	EQUIVALENT MG/ML (E.G., 2% = 20 mg/ml)	AMOUNT IN A CARTRIDGE (E.G., MULTIPLY BY 1.7)
0.5%	5 mg/ml	8.5 mg
1%	10 mg/ml	17 mg
2%	20 mg/ml	34 mg
3%	30 mg/ml	51 mg
4%	40 mg/ml	68 mg

AMOUNT OF VASOCONSTRICTOR (1.7 ML CARTRIDGE)

VASOCONSTRICTOR	DILUTION	AMOUNT (MG) PER CARTRIDGE
Levonordefrin (in mepivacaine)	1:20,000	0.051
Epinephrine (in lidocaine)	1:50,000	0.034
Epinephrine (in lidocaine)	1:100,000	0.017

the epinephrine (e.g., the patient may experience palpitations and feel like their heart is racing). Esters are associated with a higher incidence of allergic reactions due to their breakdown product, para-aminobenzoic acid (PABA; used in some sunscreen products). PABA is structurally similar to methylparaben, which was used in anesthetics as a preservative. Also, antioxidants (e.g., sodium bisulfite and metabisulfite) are added to local anesthetics that contain vasoconstrictors to prevent biodegradation by oxygen. These antioxidants may cause an allergic potential.

At the end of the cartridge is the diaphragm, where the needle penetrates. This diaphragm is composed of latex and there is concern about patients with latex allergy because the allergen may leach from the diaphragm. Some manufacturers do not use latex diaphragms.

Central Nervous System

Toxicity of local anesthetics is a function of systemic absorption. Depending on local tissue concentrations of local anesthetics, there may be excitatory or depressant effects on the central nervous system. At lower concentrations, a relatively selective depression of inhibitory neurons results in cerebral excitation, which may cause convulsions (seizures). At higher blood levels of the anesthetic either from inadvertent intravascular injection or too much anesthetic injected, a profound depression of brain functions occurs, which may may lead to respiratory arrest, coma, and, finally, death.

Although the main systemic effect of local anesthetics is on the central nervous system (crosses the blood–brain barrier), in high blood concentrations there are cardiovascular effects, including hypotension and cardiac depression. At toxic levels they may cause seizures and cardiac arrhythmias. Local anesthetics can initially cause CNS stimulation (e.g., tremor, restlessness) followed by sedation and depressed CNS function. Patients may also experience headache and nausea. The danger

to the systemic effects of epinephrine arises when the local anesthetic solution is injected into the blood vessels. Thus, it is imperative to use an aspirating syringe to ensure that no blood is found in the dental cartridge. However, *death from local anesthetic overdose is usually due to respiratory failure.*

The use of cocaine (an ester) as a local anesthetic was first reported in 1884. Its potential to become addictive and its toxicity precludes its use as a dental anesthetic; however, it is used for surface anesthesia (e.g., nose, ophthalmology) to obtain vasoconstriction. Cocaine, a very potent vasoconstrictor, works by inhibiting the reuptake of norepinephrine (NE), allowing for the accumulation of NE, which potentiates sympathetic nervous system activity (e.g., increased blood pressure and heart rate). It initially produces vasodilation, which is followed by an intense vasoconstriction of long duration.

Adverse reactions involving epinephrine include palpitations, tachycardia (rapid heart rate), anxiety, headache, tremor, and hypertension.

Blood Disorders

METHEMOGLOBINEMIA This is a rare and uncommon adverse reaction usually with high doses of prilocaine, but it may also occur with articaine and topical benzocaine. Normally, hemoglobin transports oxygen when the iron is in the ferrous form. When hemoglobin becomes oxidized, it is converted into methemoglobin, which does not bind to and transport oxygen. Normally, red blood cells are exposed to various oxidant stresses, so blood normally contains about 1% methemoglobin. Excessive methemoglobin levels (methemoglobinemia) reduce the amount of hemoglobin that is available for oxygen transport to the tissues. Clinical signs include blood that is dark in color, headache, weakness, confusion, chest pain, and grayness/cyanosis of lips, mucous membranes, and nail beds. When methemoglobin levels are above 70%, death may result if not treated immediately. Treatment of methemoglobinemia is with methylene blue administered with an IV over a 5-minute period. Results are typically seen within 20 minutes. Administration of methylene blue reduces methemoglobin back to hemoglobin.

> **DID YOU KNOW?**
>
> In 1888, John S. Pemberton, a pharmacist, invented a beverage that contained caffeine and cocaine. Today, this beverage is known as Coca-Cola.

Liver Disease

Since there is a decreased metabolism of local anesthetics in patients with severe liver disease (e.g., hepatitis, cirrhosis of the liver), a medical consultation with the patient's physician is required. A patient with severe liver disease still requires the standard amount of anesthetic, but the total dose must be reduced or minimized.

Treatment of Toxicity

Acute emergencies from local anesthetics are first managed by constant monitoring of cardiovascular and respiratory vital signs and the patient's state of consciousness. If there are changes in the patient's condition, oxygen should be administered. Convulsions may also occur. Emergency services should be employed.

Selection of the Local Anesthetic

Selection of the appropriate local anesthetic for the dental patient depends on:

1. Duration of the dental procedure; amount of time pain control is required
   a. Short procedure (especially involving mandibular block): solutions without vasoconstrictor such as mepivacaine or prilocaine plain
   b. Longer procedure: bupivacaine has a long duration of action
2. Anticipation of postoperative pain; choose a longer duration anesthetic to cover postoperative pain
   a. Bupivacaine
3. Contraindications (e.g., drug interaction; disease) for a specific anesthetic
   a. If epinephrine is contraindicated, use mepivacaine or prilocaine plain
4. Routine procedures
   a. Use of epinephrine is justified for most dental procedures
   b. Lidocaine, articaine, prilocaine, or mepivacaine
5. Children and pregnant patients
   a. Lidocaine

Dental Management of Medically Compromised Patients

Diseases and Disorders

HYPERTENSION   Using vasoconstrictors in hypertensive patients is only contraindicated if it is severely uncontrolled; however, precautions using lower concentrations of vasoconstrictors and cardiac monitoring are taken with patients who have controlled hypertension. Blood pressure should be monitored before and during dental treatment for any changes in blood pressure.

Patients taking a nonselective β_1/β_2-blocker such as propranolol (Inderal), metoprolol (Toprol), nadolol (Corgard), or timolol (Blocardren) may have an increased pressor response to epinephrine, but this effect is unlikely with low doses of epinephrine. Blocking vasodilating β_2-receptors in the blood vessels of skeletal and smooth muscle and the β_1-receptors, which lowers heart rate, causes epinephrine to act vascularly as a pure α_1-adrenergic stimulant, which increases heart rate. The initial dose should be minimal (1/2 cartridge), which should be injected slowly using aspiration to avoid intravascular injection. After waiting and monitoring for toxicity for a few minutes, more of the anesthetic may be injected. The maximum dose of epinephrine to be used in a patient taking nonselective β-blockers is 0.04 mg of epinephrine, equivalent to two cartridges (0.018 mg per cartridge 1:100,000) and 0.2 mg of levonordefrin (0.05 mg/cartridge 1:20,000). The benefits for maintaining adequate anesthesia (reducing the pain) outweigh the risks for toxicity. Careful monitoring for toxicity (e.g., increased blood pressure, cardiac arrhythmias including tachycardia) should be done. Epinephrine 1:50,000 should be avoided, as well as a gingival retraction cord containing epinephrine used in restorative dentistry.

> **RDH**
> ### Rapid Dental Hint
>
> Remember: To reduce the incidence of toxicity, you should administer the local anesthetic slowly and aspirate or use an aspirating syringe.

Epinephrine or levonordefrin may be used in patients taking nonselective β-blockers, but the initial dose should be kept to a minimum (e.g., 1/2 cartridge of lidocaine with epinephrine 1:100,000).

There are no major concerns in patient taking cardioselective $\beta 1$-blockers such as atenolol (Tenormin), metoprolol (Lopressor), acebutolol (Sectral), or betaxolol (Kerlone) because these drugs act only on $\beta 1$-receptors.

> **RDH**
> ### Rapid Dental Hint
>
> Epinephrine may be used in patients taking nonselective β-blockers, but the initial dose should be kept to a minimum (e.g., ½ cartridge of lidocaine with epinephrine 1:100,000).

HEART FAILURE/ANGINA/STROKE/MYOCARDIAL INFARCTION In patients with heart failure and angina pectoris, the amount of vasoconstrictor should be minimized with prudent cardiac monitoring before and during anesthesia administration. Epinephrine is contraindicated in patients that have had a stroke or heart attack within the last 6 months. Epinephrine is also contraindicated in patients that had a coronary bypass or unstable angina within the last 3 months.

DIABETES MELLITUS Patients with controlled type 1 or type 2 diabetes mellitus can generally be given vasoconstrictors without special precautions. Patients who are not well controlled with fluctuating blood glucose (sugar) levels or taking high doses of insulin should have the amount of epinephrine limited. Epinephrine is able to counteract the hypoglycemic effects of insulin by elevating blood glucose. Epinephrine mobilizes liver carbohydrate stores and stimulates the production of lactic acid from glycogen in muscle (glycogenolysis). The lactic acid may be used by the liver to manufacture new carbohydrate (glucose), elevating blood glucose. In these patients, the amount of vasoconstrictor should be minimized.

ADRENAL DISEASE Vasoconstrictors are contraindicated in patients with pheochromocytoma. Pheochromocytoma is a tumor of the adrenal medulla characterized by increased secretion of epinephrine, which leads to hypertension and cardiac arrhythmias.

THYROID DISEASE Vasoconstrictors (e.g., epinephrine) should be avoided in patients with thyrotoxicosis (hyperthyroidism). These patients should not receive dental hygiene care until controlled. Patients with excessive thyroid hormone levels develop hypertension and arrhythmias. However, in patients taking thyroid hormone replacement (Synthroid) and who are well controlled, no special precautions are needed.

BLOOD DYSCRASIAS The use of prilocaine is contraindicated in patients with methemaglobinemia.

ASTHMA Vasoconstrictor use should be minimized in asthmatic patients because the anesthetic solution contains sulfites, which may cause an allergic reaction in asthmatics.

BRONCHITIS Bronchitis and emphysema are the most common forms of chronic obstructive pulmonary disease. No special precautions are needed with administration of local anesthetics.

Drugs

COCAINE USER Many times a patient may not willfully report the use of recreational cocaine. Vasoconstrictors should not be used in the patient for at least 24 hours after the last use of cocaine to allow for metabolism and elimination of the drug.

TRICYCLIC ANTIDEPRESSANTS AND MONOAMINE OXIDASE INHIBITORS The administration of local anesthetics with vasoconstrictors to patients receiving tricyclic antidepressants (e.g., Elavil) may produce severe, prolonged hypertension. There is no evidence of a significant interaction with monoamine oxidase inhibitors (MAOIs).

Tricyclic antidepressants block the reuptake of norepinephrine back into the nerve, which causes an increase in the amount of norepinephrine within the synapse. Severe and prolonged hypertension may result when epinephrine is administered, resulting in higher amounts of NE/EPI in the synapse. According to the drug insert from the manufacturer, the combination of a vasoconstrictor and a tricyclic antidepressant should be avoided. Other sources state that these patients should be treated similarly to cardiac patients receiving local anesthetics with vasoconstrictors. The amount of epinephrine used in the local anesthetic should be limited to two cartridges of lidocaine with 1:100,000 epinephrine, equivalent to 0.034 mg epinephrine; any additional injections should be given 30 minutes apart.

Levonordefrin (contained in mepivacaine) should be avoided because of a greater chance of developing hypertension due to alpha-receptor stimulation. A gingival retraction cord containing epinephrine for tooth impressions should be avoided. The patient's cardiac condition should be monitored by taking blood pressure. If an adverse reaction occurs, it can be controlled by the use of an alpha-receptor blocker drug such as phentolamine.

SELECTIVE SEROTONIN REUPTAKE INHIBITORS (SSRIS) There are no vasoconstrictor interactions with SSRIs such as paroxetine (Paxil), fluoxetine (Prozac), and sertraline (Zoloft). Blocking serotonin reuptake has no affect on epinephrine.

ANTIPSYCHOTICS Antipsychotics such as aripiprazole (Abilify), clozapine (Clozaril), and olanzapine (Zyprexa) can block α-adrenergic receptors. Thus, the use of epinephrine may cause hypotension and tachycardia (increased heart rate). A minimal amount of EPI may be used and the patient's vital signs should be monitored.

Dental Hygiene Applications

The use of local anesthetics with vasoconstrictors in medically compromised patients generally can be given safely. In most patients, the benefits outweigh the low possible risk. The anesthetic solution should be aspirated before injecting to avoid intravascular introduction of the solution, which would result in systemic involvement. The solution should then be administered slowly.

Selection of the type of anesthetic and the decision to use a vasoconstrictor is based on patient history and type and duration of the procedure (extraction, periodontal debridement, periodontal surgery). It is ideal to use a local anesthetic without a vasoconstrictor for short procedures using a mandibular block. On the other hand, bupivacaine is best for long procedures because it has a long duration of action. Lidocaine is preferred in children and pregnant patients. For conventional dental procedures, articaine, lidocaine, mepivacaine, or prilocaine can be considered. Prilocaine, and maybe articaine and topical benzocaine, should be avoided in patients with congenital methemoglobinemia. The goal is to use the minimal amount of anesthetic/vasoconstrictor that is needed to obtain profound anesthesia.

Documentation in the treatment record must include the type and dosage of local anesthetic in milligrams. Vasoconstrictor, if any, must be noted whether in milligrams or concentration (e.g., 34 mg lidocaine 2% with 0.017 mg 1:100,000 epinephrine). Documentation must also include the type of injection given (e.g., infiltration, block).

Key Points

- Anesthetics block sodium channels in the nerve cell membrane.
- An anesthetic is less effective in inflamed, acidic tissue.
- Levonordefrin (Neo-Cobefrin) is half as potent a vasoconstrictor as epinephrine.
- Levonordefrin stimulates α-adrenergic (sympathetic) receptors with little to no effect on the β-adrenergic receptors, causing hypertension.
- Precautions are needed when using vasconstrictors in certain medically compromised patients.
- Use no more than 0.04 mg of epinephrine for patients with cardiovascular disease.
- Prilocaine, articaine, and topical benzocaine may cause methemoglobinemia, clinically characterized by cyanosis (low oxygen).
- www.ada.org/govenmental_affairs/downloads/local-anesthesia.pdf describes local anesthesia administration by dental hygienists (state chart).

Board Review Questions

1. Which of the following agents primarily stimulates α_1-receptors, causing increased blood pressure? (p. 68)
   a. Lidocaine
   b. Mepivacaine
   c. Epinephrine
   d. Levonordefrin

2. Which of the following agents is available as a topical formulation? (p. 65)
   a. Mepivacaine
   b. Lidocaine
   c. Articaine
   d. Bupivacaine

3. The concentration (in mg) of epinephrine in one (1.7 ml) cartridge of lidocaine 2% with 1:100,000 epinephrine is (p. 69)
   a. 0.018.
   b. 0.017.
   c. 0.036.
   d. 0.36.
   e. 0.054.

4. The concentration (in mg's) of epinephrine in one (1.7 ml) cartridge of lidocaine 2% with 1:50,000 epinephrine is (p. 69)
   a. 0.018.
   b. 0.017.
   c. 0.09.
   d. 0.36.
   e. 0.034.

5. Death from an overdose of a local anesthetic is usually due to (p. 69)
   a. cardiac stimulation.
   b. respiratory failure.
   c. bradycardia.
   d. tachycardia.

6. Which of the following anesthetics is an ester? (p. 65)
   a. Benzocaine
   b. Lidocaine
   c. Mepivacaine
   d. Etidocaine

7. Which of the following anesthetics is a potent vasoconstrictor? (p. 69)
   a. Cocaine
   b. Mepiviance
   c. Lidocaine
   d. Bupivacaine

8. Which of the following anesthetics contains levonordefrin as a vasoconstrictor? (p. 68)
   a. Lidocaine
   b. Procaine
   c. Bupivacaine
   d. Mepivacaine

9. According to the 2005 labeling of dental anesthetic cartridges, the volume of an anesthetic cartridge is (p. 64)
   a. 1.5 ml.
   b. 1.7 ml.
   c. 2.0 ml.
   d. 3.0 ml.

10. Which of the following local anesthetics can cause methemaglobinemia? (p. 69)
    a. Prilocaine
    b. Cocaine
    c. Lidocaine
    d. Bupivacaine

Selected References

Nava-Ocampo AA, Bello-Ramirez AM. 2004. Lipophilicity affects the pharmacokinetics and toxicity of local anaesthetic agents administered by caudal block. *Clinical and Experimental Pharmacology and Physiology* 31:116–118.

Bader JD, Bonito AJ, Shugars DA. 2002. A systematic review of cardiovascular effects of epinephrine on hypertensive dental patients. *Oral Surgery, Oral Medicine, Oral Radiology and Endodontics* 93:647–653.

Bassett KB, DiMarco AC, Naughton DK. 2010. *Local anesthesia for dental professionals.* Upper Saddle River, NJ: Pearson.

Budenz AW. 2000. Local anesthetics and medically complex patients. *J California Dental Association* 28:611–619.

Budenz AW. 2003. Local anesthetics in dentistry: Then and now. *J California Dental Association* 31:388–396.

Carroll A, Sesin GP. 2002. A case study of benzocaine-induced methemoglobinemia. *U.S. Pharmacist* 27(12):HS-44-HS-46.

Haas DA. 2002. An update on local anesthetics in dentistry. *J Can Dent Assoc* 68(9):546–551.

Hersh EV, Giannakopoulos H, Levin LM, Moore PA, Hutcheson M, Mosenkis A, Townsend RR. 2006. The pharmacokinetics and cardiovascular effects of high-dose articaine with 1:100,00 and 1:200,000 epinephrine. *JADA* 137(11):1562–1571.

Horlocker TT, Wedel DJ. 2002. Local anesthetic toxicity—Does product labeling reflect actual risk? *Regional Anesthesia and Pain Medicine* 27:562–567.

Mazoit, J-X, Dalens BJ. 2004. Pharmacokinetics of local anesthetics in infants and children. *Clinical Pharmacokinetics* 43(1):17–32.

Neal JM. 2003. Effects of epinephrine in local anesthetics on the central and peripheral nervous systems: Neurotoxicity and neural blood flow. *Regional Anesthesia and Pain Medicine* 28:124–134.

Weinberg MA, Segnick SL. 2010. Management of non-variceal upper gastrointestinal bleeding. *U.S. Pharmacist* 35(12):HS-11-HS-20.

Yagiela JA. 1999. Adverse drug interactions in dental practice: Interactions associated with vasoconstrictors. Part V of a series. *JADA* 130:701–709.

Web Sites

www.adha.org/governmental_affairs/downloads/localanesthesia.pdf
www.guideline.gov
www.ada.org/prof/resources/topics/color.asp
www.ncbi.nlm.nih/gov/entrez/query.fcgi?cmd=Retrieve&db=PubMed&list_uids=12636129&dopt=Abstract

PEARSON
myhealthprofessionskit™

Use this address to access the Companion Website created for this textbook. Simply select "Dental Hygiene" from the choice of disciplines. Find this book and log in using your username and password to access video clips of selected tests.

QUICK DRUG GUIDE

Esters

- Benzocaine 20% (Hurricaine), topical
- Tetracaine (Pontocaine), topical, injectable
- Tetracaine + benzocaine (Cetacaine), topical
- Cocaine, topical

Amides

- Lidocaine (Xylocaine, Octocaine 50, 100), topical, injectable
- Mepivacaine (Carbocaine), injectable
- Prilocaine (Citanest), injectable
- Bupivacaine (Marcaine), injectable
- Etidocaine (Duranest), injectable
- Articaine (Septocaine, Zorcaine, Ultracaine D-S Forte, Ultracaine D-S), injectable

Other

- Lidocaine and prilocaine gel (Oraqix), topical
- Lidocaine (DentiPatch), transoral

Sedation and General Anesthetics

EDUCATIONAL OBJECTIVES

After reading this chapter, the reader should be able to:

1. Summarize the concepts of minimal, moderate, and deep sedation.

2. List various pharmacological agents used for moderate sedation.

3. List the objectives in using sedation to manage dental patients.

4. Discuss the role of nitrous oxide in the dental office.

GOAL

To gain knowledge about pharmacological agents used for minimal, moderate, and deep sedation, anxiety control, and general anesthesia in the dental patient.

KEY TERMS

Minimal sedation

Moderate sedation

Deep sedation

General anesthesia

Nitrous oxide

Introduction

The management of fear and anxiety is an integral part of patient care in the dental office. Today, a wide variety of equipment and medications are available to the dental clinician to help deal with patient apprehension of dental treatment.

Many types of drugs are used in anesthesia during minor and major surgery in hospitals and dental offices. These drugs produce CNS depression and analgesia, with a reversible loss of consciousness and the absence of response to painful stimuli. Dentists must be trained to use moderate sedation and general anesthesia. Dental hygienists may administer nitrous oxide.

Terminology

Minimal sedation (anxiolysis) is a drug-induced state during which patients respond normally to verbal commands. Although cognitive function and coordination may be impaired, ventilatory and cardiovascular functions are unaffected.

Moderate sedation (previously known as conscious sedation) refers to the administration of drugs for the purpose of sedation (sleepiness), lack of awareness of surroundings (narcosis), amnesia (loss of memory), or analgesia (increased pain threshold without loss of consciousness), so the patient still responds to verbal (arousable) and physical stimuli during stressful dental/medical procedures. Moderate sedation is not expected to induce depths of sedation that would impair the patient's own ability to maintain the integrity of the airway. Thus, intubation is usually not required, but may be in order to manage the airway and support vital signs. This procedure can be performed in the hospital or dental office by qualified dentists. General anesthesia is not routinely used for dental procedures because skeletal muscle relaxation and unconsciousness is not the goal. In dentistry minimal and moderate sedation and analgesia is used.

Deep sedation and analgesia is a drug-induced depression of consciousness during which patients cannot be easily aroused, but respond purposefully following repeated or painful stimulation. The patient breathes spontaneously but maintenance of a free airway may be impaired. Optimal sedation in these circumstances would include quick onset, low cardiopulmonary depression, and rapid recovery. It is possible to move from moderate sedation to deep sedation without recognition, and the varying levels of deep sedation may overlap with general anesthesia. Patients under deep sedation require more cardiac, blood pressure, and respiratory monitoring than under conscious sedation. Deep sedation is done in a hospital setting.

General anesthesia is an induced state of unconsciousness together with a *partial* or *complete* loss of protective reflexes, including the inability to maintain an airway independently and respond to physical stimulation or verbal command. A ventilator (endotracheal intubation is performed to put a tube into the trachea) breathes for the patient during the surgical procedure. General anesthesia is primarily used for lengthy surgical procedures. Balanced anesthesia is used where low doses of several drugs, rather than one drug, with different actions are given to minimize adverse events and provide recovery of the protective reflexes within a few minutes of the end of the surgical procedure.

Routes of Administration

Different routes of administration of pharmacological agents used to induce and maintain general anesthesia/conscious sedation are available and include:

- Enteral: Absorption is through the GI tract (e.g., oral, rectal, sublingual), the most common route for moderate sedation.
- Parenteral: Absorption bypasses the GI tract (e.g., intravenous [IV] and subcutaneous [SC]). The subcutaneous route of drug administration is usually used in pediatric dentistry because of a more rapid onset of action and more profound clinical effects.
- Inhalational: Gaseous or volatile drug is introduced into the lungs.
- Transdermal: Drug is administered by a patch or iontophoresis.

Types of Anesthesia

- *Oral moderate sedation* is obtained via the enteral route. A disadvantage of this route is that a large initial dose must be given and absorption is not predictable, nor easily reversible.
- *Inhalation moderate sedation* is obtained via inhalation via the lungs. Nitrous oxide/oxygen is administered through this route only for anxiolysis (anti-anxiety), and not for anesthesia. Advantages of this route include easy adjustment of depth of sedation and rapid recovery.
- *Combined moderate sedation* is obtained via enteral and/or combination inhalation (e.g., nitrous oxide/oxygen) or enteral conscious sedation. The combined route is more effective than either route used alone.
- *Intravenous moderate sedation* is the most effective method of obtaining adequate and predictable sedation. A generalized misconception is that intravenous sedation is synonymous with general anesthesia. It is not, because the patient has a minimally depressed level of consciousness and can maintain an airway.
- *General anesthesia* is obtained via intravenous and inhalation of drugs.

Therapeutic Uses

General anesthesia is administered to patients undergoing major general surgery in the hospital in the treatment of injury, deformity, and disease. Areas of the body treated by general surgery include the stomach, liver, intestines, heart, and eyes.

Moderate sedation is administered to patients undergoing minor surgical procedures. It is used in the dental office or hospital to make the patients unaware of their surroundings and to provide analgesia (pain relief). The same agents used for general anesthesia are used to induce conscious sedation.

Patient Physical Status Classification

Every patient seen in the medical/dental office or hospital is given a physical status classification according to the American Society of Anesthesiologists. This classification is used to determine the medical status of the patient and should be done before treatment is started. Patients receiving anesthesia should be medically stable with an ASA I or II. A medical consultation from the patient's physician may be required, especially for ASA III or IV. Table 5-1 reviews the classification of a patient's physical status and should be used when administering any type of anesthesia.

Moderate Sedation in the Dental Office

The goal of moderate sedation is to achieve anxiety reduction, pain control, and amnesia in the dental patient. The patient's mood must be altered so dental treatment will be tolerated. The patient remains responsive and cooperative during the dental procedure. Additionally, the patient's airway remains open. Although dental hygienists cannot administer conscious sedation, they will be performing dental procedures on these patients and must be familiar with specific agents and their safe and effective use.

The objectives for moderate sedation differ depending on the dental case. For instance, a long periodontal surgical procedure such as dental implants or grafting in an anxious and fearful patient may require a regimen that includes analgesic and amnesic properties, whereas managing an uncooperative patient during a minor restorative or periodontal procedure may just require orally administered mood-alteration drugs or nitrous oxide.

Dentists providing moderate sedation must be qualified to recognize deep sedation, manage its consequences, and adjust the level of sedation to a moderate or minimal level.

TABLE 5-1   Patient Physical Status Classification

ASA I	Normal, healthy patient
ASA II	Patient with mild systemic disease: type 2 diabetes, hypertension
ASA III	Patient with severe systemic disease: stable angina, type 1 diabetes, chronic obstructive pulmonary disease
ASA IV	Patient with severe systemic disease that is a constant threat to life: heart attack within 6 months, unstable angina, uncontrolled diabetes or uncontrolled epilepsy
ASA V	Moribund patient who is not expected to survive without the operation: patient is not expected to survive 24 hours with or without medical intervention
ASA VI	A declared brain-dead patient whose organs are being removed for donor purposes
E	Emergency operation used to modify any of the above classifications

Source: ASA, American Society of Anesthesiologists; E, emergency.

Intravenous moderate sedation in the dental office can be administered with a combination of just a few drugs. Today, intravenous sedation is the most effective way to achieve adequate and predictable sedation in most dental patients. The most common method for achieving anxiety control in dental patients is with a combination of the following:

- Benzodiazepines such as diazepam (Valium, generics); midazolam (Versed) for its amnesia effect and reducing apprehension and fear
- Narcotic analgesics such as fentanyl (Sublimaze, generics), morphine, and meperidine (Demerol, generics) for analgesia and euphoria
- Sedative/hypnotics: Nonbarbiturates such as propfol (Diprivan)
- Sedatives: Barbiturates such as pentobarbital may also be used if the patient cannot take benzodiazepines.

IV/Oral/Inhalational Agents for Moderate Sedation

Intravenous anesthetics are mainly used for the rapid *induction* of general anesthesia or moderate sedation, which is then maintained with an appropriated inhalational drug such as nitrous oxide-oxygen, or by intermittent or continuous infusion. Intravenous anesthetics are administered first to decrease anxiety and fear. These drugs may also be used alone to produce a light level of narcosis (unawareness of the surroundings) for short surgical procedures, especially those performed with the aid of local anesthetics, which is used for an analgesic effect.

There is great individual variation in response to intravenous anesthetics. Some, but not all, of this is explained by lower tolerance of poor-risk patients or the increased requirements of those who have become tolerant to other CNS depressants such as alcohol or sleeping pills. Thus, assessment of individual requirements is necessary.

Intravenous anesthetics are administered directly into the blood and distribute to the lipid regions of the body, so the onset of action is within seconds. The higher the lipid solubility of the agent, the more readily it is redistributed to other fatty regions. The drug is then slowly metabolized and excreted over several hours. Benzodiazepines take a few minutes to distribute to the brain, whereas barbiturates take about 20 seconds. Nonbarbiturates such as propofol and etomidate are highly lipid soluble and are rapid in onset, but shorter in duration of action. These agents are metabolized rapidly, with less accumulation in fatty deposits.

Sedation of children is different from sedation of adults. Generally, sedation is restricted to uncooperative children. According to the American Academy of Pediatrics, sedative and anxiolytic medications should only be administered by or in the presence of individuals skilled in airway management and cardiopulmonary resuscitation. The American Academy of Pediatric Dentistry (reference manual, 2006) recognizes nitrous oxide/oxygen inhalation as a safe and effective technique to reduce anxiety and produce analgesia.

TABLE 5-2 Classification of Intravenous Anesthetics Used for Moderate Sedation/Analgesia
DRUG NAME
Benzodiazepines
Diazepam (Valium)
Lorazepam (Ativan)
Midazolam (Versed)
Triazolam (Halcion)
Opioids (Narcotics)
Fentanyl (Sublimaze)
Alfentanil (Alfenta)
Sufentanil (Sufenta)
Meperidine (Demerol)
Sedative/Hypnotics
Thiopental (Pentothal)
Etomidate (Amidate)
Methohexital (Brevital)
Nonbarbiturate Sedative Hypnotics
Propofol (Diprivan)
Ketamine (Ketalar)
Chloral hydrate (Noctec)
Reversal Drugs
Naloxone (Narcan): reverses narcotics
Flumazenil (Mazicon, Romazicon): reverses benzodiazepines

Table 5-2 lists intravenous anesthetic agents used for the induction of general anesthesia or moderate sedation.

Anti-Anxiety Agents: Benzodiazepines

Benzodiazepines are used to treat anxious dental patients. These drugs are sedating, reduce anxiety, induce relaxation, and produce amnesia. Some benzodiazepines used for IV sedation dentistry are diazepam (Valium) and midazolam (Versed). Diazepam, a long-acting benzodiazepine, can be irritating when administered IV and may cause pain at the injection site. On the other hand, midazolam, a short-acting benzodiazepine, causes less pain at the site of injection and is primarily used for preoperative sedation and for procedures that do not require a high level of analgesia. Midazolam has greater potential for respiratory depression in older adults than in children, and has a pregnancy category of D (warning for use in pregnant women). For an adult the dosage is IV 1–1.5 mg, which may be repeated in 2 minutes prn or IM 0.07–0.08 mg/kg 30–60 minutes before the dental procedure (Table 5-2). Diazepam oral solution is recommended for children over 6 years. Another benzodiazepine, triazolam (Halcion), has a pregnancy category of X, so it is contraindicated in pregnant women.

Respiratory status should be monitored in the dental patient taking a benzodiazepine. The effects can be reversed with flumazenil (Mazicon, Romazicon). Additionally, the dental hygienist should observe the patient for possible abuse and dependency on the drug.

Benzodiazepines are also used for oral minimal/moderate sedation of apprehensive and fearful dental patients. Orally administered benzodiazepines include lorazepam (Ativan), chlorazepate (Tranxene), alprazolam (Xanax), and triazolam (Halcion). The medication can be taken either the night before or one hour before the dental procedure. Oral benzodiazepines have the same drug interactions as injectable benzodiazepines.

Flumazenil (Mazicon, Romazicon) is a benzodiazepine antagonist and is given to patients to reverse the action of a benzodiazepine in cases of overdose.

Sedative/Hypnotics: Barbiturates

Barbiturates are used for anxiety reduction, light sedation, and general anesthesia. Barbiturates used for moderate sedation are classified as sedative hypnotics. Barbiturates produce sleep by depression of central nervous system activity with minimal cardiovascular effects at sedative doses. Their popularity over the years has been reduced by the benzodiazepines; however, they still are being used because of the ease of multiple routes of administration.

Several disadvantages include respiratory depression, irritation of rectal mucosa with rectal administration, and slow onset with oral administration. Paradoxical excitement can occur when the barbiturate instead of causing depression causes excitement, especially when used for painful procedures. Barbiturates have primarily been replaced by other drugs that cause fewer adverse effects.

For dental situations, it is recommended to use a short-acting barbiturate such as pentobarbital or secobarbital. The duration of action is about 3–4 hours. Longer-acting barbiturates such as phenobarbital are used as anticonvulsant drugs.

Sedative/Hypnotics: Nonbarbiturates

PROPOFOL Nonbarbiturates are preferred over barbiturates because they have fewer side effects, including less cardiac depression. Propofol (Diprivan) is widely used for conscious sedation because it is associated with rapid recovery without hangover and nausea and vomiting. It has a rapid induction (40 seconds) and short duration of action (5–10 minutes) with a quick recovery. It can be used for lengthy surgical procedures, unlike thiopental, because it is rapidly metabolized by the liver and excreted in the urine. Propofol is usually combined with an analgesic agent or local anesthetic because by itself it provides no analgesia. Adverse effects include twitching, jerking, coughing, and vasodilation, which can result in marked hypotension. It is available as an emulsion, which contains soybean oil and egg phosphatide.

NARCOTICS Opioids are used to produce mood changes, provide analgesia, and elevate the pain threshold. Narcotics are also used to reduce the dose of intravenous anesthetic and are usually used with benzodiazepines and as supplements to nitrous oxide. Narcotics commonly used for conscious sedation include fentanyl (Sublimaze) and meperidine (Demerol). For children, intranasal or oral transmucosal routes ("lollipop") for fentanyl (Sublimaze) and sufentanyl (Sufenta) are available and achieve both analgesia and sedation.

Narcotics have a direct effect on the gastrointestinal tract, causing constipation. Other side effects include respiratory difficulties, headache, itching, and nausea and vomiting.

Rapid Dental Hint

Remember to monitor your patients. Watch for respiratory status, state of consciousness, heart rate, and blood pressure.

Others

Chloral hydrate (Noctec) is a sedative/hypnotic with little to no analgesic properties. It has been used orally (not very palatable) or rectally for anxious children, especially under 2 years, before a dental/medical procedure or for sedation before and after surgery. Particular care must be taken in calculating and administering the proper dose because overdose and death can occur very easily. It is only given for conscious sedation and not for general anesthesia. It is readily absorbed, with an onset of action of 30–60 minutes and duration of action of 4–8 hours. It is metabolized in the liver to the active metabolite trichloroethanol. Chloral hydrate is not indicated as an analgesic for pain control and may actually cause excitement and delirium. *Sudden death can occur due to cardiac arrest.* Its use has been prohibited in California in pediatric dentistry due to deaths.

Monitoring

The dental hygienist must be trained in monitoring the safety of patients and in the recognition and management of adverse reactions and emergencies that are associated with the use of these pharmacological agents.

DID YOU KNOW?

Chloral hydrate is the oldest hypnotic depressant (sleep pill); it was first synthesized in 1832, but not used in medicine until 1869.

DID YOU KNOW?

The expression "knockout drops" or "Mickey Finn" is a drink consisting of a mixture of chloral hydrate and alcohol that is used on an unsuspecting victim to incapacitate them.

The patient should be assessed for adequate airway and gas exchange and cardiovascular response. The patient's vital signs, including pulse rate, blood pressure, and respiration rate, must be monitored and documented. Vital signs reflect changes in depth of anesthesia or physical status. A pulse oximeter is used to monitor the pulse rate and level of oxygen in the blood. An electrocardiogram (EKG) monitor can also be used to assist in monitoring the patient. The dental hygienist must also be aware of drug antagonists that are used to reverse the actions of some of these drugs. However, once some of these drugs are injected into the blood, it is not possible to reverse the actions.

Nitrous Oxide

Properties and Indications: Nitrous Oxide

First discovered in 1783 by Joseph Priestley, **nitrous oxide** (referred to as "laughing gas" because of the euphoria that it produces) is the only anesthetic gas used today, and is the least soluble in blood of all inhalational anesthetics. Dr. Horace Wells was the first dentist to use nitrous oxide for tooth extractions (on himself!). Nitrous oxide (N_2O) is a colorless, sweet-smelling gas used for induction (if used alone for moderate sedation) or maintenance (if used after intravenous general anesthetic) of anesthesia. *It is a weak general anesthetic and is generally not used alone in anesthesia; however, it has marked analgesic and amnesia properties,* is relatively nontoxic, and does not produce respiratory depression (slow breathing), bronchodilation, hypotension (low blood pressure), or heart arrhythmias. This makes it an ideal, safe sedative agent in the dental office (Table 5-3).

The following are indications for nitrous oxide:

- Fearful, anxious patient (child/adult)
- Cognitively, physically, or medically compromised child or adult
- Gag reflex interfering with oral health care
- Profound local anesthesia cannot be obtained or tolerated
- Cardiac conditions, hypertension, asthma, cerebral palsy

When used alone, nitrous oxide has a rapid action (2–3 minutes) and a rapid recovery without loss of consciousness. It is easy to administer and can be self-delivered by the patient using the demand-valve positive pressure method. Using this method, analgesia is obtained in less than 20 seconds and the patient is relaxed in 30–60 seconds. It is also acceptable for use in children. Besides its use in the dental office, nitrous oxide is used for many medical procedures, including minor painful orthopedic injuries or changing burn dressings.

Because of its analgesic properties and lack of major cardiovascular or respiratory depression, nitrous oxide is often used as a part of balanced anesthesia in combination with other anesthetic agents or drugs in low doses to reduce the requirements (MAC) of other, more potent agents. It cannot be used alone for surgical anesthesia because of its low potency.

Pharmacokinetics

Nitrous oxide is rapidly absorbed from the pulmonary alveoli into the bloodstream. The higher the concentration of nitrous oxide in the mask, the more rapidly the same concentration will

TABLE 5-3 Features of Nitrous Oxide

	ADVERSE EFFECTS	CONTRAINDICATIONS	NOTES
Nitrous oxide	Nausea and vomiting with very high concentrations, or on an empty or full stomach	Chronic obstructive pulmonary disease (COPD; bronchitis, emphysema), upper respiratory obstruction (e.g., cold, stuffy nose, blocked Eustachian tubes), epilepsy, first trimester of pregnancy, communication difficulty, fear of sedation/negative past experience	Does not cause respiratory depression, bronchodilation, or low blood pressure. Patients should avoid a large meal within 3 hours of dental visit to prevent vomiting.

develop in the lungs. When the high concentration of nitrous oxide at the mask is removed, the concentration falls and the nitrous oxide unchanged is removed from the body in the expired air at the same rate.

Method of Administration

Nitrous oxide is administered with oxygen by adjusting the concentration of nitrous oxide to titrate the patient to the desired level of sedation. There are two tanks: Oxygen is the green tank and nitrous oxide (N_2O) is the blue tank. Pure oxygen (100%) is administered with a mask for the first 2–3 minutes, and then nitrous oxide is added to the oxygen in 5–10% (up to about 20–30%) concentrations until the desired level of sedation is reached. The suggested induction dosage for patient comfort is about 50% or less (50/50). For maintenance the dosage should be 30/70. Onset of sedation is usually within 3–5 minutes. When the dental procedure is finished the patient must be administered only 100% oxygen for at least 5 minutes. Diffusion hypoxia (low oxygen levels to the tissue; headaches can develop) may result when there is not enough oxygen delivered. To prevent hypoxia, the mask should not be removed until the patient receives enough oxygen.

DID YOU KNOW?

When nitrous oxide was first discovered in 1772, it was used at social parties to produce euphoria. It wasn't until the 1860s that nitrous oxide was used for anesthesia.

Adverse Effects

The most common adverse effects include nausea and vomiting, which can be minimized by having the patient eat a light amount of food before the appointment. Chronic abuse of nitrous oxide is associated with a fall in the white-cell count and neuropathy (nerve damage including numbness of limbs). Exposure of anesthetists or other operating room personnel to nitrous oxide should be minimized.

DID YOU KNOW?

Joseph Priestley, who discovered nitrous oxide, also invented the eraser.

Megaloblastic anemia can occur with abuse of nitrous oxide. There may be an added sedative effect when a patient is also taking sedative drugs or St. John's wort.

Contraindications

Nitrous oxide should not be used in patients with:

- Chronic obstructive pulmonary disease (e.g., bronchitis or emphysema) because there is damage to the alveoli in the lungs and they do not perform gas exchange as easily or well as someone with healthy lungs would. Also, COPD patients require low oxygen concentrations in the blood as their primary stimulant for respiration. Using high-dose oxygen in these patients can cause respiration to stop.
- Respiratory obstructions (e.g., stuffy nose, blocked eustachian tubes) because the patient needs to breathe in the nitrous oxide/oxygen mixture. May not be able to breath through the mask.
- First-trimester pregnancy. Chronic exposure to pregnant women increases the incidence of miscarriages.
- Bowel obstructions because nitrous oxide use may contribute to bowel distention.
- Cognitive impairment.

DID YOU KNOW?

In the days of Joseph Priestley, nitrous oxide was administered in a leather bag.

Occupational Exposure

The National Institute of Occupational Safety and Health (NIOSH) reported nitrous oxide levels of approximately 50 ppm were achievable in the dental office. To keep occupational exposure to a minimum, the procedure time should be short and there should be ventilation and monitoring devices. Faulty equipment can pose hazards for dental/medical clinicians in the room, especially spontaneous abortion and genetic effects.

Abuse of Nitrous Oxide

Nitrous oxide has been reported to be used by medical/dental professionals for recreational use. Long-term exposure of nitrous oxide can result in numbness of extremities (neuropathy), vitamin B_{12} deficiency, and reproductive adverse effects.

General Anesthesia

History

The first time general anesthesia was used for major surgery was in 1846 by William Morton at the Massachusetts General Hospital. He used only one agent, diethyl ether, which is no longer used in developed countries because of a slow rate of induction, with many postoperative adverse effects such as nausea and vomiting. General anesthesia allowed for longer and more sophisticated procedures to be done, not just quick procedures. Modern anesthesia uses a combination of many drugs to achieve surgical anesthesia rather than only one agent, as William Morton did in the 1800s.

Indications

General anesthesia is not commonly used in dentistry except for patients who are very fearful of having dental procedures performed, are mentally or physically challenged, or are having very stressful and traumatic procedures done, such as multiple tooth extractions. General anesthesia is administered via inhalation and intravenous routes. General anesthetics are drugs that rapidly produce unconsciousness and total analgesia.

Stages

General anesthesia is a progressive process that occurs in distinct stages or levels (Guedel's signs). The most potent anesthetic agent can quickly induce all four stages, while others such as nitrous oxide are only able to induce Stage I. Most surgery requires the patient to be in Stage III, called surgical anesthesia. Pupil dilation, tachycardia (increased heart rate), hypotension, and skeletal muscle relaxation are the four signs that indicate a patient is in Stage III surgical anesthesia. The stages of general anesthesia are listed in Table 5-4.

General anesthesia involves the administration of different drugs. To achieve balanced anesthesia the following regimens are used:

1. *Premedication* is administered to reduce anxiety and obtain analgesia (for short surgical procedures premedication is not necessary). Premedication is performed before the patient goes into the operating room. The patient may be premedicated with an antibiotic, anxiolytics (e.g., midazolam), or anti-emetic (e.g., droperidol; to help prevent nausea and vomiting after the procedure; sometimes anti-emetics are administered intravenously during anesthesia rather than as premedication).

TABLE 5-4	Stage of Surgical Anesthesia: Guedel's Classification
STAGE	**FEATURES**
Stage I	Amnesia and analgesia
	• Moderate sedation
	• Nitrous oxide produces Stage I
	• Loss of pain, loss of general sensation but still awake, even though the patient does not know anything is happening; semiconscious
	• Reflexes intact
Stage II	Excitement/delirium
	• Loss of consciousness
	• Patient may resist treatment; involuntary muscle movements
	• Increase in blood pressure
	• Irregular respirations
	• IV agents may be used to calm the patient; loss of consciousness to onset of anesthesia
	• Patient may become incontinent
Stage III	Surgical anesthesia
	• Required stage for major surgical procedures
	• Loss of consciousness
	• Dilation of pupils
	• Tachycardia (increased heart rate)
	• Hypotension
	• Reflexes absent
	• Skeletal muscles relaxed
Stage IV	Medullary paralysis: anesthetic overdose
	• Paralysis of the medulla region of the brain, which controls respiratory and cardiovascular activity
	• Death can occur if heart stops
	• Stop anesthetics and administer 100% oxygen

2. *Induction* is most commonly obtained with intravenous agents. Induction refers to initiating anesthesia and is performed when the patient is in the operating room.

3. *Maintenance* of induction with inhalational agents. Maintenance occurs when the surgery is being performed and more anesthetic is required to finish the surgical procedure.

4. *Recovery* from anesthesia. Recovery begins when maintenance agent is discontinued up to the time when the patient is fully responsive and able to be dismissed. Medications may be given at this time to control pain or for nausea and vomiting.

Classification and Chemistry

A variety of drugs can be used to provide sedation and analgesia. The classification of agents is listed in Tables 5-5 and 5-6. The drugs used depend on whether the outcome is sedation, analgesia, and/or amnesia.

There are two main methods of inducing general anesthesia:

1. Intravenous agents are usually administered first to induce anesthesia quickly.

2. After the patient loses consciousness, inhaled agents are used to maintain the anesthesia.

Inhalational Anesthetics

Inhalational anesthetic agents are divided into two classifications (Table 5-5): nonhalongenated drugs and halogenated drugs. These agents are either gases or volatile liquids, and are used mainly for maintenance of anesthesia after induction with an intravenous induction agent.

Gaseous agents require suitable equipment for storage under pressure in metal cylinders, reduction to operating pressure, and monitoring of gas flow-rate. Most volatile agents are metered by calibrated vaporizers, using air or oxygen as carriers, though some can be given by direct drip onto a pad and vaporized by the patient's breath.

CHEMISTRY AND PHARMACOKINETICS Unlike orally administered drugs, the dose of an inhalational agent is not expressed in terms of milligrams or grams of the drug, but in terms of partial pressure or percentage of inspired air. The potency of an inhalational anesthetic is expressed as the inspired concentration

TABLE 5-5 Classification of Inhalational Anesthetics Used for General Anesthesia

VOLATILE LIQUID GENERAL ANESTHETICS

Desflurane (Suprane)
Enflurane (Ethrane)
Halothane (Fluothane)
Isoflurane (Forane)
Methoxyflurane (Penthrane)
Sevoflurane (Ultane)

TABLE 5-6 Injectable General Anesthetics

Alfentanil	Narcotic
Droperidol	Narcotic
Etomidate	Sedative/hypnotic
Ketamine	Dissociative anesthetic
Methohexital	Barbiturate
Propofol	Nonbarbiturate sedative/hypnotic
Succinylcholine	Neuromuscular blocking drug
Sufentanil	Narcotic
Thiopental	Barbiturate

of the inhaled anesthetic required to induce surgical anesthesia in 50% of patients. This is referred to as the minimal alveolar concentration (MAC). MAC is used to measure and compare the potency of inhalational anesthetic agents. For example, agents with MACs greater than 1 are less potent than agents with an MAC of less than 1. Agents with low MACs are used in combination with nitrous oxide to reduce the concentration of each, resulting in less adverse effects.

Metabolism is of little importance since general anesthesia is not maintained for prolonged periods of time. Recovery occurs because of redistribution of the drug away from the brain back into the lungs, where expiration occurs. Partial pressure in the lungs decreases as the administration of the gas stops, allowing for more drug diffusion from the lipid regions of the body to the blood. Recovery time for obese patients is longer because of greater distribution of the anesthetic to fat stores.

ADVERSE EFFECTS The inhalational anesthetics used in general anesthesia can cause severe reactions, including:

• Airway irritation
• Bronchodilation
• Respiratory depression
• Low blood pressure (hypotension)
• Cardiac arrhythmia
• Nausea is common for a few hours after the procedure (avoid a heavy meal 3 hours before appointment to minimize vomiting)

VOLATILE LIQUID GENERAL ANESTHETICS/HALOGENATED DRUGS Volatile liquids have replaced the older anesthetics such as diethyl ether, which was highly explosive, because these drugs have a more rapid rate of induction and recovery with less postoperative adverse effects such as nausea and vomiting. However, these drugs cause more respiratory and cardiovascular relaxation/depression, which is dose related (e.g., the more agent given, the increased incidence of side effects). It is liquid at room temperature and is converted to a vapor and inhaled. Careful monitoring of vital signs is very important with these agents. Balanced anesthesia is usually achieved when these agents are administered with nitrous oxide (often in a 2:1 ratio with oxygen), opioids, or skeletal muscle relaxants because by themselves they produce little analgesia or muscle relaxation. All of these anesthetics are volatile liquids at room temperature but are converted into a vapor and inhaled to produce their anesthetic effects. These agents are only used by dentists/anesthesiologists in a hospital setting.

SEVOFLURANE/DESFLURANE   Compared to the other halogenated agents, the newer agents sevoflurane (Ultane) and desflurane (Suprane) have a more rapid onset and shorter duration of action due to a low blood-gas solubility, which makes it easier to titrate the dose and are more widely used today. They cause little cardiac toxicity. Desflurane is less potent and requires higher concentrations to be inhaled, which may be irritating to the respiratory tract, causing coughing and breath-holding. These agents are often combined with nitrous oxide.

HALOTHANE   Halothane (Fluothane) is the prototype volatile liquid inhalational anesthetic; however, it is not used too much today. It is potent (MAC 0.75) and can be easy to overdose. It has a high blood-gas solubility (2.3), so the rate of induction and recovery is slower than the other halogenated agents. *Halothane is contraindicated in pregnancy and in patients with diminished hepatic (liver) function since it can be hepatoxic.* It is extensively metabolized in the liver to toxic metabolites. It is used for the maintenance of anesthesia in major surgery and to supplement the action of nitrous oxide and oxygen in balanced anesthesia. Halothane has poor analgesic effects but is more potent and induces deep anesthesia (unconsciousness).

ISOFLURANE   Isoflurane (Forane) has moderate potency with a moderate onset of action and is inexpensive. It causes more muscle relaxation, so additional muscle relaxants during surgery are not needed. However, isoflurane causes more respiratory depression (slow breathing), hypotension, and can induce heart rhythm abnormalities.

Injectable Anesthetics for General Anesthesia

Some drugs that were used in lower doses to produce moderate sedation are also used in general anesthesia, but in higher doses. Table 5-6 lists intravenous anesthetic agents used for the induction of general anesthesia.

SEDATIVE/HYPNOTICS: BARBITURATES   As an induction agent, thiopental has a rapid onset of 20 seconds but a long elimination time, resulting in a hangover effect and nausea and vomiting. It should not be continuously infused for long periods of time because it is slowly metabolized by the liver and can accumulate in the body. It is usually combined with nitrous oxide/oxygen to produce surgical anesthesia. Additionally, thiopental may cause bronchospasm, and was the primary agent until propofol was introduced.

Methohexital (Brevital) is an ultra short-acting barbiturate with an onset of 20–40 seconds and a duration of action of 5–10 minutes. There is a high incidence of postoperative nausea and vomiting.

PROPOFOL   Propofol is used for induction of general anesthesia or for maintenance of a balanced anesthesia technique. It provides complete anesthesia in and outside the operating room without having to transport an anesthesia machine.

NARCOTICS   Intravenous narcotics are not considered to be true anesthetics because they do not usually produce total unconsciousness, which is needed for general anesthesia. However, they have superior analgesic and sedative properties, which allow for easier endotracheal intubation and surgical incision. Sufentanil, alfentanil, and remifentanil are used most often in dentistry for deep sedation and general anesthesia. Fentanyl is combined with droperidol (a premixed vial is marketed as Innovar), an antipsychotic drug, to produce an analgesia where the patient is conscious but insensitive to pain and unaware of the surroundings.

DISSOCIATIVES   Ketamine (Ketalar) affects the senses and produces a dissociative/hallucinatory anesthesia where the patient may appear to be awake and receptive but does not respond to sensory stimulation. It has potent analgesic properties and mild respiratory depression. Ketamine is recreationally abused for intoxicating and hallucinatory effects. It is used in pediatric patients because it can be administered by intramuscular injection.

MUSCLE RELAXANTS   Neuromuscular-blocking drugs are used for the induction and maintenance of skeletal relaxation during general anesthesia. These drugs are also used during premedication to facilitate endotracheal intubation by relaxing the muscles of the trachea. Some examples include succinylcholine (Anectine) and pipecuronium (Arduan).

TYPICAL SEQUENCE OF EVENTS FOR INTRAVENOUS SEDATION   A typical sequence is to induce loss of consciousness for 2–3 minutes with propofol or other intravenous anesthetic and maintain anesthesia with nitrous oxide/oxygen (50/50) mixtures, supplemented, when necessary, with halothane or another potent inhalational anesthetic, or with a narcotic analgesic. The action of the anesthetic is enhanced by the narcotic analgesic, and overall anesthetic requirements are reduced. (This is balanced anesthesia.) Adequate muscle relaxation, if needed, is given.

Postoperative Problems: General Anesthesia

Many postoperative adverse events can occur in patients after general anesthesia. These include:

1. Respiratory
   - Airway obstruction
   - Sore throat
   - Difficulty breathing
   - Hypoxia (low oxygen)

2. CNS/Neurological
   - Pain
   - Muscle weakness
   - Sleepiness

3. Cardiovascular
   - Hypotension (low blood pressure)
   - Hypertension (high blood pressure)
   - Arrhythmias
4. Gastrointestinal
   - Constipation (with narcotics)
   - Nausea and vomiting

Dental Hygiene Applications

Nitrous oxide is used in dental offices for its anti-anxiety effects rather than its anesthetic effects. The dental hygienist should have a general knowledge of the medical status of patients who are candidates for nitrous oxide and IV sedation, as well as knowledge of the pharmacology of these agents. The patient should be instructed to eat a small amount of food before coming to the dental appointment to minimize nausea that can occur after nitrous oxide use. The dental hygienist should question the patient about medications they are taking to avoid any drug–drug interactions.

Key Points

- The goal of general anesthesia is to provide a rapid and complete loss of sensation; general anesthesia is not used in the dental office but is used in dentistry (in a hospital setting) for a certain group of patients, for example, patients who are fearful and apprehensive about having multiple tooth extractions at one time.
- General anesthesia is administered by anesthesiologists or certified registered nurse anesthetists (CRNA).
- Intravenous moderate sedation is not synonymous with general anesthesia.
- Intravenous sedation is performed by well-trained, qualified dentists in the dental office.
- The goal of minimal sedation or moderate sedation/analgesia in the dental office is to relieve patient anxiety and produce some amnesia and pain control.
- Usually a benzodiazepine and a narcotic are used for intravenous (IV) sedation in the dental office.
- Benzodiazepines are used for oral minimal sedation or moderate sedation/analgesia.
- Nitrous oxide is the only gas used for inhalational anesthesia.
- Nitrous oxide is the least potent of inhalational anesthetics and does not reduce consciousness. It has strong analgesic and amnesia properties, and is good when used with local anesthesia in the dental office.
- Nitrous oxide cannot be used in patients who have nasal obstruction, fear losing consciousness, or are mentally unstable.
- Sedation is obtained with nitrous oxide.
- The most serious danger of anesthesia is overdosage, which results in death.

- Intravenous anesthetics are primarily used for rapid induction of general anesthesia with inhalational anesthetics for maintenance.

Board Review Questions

1. Which of the following agents is considered to be a gas? (p. 79)
   a. Nitrous oxide
   b. Fentanyl
   c. Propofol
   d. Diazepam
2. Which of the following inhalational anesthetics does not cause respiratory depression and hypotension? (pp. 77, 80, 82)
   a. Nitrous oxide
   b. Enflurane
   c. Isoflurane
   d. Halothane
3. All of the following statements are true about moderate sedation *except* one. Which one is the exception? (p. 76)
   a. Complete loss of protective reflexes
   b. Total unconsciousness
   c. Patent airway
   d. Responds to physical stimulation
4. Propofol is preferred over thiopental as an intravenous anesthetic because of its (pp. 77, 78)
   a. recovery characteristics.
   b. can be taken orally.
   c. long onset of action.
   d. prolonged duration of action.
5. Which of the following side effects is common after general anesthesia? (p. 82)
   a. Diarrhea
   b. Esophageal reflux
   c. Nausea and vomiting
   d. Muscle weakness
6. Which of the following maintenance dosages of nitrous oxide/oxygen is usually used in dentistry? (p. 80)
   a. 25:25
   b. 25:50
   c. 30:70
   d. 50:75
7. Use of nitrous oxide/oxygen is contraindicated in patients with (pp. 79–80)
   a. allergies to pollen.
   b. upper respiratory infection.
   c. bacterial infections.
   d. hepatitis.
8. Which of the following ASA classification describes a patient with mild hypertension? (p. 77)
   a. I
   b. II
   c. III
   d. IV
   e. V

9. Which of the following procedures is used for anxiety reduction, pain control, and amnesia in the dental patient while remaining responsive and cooperative during the dental procedure? (p. 76)
   a. Deep sedation
   b. Local anesthesia
   c. Moderate sedation
   d. Minimal sedation
10. At which of the following stages of anesthesia is surgical anesthesia attained? (p. 81)
   a. 1
   b. 2
   c. 3
   d. 4

Selected References

American Academy of Pediatric Dentistry. 2004. Clinical guideline on use of anesthesia-trained personnel in the provision of general anesthesia/deep sedation to the pediatric dental patient. *Pediatr Dent* 26:104–105.

American Association of Oral and Maxillofacial Surgeons. 1997, Spring. *Anesthesia in the dental office.* Rosemont, IL: Author.

American Dental Association. 2003. *ADA Guide to Dental Therapeutics,* 3rd ed. Chicago: Author.

American Dental Association. 2003. *Guidelines for Teaching the Comprehensive Control of Anxiety and Pain in Dentistry.* Chicago: Author.

American Dental Association House of Delegates. October 2003.

Bell CZ, Kain N. 1997. Anesthesia and sedation away from the operating room. In *The pediatric anesthesia handbook.* St. Louis, MO: Mosby, pp. 433–452.

Byrne BE, Tibbetts LS. 2003. Conscious sedation and agents for the control of anxiety. In *ADA Guide to Dental Therapeutics,* 3rd ed. Chicago: ADA Publishing, pp. 17–53.

Nick D, Thompson L, Anderson D, Trapp L. 2003. The use of general anesthesia to facilitate dental treatment. *Gen Dent* 51:464–468.

Shampaine GS. 1999. Patient assessment and preventive measures for medical emergencies in the dental office. *Dental Clinics of North America* 43:383–400.

Standards for Sedation and Anesthesia Care from the Joint Commission. *Moderate/deep sedation stands comprehensive accreditation manual for hospitals.* February 1, 2003, update.

Web Sites

www.ada.org/prof/resources/positions/statements/anxiety_guidelines.pdf.
www.chclibrary.org
http://emedicine.medscape.com/article/1413427-overview
www.aapd.org/media/policies_guidelines/g_sedation.pdf

PEARSON **myhealthprofessionskit**

Use this address to access the Companion Website created for this textbook. Simply select "Dental Hygiene" from the choice of disciplines. Find this book and log in using your username and password to access video clips of selected tests.

QUICK DRUG GUIDE

Oral Anti-Anxiety Agents for Minimal to Moderate Sedation

Benzodiazepines
- Alprazolam (Xanax)
- Clorazepate (Tranxene)
- Diazepam (Valium)

- Lorazepam (Ativan)
- Triazolam (Halcion)

Minimal/Moderate Sedation/Deep Sedation/General Anesthesia

Intravenous Agents

Benzodiazepines
- Diazepam (Valium)
- Lorazepam (Ativan)
- Midazolam (Versed)
- Triazolam (Halcion)

Opioids
- Fentanyl (Sublimaze)
- Alfentanil (Alfenta)
- Sufentanil (Sufenta)
- Meperidine (Demerol)

Sedative/Hypnotics
- Pentobarbital
- Secobarbital

Nonbarbiturate Sedative Hypnotics
- Propofol (Diprivan)
- Ketamine (Ketalar)
- Chloral hydrate (Noctec)

Reversal Drugs
- Naloxone (Narcan)
- Flumazenil (Mazicon)

Inhalational Agents
- Nitrous Oxide-Oxygen

General Anesthesia/Inhalation Agents

Halogenated (volatile liquids)
- Desflurane (Suprane)
- Enflurane (Ethrane)
- Halothane (Fluothane)
- Isoflurane (Forane)

- Methoxyflurane (Penthrane)
- Sevoflurane (Ultane)

IV Agents
- Methohexital (Brevital)
- Thiopental

Drugs for Pain Control

EDUCATIONAL OBJECTIVES

After reading this chapter, the reader should be able to:

1. Discuss the concepts of dental pain.
2. Discuss the commonly used pharmacological agents used for the treatment of orofacial pain.
3. Identify drug–drug interactions that pertain to dental treatment.
4. Describe the classification of narcotic analgesics.
5. Discuss when a narcotic versus a nonnarcotic analgesic is indicated for dental patients.
6. Discuss screening methods to detect potential patients with a chemical dependency.

KEY TERMS

Nociceptive pain
Cyclooxygenase
Prostaglandins

Opioid
Narcotics
Drug dependency

GOALS

- To educate dental hygienists on the pathophysiology, treatment, and patient management for oral pain.
- To gain an understanding of the basic principles of drug abuse.

Introduction

Medications to selectively decrease pain perception are used extensively in dentistry. These medications are termed analgesics. Analgesics are indicated for the relief of acute and chronic dental/orofacial pain, postoperative pain, and preoperative pain to reduce expected pain after the dental procedure (e.g., periodontal surgery).

Neurophysiology of Pain

Pain Components

There are two parts to pain: sensory, which is the actual painful stimulus, and the reaction to pain, which is the emotional response to pain. The reaction to pain is more important than the actual pain stimulus in controlling pain. *The emotional response to pain originates from the central nervous system, while the stimulus comes from the peripheral nervous system.* This distinction is important because analgesics used to treat pain will target the peripheral pain, central pain, or both.

Pain can be acute or chronic, depending on when it started. Acute pain has a short time course and is usually simple to evaluate and treat. Chronic pain has an undetermined time course with a more complex evaluation. Treatment is not as successful as with acute pain.

Types of Pain

CLASSIFICATION: OROFACIAL PAIN Orofacial pain is classified into **nociceptive** and neuropathic pain and acute and chronic pain (Table 6-1).

Nociceptive Acute Orofacial Pain Pain that arises from a stimulus (e.g., injury to tissues), bone, joint, muscle, or connective tissue that is outside of the central nervous system produces nociceptive pain. Examples of nociceptive pain include pulpitis (inflammation of the pulp), pericoronitis, exposed dentin, post-periodontal surgery, post-oral surgery, and maxillary sinusitis. Nociceptive pain is classified into somatic pain, which produces sharp, localized sensations, or visceral pain, which is a generalized dull, poorly localized, throbbing, or aching pain. Visceral pain is associated with a phenomenon called referred pain, which detects the painful stimulus in areas removed from the site where the pain originated. For example, an individual

having a heart attack has pain referred to the jaw and arm. A dental patient has pain in the maxillary sinuses, which was pain referred from the maxillary molar area.

The process of pain transmission begins when *nociceptors* (located at the ends of nerves within peripheral body tissue) are stimulated by noxious stimuli such as tissue damage (e.g., gingiva, bone, pulp). This is normal pain in response to injury to the body. The nerve impulse signaling the pain is sent to the spinal cord along two types of sensory neurons, called Aσ and C fibers. The Aσ fibers signal sharp, well-localized pain and the C fibers conduct dull, poorly localized pain.

Nociceptive pain prevents an individual from using injured parts of the body because further damage can occur. The concept of blocking nociceptors with local anesthetics allows for dental procedures to be performed without causing pain. Nondental-related examples of nociceptive pain include backaches, sprains, sports/exercise injuries, broken bones, and arthritis (joint pain).

Because pain signals begin at nociceptors located within peripheral body tissues and continue through the CNS, there are several targets where medications can work to stop pain transmission. Control of nociceptive pain is usually accomplished with nonnarcotic analgesics such as aspirin, nonsteroidal anti-inflammatory drugs (NSAIDs), acetaminophen at the peripheral level, and opioids (narcotics) at the central level within the CNS.

Drug Therapy for Dental Pain

Treatment for *nociceptive dental pain* is not as complicated as it is for neuropathic pain. Nonsteroidal anti-inflammatory drugs (NSAIDs) or acetaminophen (Tylenol) is adequate for mild to moderate acute pain control. More intense nociceptive chronic pain may also respond well to narcotic analgesics.

The following sections review the fundamentals of nonnarcotic analgesics, nonsteroidal anti-inflammatory drugs (NSAIDs), opioid analgesics, anti-epileptics, and tricyclic antidepressants. Dosage adjustments may be necessary in patients with renal and hepatic impairment and in older adults.

Nonnarcotic Analgesics

Drugs used for the treatment of mild to moderate nociceptive acute dental pain include nonnarcotic analgesics (aspirin, acetaminophen) and nonsteroidal anti-inflammatory drugs (NSAIDs).

TABLE 6-1 Nociceptive and Neuropathic Orofacial Pain	
NOCICEPTIVE ACUTE PAIN	**NEUROPATHIC CHRONIC PAIN**
Toothache (pulpitis)	Trigeminal neuralgia
Dental surgery (extractions, periodontal surgery, orthodontic surgery)	Post-herpetic neuralgia
	Oral dysesthesia (burning mouth)
Mucosal lesions (aphthous ulcers, herpetic lesions)	Migraine headache
	Atypical facial pain
	Drug-induced nerve damage
Maxillary sinusitis	Fibromyalgia
Other: arthritis (joint), cancer	Peripheral neuropathy

Aspirin and NSAIDs are anti-inflammatory (reduce inflammation associated with pain) with analgesic (pain relief) and antipyretic (reduce fever) properties. Acetaminophen has no peripheral anti-inflammatory activity.

PROSTAGLANDIN SYNTHESIS PATHWAY: PERIPHERAL INFLAMMATION   Pain is provoked when a variety of substances (e.g., histamine, prostaglandins, leukotrienes, and bradykinin) are released or injected into the tissues after trauma (surgery, cut, or infection). The prostaglandin synthesis pathway explains the inflammatory events that occur locally after tissue trauma/damage (Figures 6-1 and 6-2). These events occur in all tissue cells found in the body.

Any slight trauma to a nerve fiber stimulates an enzyme called phospholipase A_2, which breaks off arachidonic acid from the phospholipids bound in the cell membrane. Arachidonic acid enters two metabolic pathways: In the first pathway, an enzyme called **cyclooxygenase** breaks down arachidonic acid into prostaglandins (PGE_2) *prostacyclin* (PGI_2) and *thromboxane* A_2. The second metabolic pathway involves arachidonic acid being metabolized by the lipoxygenase pathway into leukotrienes. Leukotrienes produce bronchoconstriction in allergic reactions. The following topics all pertain to the arachidonic–cyclooxygenase pathway.

The following substances are metabolites of arachidonic acid via the *cylcooxygenase pathway:*

- **Prostaglandins** (PGs): Prostaglandins are fatty acids found in all tissues. Prostaglandins are not stored in the cells, but are synthesized during inflammation. Once released, prostaglandins are metabolized rapidly. The biological effects of prostaglandins include:
  - PGE_2, which has *potent inflammatory properties and is involved in inflammatory periodontitis*
  - Pain (increases pain sensitivity)
  - Production of gastric mucus and reduced production of gastric acid (protective effects)

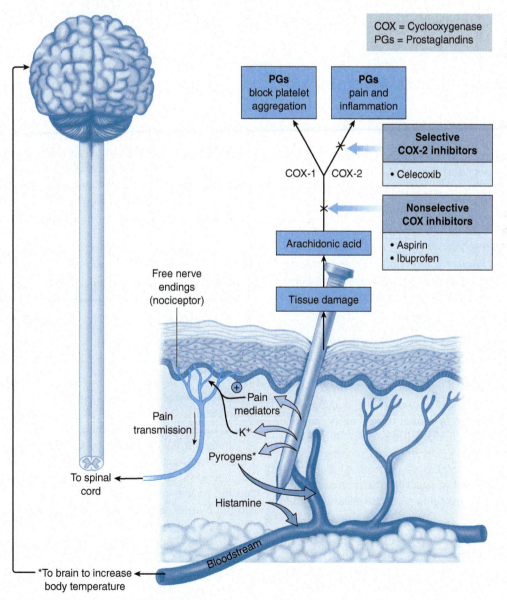

FIGURE 6-1 Pathways of arachidonic acid metabolism: Mechanisms of pain.

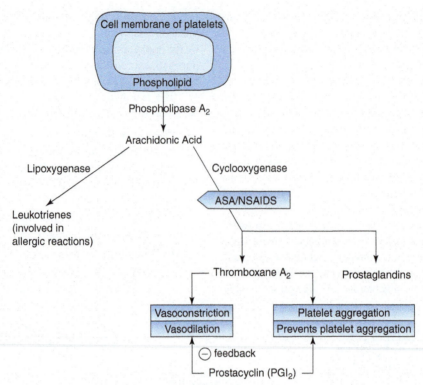

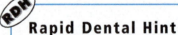

FIGURE 6-2 Aspirin and most other NSAIDs block prostaglandins.

- Uterine contractions during labor
- PGI_2 (prostacyclin) released from blood vessels and inhibiting platelet (clot) formation,
- Bronchodilation (PGE_2 and PGI_2) and bronchoconstriction ($PGF_2\alpha$)
- Increased renal blood flow
- Reduction in blood pressure
- *Prostacyclin and thromboxane A_2 play a role in regulating the aggregation of platelets. Small breaks in capillaries cause platelets to aggregate (come together), which forms clots.*

  - Thromboxane A_2 (TXA_2) is synthesized and found in platelets. When released from platelets, it is a potent vasoconstrictor of blood vessels and *induces* platelet aggregation or clumping and prevents bleeding.
  - Prostacyclin (PGI_2), which is synthesized and present in endothelial cells in blood vessel walls, has the opposite function of thromboxane A_2. It prevents platelet aggregation (clumping) and prolongs bleeding time. This is a homeostatic process whereby both thromboxane A_2 and prostacyclin balance each other without one substance being produced excessively and not the other.

Cyclooxygenase Currently, three cyclooxygenase isoenzymes are known: COX-1, COX-2, and COX-3. COX-1, an endogenous enzyme normally found in most body cells, is responsible for tissue homeostasis and is considered a "housekeeping" enzyme. COX-1 is normally found in the gastrointestinal tract, kidneys, and platelets. Under the influence of COX-1, prostaglandins maintain and protect the gastric mucosa (lining of the stomach), maintain normal platelet function (aggregation and homeostasis) through the formation of thromboxane A_2 and prostacyclin (PGI_2), and regulate renal blood flow.

Rapid Dental Hint

COX-1 is protective and COX-2 is produced only during inflammation.

On the other hand, COX-2 is produced only during inflammation and is found only in low amounts in the tissues. The objective of using anti-inflammatory drugs is to reduce the inflammation that is caused by COX-2, but ideally the drug should not affect COX-1, which is a protective substance. The analgesic properties of aspirin and other nonsteroidal anti-inflammatory drugs (NSAIDs) such as ibuprofen (Advil, Motrin, Nuprin) are due to inhibition of cyclooxygenase but these drugs are not selective for COX-2; thus, there are many adverse effects due to the inhibition of COX-1, which serves a protective role. Celebrex, an NSAID that selectively inhibits COX-2, minimizes the adverse effects seen with inhibition of the protective COX-1; thus, there is less gastrointestinal upset because the gastric mucosa is kept intact.

Nonnarcotic Analgesics

Salicylates

SALICYLIC ACID DERIVATIVES (ASPIRIN) Aspirin (acetyl-salicylic acid; abbreviated as ASA) is a component of the bark of the willow tree. In the fifth century B.C., the Greek physician Hippocrates used this substance. In 1899, Bayer marketed this substance with the trade name "Aspirin." Aspirin was introduced in the United States in 1925, and Bayer lost a lawsuit to keep Aspirin as a trade name.

According to the National Drug Code, which is part of the Centers for Disease Control and Prevention (www.cdc.gov/nchs/datawh/nchsdefs/ndc_dtc.htm, Table XI), aspirin is considered to be a nonnarcotic analgesic and not a nonsteroidal anti-inflammatory drug (NSAID) because of its common use for cardiac therapy; however, many references may include aspirin as being an NSAID because of its anti-inflammatory properties. Most of aspirin's effects are due to its interruption of prostaglandin synthesis via blockade primarily of COX-1 rather than COX-2 enzymes.

> **DID YOU KNOW?**
>
> Bayer Aspirin was the first drug to be marketed in tablet form.

Therapeutic Indications for Aspirin

- *Analgesic* (pain control):
  - Inhibits prostaglandin (PGE_2) synthesis by blocking the cyclooxygenase enzyme.
  - Acts peripherally not centrally in the brain
  - For mild to moderate pain relief (does not eliminate the pain, only decreases the sensitivity to pain)

- Onset of action 30 minutes
- *Ceiling effect:* Increasing the dose of aspirin will not increase the effects of aspirin after a certain point (Figure 6-3). For example, an average individual will take 650 mg (two 325 mg tablets) of aspirin for mild to moderate pain following periodontal debridement. Let's say that this amount of aspirin does not take the individual out of pain; however, increasing the dosage to three or four tablets will not be effective in increasing the analgesic effect and may even cause more adverse effects. Thus, if two tablets of aspirin are ineffective in the relief of pain, a more potent alternative drug should be used.

- *Anti-inflammatory*
  - Blocks the formation of PGE_2, which has a potent inflammatory effect. This attribute allows for treatment of arthritic conditions.
    - The optimal anti-inflammatory dose of aspirin is 3.6–5.4g/day, which is higher than the analgesic dose, which is a maximum of 4g/day.

- *Antipyretic*
  - Reduces abnormally high body temperature (fever) but does not alter normal body temperature.
    - Vasodilation (increased blood flow to surface by dilating blood vessels), which causes an increase in respiration. This results in an increase in the evaporation of water and increased sweating. Aspirin does not reduce heat production, but increases heat loss through sweating.

- *Uricosuric effects*
  - Increases the excretion of uric acid, which is used in the treatment of gout, an arthritic condition involving an imbalance in uric acid metabolism.

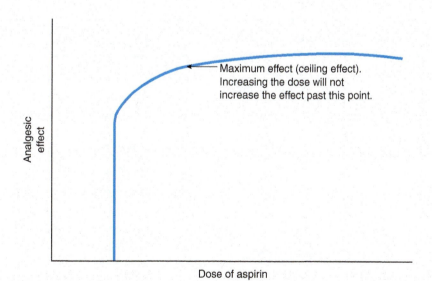

FIGURE 6-3 Ceiling effect of aspirin. A plateau is reached where increasing the dose of aspirin will not create more analgesic/anti-inflammatory effects.

- *Antiplatelet effects*
  - Clinical studies in the 1980s documented that aspirin in low doses also was a platelet aggregation (clotting) inhibitor.
  - Because of its role in prevention of clots, aspirin in low doses is used as antiplatelet therapy in the prevention of heart attack and stroke in individuals who previously have had a heart attack or stroke (secondary prevention), but whose cardiovascular disease is stabilized.
  - Action: In the gastrointestinal tract and blood, aspirin breaks down into salicylate (salicylic acid) and acetic acid. It is the acetic acid that *irreversibly* covalently binds to COX-1 in platelets, while salicylate has analgesic and anti-inflammatory actions. This binding *prevents the formation of thromboxane A$_2$, resulting in a decrease in the ability to form clots and increase bleeding time,* which lasts for the life of the platelet because the platelet is incapable of resynthesizing new cyclooxygenase enzyme. In order to make more enzymes, new platelets must be formed, which takes about 7 days. The antiplatelet effect of aspirin lasts for the lifetime of a platelet, about 7–10 days. This occurs because the effect of aspirin on cyclooxygenase enzymes in platelets is irreversible, so bleeding will occur until new platelets are formed.

Rapid Dental Hint

Low-dose aspirin used in prevention of stroke and heart attack means as low as 40 mg but up to 81 mg ("low-dose aspirin")—to 100 mg/day or 325 mg every other day.

- It may not be necessary to discontinue aspirin; however, if the patient is taking aspirin prophylactically and has no previous heart conditions, discontinuing aspirin is acceptable. Consult with the patient's physician before any action is taken. Effective local hemostatic measures should be taken.
- Research advocates continuing use of aspirin to prevent emboli. (See Jeske AH, Suchko GD. 2003. Lack of scientific basis for routine discontinuation or oral anticoagulation therapy before dental treatment. *JADA* 134:1492–1497; Ardekian G, et al. 2000. *JADA* 131(3):331–335.)

Rapid Dental Hint

Many dental patients take aspirin daily without the supervision of a physician.

At the same time aspirin inhibits the formation of thromboxane A$_2$ in the platelets via inhibiting COX-1, the synthesis of PGI$_2$ in the blood vessel walls is inhibited by COX-2. Do these seem like opposite actions? Yes, but aspirin causes inhibition of thromboxane A$_2$, causing inhibition of platelet aggregation, resulting in bleeding because it is a more potent inhibitor of COX-1 than COX-2. Low doses (as low as 40 mg but up to 81—"low-dose aspirin"—to 100 mg/day or 325 mg every other day) of aspirin inhibits platelet aggregation and prolongs bleeding time, while high doses (arthritis doses 3–6 g per day) may have no effect or shorten bleeding time because high doses prevent the formation of prostacyclin.

Rapid Dental Hint

One low-dose aspirin contains 81 mg of aspirin.

Pharmacokinetics Orally administered aspirin is absorbed rapidly, mostly from the upper small intestine, but also (a small part) from the stomach. Concentrations are found in the blood within 30 minutes, with peak concentration by 2 hours. It is metabolized in the liver to salicylic acid. Salicylates are excreted in the urine.

Rapid Dental Hint

Tell patients not to suck on aspirin tablets; this causes white lesions on the buccal mucosa.

Adverse Effects of Aspirin

- Gastrointestinal irritation
  - Gastrointestinal bleeding and peptic ulcers
    - Due to COX-1 inhibition, which decreases GI mucosal defense mechanisms and increases gastric acid secretion. This leads to ulceration. Inhibition of prostaglandins decreases gastric mucous production and increases gastric (hydrochloric) acid production. Aspirin is formulated as enteric-coated tablets to avoid these problems.

- Nausea and vomiting
- Hypoglycemia (low blood sugar), which in some diabetics taking medications (e.g., insulin) can cause a loss of control of blood sugar.
- Renal dysfunction (decreased renal elimination), especially in patients with preexisting renal disease or congestive heart failure. Aspirin inhibits renal prostaglandin production, which causes water retention and decreased renal blood flow.
- Aspirin may produce hemolytic anemia in certain racial groups (e.g., Egyptians), who do not have the enzyme glucose-6-phosphate dehydrogenase, responsible for inactivating certain metabolites of aspirin inside red blood cells.

Rapid Dental Hint

Low-dose aspirin is taken by many patients with or without it being prescribed by a physician for prevention of cardiovascular disease and stroke. Older patients should be questioned about aspirin use, including the amount taken.

Aspirin Toxicity and Treatment of Overdose   Excessive doses of aspirin produce many toxic effects. Aspirin in high doses (600–900 mg) stimulates the depth and rate of respiration (hyperventilation).

Salicylism, which is manifested as ringing in the ears or tinnitus and vertigo (loss of equilibrium/severe dizziness) occurs in doses of only 300–600 mg and can lead to deafness. Onset of chronic salicylism may be insidious especially in older adults, who may consume an increasing amount over several days to alleviate the pain of arthritis.

Shock, coma, respiratory and renal failure, and ultimately death occur after ingesting 2,000–3,000 mg.

Aspirin is more toxic to children than adults. In a child, toxicity is seen with 1 g (1,000 mg) and a lethal dose is 10 g. Treatment of an overdose is initiated by stopping absorption by gastric lavage and activated charcoal. Intravenous administration of sodium bicarbonate counteracts the metabolic acidosis. Finally, vitamin K is administered to compensate for prothrombin anemia, seen following toxicity.

Precautions/Contraindications

- Contraindicated in patients with renal disease, gastric ulcer, and bleeding tendencies.
- Certain individuals with a history of nasal polyps and asthma are at risk of developing bronchoconstriction if aspirin is taken. The association between asthma, nasal polyps, and aspirin intolerance is known as Samter's triad. Aspirin and NSAIDs should be used with caution in asthmatics and avoided in asthmatics with nasal polyps. About

10% of patients with asthma are intolerant to aspirin and NSAIDs. Asthmatic patients who take aspirin are at risk of developing severe, even fatal, exacerbations of asthma. Aspirin should be avoided in asthmatics with a history of aspirin-induced bronchospasm.

- Reye's syndrome is primarily a children's disease, although it can occur at any age. Using aspirin to treat viral illnesses, including chicken pox or flu, increases the risk of developing Reye's syndrome. Symptoms of Reye's syndrome include repetitive vomiting, lethargy, headache, fever, convulsions, and even death.

  - *The U.S. Surgeon General, the Food and Drug Administration, the Centers for Disease Control and Prevention, and the American Academy of Pediatrics recommend that aspirin and combination products containing aspirin not be given to children under 19 years of age during episodes of fever-causing illnesses.*

Rapid Dental Hint

Research has shown that patients do not need to discontinue aspirin for periodontal debridement procedures.

DID YOU KNOW?

In 1969, aspirin tablets were included in the self-medication kits taken to the moon by the *Apollo* astronauts. Aspirin was used for headaches and muscle pains that frequently resulted from long periods of immobility.

Drug–Drug Interactions

- Aspirin inhibits PGE_2, which increases insulin secretion. In diabetics, aspirin increases the hypoglycemic response of oral antidiabetic drugs (e.g., sulfonylureas). Consult with the patient's physician.
- Antacids can reduce salicylate levels.
- Aspirin interferes with the diuretic effect of thiazide or loop diuretics (furosemide) because it inhibits renal prostaglandin production, which causes water retention. This will decrease the actions and effectiveness of the diuretic.
- By inhibiting cyclooxygenase, aspirin (in doses of 300 mg/day or more) prevents the formation of prostaglandins, which have vasodilation effects. This *may* decrease the hypotensive effects of antihypertensive medications, including angiotension-converting enzyme inhibitors: ACE inhibitors (e.g., Vasotec), diuretics (e.g., hydrochlorothiazide), and beta-blockers (e.g., Tenormin, Inderal).

However, low-dose aspirin (100 mg/day) may not interfere with these antihypertensives. (Refer to Zanchetti A, Hansson L, Leonetti G, Rahn KH, et al. 2002. Low-dose aspirin does not interfere with the blood pressure–lowering effects of antihypertensive therapy. *J Hypertension* 1015–1022.)

Rapid Dental Hint

Patients may be taking vitamin E and aspirin, both blood thinners. Ask patients about all medications taken.

- There is an increased risk of bleeding when aspirin is taken with anticoagulants, due to its effect on platelet aggregation.
- Alcohol should not be taken with aspirin because both act as gastric irritants.
- The use of aspirin with other NSAIDs should be avoided because of increased risk for GI bleeding or decreased kidney function.
- Drug–herbal interactions include white willow, dong quai, chamomile, ginseng, ginger, and red clover. Taking these herbal supplements with aspirin may cause increased bleeding.

DID YOU KNOW?

Caffeine, a stimulant included in many OTC analgesics for "headaches," helps the analgesic (aspirin, acetaminophen) work better. This is a contradiction; caffeine is a common cause of headaches because caffeine is a vasodilator.

Guidelines for Patients Taking Low-Dose Aspirin

- Ask patients why they are taking aspirin (e.g., for pain, as a blood thinner to prevent heart problems).
- Ask patients if their physician knows they are taking aspirin.
- Ask patients if they are taking low-dose aspirin (81 mg) or regular-strength aspirin (325 mg).
- Determine if aspirin will cause increased bleeding during the dental procedure.
- You may need to consult with the patient's physician.
- Remind patients not to put aspirin directly on the tooth or gums because it may cause an "aspirin burn" on the tissue, which clinically looks white.

Rapid Dental Hint

Aspirin may decrease the hypotensive effects of antihypertensive medications. Limit the use of aspirin to 5 days and monitor blood pressure. However, low-dose aspirin does not have an effect blood pressure medications.

Other Salicylate-Like Drugs

Diflunisal (Dolobid) is a derivative of salicylic acid but is not converted to salicylic acid. It is a more potent anti-inflammatory than aspirin, and it is an inhibitor of cyclooxygenase. It does not have antipyretic activity because it penetrates the CNS poorly. Adverse effects are few, and it causes fewer and less intense gastrointestinal and antiplatelet effects than does aspirin. Diflunisal is useful for dental pain starting with a loading dose of 1 g followed by 500 mg twice a day. It is indicated for mild to moderate pain.

Drug Profile   Aspirin

Aspirin (acetylsalicylic acid, ASA) inhibits prostaglandin synthesis via inhibiting cyclooxygenase-1 and cyclooxygenase-2 enzymes, involved in the production of pain, fever, and inflammation. It inhibits thromboxane A_2, involved in anticoagulation (antiplatelet effect; inhibits blood clots). For this reason, aspirin is given in low doses (81 mg) to reduce the risk of mortality following heart attacks and to reduce the incidence of strokes.

Aspirin may cause gastrointestinal bleeding because of its antiplatelet effects. Aspirin should not be given to children with fever, chicken pox, or flu-like symptoms because of its association with Reye's syndrome.

Nonsteroidal Anti-Inflammatory Drugs

Although aspirin is separately classified as a nonnarcotic analgesic, there are many similarities with nonsteroidal anti-inflammatory drugs (NSAIDs). The difference between the two types of drugs is that NSAIDs do not have the same antiplatelet effect.

Ibuprofen and Ibuprofen-Like Drugs

Mechanism of Action   Similar to aspirin, ibuprofen, the prototype NSAID, and other NSAIDs function to inhibit prostaglandin synthesis (primarily PGE_2) by inhibiting the cyclooxygenase enzymes, resulting in a reduction of inflammation. They also inhibit both COX-1 and COX-2, resulting in many adverse effects because COX-1 has a protective role on the GI mucosa and kidneys. Inhibition of COX-2 in tissues is responsible for the anti-inflammatory effects of NSAIDs. Nonsteroidal anti-inflammatory drugs have a ceiling effect similar to aspirin. The following are effects of NSAIDs:

- *Analgesic:* Has an indirect analgesic effect by inhibiting the production of prostaglandins and does not directly affect hyperalgesia (increased sensitivity to pain) or the pain threshold.
- *Anti-inflammatory:* Most of the anti-inflammatory effects of NSAIDs are due to inhibition of COX-2 rather than COX-1.
- *Fever:* NSAIDs are antipyretic by suppressing the synthesis of prostaglandins, specifically PGE_2 near the hypothalamus.
- *Antiplatelet effects:* Inhibition of COX-1 also inhibits the production of thromboxane A_2, which prevents platelet aggregation. NSAIDS do not covalently bind to the cyclooxygenase enzymes and do not irreversibly inhibit platelet function as aspirin. Thus, unlike aspirin, ibuprofen and the other NSAIDS are not used to prevent heart attacks and strokes; however, they still cause increased bleeding and for this reason aspirin and NSAIDs should not be taken together.

Indications   All NSAIDs are antipyretic, analgesic (mild to moderate acute pain), and anti-inflammatory. NSAIDs are primarily used as anti-inflammatory drugs in the treatment of various forms of arthritis (Table 6-2). NSAIDs are not indicated for prophylaxis against heart attacks and strokes.

Adverse Effects   Adverse gastrointestinal effects are similar to aspirin:

- Increased stomach irritation, bleeding, and ulcer formation (Table 6-3)
  - As with aspirin, there is a high risk for ulcer development in patients taking a corticosteroid (e.g., prednisone), and previous GI problems. In these high-risk patients, concurrent administration of an anti-ulcer drug such as a proton pump inhibitor [e.g., esomeprazole (Nexium) or omeprazole (Prilosec)] may help prevent the development of gastric ulcers from NSAID use. Misoprostol (Cytotec) is a prostaglandin E_2 analog and is approved for prophylaxis against NSAID-induced ulcers.

Rapid Dental Hint

Interview your patients concerning the use of aspirin for the prevention of heart attack and stroke and the use of NSAIDs (e.g., ibuprofen) for pain relief because of increased bleeding tendencies. Many patients may not think to tell you that they are taking one or both of these drugs. It is important to fully interview patients about all OTC drugs!

- Kidney function may be depressed due to inhibition of prostaglandin synthesis, which plays a protective role in

TABLE 6-2   Analgesics Used for Dental Pain: Nonsteroidal Anti-Inflammatory Drugs—Salicylates and Other Analgesics

DRUGS	DOSAGE
Salicylates	
Aspirin (Ecotrin, Bayer, and many more)	325 mg q4–6h
Diflunisal (Dolobid)	1,000 mg initially, then 500 mg q12h
Nonsteroidal Anti-Inflammatory Drugs (NSAIDs)	
Ketorolac (Toradol)	10 mg q4–6h
Ibuprofen (Advil, Motrin)	200–600 mg q4–6h
Ketoprofen (Orudis, Actron)	50 mg q6–8h
Flurbiprofen (Ansaid)	50–100 mg bid
Naproxen (Naprosyn)	250–500 mg q12h
Naproxen sodium (Anaprox, Anaprox DS, Aleve)	Anaprox: 250–500 mg q12h
	Aleve (OTC): 220 mg q8–12h
Etodolac (Lodine)	200–400 mg q6–8h
Celecoxib (Celebrex)	100 mg bid
Other Analgesics	
Acetaminophen (Tylenol)	325 q4–6h; max: 5 tabs/24h

kidney function. This problem is reversible within 1–3 days after stopping the NSAID.

- It should be noted that there are different preparations of naproxen: naproxen (Naprosyn) and naproxen sodium (Aleve, Anaprox, Anaprox DS). The preparations containing sodium are not recommended for use in patients with hypertension.

Precautions/Contraindications   The precautions that were taken for aspirin in patients with asthma and nasal polyps are taken with the other NSAIDs. This reaction rarely occurs in children. Within 20 minutes to 3 hours of taking an NSAID, aspirin-sensitive asthmatics can develop respiratory symptoms such as bronchospasm and respiratory arrest.

Unlike with aspirin, there is no contraindication for giving an NSAID such as children's Motrin to a child with the flu or chicken pox.

TABLE 6-3   Risk Factors for NSAID-Induced Gastrointestinal Ulcers

- Older adults
- Past history of ulcers
- Higher doses of NSAID
- Concurrent use of corticosteroids

Rapid Dental Hint

Patient should be warned about the potential adverse effects/precautions of aspirin and NSAIDs and should be asked if they are using any of these products since many of these medications are available over-the-counter.

Drug Interactions

- NSAIDs may counteract the antihypertensive effects of angiotension-converting enzyme inhibitors [ACE inhibitors (e.g., Vasotec), diuretics (e.g., hydrochlorothiazide) and beta-blockers (e.g., Tenormin, Inderal)] by inhibiting formation of prostaglandins. It is important to monitor blood pressure and dosage adjustment may be necessary. This may also cause an increased risk of recurrence of heart failure. NSAIDs should not be used for more than 5 days (refer to Interactions between antihypertensive agents and other drugs. *European Society of Hypertension Scientific Newsletter: Update on hypertension management* 2003;4(17). Aspirin does not interfere with the actions of antihypertensive medications.

Rapid Dental Hint

If the patient is pregnant, contact the physician before recommending ibuprofen. It is especially important not to take ibuprofen during the last 3 months of pregnancy.

- Aspirin taken with NSAIDs increases the incidence of GI problems and bleeding; these drugs should not be taken together.
- Antacids may decrease the absorption of NSAIDs.
- Patients taking a corticosteroid such as prednisone may be at higher risk for GI ulcers if they also take aspirin or an NSAID.
- NSAIDs decrease renal excretion of lithium, which increases lithium plasma levels and can cause lithium toxicity.
- All NSAIDs are highly plasma protein bound and have the potential to displace other highly protein-bound drugs such as warfarin (NSAIDs potentiate the anticoagulant effect) and antidiabetic drugs (sulfonylureas) (NSAIDs potentiate the hypoglycemic effects).

Selective COX-2 Inhibitors

Mechanism of Action   Celecoxib exerts anti-inflammatory and analgesic effects through the inhibition of prostaglandin synthesis by binding of the sulfonamide side chain on celecoxib to a site on COX-2 that is not present on COX-1, *reversibly* blocking COX-2 activity and preventing the formation of prostacyln (PGI_2), which will induce platelet clumping and cause vasoconstriction. Celecoxib and the traditional NSAIDs are equally effective in treating pain and inflammation.

Rapid Dental Hint

Before recommending an OTC NSAID such as ibuprofen or Aleve to your patients, make sure they are not taking anti-hypertensive medications.

Guidelines for Patients Taking NSAIDs (e.g., Ibuprofen)

- Patients should take pill with a full glass of water and with food.
- Patients should not take with aspirin; can take with acetaminophen.

Celecoxib does not inhibit platelet aggregation because platelets contain the COX-1 enzyme and not COX-2. Celecoxib selectively inhibits the formation of prostacyclin (PGI_2) rather than thromboxane A2.

Safety and Adverse Effects   In 2004, the FDA issued a public health advisory in response to clinical studies that found that the COX-2 inhibitors were associated with a significantly greater incidence of thrombotic cardiovascular events (heart attack and stroke), leading to death in some cases. Data collected from clinical studies suggested that high doses and long-term use of these drugs may contribute to these risks. A black-box warning highlights the potential for increased risk of cardiovascular events, as well as serious and potentially life-threatening gastrointestinal bleeding. The government has also requested that manufacturers of over-the-counter NSAIDs such as ibuprofen (Advil, Motrin), ketoprofen (Orudis, Actron), and naproxen (Aleve) also revise their labeling to include these risks. It is advised to use the lowest effective dose for the shortest duration to avoid these potentially fatal adverse events.

Contraindications and Drug Interactions   Celecoxib is contraindicated in patients with sulfonamide (sulfa) allergy because of a sulfonamide chain on the drug molecule.

Acetaminophen

Acetaminophen (Tylenol), a nonnarcotic analgesic, is a derivative of para-amino phenol. Acetaminophen is a poor inhibitor of cyclooxygenase in the tissues, so its anti-inflammatory effects are less potent than aspirin and NSAIDs. A major difference between aspirin and acetaminophen is its lack of effect on platelet function and less (or no) gastric irritation.

DID YOU KNOW?

Physicians advise runners not to take NSAIDs (e.g., Advil) for pain control before a race because it causes nausea and may decrease kidney function.

Rapid Dental Hint

Do not recommend NSAIDs to patients with peptic ulcers or if he or she is taking warfarin (an anticoagulant).

Acetaminophen is primarily used as an analgesic and antipyretic. Studies have shown that NSAIDs are more effective than acetaminophen alone for the relief of acute dental pain. It has a pregnancy category B and is safe to use during pregnancy.

Pharmacokinetics Acetaminophen is rapidly and almost completely absorbed from the GI tract into the bloodstream. After ingestion, it reaches peak blood levels in about 30-60 minutes. It is not highly bound to plasma proteins, so there is no interaction with drugs that are highly plasma protein bound such as warfarin. It is extensively metabolized in the liver and distributed to most tissues. Little is excreted unchanged in the urine, which means that it undergoes conjugation to glucuronic acid followed by kidney excretion.

Adverse Effects Acetaminophen overdose is the leading cause of acute liver failure, even if alcohol is not taken concurrently. The maximum safe dose of acetaminophen for adults should not exceed 4 grams or 4,000 mg (e.g., eight 500 mg tablets) over a 24-hour period, with higher doses increasing the risk of liver damage. The U.S. Food and Drug Administration (FDA) is asking drug manufacturers to limit the strength of acetaminophen in prescription drug products, which are predominantly combinations of acetaminophen and opioids. This action will limit the amount of acetaminophen in these products to 325 mg per tablet, capsule. Acetaminophen has a narrow margin of safety; the difference between a therapeutic dose and a toxic one is very small. The toxic dose is only 7 grams taken all at once.

Acetaminophen is supplied as 160, 325, 500, and 650 mg tabs. Long-term use (more than 10 days) is not recommended. Acetaminophen overdose is treated with acetylcysteine (Mucomyst), which can prevent or reduce hepatotoxicity.

Effects on the GI tract are few to none. Common side effects include skin rash and allergic reactions, which can develop into

a drug-induced fever. Acetaminophen is metabolized into methemoglobin, which can result in methemoglobinemia (decreased capacity of red blood cells to carry oxygen).

There is some evidence that long-term use of acetaminophen is associated with an increased risk of renal dysfunction.

Drug Interactions A significant interaction occurs between alcohol and acetaminophen. Both ethanol and acetaminophen are metabolized by CYP2E1. If there is enough ethanol to occupy the CYP2E1 enzyme, then it is not available to metabolize acetaminophen into n-acetyl-p-benzoquinone imine or NAPQ1, which are responsible for its toxic effects. It has been reported that there is an increased risk of hepatotoxicity with excessive alcohol use (more than three drinks per day).

Carbamazepine (Tegretol) and phenytoin (Dilantin) may increase the risk of chronic hepatotoxicity.

Opioid Analgesics

Introduction

An **opioid** analgesic is a natural or synthetic morphine-like substance used for reducing moderate to severe pain that cannot be controlled with other types of analgesics. Opioids are **narcotics** that act exclusively on the central components of pain and produce analgesia and CNS depression. Several opioids are derived from opium, which was originally isolated from the dried juice of seeds of the Oriental poppy flower in the nineteenth century. Opium contains primarily morphine, codeine, and other substances. These natural substances are called opiates. *Narcotic* is a general word used to describe morphine-like drugs and can be natural (morphine) or synthetic (meperidine).

Morphine, the prototype narcotic, produces analgesia, drowsiness, and a change in mood and mental clouding without a loss of consciousness. Other sensory modalities such as touch, vision, and hearing are not impaired at doses that reduce pain. Opiates are water soluble, allowing them to be abused by the parenteral route.

Mechanism of Action

OPIOID RECEPTORS Opioids interact with binding sites in the CNS called opiate receptors, which are diffusely distributed throughout the central nervous system, with the highest concentrations in the limbic system (Table 6-4). The endogenous peptides, enkephalins, endorphins, and dynorphins are released from neurons in the brain and activate opioid receptors, thereby blocking the transmission of pain impulses. These substances are the body's natural opiates that inhibit painful stimuli.

Drug Profile **Acetaminophen**

The exact mechanism of acetaminophen's ability to reduce pain is not clear. It reduces fever by direct action in the central nervous system. Acetaminophen and aspirin are equally effective in relieving pain and reducing fever. It is good for the treatment of fever in children and for the relief of mild to moderate pain when aspirin is contraindicated.

When taken in toxic doses, acetaminophen may cause liver damage. Alcohol should not be taken with acetaminophen. It is safe to give during pregnancy.

DID YOU KNOW?

If you eat poppy seeds from a bagel, you could have a positive urine test for narcotics!

TABLE 6-4   Opioid Drugs

Short-Acting Opioid Agonists

- Morphine
- Hydromorphone (Dilaudid)
- Oxycodone (controlled-release OxyContin)
- Hydrocodone (Vicodin, Lorcet, Vicoprofen in combination with a nonnarcotic)
- Codeine
- Meperidine (Demerol)
- Fentanyl (Duragesic patch)

Long-Acting Opioid Agonists

- Methadone
- Levorphanol (Levo-Dromoran)
- Oxymorphone (Numorphan)

Other Opioid Agonists

- Dextromethorphan (used in cough syrups; Robitussin, Sucrets, Vicks, Delsym, Benylin)
- Diphenoxylate (with atropine; Lomotil)
- Loperamide (Imodium–antidiarrheal)
- Tramadol (Ultram)

Mixed Agonist/Antagonists

- Buprenorphine (Buprenex)
- Butorphanol (Stadol)
- Nalbuphine (Nubain)
- Pentazocine (Talwin)

Antagonists

- Naloxone (Narcan)
- Naltrexone (Depade, ReVia)

CLASSIFICATION OF OPIOID RECEPTORS The main opioid receptors are classified as mu (μ), delta (δ), and kappa (κ), depending on their affinity for the different opioids (Figure 6-4). For example, morphine stimulates both μ receptors and κ receptors. Other opioids such as pentazocine (Talwin) stimulate the kappa receptors and block the mu receptors. Naloxone (Narcan) is an opioid blocker and inhibits both the μ and κ receptors. Table 6-5 shows responses produced by activation of specific receptors.

Pharmacokinetics

Opioids are readily absorbed from the GI tract, nasal mucosa, and lungs. They are also absorbed after parenteral injection (e.g., subcutaneous, intramuscular, and intravenous), producing the greatest effect.

Classification

Based on their clinical effectiveness or strength (potency), opioids are classified as:

- Full agonists: strong or moderate in producing an analgesic effect

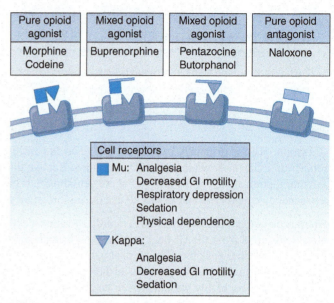

FIGURE 6-4 Opioid receptors.

- Mixed opioid agonist/antagonists: analgesic (relief of pain) effect with some antagonist activity
- Pure antagonists: no analgesic effects; used in opioid overdose

Opioid Agonists: Strong Potency

MORPHINE Morphine is the prototype narcotic analgesic that is the standard against which other narcotic analgesics are compared. The main actions of opium are due to its morphine

---

Drug Profile   Morphine

Morphine produces analgesia by binding to opioid receptors in the brain. It is indicated for severe pain and chronic pain after nonnarcotic analgesics fail. Morphine may cause dysphoria (restlessness, depression, and anxiety), constipation, nausea and vomiting, and itching.

TABLE 6-5   The Opioid Responses

RECEPTOR	MU RECEPTOR	KAPPA RESPONSE
Analgesia	+	+
Decreased GI mobility (constipation)	+	+
Euphoria	+	−
Miosis (pupil contraction)	−	+
Physical dependence	+	−
Respiratory depression	+	−
Sedation	+	+

content (9–17%). Morphine binds to the μ and κ receptors to produce strong analgesic effects. In doses of 5–10 mg severe pain will be reduced (make it less intense) or eliminated. Morphine increases the pain threshold and increases the capacity to tolerate pain by reducing the emotional component of pain. Essentially, the painful stimulus itself is recognized, but it may not be perceived as painful. The patient may say the pain is still present, but they feel more comfortable. Morphine acts not only in the brain but also in the spinal cord, where it is injected directly into the cerebrospinal fluid.

Morphine does not accumulate in tissues because it is not lipid-soluble. It is cleared from the body within 24 hours of the last dose. Excretion is 90% in the urine and 10% in the feces followed by biliary excretion.

Actions and Adverse Effects

Central actions of morphine

- Analgesia
- Drowsiness/sleep
- Cough suppression
- Vomiting (due to stimulation of chemoreceptor trigger zone in the brain)
- Hypotension
- Miosis (pupillary constriction due to stimulation of parasympathetic nerves)
- Respiratory depression (in high doses, respiratory depression becomes the major toxic effect and cause of death because no tolerance is developed to respiratory depression)
- Euphoria (ecstasy; develop tolerance rapidly to euphoric actions)
- Increased release of ADH (antidiuretic hormone), which causes urinary retention (an effect on the sphincter)

Peripheral actions

- Constipation (due to stimulation of cholinergic activity in the GI tract)
- Body warmth/flushing/itchy (due to histamine release)

Indications Morphine sulfate is used for relief of moderate to serious pain due to trauma, postsurgery, cancer, or myocardial infarction. It is usually given intramuscularly or subcutaneously. It is also used as preanesthetic medication before surgery. Morphine is not administered orally because it undergoes extensive first-pass inactivation in the liver.

Characteristics Morphine exhibits dependence and drug-seeking behavior, which is dose related. The higher the dose and the longer the individual is taking the drug and then stops the drug, the more severe the withdrawal symptoms. Cross-dependence develops between morphine and other opioids such as heroin, methadone, and meperidine. Withdrawal can be suppressed by substituting another one of these drugs for morphine. Tolerance develops to the analgesic, sedative, and euphoric effects of the drug but not miosis and constipation; as you use the drug, it becomes less effective. Normally a dose of 10 mg will produce strong analgesic effects,

but addicts often require up to 250 mg to achieve the same effect. There is a cross-tolerance where an individual will also become tolerant to other narcotics; if morphine does not work, then other narcotics like morphine will not work either. Since there is no tolerance to miosis, a characteristic sign of narcotic use is pinpoint pupils. Because of its high abuse potential, morphine is not used as an antitussive.

Drug Interactions Any drug that causes CNS depression will potentiate the effects of opioid drugs because they also are CNS depressants. Examples include antihistamines, sedative/hypnotics, alcohol, and psychiatric drugs. Herbals such as kava-kava, valerian, and St. John's wort may increase sedation.

METHADONE AND BUPRENORPHINE Methadone is a long-acting synthetic morphine derivative used orally in the treatment of opioid (usually heroin) addiction or pain. Since it is a narcotic, it can be abused; however, it is used to "wean" patients off narcotics because it does not produce euphoria. Methadone treatment is done in a methadone maintenance program, which is currently restricted to highly regulated, federally licensed programs.

Only about 20% of heroin addicts are receiving treatment with methadone, naltrexone, clonidine, or levo-alpha-acetyl-methadol (LAAM). Withdrawal syndrome is severe and uncomfortable for the individual. LAAM is similar to methadone, but it has a longer duration of action, which allows patients to visit treatment programs less frequently. Clonidine is a α_2-adrenergic agonist that decreases withdrawal symptoms by decreasing the sympathetic output responsible for many withdrawal symptoms such as sweating, diarrhea, intestinal cramping, and nausea.

Buprenorphine (www.usdoj.gov/ndic/pubs10/10123/index.htm) is the latest drug approved for the management of opiate addiction. There are two formulations: buprenorphine (Subutex), used in the initial stages of therapy, and the combination of buprenorphine and naloxone (Suboxone), used in the maintenance stage. While most commonly used to treat heroin addiction, it is also used to treat addiction to OxyContin and Percocet. It is obtained from the pharmacy and physicians must become certified by attending a special training course and submitting their qualifications to the Substance Abuse and Mental Health Services Administration (SAMHSA).

Buprenorphine is a derivative of thebaine, an extract of opium. It is a partial agonist and can produce the euphoria, analgesia, and sedation associated with opiates, but to a lesser degree than full opiate agonists such as morphine and heroin.

Buprenorphine is administered either as a transdermal patch or under the tongue via a small syringe and is absorbed through the sublingual mucous membranes. A flexible dosing schedule allows for better compliance. The naloxone contained in Suboxone prevents it from being abused because naloxone will precipitate withdrawal symptoms.

MEPERIDINE Meperidine (Demerol) is a less effective analgesic than morphine, with half the duration of action [75 mg meperidine IM (intramuscular injection) = 10 mg morphine IM]. It is sometimes used in dentistry. It is metabolized to normeperidine, which can cause convulsions. It does not have antitussive properties. Tolerance, cross-tolerance, dependence, and cross-dependence develop with meperidine. No tolerance develops to CNS stimulation. Meperidine should not be used in patients also taking antidepressant monoamine oxidase inhibitors such as selegiline (Eldepryl). There are increased CNS depressant effects when taken with alcohol, and increased sedation when taken with St. John's wort.

OXYCODONE AND HYDROCODONE   Oxycodone (OxyContin) and hydrocodone are semisynthetic morphine derivatives used in the treatment of moderate to severe pain. Vicodin is a combination of hydrocodone and acetaminophen. These have all of the adverse side effects of morphine: respiratory depression, antitussive, constipation, and dependence. They are most effective when combined with NSAIDS, aspirin, or acetaminophen. OxyContin has received much media attention because of its high abuse potential. Other opioids are listed in Table 6-4.

Often opioids are combined with nonnarcotic analgesics or NSAIDs into a single tablet to act synergistically to relieve pain, and the dose of narcotic can be kept small to avoid dependence and opioid-related side effects. Examples include hydrocodone/acetaminophen (Vicodin) and hydrocodone/ibuprofen (Vicoprofen).

FENTANYL   Fentanyl (Duragesic) is a semisynthetic opiate that is very potent and lipid soluble and crosses the blood–brain barrier very quickly; thus, it is used primarily in anesthesiology. It is also available as a patch (absorbed easily through the skin because it is lipid soluble) or injectable, and is indicated for severe chronic pain when continuous analgesia is required.

Opioid Agonists: Moderate Potency

CODEINE   Codeine is a naturally occurring narcotic agonist obtained from the opium poppy but in lesser amounts than morphine. It is much more active orally than other opioid compounds, but is a less potent analgesic than morphine (120 mg of codeine phosphate IM = 10 mg morphine IM; 200 mg codeine oral = 30–60 mg morphine orally). It causes less respiratory depressant action and constipation, and has less dependence potential. It is a prodrug because its analgesic activity is the result of a conversion to morphine by cytochrome P450 liver enzymes (CYP2D6). Some people respond well to codeine, but some do not because of a deficiency of CYP2D6.

Adverse Effects   Codeine causes less respiratory depression than morphine, but if given in high doses the same degrees of respiratory depression will occur. Additional adverse effects include (as with all narcotics) dizziness, nausea, vomiting, constipation, sedation, and itching.

Indications   Codeine is usually combined with other nonnarcotic drugs such as acetaminophen for the relief of acute nociceptive mild to moderate dental pain, and is not used for treating severe pain. It is also added to many cough syrups as an antitussive. Codeine has the same abuse potential as morphine, but is less potent. The phosphate and sulfate salt forms are available, but the phosphate form is more water soluble and is more commonly used. The oral dose of codeine is 60, 30, or 15 mg.

Drug–Drug Interactions   There may be an increase in CNS depressant effects if taken with alcohol. There may be increased sedation if taken with St. John's wort. Since codeine is metabolized by CYP2D6, any drugs that inhibit this enzyme will increase plasma levels of codeine. Some drugs that inhibit CYP2D6 include selective serotonin reuptake inhibitors (antidepressants) such as Paxil and Prozac, Celebrex, and cimetidine (Tagamet). Because of differences in responsiveness among individuals in the activity of codeine, some clinicians prefer to use hydrocodone.

PROPOXYPHENE   In November 2010, the FDA banned Darvon and Darvocet and other brand/generic drugs containing propoxyphene due to increased reports of serious heart side effects in healthy people taking normal dosages.

Other Agonists

Dextromethorphan is an opioid without any analgesic activity but high antitussive effects. It is a component of cough medicines. Some trade names are Benylin, Delsym, and Vick's.

Loperamide (Imodium) is an opioid without analgesic effects but causes increased smooth muscle tone in the gastrointestinal tract, and is used as an antidiarrheal. It is available over-the-counter.

Diphenoxylate is an opioid/anticholinergic Schedule V controlled drug that is also used as an antidiarrheal. It is combined with atropine in a product called Lomotil. It can cause severe respiratory depression, coma, and death after overdose in children.

Tramadol (Ultram) is a unique analgesic having both opiate and central acting adrenergic qualities. It is an opioid-like drug that is not a controlled substance. It is FDA approved for moderate to moderately severe pain. Tramadol can cause serious neurotoxicity, and is not the first-line drug of choice.

Mixed Agonist/Antagonists

Mixed agonist/antagonists are analgesic drugs that have combinations of full agonist, partial agonist, and antagonists. These parenterally administered drugs are used for preoperative and postoperative analgesia and for analgesia during labor and delivery. Examples include buprenorphine, butorphanol, nalbuphine, and pentazocine. Pentazocine (Talwin) is a κ receptor agonist with partial agonist activity at μ receptors. It is available in an oral and parenteral form and is used for moderate to severe pain. Butorphanol (Stadol) is available as a nasal spray for migraine headaches (Table 6-4).

Antagonists

Opioid antagonists inhibit the effects of morphine and are used in situations of narcotic overdose, reversing all opioid effects including analgesia. Naloxone (Narcan) and naltrexone

---

Guidelines for Patients Taking Codeine

- Monitor patients for dry mouth; use fluoride rinses if indicated.
- Monitor vital signs due to effects of the heart and the respiratory system.
- Causes drowsiness/sedation.

(Depade) are not used to reverse non-life-threatening effects. A new formulation combines morphine and naltrexone (Embeda), which helps to decrease the risk of abuse.

The antagonist drug binds the opioid receptors but exerts no activity (there is no analgesic or antitussive activity, nor is there respiratory depression). For example, naloxone (Narcan) binds to all three receptors and blocks the action of the opioid.

Combination Narcotic Analgesic and Nonnarcotic Analgesic

Many opioids are used in combination with a nonnarcotic analgesic such as aspirin, acetaminophen, or ibuprofen to obtain a greater analgesic effect than any of the agents alone and to use less dose of the narcotic. Table 6-6 lists the various narcotic/nonnarcotic analgesic combinations that are used for moderate to severe pain. The disadvantage of using combination therapy is that it increases the risk of adverse effects and drug interactions.

SELECTION OF AGENT AND DOSAGE   There are two criteria for the selection of a narcotic drug:

1. Potency and maximal effect: The most potent in maximal effect is morphine; meperidine (Demerol) is intermediate in activity; and codeine is the least active.
2. Duration of action: Morphine has a quick onset and short duration but it is not used orally and thus is not used in dentistry; meperidine (Demerol) has a short onset and very short duration; and methadone has a long onset and long duration.

Rapid Dental Hint

Remember: Before any drugs are prescribed to your patients, reference the drug.

Substance Abuse and Dependency

Drug (substance or chemical) dependency and abuse are major public health problems; many patients seen in the dental office or clinic are dependent on or abuse drugs or alcohol. **Drug dependency** (formerly called drug addiction) is when a patient feels the absolute need for a drug or will experience withdrawal symptoms if the drug is taken away. Tolerance may develop whereby more and more of the drug must be taken to achieve the desired effect. The individual finds it is difficult to discontinue and cannot quit. If the person does stop taking the drug, they will undergo withdrawal symptoms characterized by painful physical and/or mental suffering. Drug abuse refers to the recurrent and frequent use of a drug or substance that causes physical or mental harm or impairs social behavior (e.g., a substance abuser cannot function at work, school, or home), or drugs will be used in situations that are physically hazardous (e.g., driving a car).

TABLE 6-6	Narcotic/Nonnarcotic Combinations	
FORMULATION	**TRADE NAME**	**SCHEDULE**
Hydrocodone/ acetaminophen	Lorcet 10/650 mg	C-III
	Lorcet HD 5/500	C-III
	Lorcet Plus 7.5/650	C-III
	Lortab 2.5/500; 5/500; 7.5/500; 10/500	C-III
	Vicodin 5/500	C-III
	Vicodin ES 7.5/750	C-III
	Vicodin HP 10/660	C-III
Hydrocodone/ ibuprofen	Vicoprofen 7.5/200	C-III
Oxycodone/ acetaminophen	Percocet 2.5/325; 5/325; 7.5/500; 10/650	C-II
	Roxicet 5/325; 5/500	C-II
	Tylox 5/500	C-II
Oxycodone/ ibuprofen (5mg/400mg)	Combunox 5/400	C-II
Oxycodone HCl/ aspirin	Percodan 5/325	C-II
	Percodan-Demi 2.5/325	C-II
Acetaminophen/ codeine	Tylenol w/codeine (No. 2, No. 3, No. 4) 300/15; 300/30; 300/60	C-III
Aspirin/codeine/ carisoprodol	Soma compound w/codeine 325/16/200	C-III
Dihydrocodeine/ aspirin	Synalgos-DC 16/356 (contains 30 mg caffeine)	C-III
Acetaminophen/ butalbital/ caffeine/codeine	Fioricet w/codeine	C-III
Aspirin/butalbital/ caffeine/codeine	Fiorinal w/codeine	C-III

Recognizing Drug Abuse Patients

The dental hygienist should recognize and screen those patients who are currently abusing drugs and alcohol as well as those who are recovering from substance abuse and dependency. Some patients may not reveal that they currently have or have had a history of drug abuse. Dental hygienists should be aware of signs and symptoms of drug abuse (Table 6-7).

Patients may request a second prescription for a narcotic for many reasons, including "The pills fell into the sink" or "My dog ate them."

Central nervous system stimulants produce excitatory effects in the central nervous system, characterized by increased

TABLE 6-7 Signs and Symptoms of Drug Abusers

Symptoms of drug abuse depend on the drug being abused:

- Alcoholics may have facial (especially nose) "spider veins," odor of alcohol on their breath, liver disease, weight changes, abusive behavior, and difficulty concentrating.
- Cocaine users may have chronic sniffles due to vasconstrictive properties, increased alertness, euphoria, excitation, increased blood pressure, and pulse rate.
- Marijuana users have an increased appetite and may be disoriented.
- Depressant drug users (barbiturates, benzodiazepines) may show slurred speech, disorientation or behavior similar to an alcoholic but without the alcohol breath, shallow respiration, clammy/sweating skin, and pinpoint pupils.
- Amphetamine and LSD users have illusions and hallucinations and an altered perception of time.
- Narcotics abusers (e.g., heroin, hydrocodone, oxycodone, morphine) appear as euphoric with dilated pupils. They usually show drowsiness, respiratory depression, nausea, and clammy/sweaty skin.

wakefulness and alertness and feelings of increased initiative and ability and depression of appetite. Excessive dosage, particularly when administered intravenously, produces a delirious or psychotic state. Examples of central nervous system stimulants include amphetamines and cocaine.

Narcotic analgesics relieve pain, induce sedation or sleep, and elevate mood—particularly when it is depressed—and act as cough suppressants. A high degree of tolerance and severe physical and psychological dependence usually develops with prolonged or repeated use. There are reportedly between 1 and 2 million Americans abusing opioids, including heroin. The dental hygienist must be wary of patients requesting these types of drugs.

These drugs are taken orally, sniffed, injected subcutaneously or intravenously, and smoked (opium). Examples of more commonly abused narcotic analgesics include opium, morphine, heroin, codeine, meperidine, and methadone.

Cannabis is a drug derived from the hemp plant *cannabis sativa*. Cannabis is smoked (marijuana), occasionally ingested (hashish), or sniffed. In high doses it produces clearly hallucinogenic effects.

Common long-term adverse effects of opioids include xerostomia, constipation, and pupillary constriction. Sniffing cocaine causes irritation and drying of the nasal mucosa. Those who take intravenous opioids will have puncture marks on their arms.

Patients asking for medications that are addicting, including opiates and anti-anxiety drugs, should be evaluated for a dependency problem. Some patients may request a certain pain medication after periodontal surgery or extractions that they say works best for them. The dental hygienist should be aware that if the dental procedure is not too traumatic or painful and the patient requests a narcotic such as Percodan or Vicodin, this patient may have a drug problem. Patients who are recovering

from substance abuse should not be prescribed drugs that will have the potential for abuse or addiction. This includes alcohol-containing mouthrinses such as Listerine or chlorhexidine gluconate (Peridex, PerioGard). Nonalcoholic rinses (e.g., Rembrandt, Oral-B) are recommended.

There are alternative drugs to prescribe to patients either currently experiencing or recovering from chemical dependency for certain conditions related to dentistry including for pain control. Instead of giving a narcotic, recommend acetaminophen and/or a NSAID such as ibuprofen or naproxen.

Dental Hygiene Applications

MILD PAIN	MODERATE PAIN	SEVERE PAIN
Aspirin	APAP/codeine (Tylenol No. 3)	Morphine
Acetaminophen	APAP/hydrocodone (Vicodin)	Methadone
NSAIDs	APAP/oxycodone (Combunox)	Levophanol
+/− adjuncts	Tramadol (Ultram)	Fentanyl
	+/− adjuncts	Oxycodone (OxyContin)
		+/− adjuncts

APAP, acetaminophen
World Health Organization. 1996.
Source: Cancer Pain Relief, with a Guide to Opioid Availability.

The World Health Organization (WHO) provides a stepladder for the treatment of pain.

Dental pain is an acute nociceptive pain that in most cases can be managed as mild to moderate pain using either a NSAID or, for more moderate pain, or a short-acting narcotic/nonnarcotic combination containing oxycodone or codeine.

Aspirin and the NSAIDs have a ceiling effect whereby increased doses do not produce increased effects after a certain point. Opioids do not have a ceiling effect. The narcotic dose can be titrated (administration of small incremental doses) to achieve maximum pain relief.

Neuropathic pain—such as trigeminal neuralgia, postherpetic neuralgia, entrapment neuropathy (e.g., carpal tunnel syndrome), and phantom limb pain—is chronic, difficult to treat, and is often resistant to therapy but may respond to anticonvulsants (e.g., gabapentin), tricyclic antidepressants, or lidocaine patch. Studies are ongoing testing the efficacy and safety of opioid agonists in the treatment of neuropathic pain of nonmalignant origin. Trigeminal neuralgia is typically treated with carbamazepine (tegretol).

Samples of common prescriptions of NSAIDs and narcotics are given in Figure 6-5.

DEA #AW John Smith, D.D.S.
123 Sixth Ave
New York, NY, 10000
(212) 123-4567

Name Ann Smith Age 56
Address 123 main St Date 6/2/07

R   Ibuprofen 600mg

Disp: # 12 (twelve) tabs

Sig: Take one tab q6-8h

prn dental pain

THIS PRESCRIPTION WILL BE FILLED GENERICALLY
UNLESS PRESCRIBER WRITES 'daw' IN THE BOX BELOW

☑ Label
Refill NR Times

Dispense As Written

DEA #AW John Smith, D.D.S.
123 Sixth Ave
New York, NY, 10000
(212) 123-4567

Name Ann Smith Age 56
Address 123 main St Date 6/2/07

R (OTC)

Aleve 220mg

Take one Caplet
q8-12 hrs

THIS PRESCRIPTION WILL BE FILLED GENERICALLY
UNLESS PRESCRIBER WRITES 'daw' IN THE BOX BELOW

☑ Label
Refill NR Times

Dispense As Written

DEA #AW John Smith, D.D.S.
123 Sixth Ave
New York, NY, 10000
(212) 123-4567

Name Ann Smith Age 56
Address 123 main St Date 6/2/07

R

Celebrex 100mg

Disp: 12 Capsules

Sig: Take one Cap
bid

THIS PRESCRIPTION WILL BE FILLED GENERICALLY
UNLESS PRESCRIBER WRITES 'daw' IN THE BOX BELOW

☑ Label
Refill NR Times

Dispense As Written

DEA #AW John Smith, D.D.S.
123 Sixth Ave
New York, NY, 10000
(212) 123-4567

Name Ann Smith Age 56
Address 123 main St Date 6/2/07

R Tylenol No. 3

Disp: # 16 (sixteen) tabs

Sig: Take one tab q4-6h

prn dental pain

THIS PRESCRIPTION WILL BE FILLED GENERICALLY
UNLESS PRESCRIBER WRITES 'daw' IN THE BOX BELOW

☑ Label
Refill NR Times

Dispense As Written

FIGURE 6-5 Prescriptions for common analgesics used in dentistry.

DEA # AW John Smith, D.D.S.
123 Sixth Ave
New York, NY, 10000
(212) 123-4567

Name Ann Smith Age 56
Address 123 main St Date 6/2/07

R̶ Naproxen 250mg
Disp: # 12 tabs
Sig: Take 2 tablets
initially, then one tab
q6-8h for dental pain

THIS PRESCRIPTION WILL BE FILLED GENERICALLY
UNLESS PRESCRIBER WRITES 'daw' IN THE BOX BELOW

☑ Label
Refill NR Times

Dispense As Written

DEA # AW John Smith, D.D.S.
123 Sixth Ave
New York, NY, 10000
(212) 123-4567

Name Ann Smith Age 56
Address 123 main St Date 6/2/07

R̶ Vicodin
Disp: # 12 tabs
Sig: Take one tab
q4-6 prn dental
pain

THIS PRESCRIPTION WILL BE FILLED GENERICALLY
UNLESS PRESCRIBER WRITES 'daw' IN THE BOX BELOW

☑ Label
Refill NR Times

Dispense As Written

DEA # AW John Smith, D.D.S.
123 Sixth Ave
New York, NY, 10000
(212) 123-4567

Name Ann Smith Age 56
Address 123 main St Date 6/2/07

R̶ Anaprox 275 mg
Disp: # 12 tabs
Sig: Take two tabs Stat,
then one tab q6-8h prn
dental pain

THIS PRESCRIPTION WILL BE FILLED GENERICALLY
UNLESS PRESCRIBER WRITES 'daw' IN THE BOX BELOW

☑ Label
Refill NR Times

Dispense As Written

FIGURE 6-5 (*Continued*)

Key Points

- Prostaglandins are created by cells and act only in the surrounding area before they are broken down.
- Prostaglandins control many body functions (protective).
- COX-1 serves a protective function in the body; inhibition of COX-1 is associated with adverse GI effects and inhibition of platelet aggregation.
- COX-2 is only associated with inflammation.
- Aspirin for prevention of heart attack and stroke used in low doses (81-100 mg/day or 325 mg every other day) causes inhibition of thromboxane A_2, which results in prevention of platelet aggregation and increases bleeding.
- Aspirin in high arthritic doses (more than 6g/day) causes inhibition of prostacyclin, which has the opposite effect of thromboxane A_2 and causes platelet aggregation.
- NSAIDs and aspirin have a ceiling effect; there are no additional benefits in taking more than a certain dose.
- Some caution is necessary in administering NSAIDs to patients who are being treated for hypertension and asthma.
- Selective COX-2 inhibitors have a cardiovascular warning.
- Opioids are the drugs of choice for moderate to severe pain.

- Opioid narcotic analgesics have an abuse potential and all are controlled substances except for tramadol.
- For orofacial pain, long-term use of narcotics is not recommended because of abuse potential and many adverse effects.
- Cocaine users, or patients whom you suspect to be abusers, are at increased risk of developing myocardial infarction and cardiac arrhythmias. Avoid the use of epinephrine.
- Patients with a history of drug addiction will most likely require more analgesia.
- If possible, nonnarcotic analgesics should be prescribed/recommended to patients with addictions.
- There may be abnormal liver function in alcoholics, decreased metabolism of local anesthetics, and increased bleeding time. Avoid acetaminophen.

Board Review Questions

1. From which of the following substances are prostaglandins formed? (p. 89)
   a. Arachidonic acid
   b. Endorphins
   c. Enkephalins
   d. Norepinephrine

2. Which of the following dosages of aspirin is recommended for men to prevent stroke and heart attack (p. 92)?
   a. 81 mg/day
   b. 325 mg every 3 months
   c. 650 mg/day
   d. 3g/day

3. Opioids are recommended for patients whose nociceptive pain is considered to be (p. 97)
   a. mild to moderate.
   b. moderate.
   c. moderate to severe.
   d. intermittent.

4. Which of the following drugs is indicated for the treatment of trigeminal neuralgia? (p. 102)
   a. Phenytoin
   b. Acetaminophen
   c. Carbamazepine
   d. Lidocaine

5. Which of the following toxic effects occur with high doses of morphine? (p. 99)
   a. Cardiac failure
   b. Respiratory depression
   c. Muscle paralysis
   d. Allergic reaction

6. Which of the following opioids is considered to have moderate potency. (p. 100)
   a. Methadone
   b. Morphine
   c. Oxycodone
   d. Codeine

7. Which of the following opioids is used for heroin addiction? (p. 99)
   a. Fentanyl
   b. Hydrocodone
   c. Morphine
   d. Buprenorphine

8. All of the following are adverse effects of codeine *except* one. Which one is the exception? (p. 100)
   a. Itching
   b. Respiratory depression
   c. Antitussive
   d. Diarrhea

9. Which of the following drugs has a ceiling effect? (p. 102)
   a. Codeine
   b. Morphine
   c. Aspirin
   d. Methadone

10. Neuropathic pain usually responds well to all of the following drugs *except* one. Which is the exception? (p. 102)
    a. Anticonvulsants
    b. Tricyclic antidepressants
    c. Topical analgesics
    d. Opioids

11. Celecoxib (Celebrex) is contraindicated in patients allergic to (p. 96)
    a. sulfa.
    b. aspirin.
    c. penicillin.
    d. erythromycin.

12. Which of the following drugs should be used with some caution in a patient that is taking enalapril (Vasotec)? (pp. 93, 94)
    a. Lithium
    b. Penicillin
    c. Ibuprofen
    d. Codeine

13. Most of the COX-1/COX-2 inhibitors NSAIDs have a black box warning of increased risk of (p. 96)
    a. thrombotic cardiovascular events.
    b. duodenal and gastric ulcer formation.
    c. anaphylactic reactions.
    d. asthmatic attacks.

14. Which of the following adverse effects is commonly seen in patients taking an a NSAID? (p. 95)
    a. Gastrointestinal bleeding
    b. Hair loss
    c. Sedation
    d. Xerostomia

15. Which substance is responsible for platelet aggregation? (p. 90)
    a. PGE_2
    b. PGI_2
    c. Thromboxane A_2
    d. COX-2

Selected References

Aghabeigi B. 1992. The pathophysiology of pain. *Br Dnet J* 173:91–97.

Ardekian L, Gaspar R, Peled M, Brener B, Laufer D. 2000. Does low-dose aspirin therapy complicate oral surgical procedures? *JADA* 131(*3*):331–335.

Benoliel F, Sharav Y, Tal M, Eliav E. 2003. Management of chronic orofacial pain: Today and tomorrow. *Compendium* 24:909–927.

Berdine HJ, O'Neil CK. 2003. Neuropathic pain pathophysiology, treatment and patient management. *US Pharmacist.* Supplement.

Campbell CL, Smyth S, Montalescot G, et al. 2007. Aspirin dose for the prevention of cardiovascular disease. A systematic review. *JAMA* 297:2018–2024.

Eisenberg E, McNicol ED, Carr DB. 2005. Efficacy and safety of opioid agonists in the treatment of neuropathic pain of nonmalignant origin. *JAMA* 293:3043–3052.

European Society of Hypertension Scientific Newsletter: Update on hypertension management. 2003. 4(17).

Haas DA. 1999. Adverse drug interactions in dental practice: Interactions associated with analgesics. Part III in a series. *JADA* 130:397–407.

Jones EM, Knutson, D, Haines, D. 2003. Common problems in patients recovering from chemical dependency. *Am Fam Physician* 68:1971–1978.

Kittelson L, 2006. Substance abuse. In *ADA Guide to Dental Therapeutics,* 3rd ed. Chicago: ADA Publishing, pp. 569–578.

Lancaster T, Wareham DW, Yaphe, J. 2003. Postherpetic neuralgia. *Am Fam Physician* 67:1557–1558.

Noble, SL, King BS, Olutade J. 2000. Cyclooxygenase-2 enzyme inhibitors: Place in therapy. *Am Fam Physician* 61:3669–3676.

Page RL II. Weighing the cardiovascular benefits of low-dose aspirin. *Pharmacy Times.* ACPE Program ID Number 290-000-05-017-H01.

Ridker PM, Cook NR, Lee IM, Gordon D, Gaziano M, et al. 2005. A randomized trial of low-dose aspirin in the primary prevention of cardiovascular disease in women. *New Engl J Med* 352:1293–1304.

Rosenberg RN. 2003. *Pain Arch Neurol* 60:1520.

Sachs CJ. 2005. Oral analgesics for acute nonspecific pain. *Am Fam Physician* 71:913–918.

Schwartzman RJ, Crothusen J, Kiefer TR, Rohr P. 2001. Neuropathic central pain. *Arch Neurol* 58:1547–1551.

Weinberg MA, Segelnick SL. 2010. Management of nonvariceal upper gastrointestinal bleeding. *US Pharmacist* HS1-HS5.

Zagaria MAE. 2006. Pain assessment in older adults. *US Pharmacist* 31(5):30–36.

Zanchetti A, Hansson L, Leonetti G, Rahn KH, et al. 2002. Low-dose aspirin does not interfere with the blood pressure lowering effects of antihypertensive therapy. *Hypertens* 1015–1027.

Zuniga J. R. The use of nonopioid drugs in management of chronic orofacialpain. *J Oral Maxillofac Surg* 1998;56:1075–1080.

Web Sites

www.ncbi.nlm.nih.gov
www.pharmacytimes.com
www.uspharmacist.com
www.usdoj.gov/ndic/pubs10/10123/index.htm

QUICK DRUG GUIDE

Nonnarcotic Analgesics

Salicylates and Salicylate Derivatives

- Aspirin (Ecotrin, Bayer, Halprin, and many more)
- Diflunisal (Dolobid)
- Choline salicylate; magnesium salicylate (Trilisate)

Nonsteroidal Anti-Inflammatory Drugs (NSAIDs)

Indoles

- Indomethacin (Indocin)
- Sulindac (Clinoril)

Indole Acetic Acids

- Tolmetin (Tolectin)
- Ketorolac (Toradol)

Phenylalkoanoic Acid Derivatives

- Ibuprofen (Advil, Motrin)
- Ketoprofen (Orudis)
- Flurbiprofen (Ansaid)
- Naproxen (Naprosyn); Naproxen sodium (Anaprox, Aleve)
- Oxaprozin (Daypro)

Napthylalkanone

- Nabumetone (Relafen)

Fenamates

- Meclofenamate (Ponstel)
- Diclofenac (Voltaren)

Oxicam

- Prioxicam (Feldene)

COX-2 Selective NSAIDs

- Celecoxib (Celebrex)

Other Nonnarcotic Analgesics

- Acetaminophen

Opioid (Narcotic) Analgesics

Short-Acting

- Morphine
- Hydromorphone (Dilaudid)
- Oxycodone (controlled-release OxyContin)
- Hydrocodone (only in combination with a nonnarcotic)
- Codeine
- Meperidine (Demerol)
- Fentanyl (Duragesic patch)

Long-Acting

- Methadone
- Levorphanol (Levo-Dromoran)
- Oxymorphone (Numorphan)

Other Opioid Agonists

- Dextromethorphan (used in cough syrups; Robitussin, Sucrets, Vicks, Delsym, Benylin)
- Diphenoxylate (with atropine; Lomotil)
- Loperamide (Imodium; antidiarrheal)
- Tramadol (central analgesic) (Ultram)

Mixed Agonist/Antagonists

- Buprenorphine (Buprenex)
- Butorphanol (Stadol)
- Nalbuphine (Nubain)
- Pentazocine (Talwin)

Antagonists

- Naloxone (Narcan)

Drugs for Orofacial Pain

Tricyclic Antidepressants
- Amitriptyline (Elavil)
- Desipramine (Norpramine)

Anesthetic
- Lidocaine patch (Lidoderm 5% patch)

Anti-epileptics
- Gabapentin (Neurontin)
- Pregablin (Lyrica)
- Carbamazepine (Tegretol)
- Oxycarbazepine (Trileptal)
- Lamotrigine (Lamictal)

Narcotic/Nonnarcotic Combinations

Formulation	Trade Name	Schedule
Hydrocodone/acetaminophen	Lorcet 10/650 mg	C-III
	Lorcet HD 5/500	C-III
	Lorcet Plus 7.5/650	C-III
	Lortab 2.5/500; 5/500;	C-III
	7.5/500; 10/500	C-III
	Vicodin 5/500	C-III
	Vicodin ES 7.5/750	C-III
	Vicodin HP 10/660	C-III
Hydrocodone/ibuprofen	Vicoprofen 7.5/200	C-III
Oxycodone/acetaminophen	Percocet 2.5/325; 5/325;	C-II
	7.5/500; 10/650	
	Roxicet 5/325; 5/500	C-II
	Tylox 5/500	C-II
Oxycodone/ibuprofen (5mg/400mg)	Combunox 5/400	C-II
Oxycodone HCl/aspirin	Percodan 5/325	C-II
	Percodan-Demi 2.5/325	C-II
Acetaminophen/codeine	Tylenol w/codeine	C-III
	(No. 2, No. 3, No. 4)	
	(300/15; 300/30; 300/60)	
Aspirin/codeine/carisoprodol	Soma compound w/codeine	C-III
	325/16/200	

Formulation	Trade Name	Schedule
Dihydrocodeine/aspirin	Synalgos-DC 16/356 (Contains 30 mg caffeine)	C-III
Acetaminophen/butalbital/caffeine/codeine	Aspirin/butalbital/caffeine/codeine	
Fioricet w/ codeine	Fiorinal w/codeine	

Antibacterial Agents

GOAL

To introduce the concepts of systemic and locally applied antibiotics and antimicrobials in the treatment of bacterial infections, including dental infections. To provide an understanding of the pharmacology of drugs used to treat tuberculosis.

EDUCATIONAL OBJECTIVES

After reading this chapter, the reader should be able to:

1. List the classifications of the different antibiotics including penicillins, cephalosporins, tetracyclines, macrolides, fluoroquinolones, and nitroimidazoles.

2. Understand the concept of bactericidal versus bacteriostatic antibiotics.

3. Describe adverse effects of the various antibiotics.

4. Explain the use of antibiotics in periodontics, implants, oral surgery, and endodontics.

5. Discuss the rationale for use of topical agents used in dentistry.

6. List the various antimycobacterial drugs.

7. Discuss the dental adverse side effects of antimycobacterial drugs.

KEY TERMS

Antibiotic

Bactericidal

Bacteriostatic

Dental infection

Tuberculosis

Antimicrobial Agents

Antimicrobial Activity

Louis Pasteur's concept of symbiosis incorporates the cooperative efforts of two organisms of any kind. For example, we live in a symbiotic relationship with microorganisms in the gut (gastrointestinal tract). The opposite of symbiosis is asymbiosis, in which two organisms create substances harmful to each other.

Antibiotics are substances produced by living organisms (e.g., microorganisms) which are harmful to other organisms. Essentially, antibiotics are asymbiotic. Antibiotics are either natural or semisynthetic. There are two broad classifications of antibiotics based on whether they kill bacteria (**bactericidal**) or inhibit bacterial multiplication (**bacteriostatic**).

The *spectrum of activity* of an antibiotic indicates the range of bacteria the antibiotic affects. Narrow-spectrum antibiotics are active against some gram-positive pathogens, whereas broad-spectrum antibiotics are effective against a wider range of bacterial pathogens, including many gram-negative organisms. Extended-spectrum antibiotics act in between a narrow and broad spectrum. Ideally, antibiotics should be concentrated at the site of infection.

Adverse Effects

Ideally an antibiotic should be selective. Unfortunately, this is rarely the case. Antibiotics often have significant side effects (Table 7-1). These may include:

1. Bacterial resistance to the antibiotic
2. Superinfections
3. Gastrointestinal effects (nausea, vomiting, diarrhea)
4. Allergic reactions
5. Photosensitivity
6. Drug interactions

> **DID YOU KNOW?**
>
> In ancient times, honey from a bee was thought to have antibiotic properties and was used to heal ulcers and burns, and later to treat gunshot wounds.

ANTIMICROBIAL RESISTANCE Antibiotic use promotes development of antibiotic-resistant bacteria, rendering the antibiotic ineffective against the bacterium and allowing progression of the infection. The bacteria continue to multiply and survive despite concentrations of an antibiotic that should be lethal to them.

Normally, four situations can occur when bacteria are exposed to an antibiotic:

1. The antibiotic kills the bacteria (bactericidal).
2. The antibiotic weakens, disables, and decreases its growth (bacteriostatic), making it easier for the host's own natural defenses to kill the bacteria.
3. The bacteria will not be affected by the antibiotic (e.g., bacteria are not sensitive to the antibiotic: wrong antibiotic for the bacteria).
4. Resistance has developed.

TABLE 7-1 Penicillins

DRUG	DOSE
Natural penicillins: Narrow spectrum	Penicillin V: 500 mg qid
Penicillin V (Pen-vee K, V-cillin K, Veetids)	
Penicillin G injectable	
Aminopenicillins: Broad spectrum	Amoxicillin: 500 mg tid
Amoxicillin (Amoxil, Trimox)	
Ampicillin (Omnipen)	
Beta-lactamase inhibitors	Augmentin: 250 mg q8h or 500 mg q12h
Amoxicillin + calvulante (or clavulanic acid) (Augmentin)	
Ampicillin + sulbactam (Unasyn)	
Piperacillin + tazobactam injectable	
Penicillinase resistant	Not used in dentistry
Dicloxacillin (Dycill)	
Nafcillin (injectable)	
Oxacillin (Bactocill)	
Cloxacillin (cloxacillin)	
Antipseudomonal penicillins: Extended spectrum (all injectables)	Not used in dentistry
Carbenicillin (Geocillin)	
Ticarcillin (Ticar)	
Mezlocillin (Mezlin)	
Piperacillin (Pipracil)	

Antimicrobial resistance is an increasing problem worldwide. The danger is that when antibiotics are used unnecessarily, they will not be effective if administered later on for a serious bacterial infection. The resulting, untreated infection may result in significant morbidity and/or mortality.

The development of antibiotic resistance is both natural (inherent) and acquired. Bacteria have a certain *inherent resistance* to certain antibiotics. For example, a gram-negative bacterium may have an outer cell membrane that is impermeable to the antibiotic and the organism may lack a transport system that brings the antibiotic into the cell. This is why whenever possible a culture and sensitivity test is performed on bacterial samples from tissue specimens or spaces (e.g., periodontal pocket). When such specimens are available, it is important to use the antibiotic to which the organism is sensitive. Resistance in the microorganisms (not the host) occurs most commonly due to either inadequate amount of antibiotic or inadequate duration of therapy. Resistance among the normal inherent organisms may also occur when antibiotics are given in the absence of bacterial infection. When these organisms subsequently cause a clinical infection, the usual antibiotics will not be effective. Bacteria require high concentrations of an antibiotic to kill them if they are less sensitive to that antibiotic. Additionally, in some cases the antibiotic may kill some bacteria but some may survive; the survivors have usually developed resistance to that antibiotic.

Acquired antibiotic resistance can be produced either through a mutation or conjugation. A *mutation* is a genetic transformation that takes place under the influence of an antibiotic. A spontaneous mutation or change in the bacterial chromosome imparts resistance to a particular drug. The antibiotic kills the nonmutants, but those mutants that are resistant to the antibiotic survive and replicate.

Rapid Dental Hint

To help prevent antimicrobial resistance avoid prescribing antibiotics indiscriminately and advise the patient to take the antibiotic until all is finished even if they are feeling better.

Another form of antibiotic resistance is the transfer or exchange of resistance genes (DNA) from one bacterium to another, known as *genetic exchange.*

An *active efflux system* in some types of bacteria "pushes" the antibiotic out of the cell, allowing the bacterium to resist that antibiotic.

Adaptation is a *nongenetic transformation,* but there is genetic capability. For example, *penicillinase* is an enzyme that breaks down the antibiotic penicillin and is secreted only in the presence of penicillin. Penicillinase is produced by certain bacterial strains such as *Staphylococcus aureus.* Penicillinase breaks up the β-lactam ring on the penicillin molecule, rendering the penicillin inactive.

Treatment resistance may develop if:

1. The diagnosis was not made promptly.
2. Inadequate doses were prescribed.
3. The patient did not take the prescribed antibiotic at the prescribed dose for the prescribed amount of time.

Misuse resistance occurs when antibiotics are taken indiscriminately. Antibiotics target only bacteria, not viruses. Thus, antibiotics should not be used against the flu, the common cold, most sore throats, most episodes of "bronchitis" in children, and most cases of fever without a definite source. To help prevent antibiotic-resistant infections, patients should be encouraged to throw away any unused antibiotics, not to take an antibiotic that is prescribed for someone else, and take the antibiotic the way it was prescribed. Many cases of resistance are found in hospital settings where the patient is either immunocompromised or elderly.

SUPERINFECTIONS AND GASTROINTESTINAL PROBLEMS   Superinfections mostly occur when a broad-spectrum antibiotic causes eradication of microorganisms that are part of the normal flora (bacteria that normally live in these areas) of the gastrointestinal (GI) tract, oral cavity, respiratory tract, or vaginal area. This reduction/elimination of normal bacterial flora allows for the growth of other organisms such as fungi or bacteria. There is less incidence of superinfection with narrow-spectrum antibiotics. Oral superinfections include sore mouth (stomatitis) or tongue (glossitis). To help prevent superinfections some suggest to additionally take acidophilus in the form of yogurt or tablets/capsules/gelcaps to replace the normal flora.

Antibiotics commonly affect the GI tract either by direct irritation or indirectly by changing the normal GI flora, resulting in nausea, vomiting, and/or diarrhea. Antibiotic-associated *pseudomembranous colitis* occurs when there is an overgrowth of the bacterium *Clostridium difficile,* which secretes a toxin that causes severe inflammation of the bowel wall. It is characterized by watery diarrhea and abdominal cramping.

Rapid Dental Hint

To help the patient reduce the gastrointestinal problems and the possibility of developing a fungal infection, it is recommended to take acidophilus in the form of yogurt or tablets/caps to replace the normal flora.

If the antibiotic can be taken with food, then symptoms may be less likely to occur. Some find benefit if the antibiotic is taken with *acidophilus,* a beneficial bacteria found normally in the intestine. Antibiotic use may reduce these "good" bacteria, causing GI distress.

ALLERGIC REACTIONS   Some antibiotics may cause an allergic reaction manifested by hives, wheezing, or systemic anaphylaxis. If an allergic reaction occurs, the drug must be discontinued immediately.

PHOTOSENSITIVITY When taking some antibiotics, some individuals develop an exaggerated sunburn when exposed to the sun. Ciprofloxacin and doxycycline cause such photosensitivity.

DRUG INTERACTIONS Antibiotics may interact with other drugs (drug–drug interactions) or with foods (drug–food interactions). These interactions can either increase or decrease serum levels of the antibiotic.

DID YOU KNOW?

Fifty million unnecessary antibiotics are prescribed for viral respiratory infections each year in the United States.

SELECTION In dental practice, antibiotics are indicated for three primary purposes:

1. Treatment of acute odontogenic/orofacial infections
2. Prophylaxis against infective endocarditis
3. Prophylaxis for patients at risk for infection because of compromised host defense mechanisms

The choice of antimicrobial therapy is based on the morphology and growth of bacteria. This is true whether a dental or medical infection is being treated. Bacteria are classified according to shape (morphology) (e.g., cocci, bacilli) and growth patterns (e.g., aerobic—oxygen; anaerobic—without oxygen). Also, bacteria are classified according to whether a bacterium does or does not retain a certain stain (gram-positive or gram-negative).

In the majority of dental cases, empirical therapy is practiced, whereby the antibiotic is chosen based on knowledge of the bacterium expected to be causing the **dental infection.** This is based on previous experience by the clinician or other clinicians, and is evidence based, based on the bacteria normally found in such infections. If an unusual infection is suspected or if the patient has recently been on multiple antibiotics, thereby increasing the risk of antibiotic resistance, then culture and sensitivity tests can be performed. This will enable the clinician to choose the proper antibiotic. Samples of dental subgingival biofilms may be sent for culture and sensitivity.

Many prescriptions for antibiotics are inappropriate because they are used for conditions that most likely do not require them. For instance, a dental patient presents with a gingival abscess located on the free gingival margin. If there are no palpable lymph nodes (lymphadenopathy) and no fever, then antibiotics are not necessary. The best treatment for this case is periodontal debridement.

In the medical community, antibiotics are given inappropriately for conditions caused by viruses, such as colds, sore throats, nonspecific fevers, and "bronchitis" in children. Additionally, many broad-spectrum antibiotics (e.g., amoxicillin) are inappropriately given for dental infections. The majority of bacteria in dental infections (e.g., endodontic, periodontic) do not require these broad-spectrum drugs, and penicillin VK (narrow spectrum) is the drug of choice in most dental infections. The FDA points out that antibiotics should be used only to treat bacterial infections, and recommends counseling patients on proper antibiotic use, including taking the antibiotic for the required time.

IN PERIODONTAL THERAPY Systemic antibiotics are usually used in patients with aggressive periodontitis because the bacteria with this periodontal disease invade the soft tissue and elude mechanical debridement. Systemic antibiotics are contraindicated in chronic periodontitis and gingivitis. Topical antimicrobial agents (e.g., Atridox, Arestin) are used in patients with localized chronic periodontitis.

IN ENDODONTIC THERAPY Antibiotics are not necessary in an uncomplicated endodontic infection or if there is well-localized soft tissue swelling without systemic signs of infection such as fever, lymphadenopathy, or cellulitis. Systemic antibiotics are indicated with an endodontic lesion with soft tissue swelling that is not draining, systemic involvement, or spread of the infection. The drug of choice is penicillin VK.

IN IMPLANT DENTISTRY A systemic antibiotic as well as an antimicrobial oral rinse may be indicated for implant surgery. Postoperative infections, which usually occur on the third or fourth day after surgery, are treated with drainage and systemic antibiotics such as penicillin VK. Antibiotics are indicated in the treatment of peri-implant infections, which are associated with bone loss, suppuration, and increased pocket depths. Antibiotics are not indicated in peri-implant mucositis, which involves soft tissue inflammation around the dental implant. If necessary, an antimicrobial mouthrinse such as chlorhexidine gluconate should be used.

Bactericidal Antibiotics: Inhibitors of Bacterial Cell Wall Synthesis

Penicillins

ACTIONS Penicillin, the first antibiotic, was discovered by Sir Alexander Fleming in 1929, but it did not have a clinical application until 1939. Today, most penicillins are produced from a strain of *Penicillium chrysogenum,* while some are semisynthetically produced. Penicillin G is the prototype natural penicillin and is the most potent. Penicillins are administered orally or parenterally, but never topically because of severe allergic reactions.

MICROBIAL ACTIVITY The β-lactam ring on the penicillin molecule is responsible for the antibacterial activity (Figure 7-1). Penicillins are bactericidal or bacteriostatic depending on the concentration achieved. Penicillins act by inhibiting one or more of the penicillin-binding proteins (PBPs) located on bacterial cell walls of susceptible organisms, rendering the internal part of the bacteria cell vulnerable to the outside environment. This results in cell rupture and death (Figure 7-2). Penicillins are most effective against rapidly multiplying bacteria. Since human cells do not have a cell wall but rather cell membranes, penicillins do not affect human cells.

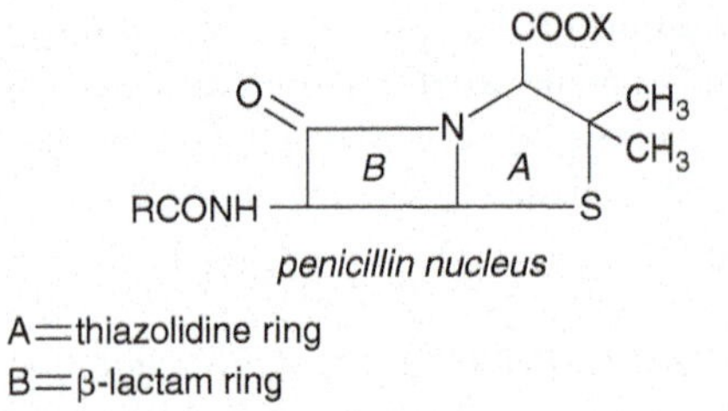

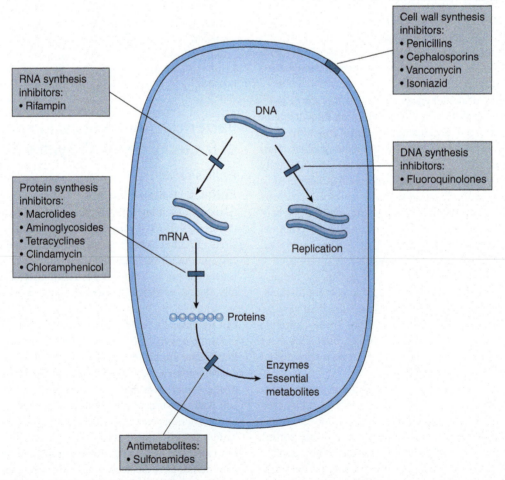

A=thiazolidine ring
B=β-lactam ring

FIGURE 7-1 Illustration of the penicillin structure. The β-lactam ring gives penicillin its antibacterial activity.

SPECTRUM OF ACTIVITY Penicillins are primarily effective against gram-positive bacteria (e.g., *Streptococcus pneumoniae*) but also some gram-negative bacteria. *Narrow-spectrum or natural penicillins* (see Table 7-1) are relatively ineffective against gram-negative bacteria because those organisms have a thick lipopolysaccharide coat that penicillins cannot penetrate. The *broad-spectrum penicillins* (Table 7-1) include the *aminopenicillins* (amoxicillin and ampicillin) and *antipseudomonal penicillins* (e.g., piperacillin, ticarcillin) and are more active against gram-negative bacteria. The *penicillinase-resistant penicillins* (e.g., oxacillin, cloxacillin, dicloxacillin) treat bacteria such as staphylococci that release penicillinase. Other penicillins include *beta-lactamase inhibitors* (e.g., amoxicillin plus clavulanate), *carbapenems,* and *monobactams.*

Guidelines for Patients Taking Penicillin VK or Amoxicillin

- Instruct patients to take the entire prescribed antibiotic even if they feel better. Take on an empty stomach (1 hour before or 2 hours after meals); amoxicillin can be taken without regard to meals.
- Monitor patients for superinfections.

Penicillins are administered orally (PO), intravenously (IV), or intramuscularly (IM). Review Table 7-1 for individual penicillins.

PENICILLIN RESISTANCE

Beta-lactamases Natural penicillins (penicillin G and penicillin V) are more potent than semisynthetic penicillins, but natural penicillins are more susceptible to destruction by β-lactamase (penicillinase). This is especially true in a hospital setting, where up to 95% of *Staphylococcus aureus* produce penicillinase.

Since amoxicillin (broad-spectrum) is sensitive to breakdown by β-lactamases, clavulanic acid (potassium clavulanate) is combined with amoxicillin to form a product called Augmentin. Clavulanic acid is a weak acid without any antibacterial activity but when

FIGURE 7-2 Mechanism of action of antimicrobial drugs.

added to the amoxicillin molecule the β-lactamase binds to the inactive clavulanic acid molecule and leaves the amoxicillin alone. Since this product contains an acid, it should be taken with food, which will lessen the adverse side effects of nausea and diarrhea.

Penicillins may also have a decreased affinity to the penicillin-binding proteins, which are enzymes essential for cell-wall synthesis.

PHARMACOKINETICS Absorption of penicillins depends on acid stability in the stomach, but they are primarily absorbed in the duodenum (small intestine). Absorption is greatest when penicillins are taken on an empty stomach (i.e., 1 hour before or 2 hours after eating). Amoxicillin is the exception and can be taken with food. All penicillins should be taken with a full glass of water to increase absorption from the GI tract.

DID YOU KNOW?

Penicillin is a naturally occurring substance and was first grown in bed pans during World War II, when Howard Florey was trying to find enough containers to grow penicillin mold.

Amoxicillin is more completely absorbed from the GI tract than ampicillin and has fewer GI effects, such as nausea and diarrhea.

Penicillins are eliminated through the kidneys. Thus, in a patient with renal failure, drug dosage must be reduced. The semisynthetic penicillins (oxacillin, dicloxacillin, cloxacillin, and nafcillin) are eliminated through the liver.

Rapid Dental Hint

Remember that amoxicillin is a broad-spectrum penicillin.

INDICATIONS Penicillin VK and amoxicillin are the only two penicillins that are used in dentistry for mild to moderate odontogenic infections (periodontal, endodontic, oral surgery). Bacteria responsible for most odontogenic infections include *Streptococci*, obligate anaerobes gram-positive cocci (e.g., *Peptostreptococcus*), and obligate anaerobic gram-negative (e.g., *Porphyromonas* or *Prevotella* sp.). Penicillin is effective against *Streptococci* species and most oral anaerobic bacteria, although some *Prevotella* species are resistant. Amoxicillin has limited activity against strep and anaerobes but is effective against *Peptostreptococus,* which is found in periodontitis sites.

ADVERSE EFFECTS

1. Allergic reaction: Allergic reactions occur in more than 10% of the population. Severity of an allergic reaction ranges from a mild rash and fever to severe anaphylaxis, which has a low incidence.

2. Pseudomembranous colitis: The offending drug is stopped and metronidazole (PO) is given to the patient. If enteral (PO) administration is not possible, vancomycin (IV) is given.

3. Gastrointestinal upset: Nausea, vomiting, and diarrhea are the most common adverse effects. These may be due to a direct irritation of penicillin in the GI tract. Most penicillins should be taken on an empty stomach. Amoxicillin can be taken without regard to meals. Augmentin should be taken with food. Oral penicillins may be taken with *Lactobacillus acidophilus* to help replace normal flora and reduce GI distress.

4. Superinfection (especially with the broad-spectrum penicillins)

5. Seizure activity: associated with high levels of penicillin

Rapid Dental Hint

Pseudomembranous colitis can occur with any antibiotic.

DRUG INTERACTIONS There are very few drug–drug interactions with penicillin.

1. Penicillin + a bacteriostatic antibiotic (e.g., tetracyclines, erythromycins): A bactericidal antibiotic requires that the bacteria be multiplying actively to be effective. If a bacteriostatic antibiotic is given concurrently, penicillin will not be as effective.

2. Oral contraceptives: Penicillins may decrease effectiveness of oral contraceptives. One theory is that estrogen (oral contraceptive) undergoes enterohepatic circulation and needs bacteria in the gut to break it down before it reabsorbs. Penicillin prevents this, thus estrogen is poorly reabsorbed and not effective.

3. Food: increases breakdown of penicillin in the stomach.

4. Probenicid (treatment of gout): decreases renal (kidney) elimination of penicillins, raising the blood level

PREGNANCY B, caution during nursing

HOW SUPPLIED Penicillin VK (Pen-Vee K, Penicillin VK): tablet; Amoxicillin trihydrate (Polymox, Trimox, Amoxil): capsule, tablet; Augmentin: tablet.

DENTAL HYGIENE APPLICATIONS Amoxicillin is the standard regimen for antibiotic premedication for infective bacterial endocarditis (IBE). Oral penicillin VK is the drug of choice for mild to moderate endodontic, periodontic, and odontogenic infections (e.g., abscess). Amoxicillin is used in skin infections, sinusitis, otitis media, and bite wound infections. For dental infections, amoxicillin should only be reserved for more serious infections. Penicillin VK is a drug of choice in the treatment of necrotizing ulcerative gingivitis (NUG). Augmentin (amoxicillin + clavulanate) is used for resistant strains of bacteria, especially for periodontal patients that are refractory to treatment or have aggressive forms of infection. While amoxicillin has a broader spectrum of activity and penetrates bone well, it is more limited against *Streptococci* and oral anaerobes than penicillin VK, a good antibiotic for oral abscesses.

If concurrent use of penicillin plus a bacteriostatic antibiotic is necessary, then the penicillin should be given a few hours before the bacteriostatic antibiotic.

Rapid Dental Hint

Female patients taking oral contraceptives who are prescribed penicillin (including amoxicillin) and tetraycyclines should be warned to discuss their options with their obstetrician/gynecologist regarding other birth control methods while on the antibiotic.

Cephalosporins

ACTIONS Cephalosporins were isolated at the same time as penicillins were discovered. They have a similar β-lactam ring, which is responsible for their antibacterial activity. Cephalosporins are bactericidal and kill bacteria by inhibiting cell wall synthesis by the same mechanism as penicillins.

INDICATIONS There are four generations of semisynthetic cephalosporins; only a few are given orally (Table 7-2). First-generation oral cephalosporins are ineffective against bacteria that produce beta-lactamase. They are generally used for skin, bone, genitourinary, and respiratory tract infections, otitis media (middle ear infection), and acute prostatitis. Cephalosporins are generally not indicated for endodontic or periodontal infections. They have a broad antimicrobial spectrum (aerobes) of activity but they are expensive.

Rapid Dental Hint

There is a 10% cross-hypersensitivity reaction with penicillins (10% of people allergic to penicillin will be allergic to cephalosporins).

ADVERSE EFFECTS

1. Allergic reaction: Anaphylaxis occurs within minutes after ingestion of the antibiotic. Clinically there is respiratory distress (e.g., bronchospasm), angioedema (swelling), rash and itching, and hypotension. Death is from airway obstruction.
2. There is a 10% cross-hypersensitivity reaction with penicillins (10% of people allergic to penicillin will be allergic to cephalosporins).
3. Morbilliform (skin) rashes: clinically these appear as raised, inflamed skin
4. Superinfection
5. Gastrointestinal: GI distress, including nausea and diarrhea

DRUG INTERACTIONS

1. Probenicid: decreased excretion of cephalosporin
2. Warfarin: may increase actions of anticoagulants; monitor blood tests (international normalized ratio [INR])

PREGNANCY B; drug enters breast milk, so caution during lactation

HOW SUPPLIED

First generation:

Cefadroxil (Duricef): tab, oral suspension

Cephalexin (Keflex): cap, oral suspension

Second generation:

Cefaclor (Ceclor): cap, oral suspension

Efprozil (Cefzil): tab, oral suspension

Cefuroxime—Axetil (Ceftin, Veftin): tab, oral suspension

Third generation:

Omnicef (Cefdinir): cap, oral suspension)

Cefixime (Suprax): tab

Cefpodoxime (Vantin): tab, oral suspension

Ceftibuten (Cedax): cap, oral suspension

Fourth generation:

Only injectable

DENTAL HYGIENE APPLICATIONS Since only a few cephalosporins are administered orally and they are expensive, they are not drugs of choice for dental infections. Additionally,

TABLE 7-2 Cephalosporins
DRUG NAME
First generation
cefadroxil (Duricef)
cephalexin (Keflex)
Second generation
cefaclor (Ceclor)
cefprozil (Cefzil)
cefuroxime—axetil (Ceftin, Veftin)
Third generation
omnicef (cefdinir)
cefixime (Suprax)
cefpodoxime (Vantin)
ceftibuten (Cedax)
Fourth generation
Only injectable

even though they are broader spectrum than penicillins, cephalosporins are effective against the anaerobic organisms that are usually found in dental infections. Cephalosporins are generally not used for an endodontic or periodontal abscess, but may be used for antibiotic premedication.

Nitroimadazoles

ACTIONS   Metronidazole is specifically effective against obligate or strict anaerobic (live in a pure nonoxygen environment) bacteria. Metronidazole is bactericidal, and its mechanism of action is to bind to and break down bacterial DNA.

INDICATIONS   Medical indications include intestinal amoebiasis, trichomoniasis, bacterial anaerobic infections, and giardiasis.

Metronidazole is used in the treatment of necrotizing gingivitis. Metronidazole in combination with amoxicillin or Augmentin may be effective against refractory and aggressive forms of periodontitis associated with *Aggregatibacter actinomycetemcomitans* and *Porphyromonas gingivalis* infection. Metronidazole is also used for peri-implant infections. Antibiotic resistance to metronidazole is rare, but there are numerous adverse side effects.

Rapid Dental Hint

Patients taking warfarin who are prescribed metronidazole, erythromycin, or clarithromycin in the dental office may have an increased international normalized ratio (INR) with an increased risk for bleeding. Consult with the patient's physician.

ADVERSE EFFECTS   Gastrointestinal upset is seen frequently, especially nausea. A metallic taste has been reported, as well as darkened urine.

DRUG INTERACTIONS

1. Consumption of alcohol, including use of alcohol-containing mouthrinses, while taking metronidazole results in a disulfirm-like reaction, which may include headache, flushing, nausea, vomiting, and cramps. The reaction usually lasts for up to 1 hour, though it may continue for a few days after discontinuation of the medication. Alcohol should not

Guidelines for Patients Taking Metronidazole

- Inform your patients that this drug is an antibiotic for his or her periodontal condition.
- Avoid alcohol, even alcohol-containing mouthrinses.
- A metallic taste may develop.
- Take the medication for the recommended time.

be consumed during metronidazole therapy and for at least 3 days after discontinuing the drug.

2. Metronidazole is contraindicated in patients taking lithium (a drug used for manic depression) and cimetidine (an anti-ulcer drug)

3. Metronidazole may decrease the metabolism of anticoagulants (e.g., warfarin), which will increase the bleeding effect of the drug.

PREGNANCY   B

HOW SUPPLIED   Metronidazole (Flagyl): cap, tab

Rapid Dental Hint

Patients may be taking metronidazole during periodontal therapy. Remind them not to use any products containing alcohol, even mouthrinses.

DENTAL HYGIENE APPLICATIONS   Many patients in the dental office may be taking metronidazole for the adjunctive treatment of refractory or chronic periodontitis. It is also used after placement of barrier membranes during periodontal surgery. Thus, patients should be counseled on the proper use of metronidazole. Alcoholic beverages are contraindicated, as are mouthrinses containing alcohol. Also, inform the patient that changes in taste perception may occur. Dry mouth and a metallic taste may develop.

Rapid Dental Hint

Review with your patients how to take his or her antibiotic, possible drug–drug, drug–food interactions, and adverse effects.

Quinolones (Fluoroquinolones)

ACTIONS   Fluoroquinolones are bactericidal because they inhibit bacterial DNA replication. Quinolones are not technically antibiotics because they are totally synthetically produced. Nevertheless, they are frequently referred to as broad-spectrum antimicrobials with good activity against facultative gram-negative anaerobes.

INDICATIONS   Acute bacterial sinusitis, acute bacterial chronic bronchitis, pneumonia, skin infections, bacterial conjunctivitis, urinary tract infections, and chronic periodontitis

ADVERSE EFFECTS   Muscle weakness, muscle pain, phototoxicity, dizziness, convulsions, headache, hallucinations, and possible joint and cartilage damage

DRUG INTERACTIONS Ciprofloxacin should be administered with care for patients taking warfarin (anticoagulant), theophylline (anti-asthma) or caffeine because it inhibits their metabolism, resulting in increased blood levels. Dairy products (calcium), sodium bicarbonate, iron and antacids (magnesium, aluminum) delay absorption, so these products should be given 4 hours before or 2 hours after oral administration of a fluoroquinolone. Food does not slow absorption.

DID YOU KNOW?

In 2001, Cipro and doxycycline were used prophylactically for exposure (inhalation) to the anthrax bacteria (biological weaponry).

PREGNANCY C

HOW SUPPLIED (ORAL PREPARATIONS)

Nonfluorinated quinolone—Nalidixic acid (NegGram): tab

Fluorinated quinolones—Ciprofloxacin HCl (Cipro): tab, oral suspension; Norfloxacin (Noroxin): tab; Enoxacin (Pentrex): tab; Lomefloxacin (Maxaquin): tab; Ofloxacin (floxin): tab; levofloxacin (Levaquin): tab;

sparfloxacin (Zagam): tab; gatifloxacin (Tequin): tab; moxifloxacin (Avelox): tab; trovafloxacin (Trovan): tab

Rapid Dental Hint

The majority of patients taking a quinolone will most likely be taking it for chronic bronchitis. The air polishing system should not be used, since sodium bicarbonate delays absorption of the drug.

Bacteriostatic Antibiotics

Macrolides

ACTIONS Macrolides are usually bacteriostatic, but they may be bactericidal at high doses. Macrolides inhibit the multiplication of bacteria by reversibly binding to the 50S ribosomal subunit of susceptible bacteria and consequently inhibit protein synthesis within the bacterial cell (Figure 7-2). Erythromycin is a type of macrolide. Erythromycins can be used when the patient is allergic to penicillin. Erythromycins are most effective against gram-positive bacteria and some gram-negative strains. Resistance to erythromycin is generally not a problem in short-term therapy. Erythromycin is produced by *Saccharopolyspora erythraea* (Table 7-3).

TABLE 7-3 Macrolide Antibiotics

DRUG	DRUG INTERACTIONS
Erythromycin base (E-Mycin, Eryc, PCE, Ery-tab) Erythromycin estolate (Ilosone) Erythromycin ethylsuccinate (EES, Eryped)	Interacts with the P450 liver cytochrome enzymes, so there are many drug interactions. Reduces metabolism resulting in toxic blood levels of: • Theophylline (for asthma) • Carbamazepine (Tegretol—for trigeminal neuralgia) • Warfarin (anticoagulant) • Triazolam (Halcion; sedative/hypnotic, anti-anxiety) • Simvastatin (Zocor)—antihyperlipidemic (cholesterol-lowering drug) • Cyclosporine (Neoral)—antirejection drug for organ transplant • Avoid: Lovastatin (Mevacor) and Simvastatin (Zocor)—antihyperlipidemic drugs • Bactericidal drugs (penicillin, metronidazole) given concurrently with bacteriostatic may interfere with the actions of the bactericidal drugs
Second-generation macrolides (Azalides) • Azithromycin (Zithromax) • Clarithromycin (Biaxin)	Azithromycin does not interact with the P450 liver cytochrome enzymes. Clarithromycin reduces metabolism resulting in toxic blood levels of: • Theophylline (for asthma) • Carbamazepine (Tegretol—for trigeminal neuralgia) • Warfarin (anticoagulant) • Triazolam (Halcion; sedative/hypnotic, anti-anxiety) • Simvastatin (Zocor)—antihyperlipidemic drug • Cyclosporine (Neoral)—antirejection drug for organ transplant • Avoid: Lovastatin (Mevacor) and Simvastatin (Zocor)—antihyperlipidemic drugs • Bactericidal drugs (penicillin, metronidazole) given concurrently with bacteriostatic may interfere with the actions of the bactericidal drugs

Azalides are second-generation semisynthetic derivates of erythromycin that have a broader spectrum of action with fewer adverse effects than the erythromycins. The two drugs in this classification are azithromycin (Zithromax) and clarithromycin (Biaxin). Dose adjustments should be considered when treating older adults with severe renal impairment.

Azithromycin has several unique features that make it useful in periodontics. It concentrates in phagocytes such as PMNs and macrophages, which contributes to its distribution into inflamed periodontal tissues (gingival connective tissue) in greater amounts than in plasma. In addition, a postantibiotic effect is seen, whereby high antibiotic levels remain after the drug is discontinued. It also has anti-inflammatory effects, and has been used in some lung diseases because of this characteristic.

Rapid Dental Hint

Azithromycin has many unique features that make it popular in the adjunctive treatment of aggressive periodontitis.

PHARMACOKINETICS Erythromycins that are orally administered are absorbed primarily in the duodenum and are widely distributed to most body tissues except the brain. Erythromycin is partly metabolized in the liver and is primarily excreted unchanged via the bile.

Erythromycin base, which is the active form of the drug, is acid-labile and breaks down in stomach acid. To prevent the disintegration or breaking down of the tablet in the stomach, the tablets are coated with a wax or cellulose film (enteric coating). These tablets are referred to as filmtabs. Additionally, the erythromycin base is dispensed as a salt (stearate) or an ester (ethylsuccinate) to decrease irritation caused by acids in the stomach.

INDICATIONS Mild upper and lower respiratory tract infections, pharyngitis, tonsillitis, community-acquired pneumonia, gonorrhea, skin infections, otitis media, acute pelvic inflammatory disease, Legionnaires' disease, Chlamydia infections. Azithromycin is used in the management of aggressive periodontal diseases.

ADVERSE EFFECTS Hepatic (liver) dysfunction (mild elevated liver function tests evident as hepatitis, usually with erythromycin estolate), gastrointestinal disturbances (abdominal pain, diarrhea, nausea, vomiting) but the second-generation macrolides have less.

DRUG INTERACTIONS Erythromycin and clarithromycin have the potential to inhibit drug metabolism in the liver through inactivation of the cytochrome P450 liver enzymes.

1. Erythromycin and clarithromycin are inhibitors of CYP3A4 enzymes. Theophylline, carbamazepine (Tegretol), cyclosporine, phenytoin (Dilantin), lovastatin (Mevacor), and simvastatin (Zocor)—cholesterol-lowering drugs—are metabolized by the CYP3A4 enzymes. Erythromycin or clarithromycin, when taken concurrently with these drugs, significantly decreases their metabolism, resulting in increased blood levels.

2. Antacids may decrease levels of macrolides.

3. Taking a bactericidal antibiotic such as penicillin with a bacteriostatic antibiotic may interfere with the action of the bactericidal antibiotic. Space the dosing of the different antibiotics so they are a few hours apart.

PREGNANCY Erythromycin, B; clarithromycin, C; azithromycin, B; telithromycin, C

HOW SUPPLIED

Erythromycin base (E-mycin, tab; ERYC, cap; Ery-Tab, tab; Ilotycin, tab; PCE, tab)

Erythromycin estolate (Ilsosone): tab, cap

Erythromycin ethylsuccinate (EES): filmtab

Erythromycin stearate (Erythrocin): stearate filmtabs

Azithromycin (Zithromax): tab, oral suspension

Clarithromycin (Biaxin): tab, tab extended release, oral suspension

DENTAL HYGIENE APPLICATIONS Many patients seen in the dental office will be taking a form of erythromycin such as azithromycin (Zithromax) or clarithromycin (Biaxin) for many types of infections, including chronic bronchitis. Since these antibiotics are bacteriostatic at usual doses, care must be taken when deciding on an antibiotic to use for prevention of infective endocarditis. For example, if a patient currently taking azithromycin will be taking amoxicillin for prevention of infective endocarditis, there is a potential drug–drug interaction. In these situations, if concurrent use is appropriate, the bactericidal amoxicillin should be given a few hours before the bacteriostatic drug. Erythromycins may be used for antibiotic premedication in patients allergic to amoxicillin.

Lincomycins

ACTIONS Clindamycin (Cleocin) is a type of lincomycin that inhibits protein synthesis by binding to the 50S ribosomal subunit on the bacteria. It is effective against most gram-positive organisms and gram-negative bacteria; aerobes (oxygen liking) are resistant to it. Clindamycin is primarily bacteriostatic, but can be bactericidal in high doses. Often dental patients will be taking clindamycin for a dental infection such as periodontal abscess or periodontal disease.

INDICATIONS Acute bacterial exacerbation of chronic bronchitis, acute bacterial sinusitis and community-acquired pneumonia, dental infections, and refractory (resistant to treatment) periodontitis (FDA off-label use)

ADVERSE EFFECTS   Pseudomembranous colitis (characterized by severe watery diarrhea or blood in the stools), visual disturbances, liver dysfunction

DRUG INTERACTIONS   No significant drug interactions

CONTRAINDICATIONS   Do not give to patients with Crohn's disease, pseudomembranous enterocolitis, or ulcerative colitis.

PREGNANCY   B

HOW SUPPLIED   Clindamycin HCl (Cleocin): cap

Rapid Dental Hint

Do not give to patients with Crohn's disease, pseudomembranous enterocolitis, or ulcerative colitis.

DENTAL HYGIENE APPLICATIONS   Since the dental patient may be taking clindamycin for a dental abscess or for refractory periodontitis, counseling is important. Many references have notoriously linked clindamycin to pseudomembranous colitis (antibiotic-associated diarrhea). Antibiotic-associated diarrhea can occur with almost any antibiotic, especially if it is broad-spectrum. The patient should observe for changes in bowel frequency and discontinue the antibiotic if there is watery diarrhea. The drug may be taken with food to minimize stomach upset, and a full glass of water to prevent esophagitis. Clindamycin may be used in antibiotic premedication.

Tetracyclines

ACTIONS   Tetracyclines as a group are bacteriostatic and broad spectrum, inhibiting bacterial growth and multiplication by inhibiting protein synthesis at the 30S ribosomal subunit (Table 7-4). Two semisynthetic analogues of tetracycline, doxycycline hyclate and minocycline HCl, are broad-spectrum antibiotics, affecting both gram-positive and gram-negative microorganisms. Doxycycline and minocycline, which are slightly more active than tetracycline, have been used in the treatment of *Aggregatibacter actinomycetemcomitans* infections in localized aggressive periodontitis and refractory periodontitis.

Anticollagenase Feature   Tetracyclines have both antibacterial and nonantibacterial properties. Besides affecting bacterial growth, they also affect the host response by inhibiting the production and secretion of collagenase by cells in the body such as polymorphonuclear leukocytes (PMNs). Collagenase is an enzyme responsible for the destruction of collagen, which makes up the connective tissue of the periodontium. This anticollagenase property does not depend on the drug's antibacterial actions. Doxycycline 20 mg (Periostat) is indicated for generalized chronic periodontitis. The use of doxycycline in 20 mg subantimicrobial doses is also called enzyme-suppression or host modulatory therapy.

Concentration in Gingival Crevicular Fluid   Another property of tetracyclines is their ability to concentrate in the gingival crevicular fluid (GCF) at two to four times blood levels following multiple doses. Doxycycline and minocycline also concentrate in higher levels in the GCF than in serum. Tetracyclines exhibit higher substantivity than other antibiotics, which allows binding to root surfaces with a slow release into the GCF. The binding of tetracyclines to calcium ions in the GCF enhances their substantivity. These properties allow the drug to maintain high therapeutic levels in the GCF. It is advantageous for a drug to concentrate in high levels in the GCF because the GCF bathes the subgingival pocket area where the periodontal pathogens live.

INDICATIONS   Chlamydia genital infections, syphilis, travelers' diarrhea, aggressive periodontitis (off-label use)

ADVERSE EFFECTS   Common adverse effects of tetracyclines include:

- Nausea, vomiting, and diarrhea. Diarrhea results because of changes in bowel flora (bacteria living in GI tract). Superinfection is common after prolonged use, especially with the broad-spectrum antibiotics. To help prevent superinfections, acidophilus in the form of yogurt or gelcaps should be taken to replace the acidophilus that was eliminated with the antibiotic. If yogurt is taken with tetracycline HCl, it must be taken 2 hours after the tetracycline dose because the calcium in the yogurt binds to tetracycline and prevents its absorption.

- Tetracyclines should be taken with a full glass of water to prevent esophagitis and esophageal ulcers and on an empty stomach (1 hour before or 2 hours after meals). This is due to a direct irritation by tetracycline of the esophagus. It must not be taken with milk.

- Doxycycline can cause dizziness. Instruct patient to be careful when upright or getting up from a chair. The patient should not drive for a few hours after taking doxycycline.

- Tetracyclines stain newly formed teeth during enamel deposition and should not be used during the last half of pregnancy or in children up to 8 years of age. A complex is formed with calcium orthophosphate that produces a yellow-gray fluorescent discoloration. Photosensitivity (with doxycycline and tetracycline) results in exaggerated sunburn when patients are exposed to the sun.

- Skin hyperpigmentation occurs with ingestion of minocycline but has not been reported for doxycycline.

TABLE 7-4   Tetracyclines
Tetracycline HCl (Sumycin)
Doxycycline hyclate 20 mg
Doxycycline hyclate (Vibramyin, Doryx)
Minocycline HCl (Minocin)

Rapid Dental Hint

Do not give tetracyclines to pregnant women or children under 8 years of age.

DRUG INTERACTIONS

1. Tetracyclines, except doxycycline and minocycline, should not be taken concomitantly with dairy products because tetracycline binds to calcium, inhibiting its absorption. Tetracycline should be taken on an empty stomach (1 hour before or 2 hours after meals) because food delays its absorption. Doxycycline and minocycline can be taken without regard to meals.

2. Absorption of all tetracyclines into the bloodstream is delayed with antacids containing aluminum and magnesium, as well as products containing iron.

3. Tetracyclines, as well as other antibiotics, interfere with the metabolism of oral contraceptives. Estrogens, a component in oral contraceptives, must be metabolized to active form in the stomach by bacteria. Most antibiotics kill or stop the growth of these bacteria, inhibiting estrogen breakdown. Patients must use other forms of birth control while taking tetracyclines.

4. Tetracyclines, or any other bacteriostatic drug, should not be given together with bactericidal antibiotics such as penicillin, metronidazole, or ciprofloxacin that would interfere with the bactericidal action of that drug.

5. Isolated cases have been reported of increased warfarin effect (bleeding) with tetracyclines.

Rapid Dental Hint

Dairy products should not be taken at the same time with tetracycline (space the dose apart about 1–2 hours), but can be taken with doxycycline.

PREGNANCY D; may cause fetal harm with pregnancy and permanent tooth discoloration during tooth development during the last half of pregnancy.

Rapid Dental Hint

Doxycycline can cause esophageal ulcers, so recommend that your patient take doxycycline with a full glass of water and not to immediately lie down. Doxycycline also causes dizziness.

HOW SUPPLIED

Tetracycline (Sumycin, Achromycin): cap

Doxycycline hyclate (Vibramycin, Vibra-Tabs, Doryx): tab, cap

Doxycycline 20 mg: tab

Minocycline HCl (Minocin): cap

DENTAL HYGIENE APPLICATIONS Some dental patients may be taking a tetracycline for a dental infection, including periodontal disease. The patient should be counseled on how to take the medication and what foods/drugs to avoid while taking it. Tetracyclines should be taken with a full glass of water to prevent esophageal irritation.

Figure 7-3 reviews the prescriptions for common antibiotics used for treating dental infections.

DID YOU KNOW?

Tetracycline stain does not respond well to dental bleaching.

Rapid Dental Hint

It is important to remind patients to take all of the antibiotic even if they are feeling better.

Miscellaneous Antibiotics

Sulfonamides

ACTIONS Sulfonamides are a synthetic analogue of para-aminobenzoic acid (PABA), which inhibits the synthesis of folic acid from PABA in bacteria. These drugs are also referred to as folate antagonists.

INDICATIONS Prophylaxis of recurrent urinary tract infection (UTI) and *Pneumocystis jiroveci* in AIDS patients.

ADVERSE EFFECTS Gastrointestinal irritation (nausea, vomiting, anorexia), skin rashes, glossitis, stomatitis, photosensitivity, allergic skin rashes in AIDS patients, changes in white blood cells. These drugs are contraindicated if an individual has hypersensitivity to sulfonamides.

DRUG INTERACTIONS Increased effects of warfarin

PREGNANCY C

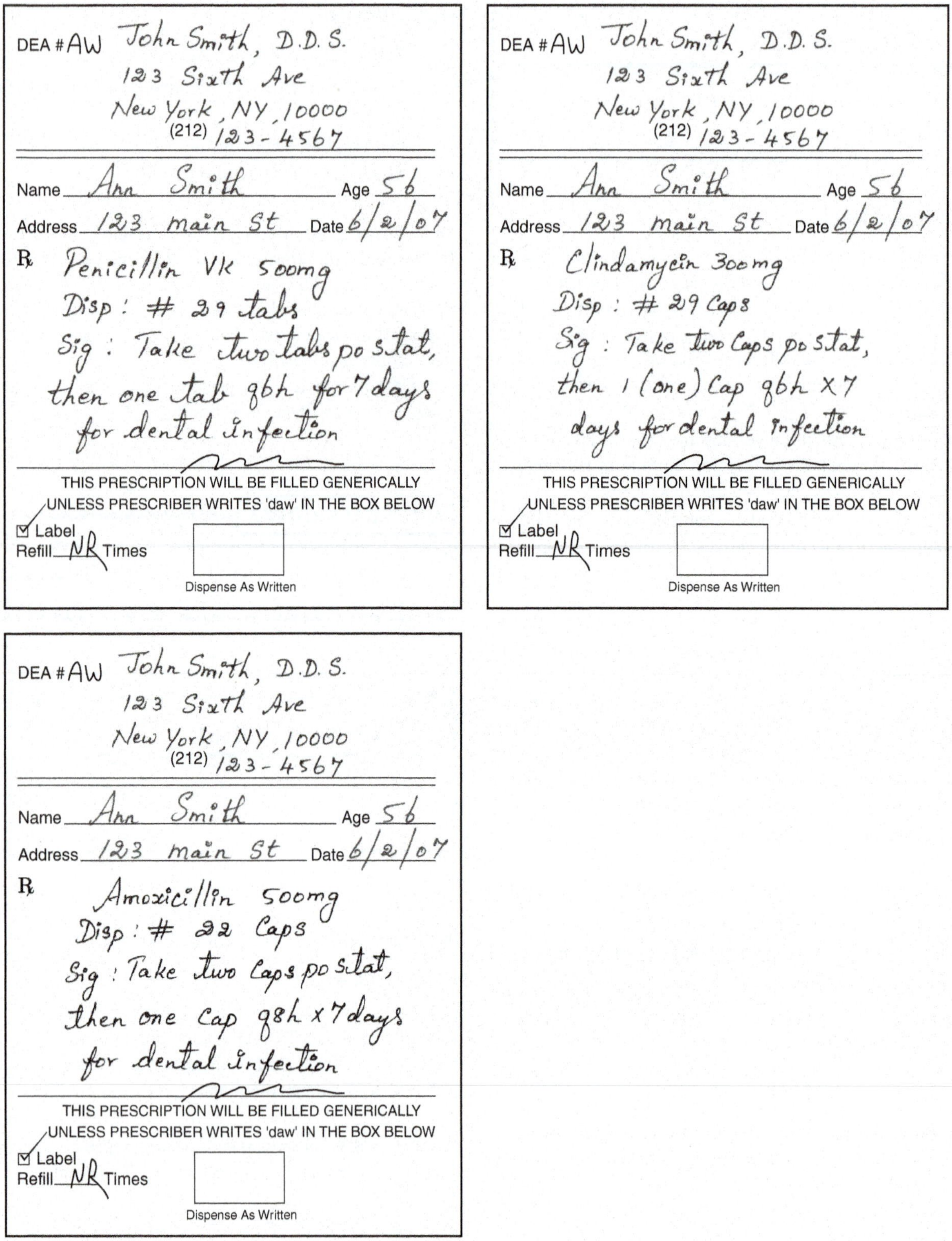

DEA # AW John Smith, D.D.S.
123 Sixth Ave
New York, NY, 10000
(212) 123-4567

Name Ann Smith   Age 56
Address 123 main St   Date 6/2/07

R̸ Penicillin Vk 500mg
Disp: # 29 tabs
Sig: Take two tabs po stat,
then one tab q6h for 7 days
for dental infection

THIS PRESCRIPTION WILL BE FILLED GENERICALLY
UNLESS PRESCRIBER WRITES 'daw' IN THE BOX BELOW
☑ Label
Refill NR Times

Dispense As Written

DEA # AW John Smith, D.D.S.
123 Sixth Ave
New York, NY, 10000
(212) 123-4567

Name Ann Smith   Age 56
Address 123 main St   Date 6/2/07

R̸ Clindamycin 300mg
Disp: # 29 Caps
Sig: Take two Caps po stat,
then 1 (one) Cap q6h X 7
days for dental infection

THIS PRESCRIPTION WILL BE FILLED GENERICALLY
UNLESS PRESCRIBER WRITES 'daw' IN THE BOX BELOW
☑ Label
Refill NR Times

Dispense As Written

DEA # AW John Smith, D.D.S.
123 Sixth Ave
New York, NY, 10000
(212) 123-4567

Name Ann Smith   Age 56
Address 123 main St   Date 6/2/07

R̸ Amoxicillin 500mg
Disp: # 22 Caps
Sig: Take two Caps po stat,
then one Cap q8h X 7 days
for dental infection

THIS PRESCRIPTION WILL BE FILLED GENERICALLY
UNLESS PRESCRIBER WRITES 'daw' IN THE BOX BELOW
☑ Label
Refill NR Times

Dispense As Written

FIGURE 7-3 Sample prescriptions of antibiotics for dental infections.

DEA # AW   John Smith, D.D.S.
123 Sixth Ave
New York, NY, 10000
(212) 123-4567

Name __Ann Smith__   Age __56__

Address __123 main St__ Date __6/2/07__

℞   Augmentin 500 mg

Disp : # 30 tabs

Sig : Take 1 tab q8h

x 10 days for dental

infection

THIS PRESCRIPTION WILL BE FILLED GENERICALLY
UNLESS PRESCRIBER WRITES 'daw' IN THE BOX BELOW
☑ Label
Refill __NR__ Times

Dispense As Written

DEA # AW   John Smith, D.D.S.
123 Sixth Ave
New York, NY, 10000
(212) 123-4567

Name __Ann Smith__   Age __56__

Address __123 main St__ Date __6/2/07__

℞   doxycycline hyclate 100mg

Disp : # 11 tabs

Sig : Take 1 tab q12h on

first day, then one tab

qd until finished

THIS PRESCRIPTION WILL BE FILLED GENERICALLY
UNLESS PRESCRIBER WRITES 'daw' IN THE BOX BELOW
☑ Label
Refill __NR__ Times

Dispense As Written

DEA # AW   John Smith, D.D.S.
123 Sixth Ave
New York, NY, 10000
(212) 123-4567

Name __Ann Smith__   Age __56__

Address __123 main St__ Date __6/2/07__

℞

Zithromax 250 mg

Disp : # 7 tabs

Sig : Take 2 tabs qd x 1 day,

then one tab qd x 5 days

THIS PRESCRIPTION WILL BE FILLED GENERICALLY
UNLESS PRESCRIBER WRITES 'daw' IN THE BOX BELOW
☑ Label
Refill __NR__ Times

Dispense As Written

HOW SUPPLIED

Sulfamethoxazole + trimethoprim (Bactrim): tab

Sulfadiazine (Microsulfon): tab

Sulfamethoxazole (Gantanol): tab

Sulfisoxazole (Gantrisin): suspension, syrup

Trimethoprim (Proloprim): tab

DENTAL HYGIENE NOTES There are no significant dental drug–drug interactions. Patients seen in the dental office taking a sulfonamide are usually taking Bactrim for *P. jiroveci.*

Vancomycin

ACTIONS Vancomycin HCl binds irreversibly to the bacterial cell wall in a manner slightly different from β-lactams (penicillins). It is primarily active against gram-positive bacteria (e.g., *Clostridium difficile*).

INDICATIONS Antibiotic-associated pseudomembranous colitis

ADVERSE EFFECTS Chills, fever, nausea, "red man syndrome" (hot, red rash)

DRUG INTERACTIONS No significant dental drug interactions

PREGNANCY B

HOW SUPPLIED Vancomycin (Vancocin): cap 125, 250 mg; oral suspension; IV

Aminoglycosides

ACTIONS Aminoglycosides have bactericidal activity against gram-negative aerobic bacteria by binding to the interface between the 30S and 50S ribosomal subunits on the bacteria. Anaerobic bacteria are resistant.

INDICATIONS Gram-negative infections: Serious infections of GI, respiratory, and urinary tract; soft tissue (burns) when other less toxic antimicrobial agents are ineffective; ophthalmic (eye) infections. Streptomycin, a type of aminoglycoside, is a secondary drug used in combination with other drugs in the treatment of tuberculosis when other drugs have failed, or there are drug-resistant organisms.

ADVERSE EFFECTS Dizziness, sensation of ringing or fullness in ears, nephrotoxicity (impaired kidney function)

DRUG INTERACTIONS Concurrent use with neuromuscular blocking agents may cause respiratory failure

PREGNANCY C

HOW SUPPLIED Neomycin: Topical for minor infections; gentamicin (Garamycin: inj. ophth., topical); tobramycin (Nebcin; inj. ophth.), amikacin (Amikin; inj.)

Prevention of Infective Endocarditis

Although its incidence is rare, infective endocarditis (IE) is a critical and potentially lethal condition. The older term, subacute

TABLE 7-5 Conditions Recommended for Prophylaxis Antibiotics

1. Artificial heart valves
2. A history of infective endocarditis
3. Certain specific, serious congenital (present from birth) heart conditions, including
   - Unrepaired or incompletely repaired cyanotic congenital heart disease, including those with palliative shunts and conduits.
   - A completely repaired congenital heart defect with prosthetic material or device, whether placed by surgery or by catheter intervention, during the first six months after the procedure.
   - Any repaired congenital heart defect with residual defect at the site or adjacent to the site of a prosthetic patch or a prosthetic device.
4. A cardiac transplant that develops a problem in a heart valve.

bacterial endocarditis (SBE), is no longer used because IE can be caused by microorganisms other than bacteria. The risk of IE associated with dental procedures makes it an important condition for the dental hygienist to be aware of. Equally important is the need for the hygienist to be thoroughly familiar with its causes and prevention. With proper knowledge of what conditions to recognize, which procedures present a risk, and how to premedicate patients at risk, the chances of a dental procedure resulting in IE may be drastically reduced.

Endocarditis most often is an infection of the valves of the heart. The heart valves are made of avascular tissue. In a healthy heart, the cusps of each valve are washed as blood passes over them with each heartbeat. However, when one of the valves is functioning abnormally, the individual may be susceptible to infection. The avascular nature of the valve tissue enables foreign microorganisms to colonize and literally hide from the immune system. Once bacteria have colonized the valve(s), they proliferate and affect the function of the valve(s). The valve affected most often is the mitral valve or bicuspid valve, on the left side of the heart. Some medical conditions create a higher risk of IE than others. In April 2007, the American Heart Association (AHA) changed the guidelines, which were last published in 1997, for patients required to take prophylactic antibiotics. These most recent guidelines are published in *Circulation* (April 23, 2007). The new guidelines are aimed at patients who have the greatest risk of a serious infection if they developed a heart infection. For patients requiring antibiotic prophylaxis, the same antibiotics and dosing as stated in the previous guidelines are to be followed. Table 7-5 lists the patients that are recommended to have antibiotic prophylaxis. Visit www.ada.org for more information. Patients with congenital heart disease can have complicated circumstances and a consultation with their cardiologist may be needed. The article can be accessed from the Infective Endocarditis link on the American Heart Association Web site at www.americanheart.org.

According to the new guidelines, patients who have taken prophylactic antibiotics in the past but no longer need them include patients with:

- Mitral valve prolapse
- Rheumatic heart disease
- Bicuspid valve disease
- Calcified aortic stenosis
- Congenital heart conditions such as ventricular septal defect, atrial septal defect, and hypertrophic cardiomyopathy.

Other conditions possibly requiring premedication prior to invasive dental treatment include (Lockart PB, Loven B, Brennan MT, Fox PC. 2007. The evidence base for the efficacy of antibiotic prophylaxis in dental practice. *JADA* 138(4):458–474.):

- Hemophilia
- Renal transplants/dialysis
- Shunts
- Immunosuppression secondary to cancer and cancer chemotherapy
- Systemic lupus erythematosus

Bacteremia may be caused by many different dental procedures, but it is important to take into account all conditions that may give rise to bacteria in the bloodstream (bacteremia). Bacteremia has been associated with poor oral hygiene and periodontal or periapical infections. The incidence and magnitude of bacteremia are directly proportional to the degree of oral inflammation and infection. It is essential for patients at risk for endocarditis to establish and maintain the best possible oral health. This is maintained through regular professional care, as well as routine home care. Table 7-6 represents the dental procedures for which prophylaxis is recommended and those for which it is not recommended.

The antibiotic regimen has not changed. Antibiotics for prophylaxis should be administered in a single dose, 30–60 minutes before the procedure. If the dosage of antibiotic is inadvertently not administered before the procedure, the dosage may be administered up to 2 hours after the procedure. The recommendations in Table 7-6 are guidelines, and are not a substitute for good clinical judgment. If it is suspected that a patient will bleed during any dental procedure, it is advisable to pretreat with a prophylactic antibiotic. Patients who have not been pretreated and those who are currently taking antibiotics for other reasons will be discussed later in more detail. It is important to note that

it is not acceptable to pretreat every patient, since prolonged use or misuse of antibiotics may lead to drug resistance. Furthermore, although it can significantly reduce the risk, antibiotic prophylaxis does not eliminate the risk of endocarditis. Clinical judgment is always necessary to evaluate each patient's risk, and close attention should be paid to the patient when risk is suspected. In the future, antibiotic prophylaxis may be eliminated.

Table 7-7 indicates recommended prophylactic antibiotic regimens for oral and dental procedures. The regimens are most effective when given around the time of dental treatment in doses that allow for adequate levels of the drug in the serum before, during, and after the procedure. In order to reduce the development of antibiotic resistance and maintain minimum serum levels for prophylaxis, the regimens are designed to give the patient adequate serum levels of the drug no longer than necessary.

The bacterium most commonly associated with endocarditis following dental and oral procedures is *Streptococcus viridans* (α-hemolytic streptococci). Amoxicillin remains the most recommended antibiotic for endocarditis prophylaxis. Agents such as ampicillin and penicillin V have an equal antimicrobial effect against these *α-hemolytic streptococci*, but amoxicillin is better absorbed in the gastrointestinal tract and provides higher, more sustained serum levels than the other penicillins.

Until 1994, the recommended adult pretreatment dose of amoxicillin for antibiotic prophylaxis was 3.0 g. However, a recent study has indicated that 2.0 g is sufficient to reach adequate serum levels for several hours. Previously, it was recommended that a second dose be given postoperatively. Currently, it has been demonstrated that not only will the initial dose of amoxicillin remain above the minimal serum level for long enough following the procedure, but the inhibitory effect of the drug is sufficient to eliminate the need for a postoperative dose.

Erythromycin, which was originally approved as an effective prophylactic agent for endocarditis in cases of penicillin allergy, is no longer among the recommended agents. Erythromycin can cause severe gastrointestinal upset, and certain formulations (e.g., erythromycin ethylsuccinate) have complicated pharmacokinetics. Instead, second-generation erythromycins, azithromycin, or clarithromycin can be used because

TABLE 7-6 Antibiotic Prophylaxis Recommendations for Dental Procedures	
HIGHER INCIDENCE	**LOWER INCIDENCE**
• Dental extractions	• Restorative dentistry (operative and prosthodontic)
• Periodontal procedures: surgery, scaling and root planing, probing and recall maintenance	• Local anesthetic injections (all except intraligamentary)
• Implant placement and reimplantation of avulsed teeth	• Placement of rubber dams
• Root canal instrumentation when beyond apex (endodontics)	• Postoperative suture removal
• Subgingival placement of antibiotic fibers or strips	• Placement of removable prosthodontic/orthodontic appliances
• Placement of orthodontic bands (not brackets)	• Taking oral impressions or radiographs
• Intraligamentary local anesthesia injection	• Fluoride treatment
• Prophylactic cleaning of teeth and implants	

		REGIMEN (TO BE TAKEN 30–60 MIN
SITUATION	DRUG	BEFORE DENTAL PROCEDURE)
Oral	Amoxicillin	Adults: 2.0 g / children: 50 mg/kg
Unable to take oral medications	Ampicillin	Adults: 2.0 g IM or IV/ children: 50 mg/kg IM or IV
	or	
	Cefazolin, or ceftriaxone*	Adults: 1 g IM or IV/ children: 50 mg/kg
Allergic to penicillins or ampicillin—oral	Cephalexin*	Adults: 2 g / children: 50 mg/kg
	or	
	Clindamycin	Adults: 600 mg / children: 20 mg/kg
	or	
	Azithromycin or clarithromycin	Adults: 500 mg / children: 15 mg/kg
Allergic to pencillins or ampicillin and unable to take oral medications	Cefazolin or ceftriaxone*	Adults: 1 g IM or IV/ children: 50 mg/kg IM or IV.
	or	
	Clindamycin	Adults: 600 mg IM or IV/ children: 20 mg/kg IM or IV

TABLE 7-7   Prophylactic Antibiotic Regimens for Oral and Dental Procedures

*Cephalosporins should not be given to an individual with a history of anaphylaxis, angioedema, or urticaria with penicillins or ampicillin.

they have better absorption and produce much less gastrointestinal upset.

Periodically, patients will present to the dental office for a routine visit during a course of antibiotic therapy with a drug used for endocarditis prophylaxis. Patients receiving antibiotics for other reasons at the time of a routine dental visit who are considered at risk for endocarditis have specific recommendations. Rather than increasing the dose of the drug currently being used, it is advisable to select an agent from a different class of antibiotic. Remember, if you have to choose another antibiotic, it must have the same bactericidal or bacteriostatic activity as the antibiotic taken for prophylaxis. For instance, if the patient is taking tetracycline (a bacteriostatic drug), he or she cannot take amoxicillin (a bactericidal antibiotic), but can take clindamycin, azithromycin, or clarithromycin, all bacteriostatic. If possible, the dental procedure is best postponed until at least 9–14 days after completion of the antibiotic. This will allow the normal oral flora to re-establish.

Since repeated use of antibiotics can lead to the emergence of antibiotic-resistant microorganisms in the oral cavity, it is recommended that there be an interval of at least 7 days between dental appointments.

Specific cardiac surgical procedures have varied implications in terms of risk for endocarditis. There is no evidence to suggest that coronary artery bypass surgery introduces risk for endocarditis (see Table 7-5). In the case of prosthetic valve placement, the risk of postoperative endocarditis increases. There is no evidence to suggest that heart transplant patients are at risk for endocarditis, but such patients are subject to an increased likelihood of valve dysfunction and are often treated as moderate-risk patients. Whenever possible, patients who plan to have any cardiac surgery should have a carefully executed dental treatment plan in order to complete any dental work necessary before the cardiac procedure. This may decrease the chance of late postoperative endocarditis.

Rapid Dental Hint

Patients with a total joint replacement need to take antibiotic prophylaxis for their lifetime.

Patients who have joint replacement surgery are at risk for developing infections of the implanted joints. Bacteria can enter the bloodstream and attach to implanted joints, causing an infection at the prosthetic joint. In 2003, the American Academy of Orthopedic Surgeons (AAOS) and the American Dental Association Advisory Statement recommended antibiotic prophylaxis for all patients within the first 2 years after total joint replacement surgery only. After 2 years, the recommendation for antibiotic prophylaxis was limited to high-risk or medically compromised/immunosuppressed patients that might place them at increased risk for total joint infection. In 2009, recommendations for antibiotic prophylaxis were updated by the AAOS. The AAOS recommends that clinicians consider antibiotic prophylaxis of all total joint replacement patients prior to any invasive procedure that may cause bacteremia. The patients should be taking antibiotic prophylaxis for their lifetime. The guidelines are available at www.aaos.org/about/papers/advistmt/1033.asp. There is some controversy regarding the 2009 guidelines. A recent article suggests that the 2009 guidelines should not replace the 2003 guidelines until further review (Little JW, Jacobson JJ, Lockhart PB. 2010. The dental treatment of patients with joint replacements. *JADA* 141(6):667-671). *It is advisable to obtain a medical consult from the patient's orthopedic surgeon.*

Table 7-8 lists recommendations for antibiotic prophylaxis in these patients. Figure 7-4 reviews the prescriptions for each of these antibiotics.

TABLE 7-8   Suggested Antibiotic Prophylaxis Regimens in Patients at Potential Increased Risk of Hematogenous Total Joint Infection

SITUATION	DRUG	REGIMEN
Standard general prophylaxis	Cephalexin or amoxicillin	2 g orally 1 h before dental procedure
Patients unable to take oral medications	Cefazolin or ampicillin	1 g IM or IV 1 h before procedure
		2 g IM or IV 1 h before procedure
Allergic to penicillin	Clindamycin	600 mg orally 1 h before procedure
Allergic to penicillin and unable to take oral medications	Clindamycin	600 mg IV 1 h before procedure

Dental Hygiene Applications

Although the majority of dental cases are treated empirically with antibiotics that the clinician has used before with good results, the concept of culture and sensitivity should be stressed. Occasionally, a patient with persistent periodontal disease who has been to many dentists and has chronically taken many different antibiotics may come to your office. In these cases, if oral hygiene is adequate, then it is more than likely necessary to culture the patient's subgingival biofilms (plaque) because there may be antibiotic resistance, since the patient is on chronic antibiotics.

Antibacterial Agents: Topical

Local delivery of antimicrobial agents is either by topical application or by controlled-release devices.

Topical application distributes the agent or drug to an exposed surface such as the teeth and gingiva. The most common route for the supragingival topical delivery of antimicrobial agents is by a mouthrinse, a dentifrice, or an oral irrigator. Subgingival topical delivery of antimicrobial agents is by oral irrigation or the use of controlled-release devices.

Controlled-release delivery devices are placed directly into the periodontal pocket and are designed to release a drug slowly over 24 hours for prolonged drug action. Antimicrobials are delivered into the periodontal pocket by gels, chips, powders, ointments, acrylic strips, or collagen films.

Oral Rinses

Mouthrinses generally are divided into two classifications: therapeutic rinses, used to treat diseases such as gingival diseases, and cosmetic rinses, used to freshen the breath. Indications for using oral rinses are as follows:

1. An addition to home care regimens that have failed to achieve plaque-control goals by other means
2. An addition to periodontal instrumentation
3. When oral hygiene may be inadequate or difficult to accomplish, as in the physically or mentally compromised
4. Following surgical procedures, when brushing and flossing are generally not practical
5. For maintenance of dental implants

Topical antimicrobial agents delivered by a rinse are effective only against supragingival bacteria; no antimicrobial rinse has been shown to be effective against periodontitis because oral rinses do not reach the subgingival area. Mouthrinses may be discontinued if oral health conditions can be maintained without their use.

ANTIPLAQUE/ANTIGINGIVITIS AGENTS   Antimicrobial agents ideally should inhibit microbial colonization on tooth surfaces and prevent the subsequent formation of plaque. They also should eliminate or suppress the pathogenicity of existing plaque. Antiseptics have a greater potential to prevent the formation of plaque than to resolve established plaque and gingivitis.

An antimicrobial agent relies on two factors for efficacy: the amount of time the agent stays in contact with the target site, and how well the agent gains access to the target site. Substantivity involves the ability of the drug to stay at the target site for longer periods of time, maintaining therapeutic levels. It is ideal to have a drug with high substantivity that will be bound in the oral cavity and released over a period of hours in order to prolong its effects. Lack of substantivity can be overcome by more frequent use of the agent, but this would likely result in noncompliance and undesirable side effects.

CLASSIFICATION OF ORAL RINSES   Topical antimicrobial oral rinses can be classified as either first- or second-generation agents (Table 7-9). First-generation agents have antibacterial properties with low substantivity and limited therapeutic value in reducing plaque and gingivitis. Examples include phenolic compounds, quaternary ammonium compounds, and peroxide. Second-generation agents have antibacterial properties in addition to substantivity. Chlorhexidine gluconate is an example of a second-generation agent and is currently the only such agent proven to prevent and control gingivitis. It is available in the United States only by a prescription. All first-generation mouthrinses are available without a prescription.

In 1986, the American Dental Association (ADA) established guidelines for evaluation of the therapeutic effectiveness of products against gingivitis. For example, studies should be conducted over a minimum of 6 months, two studies with independent investigators should be conducted, and the

TABLE 7-9   Antimicrobial Mouthrinses

- Chlorhexidine gluconate 0.12% (Peridex, Periogard)
- Phenolic compounds (Listerine)
- Cetylpyridiunium (Scope, Cepacol)
- Oxygenating agents (Glyoxide)

DEA # AW John Smith, D.D.S.
123 Sixth Ave
New York, NY, 10000
(212) 123-4567

Name _John Smith_ Age _36_
Address _123 1st Ave_ Date ____

℞ Amoxicillin 500 mg
Disp: # 4 Caps
Sig: Take four Caps po
30 min to 60 min before
dental procedure

THIS PRESCRIPTION WILL BE FILLED GENERICALLY
UNLESS PRESCRIBER WRITES 'daw' IN THE BOX BELOW
☑ Label
Refill _NR_ Times

Dispense As Written

DEA # AW John Smith, D.D.S.
123 Sixth Ave
New York, NY, 10000
(212) 123-4567

Name _Ann Smith_ Age _56_
Address _123 main St_ Date _6/2/07_

℞ Clindamycin 300 mg
Disp: # 2 (two) Caps
Sig: Take two caps
30 min to 60 min
before dental procedure

THIS PRESCRIPTION WILL BE FILLED GENERICALLY
UNLESS PRESCRIBER WRITES 'daw' IN THE BOX BELOW
☑ Label
Refill _NR_ Times

Dispense As Written

DEA # AW John Smith, D.D.S.
123 Sixth Ave
New York, NY, 10000
(212) 123-4567

Name _Ann Smith_ Age _56_
Address _123 main St_ Date _6/2/07_

℞ Clarithromycin 250 mg
Disp: # 2 (two) tabs
Sig: Take two tabs 30 min to
60 min before dental procedure

THIS PRESCRIPTION WILL BE FILLED GENERICALLY
UNLESS PRESCRIBER WRITES 'daw' IN THE BOX BELOW
☑ Label
Refill _NR_ Times

Dispense As Written

DEA # AW John Smith, D.D.S.
123 Sixth Ave
New York, NY, 10000
(212) 123-4567

Name _Ann Smith_ Age _56_
Address _123 main St_ Date _6/2/07_

℞ Azithromycin 250 mg
Disp: # 2 (two) Caps
Sig: Take two Caps
30 min to 60 min
before dental procedure

THIS PRESCRIPTION WILL BE FILLED GENERICALLY
UNLESS PRESCRIBER WRITES 'daw' IN THE BOX BELOW
☑ Label
Refill _NR_ Times

Dispense As Written

FIGURE 7-4 Sample prescriptions of antibiotics for prophylaxis against infective endocarditis.

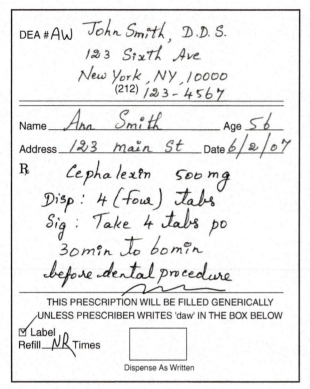

FIGURE 7-4 (*Continued*)

active product should be used as part of a normal regimen and compared with a placebo or control product.

Rapid Dental Hint

Remember to tell patients taking chlorhexidine oral rinse that there will be staining of teeth and not to brush directly before or after rinsing; wait 30 minutes.

Most mouthrinses contain alcohol as a flavor enhancer and as a vehicle for the active ingredients. There has been some concern about the association of alcohol in mouthrinses with oral cancer. Studies have yielded inconsistent findings. Some studies document that there is no reason for patients to refrain from use of alcohol-containing mouthrinses, while research from the National Cancer Institute has drawn an association between alcoholic mouthrinse to mouth and throat cancers. In vitro (laboratory) studies of acetaldehyde, a toxic compound produced by alcohol metabolism, showed that acetaldehyde caused changes in gingival fibroblasts (cells involved in oral connective tissue maintenance).

BISBIGUANIDES

Description and Mechanism of Action Chlorhexidine gluconate (Peridex, PerioGard) is a cationic (positively charged) molecule. Originally, chlorhexidine was used in medicine as an antiseptic cream for wounds, as a preoperative skin cleanser, and as a surgical scrub. In 1970, the first study on the ability of chlorhexidine

to inhibit the formation of plaque and maintain soft tissue health was released. It was not until 1986 that chlorhexidine became available in the United States by prescription at a 0.12% concentration with an alcohol concentration of 11.6%. It has the ADA seal of acceptance for the treatment of gingivitis.

After rinsing, chlorhexidine (positively charged) is attracted to and attaches to the negatively charged bacterial cell walls, causing lysis or breakage of the cell wall. The contents of the cells leak out. Chlorhexidine enters the cell through the opening, resulting in death of the bacteria. By binding to the pellicle on the tooth surface, chlorhexidine inhibits plaque attachment. Chlorhexidine exhibits substantivity, with approximately 30% of the drug binding to oral tissues and the plaque on the teeth, and showing antimicrobial activity for 8–12 hours afterward.

Indications Rinsing with chlorhexidine is indicated before, during, and after periodontal debridement to reduce plaque levels and gingival inflammation. Chlorhexidine rinses can improve wound healing and provide better plaque control after periodontal surgery when brushing and flossing is not feasible. Rinsing with chlorhexidine has been shown to decrease the severity of mucositis in patients receiving chemotherapy. Since peri-implantitis is similar to gingivitis, rinsing with chlorhexidine may be effective in implant plaque control.

Usage It is recommended to rinse twice a day for 30 seconds. The positive charge of chlorhexidine causes it to bind to the negatively charged molecules in toothpastes such as fluorides and sodium lauryl sulfate (a detergent), and thus inactivates them. Therefore, it is best to rinse either 30 minutes before or after toothbrushing or rinse very well with water after toothbrushing. Because of this inactivation of anionic compounds, chlorhexidine is not available in toothpaste. Chlorhexidine can be used as an irrigant, but it is usually diluted with water to reduce the incidence of staining. A sample prescription is shown in Figure 7-5.

Adverse Effects Chlorhexidine is relatively safe because it is poorly absorbed from the oral membranes and systemic circulation. The most common adverse side effect is a yellow, brownish extrinsic staining of the teeth, tongue, and restorations within the first few days of use. Staining is more frequent with chlorhexidine than with other agents because of its affinity for oral surfaces. The staining may be associated with food dyes found within certain foods and beverages. This staining is not permanent and can be removed mechanically during professional prophylaxis (stains may not be removed from pits of composite restorations). If the patient is compliant with oral home care, the staining is more likely on proximal tooth surfaces than facial or lingual surfaces. Other adverse side effects include a temporarily impaired taste perception and increased supragingival calculus formation.

PHENOLIC COMPOUNDS Listerine is a combination of phenolic compounds or essential oils, including thymol, eucalyptol, menthol, and methyl salicylate, in an alcohol vehicle. The mechanism of action is cell wall disruption, resulting in leakage of intracellular components and lysis of the cell. The original-formula Listerine contains 26.9% alcohol, whereas the Cool Mint, Fresh Burst Listerine, and Natural Citrus contain 21.6% alcohol.

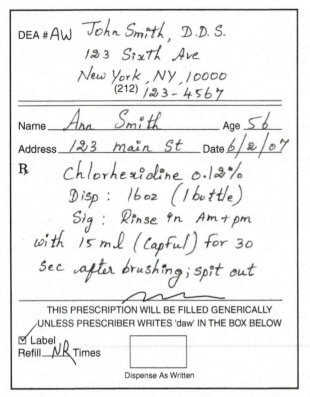

DEA # AW   John Smith, D.D.S.
            123 Sixth Ave
            New York, NY 10000
            (212) 123-4567

Name ___Ann Smith___ Age _56_

Address _123 main St_ Date _6/2/07_

℞

Chlorhexidine 0.12%
    Disp: 16oz (1 bottle)
    Sig: Rinse in Am + pm
with 15 ml (Capful) for 30
Sec after brushing; spit out

THIS PRESCRIPTION WILL BE FILLED GENERICALLY
UNLESS PRESCRIBER WRITES 'daw' IN THE BOX BELOW

☑ Label
Refill _NR_ Times

Dispense As Written

FIGURE 7-5 Sample prescription for chlorhexidine.

Because of low substantivity, effectiveness is strongly related to the duration of tooth contact. Clinical studies have shown that this product significantly reduces plaque development in patients with minimal plaque levels. Listerine has been documented to reduce plaque and gingivitis from 20 to 34%; the subjects had preexisting plaque and gingivitis, and no prophylaxis was performed at the beginning of the study.

Recommendations are to rinse for 30 seconds with 2/3 ounces, once in the morning and once at night. Possible adverse side effects include a burning sensation and bitter taste.

QUATERNARY AMMONIUM COMPOUNDS Quaternary ammonium compounds are positively charged (cationic) compounds similar to chlorhexidine. They readily bind to oral surfaces and are released more rapidly or lose their activity on binding to the surface. Substantivity is only approximately 3 hours. An increase in bacterial cell wall permeability leads to cell lysis and decreased attachment of bacteria to tooth surfaces. Cetylpyridinium chloride is the active ingredient in Scope Original and Cepacol. The alcohol concentration is 14% for Cepacol and 18.9% for Scope Original.

Clinical data on plaque reduction and gingivitis control have been relatively inconclusive because of variability in results between studies. Following an initial professional prophylaxis and suspension of all oral hygiene, chlorhexidine was found to be superior to cetylpyridinium in the reduction of plaque. Cetylpyridinium chloride may have some antiplaque action but less effect on gingivitis when used as an adjunct to conventional oral home care. Lack of substantivity limits clinical efficacy. As with chlorhexidine, to obtain the maximum effect, the patient

should rinse very well or wait 30 minutes after brushing with a dentifrice before using the rinse. Adverse side effects are similar to those of chlorhexidine, including some staining, calculus formation, and mucosal ulceration.

OXYGENATING AGENTS Oxygenating agents such as peroxides and perborates have been used in mouthrinse formulations primarily for inflammation of the gingival soft tissues. Since hydrogen peroxide liberates gaseous oxygen, it provides a cleansing action and gentle effervescence for oral wounds. However, peroxide has minimal antimicrobial action against anaerobic microorganisms. The Food and Drug Administration has approved its use as a temporary debriding agent in the oral cavity. However, antiplaque/antigingivitis claims are not well supported.

Long-term use of 3% hydrogen peroxide has resulted in gingival irritation, delayed tissue healing, and black hairy tongue, so it is not advocated to be used as an oral agent. Long-term studies do not demonstrate any additional benefit over regular home carer. Because many patients use hydrogen peroxide on a regular basis, the dental hygienist should question patients about their oral home care practices.

POVIDONE-IODINE Povidone-iodine is antibacterial and antiseptic. Its primary use is in the prevention and treatment of surface infections. Often povidone-iodine is combined with hydrogen peroxide as a subgingival irrigant for the reduction of gram-negative microorganisms. Most studies confirm that iodine may be a beneficial adjunctive treatment for the prevention and control of gingivitis when used with optimal oral hygiene self-care procedures; however, iodine can stain teeth, clothing, skin, and restorations.

FLUORIDES Fluorides have been used in dentistry primarily for prevention of dental caries by reducing demineralization and enhancing remineralization. Fluoride rinses have not been proven clinically to prevent root caries. Fluoride's role as an antiplaque/antigingivitis agent is less well documented and shows controversial results.

PREBRUSHING RINSES Plax, a prebrushing rinse, contains surfactants such as sodium lauryl sulfate (which functions as a detergent to help loosen and remove plaque), sodium benzoate (a preservative), and tetrasodium pyrophosphate (an anticalculus agent). Studies have shown limited beneficial effects of this agent over rinsing with water alone (Grossman 1988).

ALCOHOL-FREE MOUTHRINSES Most mouthrinses contain alcohol as a vehicle to carry other ingredients and as a flavor enhancer. The form of alcohol in the rinse is either ethanol (ethyl alcohol) or a specially denatured (SD) alcohol that is made synthetically. Alcohol can cause drying of the oral mucosal tissues, especially when the agent is used for extended periods of time. Indications for a nonalcoholic mouthrinse include pregnant women, former alcoholics, patients who are taking medications that would additionally dry the mouth, patients taking metronidazole, and patients who prefer to avoid alcohol.

Alcohol-free mouthrinses include:

GUM® Chlorhexidine 0.12% alcohol-free rinse

Crest Pro-Health Rinse

Rembrandt

Listerine Zero

Oral B Plaque Rinse

Listermint

BreathRX

Controlled (Sustained)-Release Drug Delivery

The development of site-specific, controlled (sustained)-release delivery systems has provided a further option for antimicrobial therapy by allowing therapeutic levels of a drug to be maintained in the periodontal pocket for prolonged periods of time. If the drug is released from the device past 24 hours, it is called a controlled-release device; if the drug is released within 24 hours, it is called a sustained-release device. Many devices are available in the United States and Europe that incorporate an antimicrobial agent into a specific material (a polymer) that is placed into the periodontal pocket. The active ingredient is then released from the material, which subsequently exerts its antibacterial activity on subgingival bacteria over several days. Then the material is absorbed (dissolves). The concentration of antimicrobials administered in a controlled (sustained)-release device does not enter the bloodstream and thus does not trigger adverse side effects. Types of materials used to incorporate antimicrobial drugs include gels, chips, collagen film, and acrylic strips. Controlled-release drug therapy is used as an adjunct to periodontal debridement and should not replace conventional mechanical therapy. In fact, the American Academy of Periodontology reported that it "would be premature to conclude that insertion of sustained-release antimicrobial systems is as effective as scaling and root planing in all populations of patients." Controlled-release antimicrobial systems are indicated for use in recurrent pockets of 5 mm or greater that continue to bleed on probing. The intended results with these devices are gains in clinical attachment levels and reductions in probing depths and bleeding on probing.

Currently in the United States, PerioChip, Atridox, and Arestin are available commercially (Table 7-10). Other controlled-release systems are available in Europe that are not approved for use in the United States.

Resorbable Controlled (Sustained)-Release Devices

CHLORHEXIDINE GLUCONATE CHIP The PerioChip is a gelatin matrix (bovine origin) containing 2.5 mg of chlorhexidine gluconate. This product received Food and Drug Administration

approval in June 1998. PerioChip is indicated for use as an adjunct to instrumentation in maintenance patients with pockets 5 mm or larger that bleed recurrently on probing. A clinical study comparing the efficacy of periodontal debridement alone with that of periodontal debridement plus PerioChip revealed statistically significant reductions in probing depth and gains in clinical attachment in the periodontal debridement plus PerioChip group. However, the magnitude of these changes was small (0.3 mm), so the results are not clinically significant. In this study, mechanical debridement was limited to only 1 hour in patients with moderately advanced periodontitis (5- to 8-mm pockets), which does not seem realistic.

After periodontal debridement, the chip is placed into the periodontal pocket. In contact with subgingival fluids it becomes sticky and binds to the epithelium lining the pocket, so no periodontal dressing is indicated. Its antibacterial action occurs when chlorhexidine is released over 7–10 days, after which it resorbs and does not have to be removed. Up to eight chips can be inserted into pockets in one visit. Another round of treatment can be done at 3 months.

DOXYCYCLINE HYCLATE GEL Atridox is composed of 10% (42.5 mg) doxycycline hyclate in a gel formulation that is biodegradable and subsequently will reabsorb. The ingredients are available in two syringes (powder and liquid) that are mixed together and injected into the pocket around the entire tooth. The gel form allows for ease of flow, readily adapting to subgingival root morphology. When the gel comes in contact with gingival fluid in the pocket, it solidifies to a wax-like substance.

Atridox is indicated as an adjunct to scaling and root planing procedures in patients with chronic periodontitis. Local anesthesia is not required. Results of therapy are to promote attachment level gain, to reduce pocket depths, and to reduce bleeding on probing. Atridox may also be used in patients who refuse to have periodontal debridement or periodontal surgery, and who are medically, physically, or emotionally compromised.

Levels of doxycycline in the pocket peaked at 2 hours after placement into the pocket, and effective drug levels were maintained at 28 days, although within a few days levels of doxycycline had peaked.

MINOCYCLINE HYDROCHLORIDE MICROSPHERES The most recent FDA-approved sustained-release device is Arestin. Arestin is a sustained-release product containing the antibiotic minocycline hydrochloride. Minocycline is a type of tetracycline but it is longer acting over a broader spectrum of antibiotic activity. Each cartridge of Arestin contains 1 mg of minocycline. Arestin is indicated as an adjunct to scaling and root planing procedures for the reduction of pocket depth in patients with chronic localized periodontitis. Studies have shown that scaling and root planing followed by the application of Arestin resulted in a greater

---

TABLE 7-10 Controlled-Release Antimicrobial Drugs Used in Dentistry

- Arestin (microspheres of minocycline HCl)
- Atridox (10% doxycycline hyclate)
- PerioChip (2.5 mg chlorhexidine gluconate)

Rapid Dental Hint

If a patient is allergic to tetracycline *do not* use Atridox or Arestin.

percentage of reduction in pocket depths (greater than or equal to 2mm) at 9 months compared to scaling and root planing alone.

Dental Hygiene Applications

When using locally applied Arestin or Atridox on selective periodontal patients, the same judgments concerning drug interactions, adverse side effects, and contraindications must be used as if these products were systemically applied. These products are an analogue of tetracycline, and as such, should not be given to pregnant women or children under 8 years of age. Additionally, one must be careful about interactions with oral contraceptives.

Alcohol-containing mouthrinses including Peridex, Periogard, and Listerine should not be used in a patient taking metronidazole (Flagyl). A severe disulfiram-like reaction occurs with nausea, vomiting, flushing, and faintness.

Key Points

- Indiscriminate use of antibiotics causes bacterial resistance to the antibiotic, whereby the antibiotic becomes ineffective in killing that bacteria.
- Bactericidal antibiotics kill the bacteria.
- Bacteriostatic antibiotics stop the growing and multiplication of the bacteria.
- Stomach problems (e.g., diarrhea) are an adverse side effect of most antibiotics; instruct the patient to take acidophilus tablets with the antibiotic.
- Most dental infections do not require broad-spectrum antibiotics.
- Chronic periodontitis does not need antibiotics as part of the treatment.
- Antibiotics primarily used in dentistry are penicillin V, amoxicillin, azithromycin, metronidazole, tetracyclines, and clindamycin.
- Many drug interactions are associated with antibiotics; review the patient's medical history and ask questions.
- Bactericidal and bacteriostatic antibiotics should not be given concurrently.
- Placement of controlled-delivery antimicrobials into the pocket: doxycycline (Atridox) and minocycline (Arestin)
- The same adverse effects, drug interactions, and contraindications that are documented with systemic antibiotics as seen with controlled-release antibiotics.

Tuberculosis

In 1993, the World Health Organization declared **tuberculosis** (TB) a worldwide emergency. Tuberculosis affects all mammals, with the most common form in humans being pulmonary tuberculosis. About 9 million people are estimated to be infected or will develop active TB disease this year.

Tuberculosis is a bacterial infection caused by *Mycobacterium tuberculosis*, a tubercle bacillus (MTB). Its name indicates its formation of firm nodules (tubercles) throughout the body. The microorganism is inhaled into the lungs through aerosol droplets from coughing, sneezing, or similar close contact with an infected individual. MTB can remain aerosolized for 8 hours. MTB is slow growing, with an optimum growing temperature of 37 degrees centigrade, which is body temperature. An individual may be "exposed" to MTB, but not clinically show signs of the disease because of the body's defense mechanism. However, inactive tubercle bacilli in the body may be activated, resulting in active TB under favorable conditions such as malnutrition, disease (diabetes mellitus, HIV/AIDS), corticosteroid or other immunosuppressive therapy, or chronic alcoholism.

About 4–6 weeks after the first contact with the infection, symptoms may develop, including fever, chills, gastrointestinal upset, and night sweats. Symptoms that develop later (active TB) include weight loss (anorexia), nausea, vomiting, night headaches, and palpitations (chest pain). A productive cough producing odorless, green-yellow sputum with blood (hemoptysis) is a feature of TB.

Testing for Tuberculosis

Screening of tuberculosis is done using the tuberculin skin test, which only indicates exposure to infection and does not differentiate between infection (presence of organisms, normal chest X-ray, no symptoms) and disease. An individual will give a positive tuberculin test about 4–6 weeks after inhaling enough organisms. The tuberculin skin test is based on a skin reaction to the intradermal injection of purified protein derivative (PPD) tuberculin, a protein fraction of TB. A positive reaction (48–72 hours after injection) causes local raised swelling and induration. The PPD test is the gold standard to detect the presence of TB.

An individual with a positive skin test (PPD+) should have a chest X-ray taken. A definitive diagnosis of TB requires sputum culture. However, typical signs and symptoms, with the typical findings on chest radiograph with a positive PPD, are enough to begin therapy.

In recent years, different assays have been developed that reduce reader variability and false readings. The FDA recently approved a whole-blood interferon-release assay. Studies are needed to determine whether the responses from this test are predicative of those who have a high risk of progression to active TB.

The Centers for Disease Control and Prevention have recommended a new, more accurate blood test for tuberculosis that yields fewer false positives. QuantiFERON-TB is a blood test that may replace the skin test in the future.

> **DID YOU KNOW?**
>
> John Henry "Doc" Holliday of Old West fame was trained as a dentist in Georgia in the 1880s. He contracted tuberculosis and could not practice dentistry. He moved to Texas, where he started to gamble and engage in gunfights, which made him very famous. On the run for many years, he died of tuberculosis in 1887 in Glenwood Springs, Colorado.

Pharmacology: Treatment of TB Infection

Drugs are available to treat the disease, but unfortunately many patients are noncompliant with the long-term regimens (6–9 months) necessary. This has led to an increase in multidrug-resistant bacterial strains, which make definitive treatment difficult. To ensure adherence, *directly observed therapy* is used, where the medication is given directly to the patient while someone is watching him or her swallow the antituberculosis drugs.

The goals of antituberculosis drug therapy are to cure the disease without relapse, prevent death, stop the spread of the disease, and prevent the emergence of drug-resistant TB.

Primary prevention efforts have focused on the Bacille Calmette-Guérin (BCG) vaccine. Although BCG vaccine is used commonly in many parts of the world, its efficacy is unpredictable in protecting individuals against developing TB.

Therapy begins with a multidrug (two or more) regimen that attempts to kill the tubercle bacilli rapidly and to prevent the development of drug-resistant *Mycobacterium tuberculosis.* Tuberculosis disease should never be treated with a single drug, due to increased risk of emergence of drug-resistant disease. Additionally, if a drug is failing, at least two drugs should be added.

Drugs that have been approved for the treatment of tuberculosis are classified as first- and second-line drugs (Table 7-11).

DID YOU KNOW?

Early therapy of tuberculosis includes rest, often at sanitaria. One of the first sanitaria was at Saranac Lake in New York State, started by Edward Livingston Trudeau (whose descendant draws the Doonesbury cartoon).

Latent Tuberculosis Infection (Prophylaxis)

Treatment of latent tuberculosis infection (Table 7-12) is recommended in individuals with a positive PPD but no symptoms and a normal chest X-ray. Treatment of those with latent TB infection helps eliminate a large reservoir of individuals at risk for progression to TB, and for spreading the disease.

Prophylaxis is started with isoniazid (INH), a first-line drug recommended by the American Thoracic Society/Centers for Disease Control and Prevention Committee on Latent Tuberculosis Infection, is to be taken for 9 months. Included in this category of latent TB infection are patients who have been infected recently or exposed to TB and individuals who are at increased risk of progression to TB following infection with *Mycobacterium tuberculosis* [e.g., immunosuppressed (HIV/AIDS)], although they are treated for longer periods of time. INH may be given to household contact of individuals with TB disease, though therapy may be stopped if the contact remains PPD negative after 3 months.

If drug-resistant tuberculosis infection is likely, the American Thoracic Society and the CDC recommend treatment with at least two drugs to which the organism is likely to be susceptible. These drugs are rifampin (Rifadin) and pyrazinamide (PZA), which are taken for 2 months, or rifampin alone for 4 months. This treatment

TABLE 7-11 First- and Second-Line Drugs for the Treatment of TB

First-Line Drugs (drugs of choice that are used first)
- Isoniazid (INH) adverse effects: nausea, vomiting, diarrhea, dizziness, heartburn, abdominal pain, low vitamin B_6 levels
- Rifampin adverse effects: red-orange discoloration of urine, feces, saliva, skin, sputum, sweat, or tears
- Rifapentine adverse effects: red-orange discoloration of urine, feces, saliva, skin, sputum, sweat, or tears
- Pyrazinamide adverse effects: arthralgia, myalgia
- Ethambutol adverse effects: decrease in visual acuity and loss of ability to perceive red and green

Second-Line Drugs*
- Cycloserine
- Ethionamide
- P-Aminosalicylic acid
- Streptomycin
- Capreomycin
- Ciprofloxacin

Note: Only drugs that are approved by the Food and Drug Administration are listed.

should not be used in HIV-positive patients. With INH and rifampin resistance, the CDC recommends ethambutol (Myambutol) with PZA. A major limitation in treating latent TB infections is poor adherence; therapy must be long enough to eradicate the organism.

The primary risk or adverse effect of isoniazid is hepatitis, characterized by abdominal pain and jaundice. Risk of hepatotoxicity is increased with alcohol and acetaminophen (Tylenol) usage and is unusual before age 35. INH also causes gastrointestinal problems, peripheral neuropathy (disease involving the nerves—muscle weakness, numbness of fingers and toes), and anemia. INH causes a pyridoxine (Vitamin B_6) deficiency,

TABLE 7-12 Treatment Regimens for Tuberculosis

DRUG NAME
Latent Tuberculosis Infection (Prophylaxis)
Isoniazid (isonicotinic acid hydrazide; INH)
Rifampin (Rifadin)
Active Tuberculosis
Two or more drugs are needed to treat active TB to reduce emergence of resistant bacterial strains. One drug alone should not be used.
Initial Phase (four-drug regimen)
Isoniazid, rifampin, pyrazinamide, and ethambutol
Pyrazinamide (PZA)
Ethambutol (Myambutol)
Continuous Phase
Isoniazid and rifampin

which is responsible for the peripheral neuropathy. Thus, pyridoxine may be given together with INH, depending on the adequacy of the patient's diet.

DID YOU KNOW?

In colonial times, maple syrup was used to cure tuberculosis.

Treatment of Active Tuberculosis

Diagnosis of active tuberculosis must be made before treatment is started. Multiple drug therapy is used to treat adequately and to prevent drug-resistant strains from developing. A single drug should not be added to a regimen that is failing. Therapy must be long enough to eradicate the organism. There are two phases of treatment for patients with TB. The initial bactericidal phase consists of 2 months of therapy followed by the continuation phase (subsequent sterilizing phase), which lasts 4–7 months for patients with drug-susceptible disease in the absence of HIV infection (Table 7-12).

A four-drug regimen should be started in patients with active TB, including isoniazid, rifampin, pyrazinamide, and ethambutol. If the sensitivity of the organism becomes known, this may alter the drug regimen. After 2 months of therapy with these four drugs, the patient enters the continuation phase, where pyrazinamide and ethambutol are discontinued and isoniazid and rifampin are continued for another 4 months. Obviously, if the organism is resistant to INH and/or rifampin, this will be altered. This completes 6 months of therapy. If the patient is considered at high risk for relapse (positive TB cultures after 2 months of therapy), therapy should continue for an additional 3 months. These medications should be given together. They may be taken with food if GI upset occurs.

Special Situations

Generally, patients with tuberculosis and HIV infection are treated with the same drugs as patients without HIV infection; however, there is a higher risk for TB resistance. One exception is that during the continuation phase the patient should receive higher doses of INH and rifampin to prevent relapse with resistant organisms, and the recommended time of treatment is longer.

Children with tuberculosis infection have a high risk of disseminated disease, so treatment should be initiated as soon as the diagnosis is suspected. However, it is also important to remember that it is very rare for young children to spread tuberculosis. Development of drug resistance is lower in children; treatment usually starts with INH, pyrazinamide, and rifampin. Ethambutol is not routinely given to children under 13 years of age because it can cause decreased visual acuity and a temporary loss of vision. It may be difficult to detect those changes in young children. If the drug sensitivities of the source case are known, the child's therapy can be altered.

If there is INH resistance, the regimen consists of rifampin, PZA, and ethambutol; with rifampin resistance, the patient is given INH, PZA, and ethambutol.

Dental Hygiene Applications

Adults presenting to the dental office for treatment who are currently taking isoniazid (INH) should have a physician's consultation regarding liver function studies. Patients with *active* TB should not have elective dental treatment done. Otherwise, standard precautions should be taken and the use of aerosols should be avoided.

Key Points

- It is important to determine if the patient has latent or active TB infection.
- Isoniazid (INH) is the drug of choice for the treatment of latent TB infection (9 months).
- INH may cause liver problems.
- Rifampin causes red/orange saliva.
- A major problem with tuberculosis is multiple antimicrobial resistance.
- A four-drug regimen should be started in patients with active TB, including isoniazid (INH), rifampin (Rifadin), pyrazinamide (PZA), and ethambutol (Myambutol).
- There are many drug interactions with rifampin.
- Treatment is long term and patient adherence is critical.

Board Review Questions

1. Which of the following antibiotics can be used for prophylaxis against infective endocarditis if a patient is allergic to penicillin? (p. 127)
   a. Ampicillin
   b. Erythromycin
   c. Azithromycin
   d. Doxycycline
2. A patient with localized aggressive periodontitis has little plaque and calculus. Treatment involves initial therapy and an antibiotic. Which of the following antibiotics is taken up by PMNs and has a postantibiotic effect? (p. 119)
   a. Penicillin
   b. Amoxicillin
   c. Metronidazole
   d. Azithromycin
3. Which of the following antibiotics is used to treat *Pneumocystis jiroveci* infection in AIDS patients? (pp. 124, 125)
   a. Metronidazole
   b. Trimethoprim + sulfamethoxazole
   c. Penicillin
   d. Doxycycline
4. A primary concern for using antibiotics for infections that are not bacterial in nature is that (p. 111)
   a. drug-resistant microorganisms could develop.
   b. drug–drug interactions increase.
   c. drug dependence will develop.
   d. significant blood diseases could occur.

5. A patient is taking clarithromycin (Biaxin) for chronic bronchitis. Which of the following procedures should be followed if the patient has to take amoxicillin for prophylaxis against infective endocarditis? (pp. 125–127)
   a. Discontinue the clarithromycin for 4 days before the dental appointment.
   b. Prescribe another drug for chronic bronchitis.
   c. Space the two antibiotics apart a few hours.
   d. Don't take amoxicillin and double the dose of clarithromycin.

6. Which of the following drugs is contraindicated while a patient is taking metronidazole? (p. 117)
   a. Penicillin
   b. Alcohol
   c. Aspirin
   d. Mushrooms

7. All of the following antibiotics have been used in the treatment of aggressive periodontal disease *except* one. Which one is the exception? (p. 113)
   a. Clindamycin
   b. Ciprofloxacin
   c. Erythromycin base
   d. Doxycycline hyclate

8. Which of the following antibiotics is contraindicated in children under 8 years old? (p. 120)
   a. Clindamycin
   b. Azithromycin
   c. Tetracycline
   d. Penicillin VK

9. Which of the following antibiotics cannot be taken concurrently with milk? (p. 120)
   a. Tetracycline
   b. Amoxicillin
   c. Metronidazole
   d. Penicillin

10. A 56-year-old patient came for his scheduled periodontal maintenance appointment. He missed two previous appointments before due to family matters. Probing revealed generalized 5–7 mm probing depths with generalized bleeding on probing. The patient does not want surgery because he cannot afford it. Which of the following medications can be used as an adjunct to periodontal debridement? (p. 120)
    a. Tetracycline 250 mg caps
    b. Azithromycin 250 mg tabs
    c. Amoxicillin 500 mg cap
    d. Doxycycline 20 mg tab

11. Which of the following defines antimicrobial activity of an antibiotic that kills sensitive bacteria? (p. 111)
    a. Narrow-spectrum
    b. Broad-spectrum
    c. Bactericidal
    d. Bacteriostatic

12. All of the following are adverse reactions to antibiotics *except* one. Which one is the exception? (pp. 111, 112)
    a. Superinfections
    b. Gastrointestinal (nausea, vomiting, diarrhea)
    c. Allergic reactions
    d. Inhibits bacterial growth
    e. Photosensitivity

13. Antibiotics are effective against which of the following? (p. 111)
    a. Yeasts
    b. Bacteria
    c. Viruses
    d. Influenza

14. Which of the following symptoms occur in the oral cavity as a result of fungal overgrowth during antibiotic use? (p. 112)
    a. Stomatitis
    b. Hypersensitivity
    c. Caries
    d. Gingivitis

15. An overgrowth of which of the following organisms is responsible for antibiotic-associated diarrhea? (p. 112)
    a. *Streptococci mutans*
    b. *Mucobacterium tuberculosis*
    c. *Clostridium difficile*
    d. *Staphylococci aureus*

16. Which of the following active ingredients is found in Atridox? (p. 132)
    a. Chlorhexidine
    b. Tetracycline
    c. Doxycycline
    d. Minocycline

17. Which of the following active ingredients is found in Arestin? (p. 132)
    a. Chlorhexidine
    b. Tetracycline
    c. Doxycycline
    d. Minocycline

18. For which of the following patients is Atridox contraindicated? (p. 132)
    a. Alcoholics
    b. Diabetics
    c. Pregnant women
    d. Teenagers

19. Which of the following agents should not be taken/used immediately after using chlorhexidine oral rinse? (pp. 128, 130)
    a. Fluoride
    b. Alcohol
    c. Arestin
    d. Antacid

20. The percentage (%) of alcohol in chlorhexidine oral rinse? (p. 128)
    a. 0.05
    b. 0.12
    c. 11.6
    d. 21.6

21. Which of the following serum-level parameters should be monitored in the tuberculosis patient taking INH? (pp. 133–135)
    a. Liver enzymes
    b. Sodium chloride
    c. Calcium ions
    d. Potassium

22. Which of the following drugs is also referred to as INH? (pp. 133–135)
    a. Rifampin
    b. Isoniazid
    c. Ethambutol
    d. Fluroquinolone
    e. Pyrazinamide

23. Which of the following TB drugs causes red/orange saliva? (p. 133–135)
    a. Rifampin
    b. Isoniazid
    c. Ethambutol
    d. Fluroquinolone
    e. Pyrazinamide

24. Which of the following TB drugs causes drug-induced hepatitis? (p. 134)
    a. Rifampin
    b. Isoniazid
    c. Ethambutol
    d. Fluroquinolone
    e. Pyrazinamide

25. A major problem with antituberculosis drugs is (p. 135)
    a. many drugs are toxic to normal cells in the body.
    b. many drugs are not specific enough to kill the bacteria.
    c. drug resistance.
    d. drug dependence.

Selected References

American Academy of Periodontology position paper: Systemic antibiotics in periodontics. 2004. *J Periodontol* 75:1553–1565.

Blumberg HM, Leonard Jr. MK, Jasmer RM. 2005. Update on the treatment of tuberculosis and latent tuberculosis infection. *JAMA* 293:2776–2784.

Dijani AS, Taubert KA, Wilson W, Bolger AF, Bayer A, et al. 1997. Prevention of bacterial endocarditis: Recommendations by the American Heart Association. *JAMA* 227:1794–1801.

Dye C, Watt CJ, Bleed DM, et al. 2005. Evolution of tuberculosis control and prospects for reducing tuberculosis incidence, prevalence, and deaths globally. *JAMA* 293:2767–2775.

Friedrich MJ. 2005. Basic science guides design of new TB vaccine candidates. *JAMA* 293:2703–2705.

Gums JG. 2004. Redefining appropriate use of antibiotics. *American Family Physician* 69:35–36.

Hanes PJ, Purvis JP. 2003. Local anti-infective therapy: Pharmacological agents—A systematic review. *Ann Periodontol* 8:79–98.

Hooton RM, Levy SB. 2001. Antimicrobial resistance: A plan of action for community practice. *Am Fam Physician* 63:1087–1098.

Newman MG, van Winkelhoff AJ. 2001. *Antibiotic and antimicrobial use in dental practice,* 2nd ed. Chicago: Quintessence.

Osborne NG. 2002. Antibiotics and oral contraceptives: Potential interactions. *Journal of Gynecologic Surgery* 18(4):171–172.

Potter B, Kraus CK. 2005. Management of active tuberculosis. *Am Fam Physician* 72:2225–2232.

Screening for tuberculosis and tuberculosis infection in high-risk populations: Recommendations of the Advisory Council for the Elimination of Tuberculosis. 1995. *Morb Mortal Wkly Rep* 44:19–34.

Segelnick SL, Weinberg MA. 2008. Recognizing doxycycline-induced esophageal ulcers in dental practice. *J Am Dent Asoc* 139(5):581–585.

Segelnick SL, Weinberg, MA. 2010. Doxycycline-induced dizziness in a dental patient. *NY State Dent J* 76(5):28–32.

Vanden Eng J, Marcus R, Hadler JL, Imhoff B, Vugia DJ, Cieslak PR, et al. 2003. Consumer attitudes and use of antibiotics. *Emerg Infect Dis* 9:1128–1135.

Wilson W, Taubert KA, Gewitz M, et al. 2007. Prevention of infective endocarditis. Guidelines from the American Heart Association Rheumatic Fever, Endocarditis and Kawasaki Disease Committee, Council on Cardiovascular Disease in the Young, and the Council on Clinical Cardiology, Council on Cardiovascular Surgery and Anesthesia, and the Quality of Care and Outcomes Research Interdisciplinary Working Group. *Circulation Journal of the American Heart Association* 116:1736–1754.

Web Sites

www.ncbi.nlm.nih.gov
www.fda.gov/bbs/topics
www.uspharmacist.com
www.ada.org
www.pharmacytimes.com
www.cdc.gov
www.perio.org

QUICK DRUG GUIDE

Bactericidal Antibiotics

Penicillins

Natural Penicillins: Narrow-Spectrum

- Penicillin V (Pen-vee K, V-cillin K, Veetids)
- Penicillin G (injectable)

Broad Spectrum: Aminopenicillins

- Amoxicillin (Amoxil, Trimox)
- Ampicillin (Omnipen)

Beta-Lactamase Inhibitors

- Amoxicillin + clavulanate (Augmentin)
- Ampicillin + sulbactam (Unasyn)
- Piperacillin + tazobactam (injectable, Zosyn)

Penicillinase-Resistant

- Dicloxacillin (Dycill)
- Nafcillin (injectable)
- Oxacillin (Bactocill)
- Cloxacillin (Cloxacillin)

Antipseudomonal Penicillins: Extended-Spectrum (all are injectables)

- Carbenicillin (Geocillin)
- Ticarcillin (Ticar)
- Mezlocillin (Mezlin)
- Piperacillin (Pipracil)

Cephalosporins

First generation

- Cefadroxil (Duricef)
- Cephalexin (Keflex)

Second generation

- Cefaclor (Ceclor)
- Cefprozil (Cefzil)
- Cefuroxime—axetil (Ceftin, Veftin)

Third generation

- Omnicef (cefdinir)
- Cefixime (Suprax)
- Cefpodoxime (Vantin)
- Ceftibuten (Cedax)

Fourth generation (only injectable)

Nitroimadazoles

- Metronidazole (Flagyl)

Fluoroquinolones

First generation

- Nalidixic acid (NegGram)

Second generation

- Ciprofloxacin (Cipro)
- Ofloxacin (Floxin)

Third generation

- Levofloxacin (Levaquin)
- Sparfloxacin (Zagam)
- Gatifloxacin (Tequin)
- Moxifloxacin (Avelox)

Fourth generation

- Trovafloxacin (Trovan)

Bacteriostatic Antibiotics

Tetracyclines

- Tetracycline HCl (Sumycin, achromycin)
- Doxycycline hyclate (Vibramyin, Doryx)
- Doxycycline hyclate 20 mg
- Minocycline HCl (Minocin)

Erythromycins (macrolides)

- Erythromycin base (E-Mycin, Eryc, PCE, Ery-tab)
- Erythromycin estolate (Ilosone)
- Erythromycin ethylsuccinate (EES, Eryped)

Second-generation Macrolides (Azalides)

- Azithromycin (Zithromax)
- clarithromycin (Biaxin)

Third generation (Ketolides)

- Telithromycin (Ketek)

Lincomycins

- Clindamycin (Cleocin)

Other Antimicrobials

Sulfonamides

- Sulfamethoxazole + trimethoprim (Bactrim)
- Sulfadiazine (Silvadene)
- Sulfamethoxazole (Gantanol)
- Sulfisoxazole (Gantrisin)
- Trimethoprim (Proloprim)

Glycopeptide Antibiotic

- Vancomycin (Vancocin)

Aminoglycosides

- Neomycin (Bacitracin zinc–neomycin–polymyxin B sulfate)
- Gentamicin (Garamycin)
- Tobramycin (Nebcin)
- Amikacin (Amikin)

Antimycobacterial Drugs: Tuberculosis (TB)

First-Line Anti-TB Drugs

- Isoniazid (isonicotinic acid hydrazide; INH)
- Rifampin (Rifadin)
- Pyrazinamide (PZA)
- Ethambutol (Myambutol)

Second-Line Anti-TB Drugs

- Cycloserine (Seromycin)
- Ethionamide (Trecator-SC)
- Para-aminosalicylic acid (Paser)
- Streptomycin (Streptomycin)
- Capreomycin (Capastat sulfate)

Antiviral and Antifungal Agents

GOAL

To gain knowledge of the various treatments for herpes simplex virus infection and oral and systemic fungal infections. To provide an understanding of the pharmacology of drugs used to treat HIV/AIDS.

EDUCATIONAL OBJECTIVES

After reading this chapter, the reader should be able to:

1. Illustrate the pathophysiology of herpes simplex viruses.

2. List various antiherpetic drugs.

3. Describe the appropriate dental management of patients with herpes labialis.

4. Describe the pharmacology of currently approved drugs used in the treatment of HIV infection.

5. Describe selected drugs with adverse side effects related to dentistry and how to manage them.

6. Explain dental implications of patients taking anti-HIV drugs.

7. List the patients that are higher risk for fungal infections.

8. List common antifungal agents used to treat oral infections.

9. List common drug interactions of systemic antifungal agents.

KEY TERMS

Herpes simplex virus

Cold sore

Antiviral agents

Human immunodeficiency virus

Acquired immune deficiency syndrome

Antiretroviral therapy

HAART

Oral candidiasis

Antifungal agents

Introduction

Although dental hygienists do not treat and prescribe medications for oral conditions, they are probably the first to see changes of the patient's oral mucosa during an intraoral examination. The dental hygienist should be aware of the various common herpetic oral lesions and the medications used to manage them.

Antivirals for Herpes Simplex

- Antiviral drugs are used in the treatment of viral infections.
- There are mainly two serotypes of **herpes simplex virus (HSV):**
  - Herpes virus type 1 (HSV-1) primarily causes oropharyngeal disease (including eyes, vermillion border of the lips, mouth, and face) and;
  - herpes virus type 2 (HSV-2) primarily causes genital disease, which is considered a sexually transmitted disease.
- Herpes simplex virus infections occur in healthy as well as in immunocompromised patients. There is transmission of HSV-1 to the genitals, and HSV-2 can cause oral herpes.

Primary Herpes Infection and Treatment

- Herpes simplex type 1 (HSV-1) can occur either as a primary or recurrent infection.
- *Primary herpes simplex virus* or *primary herpetic gingivostomatitis* infections occur with the first exposure to HSV-1 or HSV-2. It can occur in infants, children (between 2 and 3 years of age), or adults, and is characterized by high fever, malaise, fatigue, nausea and vomiting, and oral vesicles.
  - Adults may have less typical clinical features, making a diagnosis more difficult.
- After primary exposure, herpes simplex virus may persist in a latent state in the trigeminal ganglion until it is disturbed and then reactivated in adulthood.
- Herpes infection is transmissible from human to human. An important part of the transmission is intimate contact between an infected shedding person (the host) and another susceptible person. Common stimuli that disturb the host's immune system include fever, menstruation, prolonged illness, exposure to sunlight, prolonged use of steroids, or surgery. By adulthood, up to 90% of individuals will have antibodies to HSV-1.
  - Painful intraoral vesicles on the oral mucosa rapidly rupture to form small ulcers with erythematous (red) haloes.

DID YOU KNOW?

About 45 million Americans are infected with genital herpes (HSV-2).

Rapid Dental Hint

Patients with oral viral lesions should not use alcohol-containing mouthrinses.

HSV-1 is transmitted by contact with infected saliva. Lesions appear 12–36 hours after the first symptoms. Lesions are self-limiting and will resolve within 10–14 days. There is also a generalized severe gingivitis and cervical lymphadenopathy present.

- Treatment is palliative, including fluids and analgesics/antipyretics such as acetaminophen (Tylenol). Early treatment with acyclovir (Zovirax) or famciclovir (Famvir) may significantly shorten the duration of all clinical manifestations and infectivity of affected children. Antibiotics are not used in the treatment of primary herpes because they are used in bacterial infections, not viral; however, they may be helpful in preventing secondary infection.

Rapid Dental Hint

Patients should discard their toothbrush during periods of viral infection.

Recurrent Herpes Infection and Treatment

- *Recurrent herpes simplex virus infection* is also caused by HSV-1 and occurs in individuals who previously had primary herpes.
- This infection occurs in and around the mouth and is referred to as herpes labialis, a "**cold sore**" or "fever blister" when it occurs on the vermillion border of the lip (Figure 8-1).

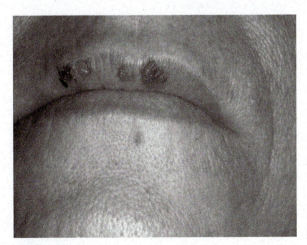

FIGURE 8-1 Herpes labialis on the vermillion border of the lip. (Courtesy of *U.S. Pharmacist*).

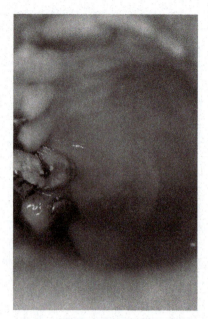

FIGURE 8-2 After multiple injections of a local anesthetic, the patient developed herpetic lesions. (Courtesy of Dr. David Lefkovitz; *U.S. Pharmacist*)

- Recurrences of these lesions are thought to be due to stress, sunlight, fever, immunocompromised patients (HIV infection/AIDS), trauma (e.g., after a dental procedure), or other irritants (Figure 8-2). Usually there is a prodromal burning and itching at the site 12–35 hours preceding eruption of the vesicles (raised blisters).

- Clinically, a small, well-localized cluster of small vesicles appears on heavily keratinized oral mucosa (gingiva, palate, tongue, alveolar ridges, and vermillion border of lips). The

vesicles subsequently rupture, ulcerate, and crust within 24–48 hours. Lesions have the potential to last more than 14 days if left untreated.

> **DID YOU KNOW?**
>
> Incidence of ocular (eye) herpes infection is approximately 0.15%.

- Antibiotics and topical corticosteroids should not be used, which will further suppress the immune system, prolonging the infection. A 50:50 suspension of diphenydramine and Kaopectate and/or lidocaine viscous 2% will help with the pain.

- Table 8-1 lists the commonly used **antiviral agents** in the treatment of recurrent oral herpes simplex infection. Antiviral drugs inhibit viral DNA synthesis. These antiviral agents do not cure the condition but may reduce healing time, reduce viral shedding, and reduce frequency of recurrences.

- Acyclovir is almost completely restricted to the herpes viruses (HSV-1, HSV-2, varicella zoster, and Epstein Barr). Acyclovir (Zovirax) 5% cream/ointment is used in adults and adolescents age 12 and older with recurrent herpes labialis. It is applied five times a day for 4 days.

- Oral acyclovir is recommended in immunocompromised (HIV+) individuals with HSV-1 and in HSV-2 infection in immunocompetent (normal immune system) patients. It has not been approved

TABLE 8-1 Antiherpetic Drugs

DENTAL NOTES	INDICATIONS	DOSAGE
Acyclovir sodium (Zovirax) 200 mg caps, 400 or 800 mg tabs, suspension, topical ointment, cream 5%, injectable; generic available (Rx)	Topical: Recurrent herpes labialis Oral: herpes labialis, genital herpes (HSV-2) Adverse effects: renal (kidney) impairment, changes in blood count, nausea, vomiting, rash, headache	Apply ointment every 3 hours up to six times a day for 7 days Oral: 200 mg 5 times a day
Docosanol (Abreva) cream 10% (OTC)	Over-the-counter for herpes labialis	Apply five times a day at first sign of cold sore; use until lesion is healed
Penciclovir (Denavir) cream 1% (Rx)	FDA approved for recurrent oral HSV; adverse effects: headache	Apply every 2 hours while awake for 4 days
Valacyclovir (Valtrex) tabs 500 mg, 1 gm (Rx)	For herpes labialis; genital herpes; well tolerated; adverse effects: may cause anemia in immunocompromised patients	For cold sores: take 2 grams orally twice a day at a 12-hour interval for only one day
Famciclovir (Famvir) tabs 125, 250, 500 mg (Rx)	For primary and recurrent genital herpes; adverse effects: headache, nausea, and diarrhea	250 mg tid × 7–10 days (primary infection); 125 mg bid × 5 days (recurrent infection)
Ganciclovir (Cytovene) injectable (Rx)	Neutropenia (low white blood cells); treatment of HSV in immunocompromised patients	Not significant

by the FDA for treatment of HSV-1 infections in immunocompetent patients, although many clinicians prescribe it.

- Penciclovir 1% (Denavir) cream is highly recommended in immunocompetent (immune system is not compromised and the patient is healthy) patients. The cream should be applied during the prodromal (feeling before active disease) stage.

Rapid Dental Hint

Patients should use a cotton-tip applicator when applying Orabase products and remember to dab it, not rub it, on the lesion.

Rapid Dental Hint

Patients should apply topical acyclovir and penciclovir with a cotton-tip applicator.

Rapid Dental Hint

There are no clinically significant dental implications with these drugs. To prevent reinfection or spread of infection, patients should not touch the lesion and should discard toothbrushes used during the infection.

- Other products available OTC for the symptomatic treatment of herpes labialis include petroleum and cocoa butter to keep lesions moist and prevent cracking, which would make them more susceptible to secondary infection. Docosanol (Abreva), a 10% OTC cream, is applied five times a day until the infection heals. It works by inhibiting the fusion of the virus with the human cell membrane, thereby blocking entry and subsequent viral replication.
- If it is too late after the first symptoms appear to apply an antiviral agent, a topical anesthetic such as 20% benzocaine (Orabase-B) may reduce the pain, burning, and itching. Patients who are allergic to para-aminobenzoic acid (PABA) or sulfonamides may also be allergic to benzocaine and tetracaine. Products containing camphor (not greater than 3%) and menthol (not greater than 1%) act as an analgesic to relieve the pain and itching (Table 8-2). Natural products such as bioflavonoids or acidophilus are not FDA approved. Examples of prescriptions are shown in Figure 8-3.

Antiretroviral Agents: HIV/AIDS

Since the first cases were reported in the United States in 1981, the AIDS epidemic has been the subject of much clinical research. The end stage of infection with **human immunodeficiency virus** (HIV) is **acquired immune deficiency syndrome** (AIDS). HIV (Figure 8-4) attacks the body's immune system, resulting in life-threatening infections and cancers. Once one has developed AIDS, the immune system is weakened enough to allow for unusual or prolonged infections.

AIDS is caused by a transmissible RNA retrovirus known as HIV type 1. A related but antigenically distinct retrovirus, HIV type 2, causes some cases of AIDS in western Africa but is rare in the United States. The primary immune cells involved are the T-lymphocytes (CD4). HIV "hunts" for CD4 cells and fuses to the cell membrane allowing viral RNA from the HIV to be released into the CD4 cell. Once inside the cell, the HIV converts viral RNA into proviral DNA by an enzyme called *reverse transcriptase,* which then incorporates into the host cell (CD4) DNA. The proviral DNA enters the nucleus of the host cell and inserts into the cell's DNA. The cell then makes copies of HIV (Figure 8-5).

TABLE 8-2 Over-the-Counter (OTC) Analgesic Medications for Treatment of Herpes Labialis	
ANALGESIC (CHEMICAL NAME)	**PRODUCT NAME**
Allantoin	Herpecin-L
Benzocaine	Anbesol, Orabase (dental paste) with benzocaine 20%
Benzyl alcohol	Zilactin
Camphor and phenol	Campho-Phenique Cold Sore Gel, Blistex, Carmex, ChapStick Medicated
Dyclonine	Tanac Medicated Gel, Orajel CoverMed
Lidocaine	Zilactin L

Source: Mackowiak E. 2003. Prevention and treatment of cold sores. *U.S. Pharmacist* 28:77–84.

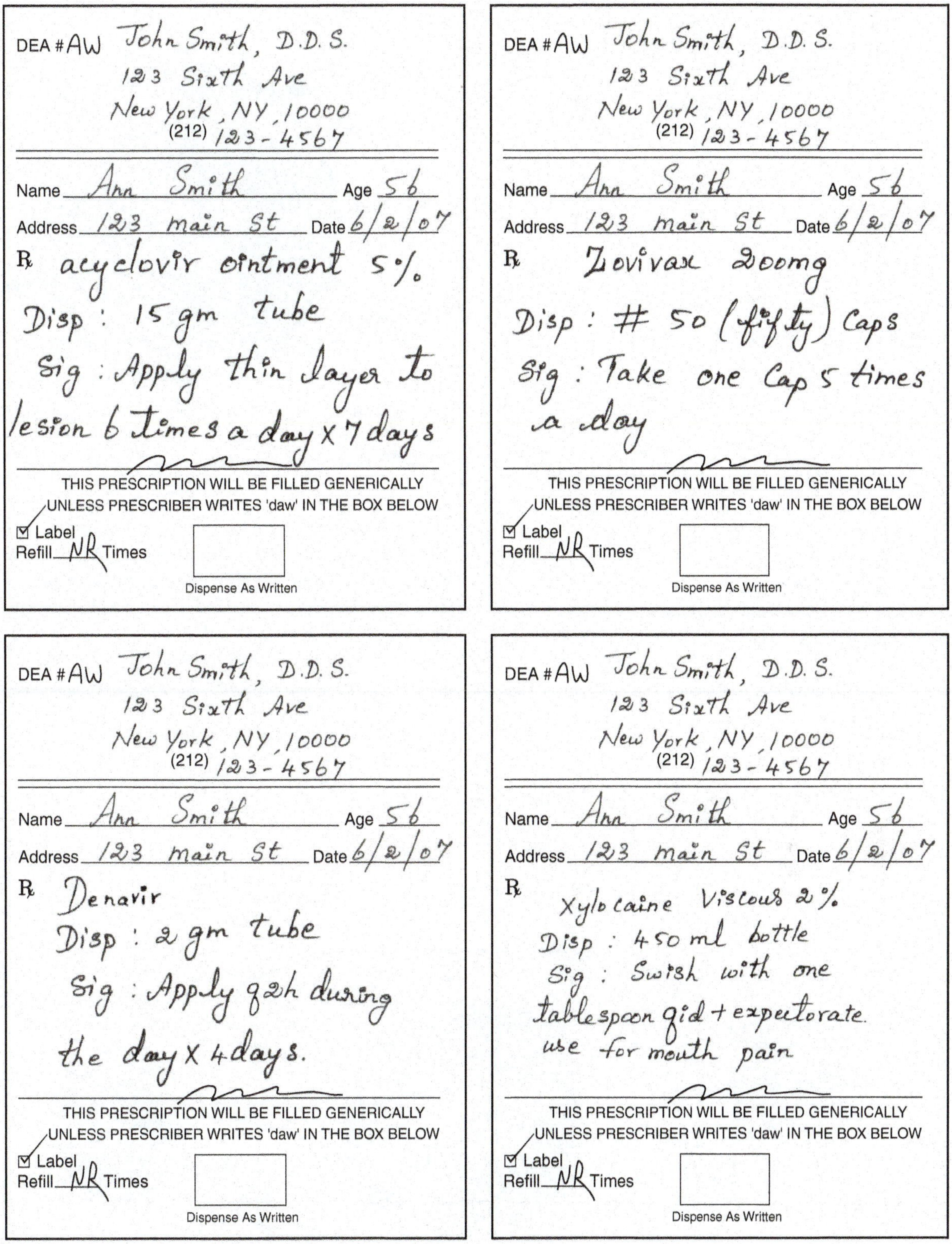

DEA #AW   John Smith, D.D.S.
123 Sixth Ave
New York, NY, 10000
(212) 123-4567

Name   Ann Smith   Age 56
Address 123 main St   Date 6/2/07

℞   acyclovir ointment 5%.

Disp : 15 gm tube

Sig : Apply thin layer to
lesion 6 times a day X 7 days

THIS PRESCRIPTION WILL BE FILLED GENERICALLY
UNLESS PRESCRIBER WRITES 'daw' IN THE BOX BELOW

☑ Label
Refill NR Times

Dispense As Written

DEA #AW   John Smith, D.D.S.
123 Sixth Ave
New York, NY, 10000
(212) 123-4567

Name   Ann Smith   Age 56
Address 123 main St   Date 6/2/07

℞   Zovirax 200mg

Disp : # 50 (fifty) Caps

Sig : Take one Cap 5 times
a day

THIS PRESCRIPTION WILL BE FILLED GENERICALLY
UNLESS PRESCRIBER WRITES 'daw' IN THE BOX BELOW

☑ Label
Refill NR Times

Dispense As Written

DEA #AW   John Smith, D.D.S.
123 Sixth Ave
New York, NY, 10000
(212) 123-4567

Name   Ann Smith   Age 56
Address 123 main St   Date 6/2/07

℞   Denavir
Disp : 2 gm tube

Sig : Apply q2h during

the day X 4 days.

THIS PRESCRIPTION WILL BE FILLED GENERICALLY
UNLESS PRESCRIBER WRITES 'daw' IN THE BOX BELOW

☑ Label
Refill NR Times

Dispense As Written

DEA #AW   John Smith, D.D.S.
123 Sixth Ave
New York, NY, 10000
(212) 123-4567

Name   Ann Smith   Age 56
Address 123 main St   Date 6/2/07

℞   Xylocaine Viscous 2%
Disp : 450 ml bottle
Sig : Swish with one
tablespoon qid + expectorate.
use for mouth pain

THIS PRESCRIPTION WILL BE FILLED GENERICALLY
UNLESS PRESCRIBER WRITES 'daw' IN THE BOX BELOW

☑ Label
Refill NR Times

Dispense As Written

FIGURE 8-3 Sample prescriptions of drugs for oral herpes infection.

DEA #AW John Smith, D.D.S.
123 Sixth Ave
New York, NY, 10000
(212) 123-4567

Name _Ann Smith_____ Age _56_

Address _123 main St_ Date _6/2/07_

℞ Benadryl Syrup 4oz
mix equal parts of Kaopectate
liquid (12 oz) or maalox (12 oz)
Sig: Rinse for 1 minute with
teasp & expectorate, Repeat
q2h or at meal times

THIS PRESCRIPTION WILL BE FILLED GENERICALLY
UNLESS PRESCRIBER WRITES 'daw' IN THE BOX BELOW

☑ Label
Refill _NR_ Times

Dispense As Written

FIGURE 8-3 (*Continued*)

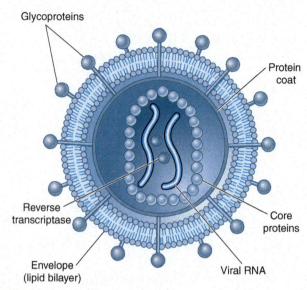

FIGURE 8-4 Structure of HIV.

A decreased CD4 T-cell count occurs as the disease progresses and serves as a good predictor of risk of opportunistic infections. These opportunistic infections include tuberculosis, fungal infections (oral candidiasis, esophageal candidiasis), *Pneumocystis jiroveci* (formerly *Pneumocystis carinii*) pneumonia (PCP), recurrent bacterial pneumonia, diarrhea, meningitis, and cancers such as Kaposi's sarcoma and non-Hodgkin's lymphoma. Additionally, the wasting syndrome occurs, where there is a tremendous amount of weight loss.

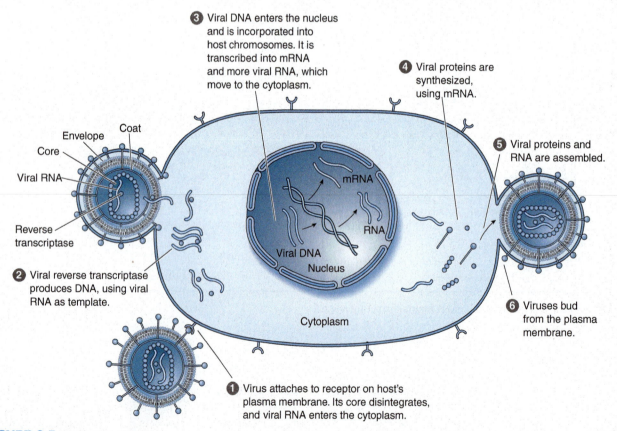

FIGURE 8-5 Replication of HIV.

Diagnosis

The Centers for Disease Control and Prevention (CDC) defines AIDS as a CD4 count of under 200/μL or CD4+ T under 14% of total lymphocytes in the presence of HIV infection. As the amount of virus in the plasma (viral load) increases, the CD4+ count decreases. A combination of CD4+ T counts and plasma HIV RNA (viral) loads is the best overall disease marker. A medical consult is necessary for this type of patient.

Antiretroviral Pharmacology

The objective of **antiretroviral therapy** is to reduce the viral (RNA retrovirus) load, thereby improving survival. HIV viral load is the most sensitive marker for disease control and should be monitored, as well as CD4+ counts. Past guidelines for the initiation of treatment in asymptomatic patients depended on the CD4+ count. However, new information indicates that quantitation of HIV RNA in plasma (viral load) is a better indicator for the start of drug therapy. Drug therapy should be started if the patient is symptomatic or if the asymptomatic patient has a CD4+ count of under 500 per mm^3 or a viral load of more than 30,000 copies per mL. Lack of adherence to drug treatment is a major cause of failure of treatment and the emergence of resistant strains of the virus, which makes it more difficult to treat.

Antiretroviral Drugs

Four classes of drugs are currently available for the treatment of HIV infection (Table 8-3):

- Nucleoside/nucleotide reverse transcriptase inhibitors (NRTI/NtRTIs)
- Nonnucleoside reverse transcriptase inhibitors (NNRTIs)
- Protease inhibitors (PIs)
- Fusion (entry) inhibitors

Three-drug combinations for initial therapy are termed highly active antiretroviral therapy (**HAART**) and are the preferred initial regimen. The purpose of HAART is to improve both survival and quality of life with a regimen using three or four drugs to suppress viral replication and management or prevention of opportunistic infections. The goal of therapy is to use a HAART that reduces plasma levels of HIV RNA to below detectable limits (fewer than 50 copies/mL). There are currently 20 FDA-approved drugs in the United States used to treat HIV. Drug toxicity and HIV resistance toward these drugs makes adherence a critical issue. Approximately 78% of patients are becoming resistant to at least one HIV drug. Current treatment guidelines recommend the use of two or more of these drugs to suppress viral replication and management or prevention of opportunistic infections. Usually, two nucleoside reverse transcriptase inhibitors (NRTI) or nucleoside analogs and a highly active protease inhibitor drug are used. Alternative regimens include two NRTIs and a nonnucleoside reverse transcriptase inhibitor (NNRTI), or two NRTIs and a protease inhibitor.

To understand the actions of these drugs, refer to Table 8-3; all of these drugs are related to the events of the HIV on the CD4+ cell. For example, NNRTIs bind to a different site on the reverse transcriptase than NRTIs, preventing the virus from transcribing viral RNA into viral DNA.

NRTIs, the first drugs approved by the FDA in the 1980s, embed themselves into viral DNA and inhibit the conversion of RNA to DNA by binding to the reverse transcriptase enzyme. Since NRTIs do not undergo extensive liver cytochrome P450 metabolism, other drugs that are metabolized that way are not affected by NRTIs.

> **DID YOU KNOW?**
>
> The first antiretroviral drug, zidovudine, is no longer given by itself except as prophylaxis in exposed newborns; it loses its effectiveness against HIV over time.

The protease inhibitors (*PIs*) prevent breakdown of proteins produced by the virus into infectious mature viruses and are the most potent of the antiretroviral drugs. These drugs are extensively metabolized by the cytochrome P450 enzymes, so there are many potential drug interactions. For example, rifampin should not be given concurrently with any PI except for ritonavir.

The *fusion (entry) inhibitors* interfere with the entry of HIV-1 into hosts (lymphocytes) by inhibiting fusion of the virus and cell membranes. For HIV-1 to enter and infect the CD4+ cell, the viral glycoprotein must bind the cell membrane. Then the glycoprotein changes its shape, which helps in the fusion of the viral membrane with the cell. Enfuvirtide (Fuzeon) works by binding to the viral glycoprotein and preventing a change in the shape of the glycoprotein required for membrane fusion and viral entry into the target cell.

Pharmacological Treatment of Systemic Opportunistic Infections

There may be an association between CD4 count and the increased incidence of specific opportunistic infections in HIV+ patients.

HIV/AIDS patients may also be taking medications to prevent or treat opportunistic infections. If the patient has or had *Pneumocystis jiroveci* pneumonia, he or she will most likely be taking trimethoprim/sulfamethoxazole. The drug of choice for various forms of systemic candidiasis includes fluconazole (Diflucan).

Rapid Dental Hint

Many HIV-infected patients present with oral lesions. Monitor those patients.

Pharmacological Treatment of Oral Opportunistic Lesions/Conditions

Table 8-4 lists common opportunistic oral lesions/conditions associated with HIV, with the appropriate treatment. Many oral infections develop in the immunocompromised patients, including:

TABLE 8-3 Antiretroviral Drugs Used for the Treatment of HIV/AIDS

DRUG NAME	ADVERSE EFFECTS
Nucleoside Reverse Transcriptase Inhibitors (NRTIs)	Extensive adverse effect profile. All can cause potentially life-threatening lactic acidosis (a condition caused by the buildup of lactic acid in the body) and hepatomegaly (enlarged liver).
Abacavir (Ziagen)	Potentially fatal hypersensitivity reaction
Didansosine (ddL, Videx)	Anemia, pancreatitis, GI distress (diarrhea, abdominal pain), peripheral neuropathy (numbness and tingling of toes, fingers), *xerostomia*
Emtricitabine (Emtriva)	Nausea, diarrhea, rash, hyperpigmentation of palms and soles of feet
Lamivudine (3TC, Epivir)	Better tolerated than the other drugs; fatigue, headache, GI distress, neuropathy, insomnia
Stavudine (d4T, Zerit) Zidovudine (Retrovir)	Bone marrow suppression, resulting in severe anemia (low blood iron), granulocytopenia (low neutrophils/white blood cells), thrombocytopenia (low platelets), myopathy (muscle weakness), and hepatitis
	Minor side effects: headache, anorexia, nausea, vomiting, dizziness, insomnia
Tenofovir disoproxil fumarate (Viread)	Lactic acidosis and hepatomegaly (enlarged liver)
Zalcitabine (ddC)—HIVID	Peripheral neuropathy; no GI or blood problems, *oral ulcerations (stomatitis, aphthous ulcers)*
Non-nucleoside Reverse Transcriptase Inhibitors (NNRTI)	
Efavirenz (Sustiva)	Dizziness, headache, rash, insomnia, hallucinations, nightmares, altered concentration
Nevirapine (Viramune)	Rash is very common, fatal liver damage
Delavirdine (Rescriptor)	Less incidence of rash compared to other NNRTIs, headaches, increase in liver enzymes
Protease Inhibitors (PIs)	
Amprevavir (Agenerase)	*Oral paresthesia* (numbness), rash
Atazanavir (Reyataz)	*Dental pain, taste changes*
Fosamprenavir (Lexiva)	*Perioral paresthesia* (numbness around the mouth), *taste disorders,* skin rash, nausea, vomiting, diarrhea
Indinavir (Crixivan)	*Metallic taste in mouth,* blurred vision, thrombocytopenia, alopecia
Lopinavir + Ritonavir (Kaletra)	Potentially fatal hypersensitivity reaction
Nelfinavir (Viracept)	Paresthesias
Ritonavir (Norvir)	Pancreatitis, hepatitis, *taste impairment,* paresthesias
Saquinavir (Fortovase; formerly Invirase)	Increase in liver enzymes
Fusion (Entry) Inhibitors	Injection only; hypersensitivity, skin reactions
Enfuvirtide (Fuzeon)	

- Fungal infections: oral candidiasis, angular cheilitis
- Viral infections: herpes simplex, human papilloma virus, hairy leukoplakia
- Bacterial infections: periodontal infections (including NUG, NUP, linear gingival erythema). It is important to emphasize that not all patients with HIV disease necessarily have gingival or periodontal infections. These infections are associated with immunodeficiency.
- Hairy leukoplakia: caused by the Epstein-Barr virus
- Intraoral pain: intraoral pain from the lesions can be so severe that eating becomes difficult, resulting in weight loss
- Aphthous ulcers
- Xerostomia: common, may predispose to fungal infections
- Oral neoplasms: Kaposi's sarcoma (KS) is a neoplasm that causes both intraoral and skin lesions
- Infections of unknown etiology

Rapid Dental Hint

There are no contraindications for using local anesthetics in HIV-infected patients.

Dental Hygiene Applications

Certain laboratory tests and values associated with HIV infection may be useful in the dental management of the patient. CD4+ lymphocyte counts range from 500 to 1,600 cells/mm^3 in the HIV-negative patient, whereas initial signs and symptoms of immune suppression occur at CD4+ counts of under 500 cells/mm^3. When the CD4 counts fall to this level, many major and life-threatening opportunistic infections and malignancies develop. Patients with CD4+ lymphocyte counts above

TABLE 8-4 Common Oral Lesions/Conditions Associated with HIV Infections and Treatment Guidelines	
CONDITION	**TREATMENT (COMMON DRUGS)**
Fungal Infections	Antifungal agents: choose one of the following regimens
Candidiasis (oral, pharyngeal)	Clotrimazole (Mycelex) troches, 10 mg: dissolve 1 troche in mouth 5 times a day
	Nystatin pastilles, 200,000 units: dissolve one pastille in mouth 5 times a day
	Nystatin (Mycostatin) vaginal troches, 100,000 units: dissolve 1 troche in mouth 6–8 times per day
	Nystatin oral suspension: take 4–6 ml 4 times a day; retain in mouth as long as possible before swallowing
	Ketoconazole (Nizoral) tab 200 mg: take 2 tabs orally on the first day, followed by 1 tab per day for 14 days
	Fluconazole (Diflucan) tab 100mg: take two tabs orally on the first day, followed by one tab per day for 14 days
Angular cheilitis	Clotrimazole topical (Lotrimin, Gyne-Lotrimin) cream 1%: apply to lesion 4 times a day
	Ketoconazole cream 2%: apply to area 4 times a day; Nystatin ointment 100,000 units: apply to area 4 times a day
Viral Infections	Acyclovir topical ointment 5%; acyclovir cap 800 mg, 1 cap 5 times a day
Herpes simplex lesions	Treatment is elective: acyclovir cap 800 mg—1 cap 4 times a day
Hairy leukoplakia (Epstein-Barr virus infection)	
Bacterial Infections	Periodontal debridement
Linear gingival erythema (LGE)	Chlorhexidine gluconate 0.12% (Peridex, Periogard): rinse with 20 ml of rinse for 30 seconds twice a day
Necrotizing ulcerative gingivitis (NUG)	Periodontal debridement
	Chlorhexidine gluconate 0.12% oral rinse plus
	Systemic antibiotic:
	Metronidazole 250 mg qid or
	Amoxicillin 500 mg tid or
	Clindamycin 300 mg tid
Necrotizing ulcerative periodontitis (NUP)	Chlorhexidine gluconate 0.12% oral rinse
	Systemic therapy:
	Metrondiazole 250 mg qid or
	Amoxicillin 500 mg tid or
	Clindamycin 300 mg tid
Other Oral Conditions	Fluocinonide gel (Lidex) 0.05% mixed with equal parts of Orabase (a methylcellulose inert ingredient that is a vehicle to carry the gel; Colgate Oral Pharmaceuticals): apply to ulcer 4 times a day. Orabase; Lidocaine viscous 2%: swish with solution until the pain goes away and spit out (expectorate) (shake well before use).
Minor aphthous ulcers (canker sores)	
Oral pain: acute due to oral lesions	Lidocaine viscous 2% (mild to moderate pain) or NSAIDs
	For severe pain: narcotic analgesics
Chronic neurological pain	Psychotropic drugs (e.g., tricyclic antidepressants)
Xerostomia	Chew or suck on sugarless candy; avoid alcohol, which further dries the mucosa
	Saliva substitutes (carboxymethylcellulose or hydroxyethylcellulose): Biotene Dry Mouth Relieving Gel, Optimoist, Salivart, Salix, Xero-Lube, Moi-Stir® Oral Swabsticks, MouthKote)
	Systemic:
	Cevemeline (Evoxac) 30 mg 3 times a day
	Pilocarpine (Salagen) 5 mg 3–4 times a day

Source: Dental management of the HIV-infected patient. 1995. Supplement to *JADA.* American Dental Association and American Academy of Oral Medicine.

200 cells/mm^3 usually have their immunological status assessed every 6 months by their physician, whereas patients with counts of under 200 cells/mm^3 usually are assessed every 3 months.

Thrombocytopenia (under 150,000 platelets/mm^3) is often seen with HIV infection. Platelet counts are used to assess the patient for bleeding tendencies. Oral signs usually present as small, blood-filled petechiae or larger ecchymoses. Excessive bleeding during surgery may occur in these patients. Anemia is common in HIV-infected patients, either due to the medications or the infection; it is important to obtain laboratory blood values from the patient's physician.

Local anesthesia has not been associated with increased risk of intraoral infections. However, deep block injections can result in medical complications in patients with a recent history of increased bleeding tendencies. In these cases, use infiltration anesthesia.

There are generally no special restorative treatment precautions for the immunocompetent HIV-infected patient.

HIV-infected patients may be taking many different types of medications for the HIV infection itself as well as for opportunistic infections. Thus, many drug–drug interactions can occur. Many antiretroviral drugs have oral adverse effects; for instance, indinavir causes a metallic taste, ritonavir causes taste impairment, and amprenavir causes oral paresthesias. Additionally, many opportunistic infections are found in the mouth.

Antibiotic prophylaxis may be necessary, although not definitive, when the CD4+ count falls below 200 cells/mm^3. HIV infection itself is not a contraindication to procedures likely to cause bleeding. However, due to the systemic nature of the disease, the need for antibiotic prophylaxis should be assessed.

Meticulous oral hygiene should be reinforced with the HIV + patient at every office visit. At least twice a year the patient should have a recall; if oral lesions are present, more frequent visits are necessary. Patients should be placed on a topical fluoride supplement such as PreviDent 1.1% neutral sodium fluoride to prevent dental caries. Chlorhexidine gluconate as an oral rinse is effective as an antiplaque and anticaries agent by reducing *lactobacillus* counts.

Key Points

- Herpes labialis is a herpes simplex type 1 viral infection.
- Antiviral drugs should be applied at the first sign of a cold sore.
- Antiviral drugs are noncurative and only palliative.
- Acyclovir, famciclovir, and valacyclovir are systemic drugs used for herpes infections.
- Topical acyclovir and penciclovir are indicated for the management of herpes labialis.
- Docosanol (Abreva) is a cream that is available OTC.
- HIV-infected patients have many opportunistic infections, including oral lesions, that may be treated in the dental office with various medications.
- While the patient is being treated in the dental office, monitor the white blood cell counts.

Antifungal Agents

Fungal infections are caused by molds or yeasts. Some molds convert into yeasts once they infect the host (called dimorphic fungi). There are many types of fungal infections caused by different species of fungi.

The majority of healthy individuals have *Candida* species in the oropharyngeal (mouth) area. There are eight species of *Candida* that are regarded as clinically important pathogens in human disease. *Candida* is part of the normal flora in the gastrointestinal and vaginal tracts. Usually, *Candida* causes a localized superficial infection that is kept in check by the body; however, in certain circumstances such as immunocompromised hosts, the infection spreads.

The incidence of *Candida* infections has escalated over the years, in more immunocompromised individuals with AIDS. Histoplasmosis, a specific type of fungal infection caused by inhalation of dust-borne microorganisms, is commonly found in the AIDS patient. These patients are also more prone to developing oral fungal infections.

Mycosis

Fungal infections (mycosis) are classified into three groups: (1) systemic mycosis (e.g., soft tissue, meningitis, urinary tract infection); (2) superficial or mucocutaneous mycoses (e.g., nails, skin, and mucous membranes); and (3) subcutaneous mycoses (e.g., infections from contaminated soil).

Dental clinicians are usually most concerned and are involved in the treatment of mucocutaneous mycoses of the mouth. Candidiasis may also present as vaginal candidiasis (vulvovaginitis, usually after antibiotic therapy) or as a diaper rash in infants. Other categories of mucocutaneous candidiasis include esophageal candidiasis and gastrointestinal candidiasis. The diagnosis of oral candidiasis is based on the clinical appearance of the lesions and by scraping of lesions.

Oral candidiasis usually responds to topical therapy if there are no systemic complications. Systemic antifungal agents are used primarily for fungal infections *not* involving the oropharyngeal area, but can be used for severe mucocutaneous candidiasis infections.

Many fungal infections tend to recur after discontinuing drug treatment; antifungal drugs should be used for about 2 days after oral lesions disappear. Topical antifungal agents that can be applied to the oral mucosa include oral suspension, vaginal cream, or ointment. Other formulations used in treating oral candidiasis include troches/pastilles or vaginal suppositories, which are "sticky" and adhere to the oral mucosa, so they remain in the mouth for an extended period. Suppositories are less costly and have no sugar content, but may require psychological adjustment.

Nystatin (Mycostatin) is usually given as an oral suspension that is swished around in the mouth and then swallowed, or as a lozenge (pastille) that dissolves slowly in the mouth. Nystatin functions to cause fungal cell lysis (break apart). Clotrimazole (Mycelex) is given as a 10 mg troche that is slowly dissolved in the mouth. Patients with a high caries index should not be given troches or nystatin oral suspension because of their high sugar content. An alternative choice is a systemic tablet.

Severe and extensive oropharyngeal candidiasis can be treated with fluconazole (Diflucan), 100–200 mg orally twice a day. Prophylactic fluconazole is recommended for *Candida* suppression in HIV disease. Table 8-5 reviews common **antifungal agents** used to treat oral candidiasis. Systemic antifungal agents are reviewed in Table 8-6. Figure 8-6 shows sample prescriptions for antifungal agents used in the management of oral fungal infections.

Rapid Dental Hint

Miconazole 50 mg buccal tablet is a new once-daily formulation for the treatment of oral thrush. It is applied to the gingiva around the canine area and is slowly dissolved throughout the day for 14 days.

CANDIDIASIS: ACUTE PSEUDOMEMBRANOUS CANDIDIASIS (THRUSH) Acute pseudomembranous candidiasis or oral *thrush* appears on the oral mucous membranes as a white plaque that wipes off easily with gauze, leaving a raw, red, bleeding connective tissue

DID YOU KNOW?

Cryptococcus neoformans, a fungus discovered in the nineteenth century, can lead to brain infection and death in people with compromised immune systems (e.g., HIV).

surface. It is caused by an overgrowth of *Candidia albicans,* which may be caused by factors that reduce natural resistance, including:

- Systemic disease (uncontrolled diabetes mellitus)
- Immune-compromised patients (e.g., HIV/AIDS, chemotherapy, organ transplants)
- Use of broad-spectrum antibiotics
- Patients with poorly fitting dentures and who do not take them out at night (and are not immunocompromised)
- Older adults and pregnant women
- Newborns are especially susceptible to an overgrowth of *Candida albicans* because they do not have an established oral flora or fully developed immune system

TABLE 8-5 Antifungal Agents: Mucocutaneous Candidiasis

DRUG NAME	INDICATIONS AND ADVERSE EFFECTS	DENTAL APPLICATIONS
Topical	Indication: For mucocutaneous (superficial) mycoses; oral candidiasis (thrush) and skin/nail lesions	Dentures should be soaked at night. Replace toothbrush after infection is cleared up.
Clotrimazole (Mycelex) Troche 10 mg (Lotrimin) cream	Troche: for oral (oropharyngeal candidiasis) lesions; to prevent oropharyngeal candidiasis in immunocompromised conditions (e.g., chemotherapy, radiotherapy) Adverse effects: Nausea and vomiting (with oral troche), rash, stinging, peeling with skin application	Dissolve slowly (over 15–30 minutes) one troche (lozenge) 5 times a day (every 3 hours) for 14 days The troche contains carbohydrates and should not be used on a long-term basis in patients with xerostomia because of increased incidence of caries.
Miconazole (Monistat) cream, solution, powder, spray, buccal 50 mg (Oravig) tablet	If necessary can use for oral lesions (cream), but other products such as troches are better; for vaginal candidiasis and tinea pedis (althlete's foot) Adverse effect: burning	Dentures should be soaked at night. Replace toothbrush after infection is cleared up. Oravig is supplied as a 50 mg tablet. The tablet is flat on one side (marked with the letter "L") and a rounded side. The rounded side is applied to the gingiva in the depressed area above the lateral incisor. Once in place, use slight pressure on the outside of the lip for 30 seconds. The tablet will slowly dissolve throughout the day. It is used only once a day. Use alternating sides each time (www.oravig.com).
Nystatin (Mycostatin) oral suspension, pastilles (lozenge), vaginal tabs, cream, ointment, powder	Oral suspension and pastille are effective for oral candidiasis Adverse effects: nausea, vomiting, diarrhea, abdominal pain, bad taste in mouth with lozenge and oral suspension Vaginal tablets can be used orally since they are "sticky" to the oral mucosa Cream or powder is used for skin infections such as tinea pedis (althlete's foot)	The oral suspension should be swished around in mouth for a few minutes and then swallowed. Use after meals and before bedtime. Do not eat or drink for 30 minutes after; suck on the vaginal tablet or troche until it dissolves. Dentures should be removed before using the oral suspension, lozenge, or vaginal tablets. Remove dentures at night; the cream can be used orally by rubbing on to the affected area. The lozenge contains carbohydrates and should not be used on a long-term basis in patients with xerostomia because of increased incidence of caries.

TABLE 8-6   Systemic Antifungal Agents

Fluconazole (Diflucan) tab	For *severe oral lesions* or esophageal candidiasis: Oropharyngeal candidiasis: 200 mg on day one followed by 100 mg every day for a minimum of 3 weeks and 2 weeks after symptoms resolve; liver function tests need to be done monthly
	Systemic fungal infections (vaginal candidiasis, coccidioidal meningitis)
	Adverse effects: elevation of liver enzymes, nausea, vomiting, diarrhea
Itraconazole (Sporanox) tab	For severe lesions (e.g., nail, vulvovaginal candidiasis) other than oral
	Do not give to patients with heart failure or liver failure
	Well tolerated
	Some nausea, vomiting, headache, dizziness, hypertension
Ketoconazole (Nizoral) tab	For severe lesions other than oral
	Well tolerated
	Adverse effects: nausea, vomiting, stomach discomfort
Nystatin (Mycostatin) tab	Oral tablets are indicated for gastrointestinal candidiasis and not for dental fungal infections
	Adverse effects: diarrhea, nausea, vomiting, GI upset, rash
Griseofulvin (Fluvicin, Grisactin, Griful-vin) tab	For severe lesions other than oral; not effective against *Candida*
	For scalp and hair ringworm; high rate of hepatitis
	Adverse effects: photosensitivity (increased incidence of burning when exposed to sun)
	Other drugs are more effective
Amphotericin B (Fungizone) Parenteral	For severe skin fungal infection, oral suspension for oral candidiasis, parenteral and topical administration
	Adverse effects: hypertension, fever, chills, hypokalemia (low potassium levels), hypomagnesimia, GI discomfort, anemia, nephrotoxicity (kidney damage)

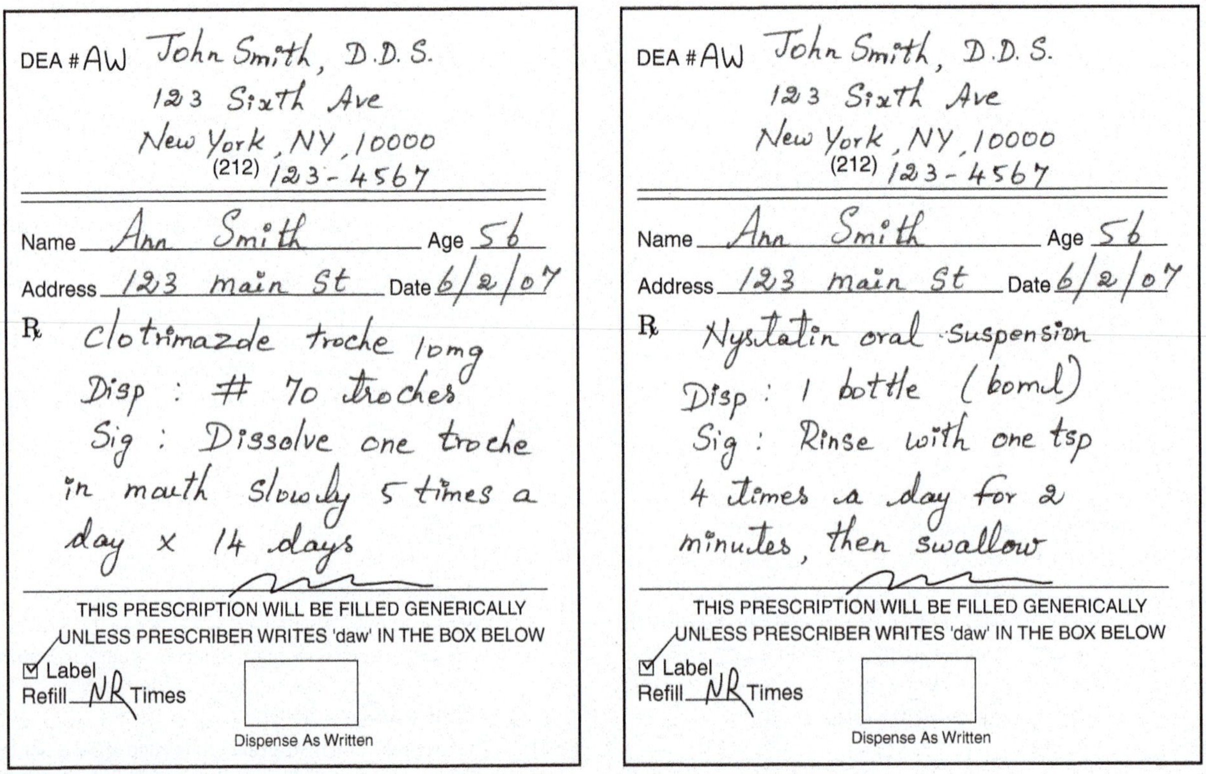

FIGURE 8-6 Sample prescriptions of drugs for oral fungal infections.

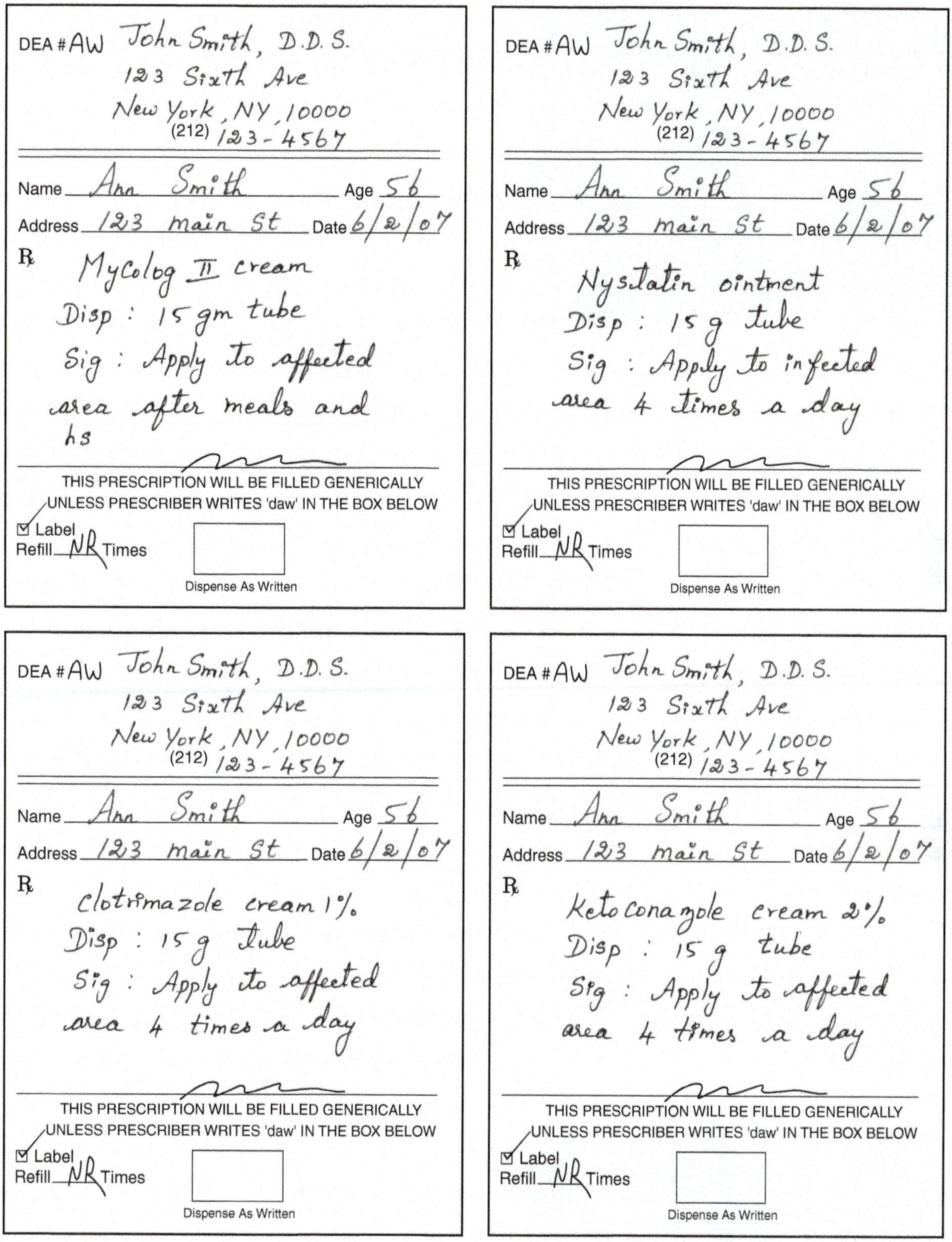

DEA #AW   John Smith, D.D.S.
123 Sixth Ave
New York, NY, 10000
(212) 123-4567

Name   Ann Smith   Age 56
Address   123 main St   Date 6/2/07
℞

MyColog II cream
Disp : 15 gm tube
Sig : Apply to affected
area after meals and
hs

THIS PRESCRIPTION WILL BE FILLED GENERICALLY
UNLESS PRESCRIBER WRITES 'daw' IN THE BOX BELOW
☑ Label
Refill NR Times
Dispense As Written

DEA #AW   John Smith, D.D.S.
123 Sixth Ave
New York, NY, 10000
(212) 123-4567

Name   Ann Smith   Age 56
Address   123 main St   Date 6/2/07
℞

Nystatin ointment
Disp : 15 g tube
Sig : Apply to infected
area 4 times a day

THIS PRESCRIPTION WILL BE FILLED GENERICALLY
UNLESS PRESCRIBER WRITES 'daw' IN THE BOX BELOW
☑ Label
Refill NR Times
Dispense As Written

DEA #AW   John Smith, D.D.S.
123 Sixth Ave
New York, NY, 10000
(212) 123-4567

Name   Ann Smith   Age 56
Address   123 main St   Date 6/2/07
℞

Clotrimazole cream 1%
Disp : 15 g tube
Sig : Apply to affected
area 4 times a day

THIS PRESCRIPTION WILL BE FILLED GENERICALLY
UNLESS PRESCRIBER WRITES 'daw' IN THE BOX BELOW
☑ Label
Refill NR Times
Dispense As Written

DEA #AW   John Smith, D.D.S.
123 Sixth Ave
New York, NY, 10000
(212) 123-4567

Name   Ann Smith   Age 56
Address   123 main St   Date 6/2/07
℞

Ketoconazole cream 2%
Disp : 15 g tube
Sig : Apply to affected
area 4 times a day

THIS PRESCRIPTION WILL BE FILLED GENERICALLY
UNLESS PRESCRIBER WRITES 'daw' IN THE BOX BELOW
☑ Label
Refill NR Times
Dispense As Written

FIGURE 8-6 (*Continued*)

Treatment depends on the age of the patient. Nystatin oral suspension is recommended for infants. For adults, treatment is with topical or systemic antifungal agents such as fluconazole (Diflucan) or ketoconazole (Nizoral).

CHRONIC ATROPHIC CANDIDIASIS (DENTURE SORE MOUTH)
This condition is seen in patients with maxillary dentures. When the denture is removed the palatal tissue appears as either small, localized asymptomatic (not painful) red spots (in the mild form) and (in a more severe form) the entire tissue is red (outlining the shape of the denture) (Figure 8-7). This usually appears in patients who wear the denture continuously without removing it to clean it. It is a fungal infection caused by *Candida albicans*.

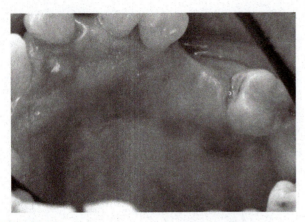

FIGURE 8-7 Denture sore mouth in a patient who never removed partial dentures at night. (Courtesy of *U.S. Pharmacist*).

Since it is a fungal infection, topical antifungal agents are generally used. Nystatin (Mycostatin) pastilles/oral suspension/ointment, miconazole cream 2%, ketoconazole cream 2%, and clotrimazole (Mycelex) cream 2%/troches are some antifungal agents. The cream should be applied to the inner surface of the denture and a reline of the denture may be indicated. Patients with a high caries rate should not be given a suspension, troches, or pastilles because of the sugar content. The patient should be instructed not to wear the denture at night.

ANGULAR CHEILOSIS   Angular cheilosis (or angular cheilitis) appears at the commissures of the lips (Figure 8-8). It is thought that this is a fungal infection caused by *Candida albicans* or a B-vitamin complex deficiency. Moist skin folds due to drooling and overclosure (decrease vertical dimension) are added factors in the development of these lesions.

Since it is a fungal infection, topical antifungal creams/ointments are the drugs of choice (Table 8-5).

Drug Interactions

There are many drug–drug interactions that are important with systemic agents and must be recognized. Since systemic antifungal drugs are metabolized by the P450 cytochrome liver enzymes, many other drugs that also are involved in this system will interfere. Topically applied antifungal agents are not involved in this metabolism.

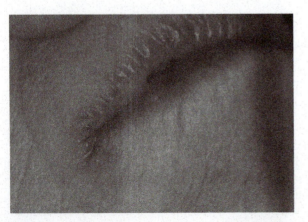

FIGURE 8-8 Angular cheilitis. (Courtesy of *U.S. Pharmacist*).

Ketoconazole inhibits the metabolism of several drugs by inhibiting the CYP3A4 isoenzyme, which increases the blood level of the following drugs:

- Benzodiazepines
- Calcium channel blockers (e.g., diltiazem, verapamil)
- Erythromycin

Fluconazole is an inhibitor of CYP2C9, so the following drugs will have increased blood levels:

- Warfarin
- Calcium channel blockers

Subcutaneous and Systemic Mycosis

These fungal infections are not related to dentistry, and thus will not be discussed in depth. Sportrichosis is an example of subcutaneous mycoses seen especially in diabetics, and occurs usually after a splinter or a thorn from a plant that enters the skin.

Systemic or deep mycoses usually occur commonly after inhalation of the offending organism including *Aspergillus, Cryptoccocus* (from bird feces), *Blastomyces,* and *Candida.* Treatment of cryptococcosis is with amphotericin B, which is administered parenterally and which can cause serious adverse effects.

Rapid Dental Hint

Be aware of fungal infections in patients who wear dentures and do not practice good oral hygiene. Management: cleanse the denture; may require relining or a new denture; use an antifungal agent.

Dental Hygiene Applications

In dentistry, mucocutaneous mycoses commonly present as infections of the oral mucous membranes. Thus, these infections will be managed by the dentist. Various causes of oral candidiasis (thrush), which is caused by the yeast *Candida albicans,* include broad-spectrum antibiotics, diabetes, inhalation corticosteroids, newborns, and in immunocompromised patients receiving immunosuppressive drugs that suppress the immune system and encourage fungi to overgrow.

Patients taking a broad-spectrum antibiotic (e.g., tetracycline, doxycycline, minocycline, amoxicillin) should be instructed to take supplemental acidophilus (found in the vitamin section of the pharmacy) or yogurt (not in combination with tetracycline) to help reduce the chances of developing a superinfection. Patients using a corticosteroid inhaler for asthma should be instructed to brush the teeth and rinse the mouth with water after each use to prevent development of oral candidiasis. Patients presenting with an oral infection (thrush) are best treated with a topical antifungal agent, which may be in the form of a troche, vaginal suppository, or oral suspension. Topical therapy has fewer side effects and a lower cost to the patient than systemic agents. If the oral infection is severe (oral and esophageal) such as in HIV disease, systemic antifungal agents may be used such as fluconazole (Diflucan).

Rapid Dental Hint

Remember to recommend to patients taking an antibiotic (e.g., tetraycycline, amoxicillin) to also take yogurt (except not to take it at the same time with tetracycline) or acidophilus to avoid developing a fungal infection.

Key Points

- Oral candidiasis or thrush is caused by *Candida albicans*.
- Treatment of oral candidiasis is usually adequate with topical antifungal agents.
- Topical therapy for oral candidiasis is with nystatin oral suspension or clotrimazole troches.
- Many drug–drug interactions occur with systemic antifungal agents because these drugs are metabolized by the P450 cytochrome liver enzymes.

Board Review Questions

1. Which of the following antiherpetic drugs is recommended for herpes labialis? (pp. 140–142)
   a. Ganciclovir
   b. Famciclovir
   c. Valacyclovir
   d. Penciclovir

2. Which of the following drugs is contraindicated for treating herpes labialis? (p. 141)
   a. Penicillin
   b. Docosanol
   c. Penciclovir
   d. Acyclovir

3. Herpes simplex virus 1 causes oral herpes. There is cross-infection where both HSV-1 and HSV-2 are transmitted by intimate contact. (p. 140)
   a. Both statements are true.
   b. First statement is true and second is false.
   c. First statement is false and second is true.
   d. Both statements are false.

4. Which of the following antiviral agents is available over-the-counter for treating herpes labialis? (p. 141)
   a. Valacyclovir
   b. Docosanol
   c. Penciclovir
   d. Acyclovir

5. What is the major ingredient in Anbesol? (p. 142)
   a. Lidocaine
   b. Camphor
   c. Benzocaine
   d. Benzyl alcohol

6. Which of the following terms is used for acute pseudo-membranous candidiasis? (p. 149)
   a. Esophagitis
   b. Thrush
   c. Vaginitis
   d. Cryptococcosis

7. Which of the following drugs interacts with systemic fluconazole (Diflucan)? (p. 152)
   a. Erythromycin
   b. Penicillin
   c. Acetaminophen
   d. Ibuprofen

8. Which of the following is the treatment of choice in the therapy of oral candidiasis? (pp. 149–152)
   a. Nystatin suspension
   b. Ketoconazole tablets
   c. Fluconazole tablets
   d. Miconazole ointment

9. Which of the following is the cause of angular cheilitis? (p. 152)
   a. Viral
   b. Bacterial
   c. Fungal
   d. Vitamin C deficiency

10. Which of the following agents is best for severe oropharyngeal candidiasis when topical therapy is inadequate? (p. 151)
    a. Griseovulvin
    b. Fluconazole
    c. Clotrimazole
    d. Nystatin

11. During an oral examination of a patient with a maxillary denture the hygienist notes that the palatal tissue is very red and shiny following the outline of the denture. How should the hygienist manage this problem? (p. 151)
    a. Tell the patient everything is fine.
    b. The patient should remove the denture and clean it and a topical antifungal medication may be needed.
    c. The patient requires an antibiotic because it is a bacterial infection.
    d. An antiviral agent is necessary because it is a herpetic infection.

12. Which of the following antiretroviral drugs may cause taste impairment? (p. 146)
    a. Enfuvirtide
    b. Nelfinavir
    c. Ritonavir
    d. Saquinavir

13. A patient with HIV/AIDS presents to the dental clinic and is taking many drugs. His chief complaint is a metallic taste in the mouth. Which of the following antiretroviral drugs may cause this problem? (p. 146)
    a. Fosamprenavir
    b. Atazanavir
    c. Amprevavir
    d. Indinavir

14. Which of the following antiretroviral drugs may cause numbness in the mouth? (p. 146)
    a. Fosamprenavir
    b. Ritonavir
    c. Indinavir
    d. Saquinavir

15. Which of the following antiretroviral drugs can cause dental pain? (p. 146)
    a. Fosamprenavir
    b. Atazanavir
    c. Indinavir
    d. Nelfinavir

Selected References

Abu-Elteen KH, Abu-Elteen RM. 1998. The prevalence of *Candida albicans* populations in the mouths of complete denture wearers. *New Microbiol* 21:41–48.

Akpan A, Morgan R. 2002. Oral candidiasis. *Postgraduate Medical Journal* 78:455–459.

Amir J. 2002. Primary herpetic gingivostomatitis: Clinical aspects and antiviral treatment. *Harefusah* 141:81–84, 124.

Arduino PG, Porter SR. 2006. Oral and perioral herpes simplex virus type 1 (HSV-1) infection: Review of its management. *Oral Dis* 12:254–370.

Birek C, Ficarra G. 2006. The diagnosis and management of oral herpes simplex infection. *Curr Infect Dis Rep* 8:181–188.

Canker sores and cold sores 2005. *J Am Dent Assoc* 136(3):415.

Chesebro MJ, Everett WD. 1998. Understanding the guidelines for treating HIV disease. *Am Fam Physician* 57:315–322.

Choi SY, Kahyo H. 1991. Effect of cigarette smoking and alcohol consumption in the aetiology of cancer of the oral cavity, pharynx and larynx. *Int J Epidemiol* 20:878–885.

Engle JP. 2002. Oral pain and discomfort. In *APhA handbook of nonprescription drugs: An interactive approach to self-care,* 13th ed. Washington, DC: American Pharmaceutical Association.

Fotos PG, Vincent SD, Hellstein JW. 1992. Oral candidosis. Clinical, historical and therapeutic features of 100 cases. *Oral Sug Oral Med Oral Pathol* 74:41–49.

Golecka M, Oldakowska-Jedynak U, Mierzwinska-Nastalska E, Adamczyk-Kanli A, Demirel F, Sezgin Y. 2005. Oral candidosis, denture cleanliness and hygiene habits in an elderly population. *Aging Clin Exp Res* 17:502–507.

Guidelines for the Use of Antiretroviral Agents in HIV-Infected Adults and Adolescents. February 4, 2002. Department of Health and Human Services (DHHS) and the Henry J. Kaiser Family Foundation.

Gulick RM, Ribaudo HJ, Shikuma CM, Lalama C, Schackman BR, et al. 2006. Three- vs. four-drug antiretroviral regimens for the initial treatment of HIV-1 infection. *JAMA* 296:769–781.

Hammer SM, Saag MS, Schechter M, Montaner JSG, Schooley RT, et al. 2006. Treatment for adult HIV infection. *JAMA* 296:827–843.

Heaton ML, Al-Hashimi I, Plemons J, Rees T. 2006. Experimental chairside test for the rapid diagnosis of oropharyngeal candidiasis. *Compendium* 27:364–370.

Koda-Kimble MA, Young LY, Dradjan WA, Guglielmo BJ. 2002. Infectious diseases: Pharmacotherapy of Human Immunodeficiency Virus infection. In *Handbook of applied therapeutics,* 7th ed. Philadelphia: Lippincott Williams & Wilkins, pp. 1–20.

Kolokotronis A, Doumas S. 2006. Herpes simplex virus infection, with particular reference to the progression and complications of primary herpetic gingivostomatitis. *Clin Microbiol Infect* 12:202–211.

Mackowiak E. 2003. Prevention and treatment of cold sores. *U.S. Pharmacist* 28:77–84.

Ohman SC, Dahlen G, Moller A, Ohman A. 1986. Angular cheilitis: A clinical and microbial study. *J Oral Pathol* 15:213–217.

Raborn GW, Martel AY, Lassonde M, Lewis MAO, et al. 2002. Effective treatment of herpes simplex labialis with penciclovir cream: Combined results of two trials. *J Am Dent Assoc* 133:303–309.

Reznik DA. 2005. Oral manifestastions of HIV disease. *Top HIV Med* 13:143–148.

Rooney JF, Straus SE, Mannix ML, Wohlenberg CR. 1993. Oral acyclovir to suppress frequently recurrent herpes labialis: A double-blind, placebo-controlled trial. *Ann Intern Med* 118:268–272.

Seelig MS. 1966. Mechanism by which antibiotics increase the incidence and severity of candidiasis and later the immunological defenses. *Bacteriol Rev* 30:442–459.

Sosinska E. 2006. Candida-associated denture stomatitis in patients after immunosuppression therapy. *Transplant Proc* 38:155–156.

Wong-Beringer A, Kriengkauykiat J. 2003. Systemic antifungal therapy: New options, new challenges. *Pharmacotherapy* 23(*11*):1441–1462.

Worrall G. 2004. Herpes labialis. *Clin Evid* 12:2312–2320.

Web Sites

www.medscape.com
www.outlineMed.com
www.emedicine.com
www.jada.ada.org/cg/reprint/134/7/853.pdf

QUICK DRUG GUIDE

Antiherpetic Drugs

- Acyclovir sodium (Zovirax)
- Famciclovir (Famvir) tabs
- Valacyclovir (Valtrex) tabs
- Penciclovir (Denavir) cream
- Docosanol (Abreva)
- Ganciclovir (Cytovene)

Antiretroviral Drugs: HIV/AIDS

Nucleoside Reverse Transcriptase Inhibitors (NRTIs)

- Abacavir (Ziagen)
- Didansoine (ddl, Videx)
- Emtricitabine (Emtriva)
- Lamivudine (3TC, Epivir)
- Stavudine (d4T, Zerit)
- Tenofovir (Viread)
- Zalcitabine (ddC, Hivid—HIVID)
- Zidovudine (Retrovir): formerly azidothymidine (AZT)

Non-nucleoside Reverse Transcriptase Inhibitors (NNRTI)

- Delavirdine (Rescriptor)
- Efavirenz (Sustiva)
- Nevirapine (Viramune)

Protease Inhibitors (PIs)

- Amprevavir (Agenerase)
- Atazanavir (Reyataz)
- Fosamprenavir (Lexiva)
- Indinavir (Crixivan)
- Lopinavir + Ritonavir (Kaletra)
- Nelfinavir (Viracept)
- Ritonavir (Norvir)
- Saquinavir (Fortovase)

Fusion Inhibitors

- Enfuvirtide (Fuzeon)

Antimycobacterial Drugs: Tuberculosis (TB)

First-Line Anti-TB Drugs

- Isoniazid (isonicotinic acid hydrazide; INH)
- Rifampin (Rifadin)
- Pyrazinamide (PZA)
- Ethambutol (Myambutol)

Second-Line Anti-TB Drugs

- Cycloserine (Seromycin)
- Ethionamide (Trecator-SC)
- Para-aminosalicylic acid (Paser)
- Streptomycin (Streptomycin)
- Capreomycin (Capastat sulfate)

Antifungal Drugs

Topical

- Clotrimazole (Mycelex Lotrimen)
- Miconazole (Monistat)
- Nystatin (Mycostatin)

Systemic

- Fluconazole (Diflucan)
- Itraconazole (Sporanox)
- Ketoconazole (Nizoral)
- Griseofulvin (Fluvicin, Grisactin, Grifulvin)
- Terbinafine (Lamisil) tabs
- Amphotericin B (Fungizone)

Antineoplastic, Immunosuppressant, and Bisphosphonate Drugs

GOAL

To provide knowledge of commonly used drugs used in the treatment of cancer and organ rejection and their oral complications.

EDUCATIONAL OBJECTIVES

After reading this chapter, the reader should be able to:

1. Discuss the role of antineoplastic agents in the treatment of neoplasms.

2. List the commonly used antineoplastic agents.

3. Discuss the common oral adverse effects of antineoplastic agents.

4. Describe the adverse effects and drug interactions of immunosuppressant drugs.

5. Review recommendations and guidelines for dental patients taking bisphosphonates for hypercalcemia.

KEY TERMS

Antineoplastic drugs

Chemotherapeutic drugs

Xerostomia

Oral mucositis

Oral candidiasis

Bisphosphonates

Osteonecrosis of the jaw (ONJ)

Immunosuppressant drugs

Antineoplastic Drugs

Actions

Antineoplastic or **chemotherapeutic drugs** are used to treat various types of cancers or neoplasms (abnormally growing cells) that cannot be treated by surgery, or are used in conjunction with surgery and radiation therapy. Neoplasms can be benign (where cells do not invade the tissues) or malignant (where cells invade and spread or metastasize to all areas of the body, including areas not affected by the cancer).

Antineoplastics, the most toxic drugs in use today, act by killing cancer cells through damaging cell DNA or interfering with DNA synthesis. Unfortunately, while killing cancer cells, most drugs also affect normal cells, which contribute to a high incidence of adverse serious side effects, toxicity, and teratogenicity, even with usual dosing. The two most common adverse side effects are nausea and vomiting. Other toxic effects include bone marrow suppression (inhibition of blood cell replication in the bone marrow), resulting leukopenia (decrease in neutrophils or white blood cells), which predisposes patients to serious infections, and thrombocytopenia (decrease in platelets), which may lead to serious bleeding problems.

Some agents primarily affect cells that are actively multiplying (Table 9-1). These agents are called cell cycle-specific (CCS) antineoplastic agents. Examples include antimetabolites. Other agents, called cell cycle-nonspecific (CCNS), kill cells that are actively multiplying or at rest. These agents are more toxic to normal cells than the CCS agents, but are good for slow growing neoplasms. Examples of these include alkylating agents and antitumor antibiotics. A major cause of cancer treatment failure is drug resistance, resulting in drugs that do not work on the cells. Antineoplastic drugs are divided into the following categories:

- Alkylating agents
- Antimetabolites
- Hormones
- Antitumor antibiotics
- Immunomodulators
- Plant extracts (mitotic inhibitors)

Cetuximab (Erbitux) was FDA approved in 2006 for use in combination with radiation therapy to treat patients with squamous cell cancer of the head and neck that cannot be removed by surgery.

Some cancer cells are becoming resistant to the drugs being administered because sometimes chemotherapy has to be stopped due to low white blood cells and/or infection. The oncologist's approach is to "hit hard and fast" with chemotherapy to prevent resistant cancer cells from developing.

Different agents are used to treat the various types of cancers. It is not within the scope of this textbook to review all adverse side effects particular to each drug, or to review specific

TABLE 9-1 Common Antineoplastic Drugs

DRUG NAME

Alkylating Agents (DNA Alkylating Drugs)	Antimetabolites (DNA Synthesis Inhibitors)	Vinorelbine (Navelbine)
Cyclophosphamide (Cytoxan)	Cladribine (Leustatin)	*Taxanes*
Altretamine (Hexalen)	Cytarabine (Cytosar-U)	Docetaxel (Taxotere)
Busulfan (Myleran)	Floxuridine (FUDR)	Paclitaxel (Taxol)
Chlorambucil (Leukeran)	Fludarabine phosphate (Fludara)	*Topoisomerase Inhibitors*
Melphalan (Alkeran)	Fluorouracil Gemcitabine (Gemsar)	Topotecan (Hycamtin)
Carboplatin (Paraplatin)	Mercaptopurine (Purinethol)	Etoposide (VePesid)
Cisplatin (Platinol)	Methotrexate (Mexate)	Teniposide (Vumon)
Cyclophosphamide (Cytoxan)	Pentostatin (Nipent)	Irinotecan (Camptosar)
Dacarbazine (DTIC-Dome)	**Antitumor Antibiotics**	**Hormones and Antagonists**
Ifosfamide (Ifex)	Bleomycin (Blenoxane)	Flutamide (Eulexin)
Mechlorethamine HCl (Mustargen)	Daunorubicin HCl (Cerubidine)	Leuprolide (Lupron)
Mitomycin (Mutamycin)	Doxorubicin HCl) (Adriamycin)	Prednisone
Carmustine (BiCNU)	Idarubicin HCl (Idamycin)	Tamoxifen (Novadex)
Lomustine (CeeNU)	**Plant Alkaloids or Extracts**	**Immunomodulators (Cytokines)**
Procarbazine HCl (Matulane)	*Mitotic Inhibitors*	Aldesleukin (Proleukin)
Streptozocin (Zanosar)	Vinblastine (Velban)	Interferon alfa
Thiotepa (Thioplex)	Vincristine (Oncovin)	

features. The emphasis of this chapter will be on chemotherapeutic drugs and oral adverse side effects.

Treatment

Cancer may be treated using surgery, radiation therapy, and drugs. Radiation therapy is effective in killing tumor cells through nonsurgical methods. High doses of ionizing radiation are aimed directly at the tumor and confined to this area as much as possible. Radiation therapy is frequently used for head and neck cancers such as squamous cell carcinoma. Cancer chemotherapy is very complex, involving the use of chemical agents that act by different mechanisms.

Adverse Effects

Chemotherapeutic drugs attack the faster growing cells in tissues including bone marrow, gastrointestinal tract, and skin. Many adverse reactions occur throughout the body, as described below.

BLOOD Bone marrow suppression is influenced by the type of drug used, the patient's age, bone marrow reserve, the patient's nutritional status, and liver and kidney function. Bone marrow suppression causes anemia (low red blood cell count), neutropenia (low neutrophil count), and thrombocytopenia (low platelet count), which can be prevented by colony-stimulating factors.

To decrease the incidence of infection (manifested by febrile neutropenia) in patients receiving myelosuppressive anticancer drugs or associated with bone marrow suppression, patients may be taking filgrastim (Neupogen), which increases neutrophil proliferation and differentiation within the bone marrow.

> **DID YOU KNOW?**
>
> Green tea is a natural antioxidant that is thought to have a protective effect against cancer.

Epoetin alfa (human recombinant erythropoietin) is indicated in patients with chemotherapy-induced anemia and zidovudine-induced anemia in patients with HIV infection. Epoetin stimulates production of red blood cells (erythropoiesis).

GASTROINTESTINAL TOXICITIES Nausea and vomiting. Treatment is with antimetics before chemotherapy and after for several days.

DERMATOLOGICAL TOXICITIES Inhibition of epidermal mitotic activity causes alopecia (loss of hair), nail changes, dry skin, and blistering.

OTHER TOXICITIES Chemotherapeutic drugs cause neurotoxicity, cardiac toxicities, nephrotoxicity, pulmonary toxicities, and hepatotoxicity.

ORAL TOXICITIES: DENTAL COMPLICATIONS Patients taking antineoplastic agents should have a medical consultation before dental treatment is started. Complications of the oral cavity occur in about 40% of patients treated with chemotherapy and all patients receiving radiation. Oral complications include mucositis, xerostomia, caries, bleeding, and oral candidiasis (Table 9-2).

Rapid Dental Hint

Monitor chemotherapy patients for oral conditions.

Xerostomia and Caries **Xerostomia** may occur due to suppression of salivary function, but it is usually not permanent, so treatment is usually palliative. Patients can become uncomfortable because there is no salivary lubrication and the mucosal tissues get "sticky." Dry mucosa may also be more prone to bleeding. Due to xerostomia, there is an increased incidence of candidiasis and dental/root caries. For prevention of caries patients should be placed on a neutral sodium fluoride rinse, such as Prevident rinse, or an acidulated phosphate rinse such as Phos-Flur. Amifostine (Ethyol), an organic thiophosphate chemoprotectant agent, is approved to reduce the incidence of moderate to severe xerostomia in patients undergoing postoperative radiation treatment for head and neck cancer.

Mucositis **Oral mucositis** (OM) is an inflammation leading to ulcerations or mouth sores on the buccal, labial, and soft palate mucosa, along with the ventral surface of the tongue and floor of the mouth. Pain usually occurs in 5–7 days following the start of therapy. Small areas of ulceration or petechaie quickly become large areas due to the direct toxic effects of the antimetabolites; antimetabolites and antitumor antibiotics are directly toxic to the mucosa. Mucosal toxicity is caused by the suppression of epithelial cell growth, and the highest incidence is found during periods of the lowest levels of white blood cells. It is difficult to prevent as well as treat mucositis; however, it is not permanent. Patients usually also have xerostomia. Maintenance of excellent oral care before and during cancer treatment is important to help reduce the frequency and severity of OM. Chlorhexidine is used because it is substantive and stays on the soft tissue. Refer to Table 9-3.

Rapid Dental Hint

Assess your patients for mucositis; it is difficult to prevent and treat.

TABLE 9-2 Dental-Related Adverse Effects in Patients Undergoing Cancer Treatment

SITUATION	RESULTS	TREATMENT
Suppressed white blood cell count (neutropenia) (< 1000 mm^3)	Infection (may be life threatening)	Contact patient's physician; use of antibiotics to prevent bacteremia (infective endocarditis)
Thrombocytopenia < 100,000 mm^3	Bleeding (gingival bleeding and mucosal surface bleeding)	Contact patient's physician before any dental treatment, including extractions If localized bleeding occurs during dental treatment, apply a hemostatic agent such as topical thrombin solution (apply with gauze and hold in place using pressure for 30 minutes—do not remove clots that have formed).
Oral mucositis: Involves gingival tissue inflammation as well as uclerations	Pain and burning of the oral mucosa; difficult to maintain oral hygiene	Difficult to prevent and treat; treatment is palliative. Excellent oral hygiene helps reduce the frequency and severity of OM. Rinses: Chlorhexidine rinse (has substantivity so it binds to oral tissue) Saline (salt) water, sodium bicarbonate solutions Other medications: viscous lidocaine 2% solution (swish in mouth until pain disappears and then spit out) Diphenhydramine elixir 15.5 mg mixed with kaopectate (50% mixture by volume); rinse with one teaspoonful every 2 hours Nystatin 1 ml mixed with Maalox (Ω120 ml), swish and spit out If the mucositis is localized to a specific area, use Benzocaine in Orabase (OTC–Colgate Oral) (apply by dabbing on the affected area; do not rub it on) Additional treatment: • Remove dentures and orthodontic appliances • Gentle toothbrushing with soft brush • Avoid mouthrinses that contain alcohol • Lubricants, such as artificial saliva, may loosen mucous and prevent membranes from sticking together • Avoid spicy, acidic, and salted foods • Use sugar-free gum or candy to stimulate saliva
Xerostomia: Usually not permanent	Increased caries, difficult to eat	Palliative treatment: sugarless candies, increase water intake, avoid alcohol, which further dries the mucosa Saliva substitutes (carboxymethylcellulose or hydroxyethylcellulose): Biotene Dry Mouth Relieving Gel, Optimoist, Salivart, Salix, Xero-Lube, Moi-Stir, Oral Swabsticks, MouthKote Systemic: Cevimeline (Evoxac) 30 mg tid Pilocarpine (Salagen) 5 mg 3–4 times a day
Oral candidiasis (thrush)	Increased growth of opportunistic fungi	Use topical/systemic antifungal agents: nystatin, clotrimazole, fluconazole
Oral biofilm accumulation	Gingival inflammation	Chlorhexidine oral rinse as an adjunct to meticulous oral hygiene

Esophagitis Esophagitis is caused by damage to the mucosal lining and usually presents as dysphagia (difficulty in swallowing). Treatment involves adequate fluid intake, avoiding acidic foods, and use of drugs such as proton pump inhibitors. Esophagitis usually resolved about 1–2 weeks after bone marrow recovery.

Oral Candidiasis Oral candidiasis (thrush) is common due to an overgrowth of fungi because of reduced white blood cell count (leukopenia). *It may be more important to prevent rather than treat oral candidiasis.*

Bacterial Infections The primary concern with high bacteria levels is the increased incidence of bacteremia. Most patients require central line placement for administering chemotherapy. Thus, the

TABLE 9-3 Immunosuppressant Drugs

DRUG NAME
Azathioprine (Imuran)
Cyclosporine (Sandimmune, Neoral)
Tacrolimus (Prograf)

patient may be placed on antibiotics as a prophylaxis for infective endocarditis. Bacterial infections are seen due to bone marrow suppression, which reduces the white blood cell count (remember that white blood cells such as neutrophils have a protective function to engulf and kill invading bacteria). Chlorhexidine gluconate oral rinse is helpful in reducing bacterial levels and helps with oral hygiene.

Taste   Alterations in taste are commonly seen in cancer patients, which may occur due to a drug's ability to affect sensitive taste-buds. Patients lose the ability to differentiate between sweet and salty foods, and are at increased risk for dental/root caries.

Bleeding and Impaired Healing   Oral ulceration, petechiae, and bleeding are usually due to thrombocytopenia (low platelet count). This generally resolves after bone marrow recovery. Impaired wound healing occurs due to neutropenia.

Limitations to Dental Treatment

There are limitations in treating patients undergoing treatment for cancer (Table 9-2). The majority of patients will have depressed white blood cells (neutrophils), which may increase the incidence of infections (signs of infection may be fever, malaise), and patients may also have low platelets, which may increase the incidence of bleeding. Antibiotics may be necessary when white blood cell counts fall below 1,500 mm^3 because of impaired healing. Bleeding becomes significant when platelets fall below 100,000 mm^3. There are some drug interactions with antineoplastic agents, but there are no dental drug interactions. Nausea and vomiting may complicate treatment of patients.

Bisphosphonates

In the mid-1990s **bisphosphonates** were first introduced and prescribed as alternate drugs for hormone replacement therapies (HRTs) for osteoporosis and to treat osteolytic tumors and possibly to slow tumor development. In 1996, alendronate (Fosamax) was the first bisphosphonate drug approved for osteoporosis (low bone mass and reduced bone strength that leads to fractures of the spine, wrist, and hip) in postmenopausal women. Over the past 5 years there has been major dental concerns regarding a rare adverse reaction of osteonecrosis of the jaw (ONJ) induced by bisphosphonates.

Bisphosphonates act by inhibiting bone resorption by decreasing the action of osteoclasts. The osteoclastic resorption of mineralized bone and cartilage is blocked through its binding to bone, which keeps the bone more dense. Also, bisphosphonates inhibit the increased osteoclastic activity and skeletal calcium release into the bloodstream induced by various stimulatory factors released by tumors. Oral bisphosphonates have an extremely long half-life (e.g., alendronate has a half-life that can exceed 10 years).

Hypercalcemia of Malignancy

In patients with hypercalcemia of malignancy (HCM), intravenous bisphosphonates decreased serum calcium and phosphorous and increased urinary calcium and phosphorous excretion. The following bisphosphonates are used in cancer therapy:

- clodronate (Bonefos)
- pamidronate (Aredia)
- zoledronate (Zometa)

Generally, hypercalcemia with malignancy occurs in patients who have breast cancer, squamous cell tumors of the head and neck or lung, renal cell carcinoma, and some blood malignancies such as multiple myeloma. Excessive release of calcium into the blood (hypercalemia) occurs as bone is resorbed.

Patients receiving intravenous bisphosphonates for cancer that has spread to the bone and undergoing extensive dental treatment can develop a condition called **osteonecrosis of the jaw (ONJ)**. The following are local dental risk factors for ONJ in patients taking intravenous or oral bisphosphonates:

- Periodontal surgery
- Extractions
- Dental implant surgery
- Ill-fitting dentures that is irritating to the tissues
- Less likely with endodontic therapy, orthodontics, scaling and root planing

Clinical features of osteonecrosis of the jaw include areas of exposed bone that occur after dental surgery or spontaneously that have not healed after 6 weeks. This condition is caused by a decrease in blood flow to the area. Bisphosphonates are indicated for cancer patients at high risk of hypercalcemia due to malignancy or skeletal-related events. The FDA and the drug companies have issued precautions for dentists to follow in patients receiving intravenous Acredia and Zometa. It is recommended that dental procedures requiring bone healing be done before patients are placed on bisphosphonates. Additionally, meticulous oral hygiene is important. Current treatment of ONJ includes antibiotics, oral rinses, pain control, and limited periodontal debridement (Novartis Pharmaceuticals Corporation. Updated Recommendations for the Prevention, Diagnosis and Treatment of Osteonecrosis of the Jaw in Cancer Patients, May 2006). It is advised that patients have a dental examination and all dental procedures be completed prior to the start of bisphosphonate therapy. Careful medical history is needed to determine if a patient will require or is currently on bisphosphonates. Patients should go for routine dental maintenance visits at least every 6 months and maintain good oral hygiene. Routine restorative and dental hygiene procedures may be performed. Elective dental procedures are not advised for patients on IV bisphosphonates.

Immunosuppressant Drugs

Immunosuppressant drugs are used in patients after receiving an organ transplant from another human being to prevent rejection of the organ (e.g., kidney, heart, lung, or liver) or in the treatment of vesicular bullous conditions such as bullous

TABLE 9-4 Oral Care of Cancer Patients Before, During, and After Therapy		
BEFORE	**DURING**	**AFTER**
• Extract all questionable/hopeless teeth • Instruct patients on proper oral home care regimens • Treat any infections	• Medical consultation before any dental treatment • May require antibiotic coverage • Treatment depends on neutrophil count (treatment only if below 1,000 mm³) • Examine and monitor patients' oral status: development of ulcerations	• Resume normal dental care

pemphigoid, lupus erythematosis (LE), and rheumatoid arthritis. These drugs are usually given together with glucocorticosteroids. Immunosuppressant drugs include azathioprine, cyclosporine, and tacrolimus. Patients taking an immunosuppressant will most likely develop hypertension and subsequently will also be taking an antihypertensive drug such as a calcium channel blocker (e.g., nifedipine), which may also cause gingival enlargement.

Rapid Dental Hint

Patients taking cyclosporine may have gingival enlargement. Management should include meticulous oral care. Referral to a periodontist for possible surgical removal of tissue to help with plaque control is recommended.

Azathioprine is a prodrug used in the treatment of bullous disorders, which must be metabolized in the liver into an active form that will enter the bloodstream. In the majority of patients taking cyclosporine, the drug of choice for organ transplant recipients, gingival enlargement occurs. Gingival enlargement can be controlled by frequent gingivectomy/gingivoplasty procedures and meticulous oral home care. Cyclosporine serum levels must be monitored because oral absorption is widely variable. This drug is also used in the treatment of rheumatoid arthritis. Drugs that alter cytochrome P450 isoenzymes in the liver may alter the plasma levels of cyclosporine (Table 9-3). Blood pressure should be monitored in patients taking cyclosporine.

Pretransplant dentistry plays a critical part in getting on a transplant list. The patient needs to be evaluated for dental infections before being placed on the list.

Dental Hygiene Applications

Many patients will present in the dental office immediately before starting cancer treatment. It is important that patients seek dental care before treatment to minimize adverse effects and be provided preventative therapy (e.g., fluoride-reducing tooth erosion caused by nausea/vomiting). It is best for patients

to achieve a stable periodontium and for the dentist to extract any teeth that are hopeless or will present with problems later on during treatment (Table 9-4).

Lab values should be monitored and the patient's oncologist should be contacted if dental treatment is needed during therapy. Prior to cancer chemotherapy white blood cell and platelet counts are generally normal and will not present with any complications following dental treatment. Neutrophil counts below 500–1,000 mm³ place patients at risk for life-threatening infections. Platelet counts below 20,000 mm³ can lead to bleeding, usually from the gastrointestinal tract.

It is important prior to cancer chemotherapy to review with the patient home care regimens that will be followed during treatment. The dental clinician should monitor for the development of xerostomia, caries, oral candidiasis, and mucositis. It is important to schedule maintenance appointments with patients during treatment and monitor the patient's gingival and tooth conditions.

Key Points

- Complications of the oral cavity occur in about 40% of patients treated with chemotherapy and all patients receiving radiation.
- Oral adverse effects include mucositis, xerostomia, caries, and bleeding.
- Cyclosporine, a drug used to prevent rejection of an organ transplant, causes gingival tissue enlargement.
- Meticulous oral hygiene is important in these patients.
- Many cancer patients with pain may be taking a bisphosphonate and can develop osteonecrosis of the jaw after dental procedures.

Board Review Questions

1. Which of the following treatments should be started for patients who complain of oral mucositis? (p. 159)
   a. Rinse with warm water
   b. Chew sugarless gum
   c. Rinse with viscous lidocaine
   d. Suck on xylitol-containing lozenges

2. Which of the following drugs may cause gingival enlargement? (p. 161)
   a. Azathioprine
   b. Methotrexate
   c. Cyclosporine
   d. Bleomycin

3. All of the following are adverse effects of antineoplastic treatment *except* one. Which one is the exception? (p. 157)
   a. Mucositis of dorsum of tongue
   b. Gingival bleeding
   c. Xerostomia
   d. Stomatitis
   e. Thrush

4. Which of the following signs should be monitored in the dental office in a patient taking cyclosporine? (p. 159)
   a. Temperature
   b. Dilatation of pupils
   c. Respiration
   d. Blood pressure

5. A patient is taking zoledronate (Zometa) for pain from multiple myeloma (a cancer). Which of the following conditions can develop after periodontal debridement? (p. 160)
   a. Orthostatic hypotension
   b. Malignant hypertension
   c. Osteonecrosis of the jaw
   d. Multiple periodontal abscesses

Selected References

American Association of Endodentists. 2007, Winter. *Bisphosphonate-associated osteonecrosis of the jaw.* Chicago: Author.

American Association of Oral and Maxillofacial Surgeons. 2006, September 25. Position paper on bisphosphonate-related osteonecrosis of the jaws. September 25, 2006. Rosemont, IL: Author.

Brenner GM. *Pharmacology.* 2000. Philadelphia: W.B. Saunders.

Clarkson JE, Worthington HV, Eden OB. 2004. Interventions for treating oral candidiasis for patients with cancer receiving treatment. *Cochrane Review Abstracts.*

Corgel JO. 2007. Implants and oral bisphosphonates. *J Periodontol* 78:373–376.

Durie BGM, Katz M, Crowley J, Woo S-B, Hande K, Richardson PG, Maerevoet M, Martin C, Duck L, Tarassoff P, Hei Y-J. 2005. Osteonecrosis of the jaw and bisphosphonates. *N Engl J Med.* 353:99–102.

Markiewicz MR, Margarone III JE, Campbel JH, Aguirre A. 2005. Bisphosphonate-associated osteonecrosis of the jaws. A review of current knowledge. *JADA* 136:1669–1674.

Marx RE. 2003. Pamidronate (Aredia) and zoledronate (Zometa)-induced avascular necrosis of the jaws: A growing epidemic. *J Oral Maxillofac Surg* 61:1115–1117.

Marx RE, Sawatari Y, Fortin M, Broumand V. 2005. Bisphosphonate-induced exposed bone (Osteonecrosis/osteopetrosis) of the jaw: Risk factors, recognition prevention, and treatment. *J Oral Maxillofac Surg* 63(11):1567–1575.

Melo MD, Obeid G. 2005. Osteonecrosis of the jaws in patients with a history of receiving bisphosphonate therapy: Strategies for prevention and early recognition. *JADA* 136:1675–1681.

Migliorati CA, Schubert MM, Peterson DE, Seneda LM. 2005. Bisphosphonate-associated osteonecrosis of mandibular and maxillary bone: An emerging oral complication of supportive cancer therapy. *Cancer* 104:83–93.

Ramachandran A. 2000. *Pharmacology recall.* Baltimore: Lippincott Williams & Wilkins.

Ruggiero S, Gralow J, Marx RE, Hoff AO, Schubert MM, Huryn JM, et al. 2006. Practical guidelines for the prevention, diagnosis, and treatment of osteonecrosis of the jaw in patients with cancer. *J Oncology Practice* 2(1):7–14.

Ruggiero, SL, Mehrotra B, Rosenberg TJ, Engroff SL. 2004. Osteonecrosis of the jaws associated with the use of bisphosphonates: A review of 63 cases. *J Oral Maxillofac Surg* 62:527–534.

Ruggiero S, Rosenberg TJ. 2004. Osteonecrosis of the jaws associated with the use of bisphosphonates. *J Oral Maxillofac Surg* 62:527–534.

Web Sites

www.medscape.com

www.cancer.gov/cancertopics/pdq/supportivecare/oral complications/patient

QUICK DRUG GUIDE

Alkylating Agents (also called DNA alkylating drugs)

- Cyclophosphamide
- Altretamine (Hexalen)
- Busulfan (Myleran)
- Chlorambucil (Leukeran)
- Melphalan (Alkeran)
- Carboplatin (Paraplatin)
- Cisplatin (Platinol)
- Cyclophosphamide (Cytoxan)
- Dacarbazine (DTIC-Dome)

- Ifosfamide (Ifex)
- Mechlorethamine HCl (Mustargen)
- Mitomycin (Mutamycin)
- Carmustine (BiCNU)
- Lomustine (CeeNU)
- Procarbazine HCl (Matulane)
- Streptozocin (Zanosar)
- Thiotepa (Thioplex)

Antimetabolites (also called DNA synthesis inhibitors)

- Cladribine (Leustatin)
- Cytarabine (Cytosar-U)
- Floxuridine (FUDR)
- Fludarabine phosphate (Fludara)
- Fluorouracil (Adrucil)

- Gemcitabine (Gemsar)
- Mercaptopurine (Purinethol)
- Methotrexate (Mexate)
- Pentostatin (Nipent)

Antitumor Antibiotics

- Bleomycin (Blenoxane)
- Daunorubicin HCl (Cerubidine)

- Doxorubicin HCl (Adriamycin)
- Idarubicin HCl (Idamycin)

Plant Extracts (Mitotic Inhibitors)

- Docetaxel (Taxotere)
- Paclitaxel (Taxol)
- Vinblastine (Velban)

- Vincristine (Oncovin)
- Vinorelbine (Navelbine)

Hormones and Antagonists

- Flutamide (Eulexin)
- Leuprolide (Lupron)

- Prednisone
- Tamoxifen (Novadex)

Immunomodulators (Cytokines)

- Aldesleukin (Proleukin)

- Interferon alfa

Antibody

- Cetuximab (Erbitux): newest drug for head and neck cancer

Immunosuprressants

- Azathioprine (Imuran)
- Cyclosporine (Neoral, Sandimmune)
- Tacrolimus (Prograf, Protopic)

Bisphosphonates (Used in the management of cancer)

- Clodronate (Bonefos)
- Pamidronate (Acredia)
- Zoledronate (Zometa)

Fluorides

GOAL

To provide an overview of the pharmacology of fluorides and their benefits in community and dental office fluoride use.

EDUCATIONAL OBJECTIVES

After reading this chapter, the reader should be able to:

1. Describe the chemical composition, metabolism, and systemic intake of fluoride.

2. Describe the various types of fluoride available in dentistry.

3. Explain acute and chronic fluoride toxicity and how it relates to systemic and topical use.

KEY TERMS

Fluoride	Safely tolerated dose (STD)
Hydroxyapatite	Certainly lethal dose (CLD)

Chemical Composition

Fluorine is a natural occurring element found in living and non-living things. Its atomic number is 9, and it is found in the halogen group (VIIa) of the periodic table. In its standard state, fluorine is a pale yellow corrosive gas. It is the most electronegative and reactive of all elements. When a fluoride ion combines with a sodium ion, the compound sodium fluoride (NaF) is formed. The chemical formula NaF represents the salt of hydrofluoric acid. The compounds of potassium **fluoride** (KF) and hydrogen fluoride (HF) are also commonly found in dentistry.

Bone consists primarily of two compounds. About 70% of bone is an inorganic ionic compound of **hydroxyapatite** $[Ca_{10}(PO_4)_6(OH)_2]$, whereas the other 30% is organic, consisting of protein collagen fibers. Fluoride ions can react with hydroxyapatite to create fluorapatite. A chemical reaction takes place where the negative hydroxide ion (OH^-) is replaced by the highly negative fluoride ion (F^-). The fluoride ions have a stronger chemical bond to the apatite matrix, making it more difficult to chemically change the matrix again. This confers increased strength and density to bone.

$$Ca_{10}(PO_4)_6(OH)_2 + 2F^- \rightarrow Ca_{10}(PO_4)_6F_2$$

Hydroxyapatite   Fluorapatite

Fluoride can be added in ratios or parts per million (ppm) to water, dentifrices, mouth washes, gels, or to tablets as supplements for ingestion. One ppm is one part in 1,000,000, 1 milligram (mg) per kilogram (kg) of weight, or 1 cent in $10,000. Depending on the sources, time of use, or ingestion, fluoride can chemically react with and be incorporated into the enamel and dentinal structures. This makes the tooth harder, denser, and structurally sounder.

Pharmacokinetics

Fluoride in its mineral compound state is considered a nonessential nutrient for daily consumption because there are no known essential metabolic reactions in its functions. There are no recommended daily intake values. However, many studies have indicated its effectiveness when retained in teeth and bones. When taken orally, fluoride is adsorbed and taken up into the plasma of the bloodstream. The plasma then circulates throughout the body to bathe bone. Fluoride in the saliva can remain chemically active for up to 3 hours, effectively bathing the teeth.

DID YOU KNOW?

Fluorine, from which fluoride is derived, is the 13th most abundant element. (Contributed by William James Maloney, DDS)

Fluoride is retained by the body in hard, calcified tissue such as bone and teeth and is excreted through the kidneys in the form of urine. The timing of ingestion, age, and tooth or bone formation determine the concentrations of the fluoride stored. Fluoride is not appreciably found in breast or cow's milk; the concentrations are 0.01 ppm and 0.05 ppm, respectively.

Sources

Fluoride is found naturally in tea, seafood, chicken, and in some water sources. Raw tea leaves can have up to 400 parts per million (ppm) of fluoride, while brewed tea would have 3 ppm. Often fluoride is added to water supplies, dentifrices, and school water systems. This can be of concern when foods are commercially prepared in areas that fluoridate their water because the fluoride ions will remain in these foods. This is important when considering fluoride content in processed foods such as baby foods, seafood products, fruit juices or other beverages, and—most important—infant formulas reconstituted with fluoridated water, which can often be forgotten. Ready-to-eat formula may contain 0.1–0.2 mg/L of fluoride. Grape juice, especially white grape juice, and baby food with processed chicken have higher levels of fluoride. Unless the manufacturing location or the amount of fluoride in the water used to reconstitute the product is known, this can make it very difficult for the consumer to evaluate the amount of fluoride in a product. Moreover, some countries such as France, Switzerland, and Jamaica add fluoride to table salt.

If water is naturally fluoridated it may contain greater than the acceptable concentration of fluoride. When potable water sources are found to have over the acceptable level of 0.7–1.2 ppm of fluoride content, the water source is defluoridated to ensure fluorosis does not occur. Another potable water source, bottled water, generally contains less than 0.3 ppm fluoride. It is usually distributed as spring or natural water or distilled, drinking, or mineral water; this labeling is regulated by the Food and Drug Administration (FDA). Any bottled water with fluoride added, such as bottled water for children, is required to state *with or added fluoride*. There are water purification systems available to make it possible for consumers to purify home water sources. These systems may work by reverse osmosis, activated charcoal, or ozonation. Most purification systems are done by filtration, which does not appreciably remove fluoride; however, distillation and reverse osmosis do remove fluoride. Due to the perception that municipal water sources are not palatable or healthy, the use of water purification devices along with the growing trend to drink bottled water have become a great concern in caries prevention, and undermine the health benefits of community water fluoridation. In order to project someone's total fluoride intake, one must consider the amount of processed foods ingested, especially reconstituted foods; use of bottled water; and water purification devices.

Uses

Diseases that affect oral health are not localized, but can affect individuals systemically. With many people living longer due to advances in medicine, they are looking at quality of life. Poor dentition can cause decreased mastication, leading to malnutrition. Poor gingival health can cause oral infections, which may spread systemically through the blood supply and cause bacteremia or endocarditis. In *Healthy People 2010*, the national goal is stated to "prevent and control oral and craniofacial diseases, conditions, and injuries and to improve access to related services." The oral health objectives in *Oral Health in America*, a report of the Surgeon General, are intended to prevent, decrease, or eliminate oral health disparities in the U.S. population. In the United States, reports indicate that by age 6 only 5.6% of schoolchildren have tooth decay in their permanent teeth but by age 17, 84% of individuals have an average of eight permanent tooth surfaces affected. This indicates that despite the great strides the United States has made in the decline of dental caries, it is still the most common dental disease affecting its children and adults.

Caries are an infectious bacterial-based disease caused by *Streptococcus mutans* and *Lactobacilli* that colonize in the biofilms, which line the oral cavity. These bacteria produce organic acids as byproducts of their metabolism. These acids can diffuse across the biofilm and into the tooth structure. The acids will erode the enamel and dentin and cause weakening of the hydroxyapatite matrix structure of the tooth, thereby causing caries. Fluoride can help in disease modification and prevention. When fluoride is exposed during or after enamel formation, fluoride ions will displace the hydroxide ions in hydroxyapatite, creating fluoroapatite. This new matrix is much more stable, less soluble, and more resistant to the acid attack of the bacterial metabolic byproducts.

Fluoride has antimicrobial properties. It can inhibit enolase and ATPases, enzymes found in the bacteria's metabolic pathway. When found in saliva, fluoride can diffuse out and through dental plaque to depress the metabolic activity of bacteria. Decreased saliva production causes dry mouth, or xerostomia. This can occur in patients who have been irradiated for head and neck cancer or individuals with Sjögren's autoimmune disease. With decreased saliva, bacteria will grow exponentially. Fluoride, when used in mouthrinses, pastes, or when ingested, decreases the bacterial count very effectively in individuals who are at increased risk of caries.

Osteoporosis is a clinical condition of age related to decline in bone mass whereby the bones can become brittle and porous. This condition is important for the mandible and maxillae, bones that support the teeth. Treatment for this condition may include bisphosphonates, calcium supplements, and weight-bearing exercise. In addition, treatment with sodium fluoride is under investigation. Sustained-release sodium fluoride has been shown to augment spinal bone mass and reduce spinal fractures in older women with osteoporosis. Greater fluoride absorption occurs as the bones are forming and plateaus at about 50–60 years of age. In later years, more fluoride is excreted in urine than stored in bones.

Deliveries

Fluoride can be delivered to the teeth through systemic or topical measures or a combination of both means. If fluoride is ingested during tooth development stages from birth to adulthood third molars, it can be incorporated into the tooth structure in the form of fluorapatite. This delivery of fluoride is systemic, meaning that the fluoride absorbed from the gut, then transferred to plasma, is exposed to all parts of the body where blood plasma will flow. Any method of ingested fluoride such as fluoridated water, fluoride tablets, or drops or vitamins with fluoride, natural foods, and ingested toothpaste are considered systemic delivery of fluoride.

Topical delivery of fluoride means the surface of the tooth is bathed with fluoride-containing solutions. It may be from saliva (a systemic source) or applied to the teeth but after eruption. The fluoride is incorporated into the tooth surface by replacing the hydroxyl ion. The concentration of the delivered fluoride will vary depending on the methods used; the amount of fluoride incorporated to the tooth will vary. The more fluoride incorporated, the longer the teeth will withstand an acid attack, therefore allowing greater caries resistance.

Systemics

Sources of naturally occurring fluoride are water and food. Fluoride can be added to water, referred to as water fluoridation. The amount of fluoride added is 0.7–1.2 ppm in order to have the maximum reduction in dental decay, without causing fluorosis or altered enamel formation. Fluorosis can have an effect on the tooth structure and also cause tooth staining. Water concentrations in moderate climates are at 1 ppm, in colder climates at 1.2 ppm. As climate warmth increases, individuals are more likely to drink increased amounts of water; in warmer climates the water is fluoridated between a 0.6 and 0.8 ppm ratio.

Approximately 65% of the population on public systems in the United States has fluoridated water; this comprises about 57% of the total U.S. population. As of 2003, 42 of the largest cities in the United States had fluoridated water.

Community Water Fluoridation

Fluoride is added to the water source in such compounds as hydrofluorosilic acid, sodium fluoride, or sodium silicofluoride. The fluoride must be soluble in order to be released in the ionized form and become available for uptake into the bloodstream. The compound must also be relatively inexpensive, safe, and easily regulated in distribution. The results of community water fluoridation may result in 40–65% fewer caries in children exposed to water fluoridation. There is also a 50% reduction of root caries in populations who have been exposed to water fluoridation over a lifetime. One cup (8 oz) provides approximately 0.2 mg of fluoride.

School Fluoridation

By adjusting the fluoride content in a school water source, the amount can be raised to over 4.5 times the amount of fluoride in natural water. This has and can be done to compensate for the limited hours per day the child is in school and the amount of water consumed. The results show a 20–30% reduction in caries over the 12 years in school. The cost and practicality of added fluoride in this manner is weighed against the more effective community water fluoridation.

Prescriptions and Supplements

Supplements given orally can come as liquid drops, tablets, or in a combination form with vitamins. The clinician must consider the age of the child and the amount of active fluoride in drinking water when prescribing the dosage of fluoride to be taken in supplement form. The clinician should do a 3-day intake diary of the child's food and drinks to get a more accurate fluoride intake history. The clinician should also factor in other sources of fluoride such as natural foods or teas, prepared foods, beverages, or formulas prepared with fluoridated water, and deficiency, if there is too little fluoride such as in well water or bottled water use. The chart by the ADA (Table 10-1) gives the usual amount of concentration and age. The method of fluoride delivery must also be considered when prescribing for children. The child's ability to chew a tablet needs to be assessed or, if unable, liquid may be added to the formula or other beverages as an alternative method of supplementation. Milk or other calcium products should not be consumed within an hour, as the calcium will bind with the newly released fluoride ion, making it insoluble and not bioavailable.

Naturally Fluoridated Water

Water can naturally contain trace amounts of fluoride. About 10 million people in the United States live in communities where water is fluoridated naturally at 0.7 ppm or higher. In communities where natural fluoridination occurs at high levels, people are at an increased risk of dental fluorosis, a hypomineralization of the enamel. Partial defluoridation can be accomplished to reduce the level to the acceptable 0.7–1.2 ppm by diluting the water with nonfluoridated water or by chemically removing enough fluoride to bring it to the recommended level.

Fluorosis

Dental fluorosis or mottled enamel can only occur with systemically ingested fluoride. This is different from fluoride toxicity, when there has been a one-time lethal dose of fluoride ingestion.

Fluorosis has its effect on ameloblasts, which occur in tooth architecture during development. Most tooth development occurs from 6 months to 6 years; fluoride ingestion must be actively monitored during this time. Studies indicate that the maxillary centrals are at the greatest risk in males from 15 to 24 months, and in females from 21 to 30 months. Any combination of systemic fluoride over the total acceptable level of 0.7–1.2 ppm can cause fluorosis. Therefore, it is very important for the dental clinician to evaluate all sources of fluoride in order to prevent this unwanted effect. Once the crown is formed, no amount of ingested fluoride can cause additional fluorosis damage to teeth.

Clinically, mild fluorosis will appear as chalky, with striations barely visible. It may be seen just at the incisal edge, involving less than one-third of the crown; this is referred to as "snow capping." A score of 0–7 is used to quantify the amount of tooth involvement from excess fluoride.

Teeth with fluorosis are less susceptible to caries; however, as the effect increases, the enamel becomes more pitted and irregular, making teeth not aesthetically pleasing. Staining can occur if the intact enamel or the dentin are visible. This is like a floor tile with a crack in it; the stain becomes more visible in the crack than the rest of the tile. Large areas of enamel may be missing.

Dental hygienists must be aware of patients' systemic fluoride intake to reduce the risk of fluorosis in formulating teeth.

Rapid Dental Hint

For esthetic purposes, prosthetics such as veneers or crowns are commonly used for severe fluorosis.

Topicals

Topical fluoride can be applied to erupted teeth. The fluoride delivered in this method is absorbed into the tooth surface from the topically applied solution. The fluoride found in saliva that bathes the tooth acts in this method. Topical sources of fluoride may appear to overlap systemic, affecting the erupted teeth and ideally not the developing teeth. Many sources of topical fluoride are self-applied by the patient, or can be applied in an office setting by the dental clinician. The home or self-applied

TABLE 10-1	Fluoride Supplement Dosage Schedule		
AGE	FLUORIDE ION LEVEL IN DRINKING WATER (PPM)*		
	<0.3 ppm	0.3–0.6 ppm	>0.6 ppm
Birth–6 months	None	None	None
6 months–3 years	0.25 mg/day**	None	None
3–6 years	0.50 mg/day	0.25 mg/day	None
6–16 years	1.0 mg/day	0.50 mg/day	None

This schedule has been approved by the American Dental Association, American Academy of Pediatrics, and American Academy of Pediatric Dentistry.

*1.0 ppm = 1 mg/liter; **2.2 mg sodium fluoride contains 1 mg fluoride ion.

fluorides are less concentrated and are to be used over a longer time period compared to office treatments, which are a more concentrated form and are applied once or twice a year.

In May 2006, evidence-based clinical recommendations were developed by the American Dental Association Council on Scientific Affairs (CSA) that evaluated the effectiveness of professionally applied topical fluoride for caries prevention. The complete article and table, "Professionally Applied Topical Fluoride: Evidence-Based Clinical Recommendations," is available online at www.ada.org/goto/ebd.

The most common active forms of fluoride found in topical fluoride delivery systems are sodium fluoride and acidulated phosphate fluoride; stannous fluoride is also available. Many of these products can be found over the counter. A prescription may be needed if the percentage of fluoride indicated is greater than over-the-counter FDA regulations. Stannous fluoride (GelKam 0.4%) is used primarily in the management of dentinal hypersensitivity, not for caries prevention, and can be purchased over the counter without a prescription. Table 10-2 reviews the more commonly used fluoride products.

Self-Applied Dentifrices

Dentifrice (toothpastes/gels and powders) are the most commonly used method of self-applied topical fluoride. A 30% decrease in

TABLE 10-2 Common Fluoride Products			
	PREPARATION	GENERIC/BRAND NAMES	NOTES
Systemic Fluorides	Community water fluoridation	—	Estimated daily consumption of water is 0.7–1.2 ppm
	Dietary Supplements		
	Chewable tablets with/without vitamins	Poly-Vi-Flor, Tri-Vi-Flor; Vi-Daylin/F, Luride Lozi-Tabs, generics	0.25, 0.5, and 1 mg sodium fluoride (NaF); recommended up to age 16 in areas where drinking water is less than the recommended levels
	Drops with vitamins	Luride, Thera-Flur, Pediaflor drops, Poly-Vi-Flor, generics	NaF; recommended up to age 16 in areas where drinking water is less than the recommended levels
Topical Fluorides	**Self-Applied**		
	Rinse	Phos-Flur (OTC)	4.4 mg acidulated phosphate fluoride (APF); sodium fluoride (NaF)
		Fluorigard (OTC)	0.05% (5 mg) NaF
		ACT (OTC)	0.05% (5 mg) NaF
		Gel-Kam Oral Care Rinse (Rx)	0.2% NaF
			0.63% stannous fluoride; for dentinal sensitivity
		PreviDent Rinse (Rx)	
		PreviDent 5000 Plus (Rx)	
		Listerine Total Care	0.0221% NaF
	Gel	PreviDent Gel (Rx)	1.1% NaF
		Oral-B NeutraCare (Rx)	1.1% neutral NaF
		Phos-Flur Gel (Rx)	1.1% NaF/APF
		PreviDent 500 Sensitive (Rx)	5% potassium nitrate; for dentinal hypersensitivity
		PreviDent 5000 Booster (Rx)	
Topical Fluorides	**Office-Applied**		
	Gel, foam	Oral-B Minute Foam	1.23% fluoride ion
		Oral-B Neutra-Foam	2.0% neutral NaF
		Oral-B Minute-Gel	1.23% APF
		Fluoro-Foam	
	Varnish	Duraphat (Rx)	5% NaF (for dentinal sensitivity)
		Duraflor (Rx)	5% NaF (for dentinal hypersensitivity)
		PreviDent Varnish (Rx)	5% NaF (for dentinal hypersensitivity)

dental caries can be achieved from the twice daily use of fluoridated dentifrice. Sodium fluoride at 0.22% (1,100 ppm) or sodium monofluorophosphate at 0.76% (1,100 ppm) are the common active forms of fluoride seen in dentifrices. This would indicate that a single ribbon of toothpaste on the brush will yield about 1 mg of fluoride when released. It is extremely important for young children to limit the amount of fluoride on the brush to no more than a pea and to expectorate (spit out) the paste. A child can ingest up to 0.3 mg of fluoride in a single brushing session. Even more can be ingested if the child continues to refill the brush and swallow the paste, or has not formed the ability to properly spit out upon request. This extra ingestion of fluoride could lead to fluorosis.

Extra-strength toothpaste at 1,500 ppm will release increased amounts of bioavailable fluoride ion for remineralization. As with toothpaste, this should be kept out of the reach of children and if used by a child should only be done so under adult supervision paying close attention to the amount used.

Toothpastes are given an ADA seal of approval for therapeutic caries preventative action based on the amount of bioavailable fluoride and the toothpaste's degree of caries reduction. The other components found in toothpaste may be assessed for varying amounts of abrasivity, calculus reduction, gingivitis reduction, desensitizing action, or whitening, or combined effects. These separate effects should be understood when recommending a toothpaste.

Mouthrinses

Mouthrinses may be cosmetic or therapeutic. Mouthrinses that contain fluoride must be studied for their effectiveness. If they have been proven in caries prevention, they may then be included in the home care regimen. The most common fluoride used in mouthrinses is sodium fluoride (NaF) at concentrations of 0.05% for daily use. This delivers 264 mg of NaF or 120 mg free fluoride. A 500 mL bottle of 0.05% NaF contains 100 mg of fluoride; therefore, the bottle must be kept out of the reach of children and packaged with a childproof cap. Children over 6 years of age who can rinse and spit the solution out properly may be instructed on how to use the mouth-rinse. Several of these low-potency mouthrinses are available over the counter, such as Act, Fluorigard, and Reach.

Higher concentrations and less frequency solutions of fluoride are available at 0.2% sodium fluoride solution (1,000 ppm). These prescription products can be found under product label names such as Fluorinse, Phos-Flur, or Point Two. These may be used in a pediatric population under supervision, such as in a school rinse program or at-home use with parents. When used appropriately, both prescription and nonprescription concentrations have been shown to result in a 35% caries reduction.

Brush-On Gels

Home-use brush-on gels may be over the counter or prescription depending on the concentration and use. Daily gels such as Stop, Gel-Kam, or Omni-Gel may contain 0.4% stannous fluoride (1,000 ppm). Prescription fluoride gels such as Prevident or Karigel may contain 1.1% sodium fluoride (5,000 ppm) or 0.05% acidulated phosphate fluoride 5,000 ppm prescription gel to be used once daily. These gels may be applied with a custom tray or brush-on technique after using conventional toothpaste.

Consideration of the dentition and restorations should be given when determining if stannous, neutral, or acidulated phosphate fluoride is selected.

Rapid Dental Hint

The dental hygienist should consider the staining effect of stannous fluoride or the etching effect of an acidulated phosphate fluoride for veneers or laminates.

Professionally Applied Fluoride

Professionally applied fluorides decrease caries by 30–40% when applied during the eruptive stages of the tooth. They are delivered in solutions, gels, foams, or varnishes and vary in the percentage of fluoride they contain. They can be applied in trays or painted on and are in one-minute or four-minute application delivery systems.

Neutral sodium fluoride at 2% delivers 9,000 ppm of fluoride in concentration and is applied twice a year or as the caries risk assessment indicates. Four applications are given one week apart during the ages of 3, 7, 10, and 13. It does not discolor teeth or cause gingival irritation. Also, a basic pH of 9.2 makes this type of fluoride treatment recommended for adults who have anterior restorations or laminates.

A 1.23% acidulated phosphate fluoride in 12,300–12,500 ppm concentration is another treatment option for those with a high risk of caries formation. It is applied twice yearly or as indicated. This combination or 2.0% NaF and 0.34% hydrofluoric acid can be delivered as a gel or aqueous solution. Since this treatment is at 3.0–3.5 pH, a side effect may be pitting or etching of porcelain or composite restorations. A full dental history should be taken when deciding to use these methods.

Stannous fluoride at 8% contains 20,000–25,000 ppm of bioavailable fluoride. It is rarely used now due to the bitter taste it has and its propensity to cause extrinsic brown staining. Its pH is 2.4 to 2.8, making it very acidic, and it may cause gingival irritations.

Choosing Treatment Methods

Determining which fluoride delivery system and frequency depends on client risks, age, natural intake of fluoride, eruption of teeth, presence of exposed cementum, types of restorations, and overall dietary issues. Children and adults should be considered for fluoride if the risk factors assessment indicates that there is a need. Children who do not receive the recommended levels of fluoride from common sources should be considered for systemic and topical deliveries. Adults at risk of caries from dietary changes, recessions, cancer therapies, xerostomia, or medications that can affect salivary flow should be considered for fluoride treatments.

The age of the child must be considered when determining which delivery method to recommend, such as the tray, paint-on, or rinse. The ability not to swallow the solutions and spit the excess or rinse without swallowing must be considered when planning an intervention. Mainly children by the age of 6 will have the capacity fully to understand what it means not to swallow. Moreover, consideration of the child's inadvertent swallowing of toothpaste as a source of fluoride must be included when tabulating the daily fluoride intake of the patient.

Toxicology

Acute toxicity refers to the rapid intake of an excess dose of fluoride over a short time. Depending on the dose ingested, this can result in mild nausea or upset stomach to death. Upon ingestion of the fluoride compound a chemical reaction takes place where the atoms dissociate into hydrogen and fluoride, making hydrofluric acid (HF). This is one of the strongest acids that can be made and is highly irritating to the stomach mucosa. Pain and vomiting will result even if the quantities ingested are small. A dose of on average 4–5 grams is such a lethal level that there will be systemic symptoms. These symptoms include muscular weakness, spasms, paresthesia, central nervous system depression, bronchospasm, ventricular fibrillation, and cardiac arrest. Death can occur within 4 hours after the lethal dose is ingested if emergency actions are not taken. The blood toxicity can reach its maximum level within 30 minutes, meaning symptoms can begin soon after ingestion.

Rapid Dental Hint

While formulating the care plan, the dental hygienist considers all benefits for fluoride for all age groups and all systemic conditions, not just children during tooth eruption years.

If under 2.3 mg fluoride/lbs body weight have been ingested, give calcium (milk). If more than 2.3 mg fluoride/lbs body weight have been ingested, induce vomiting and give orally soluble calcium (e.g., a mild 5% calcium gluconate or calcium lactate solution) and seek immediate assistance.

The lethal dose of fluoride is the amount of fluoride that is likely to cause death if not intercepted with emergency treatment. When computing this amount, the person's weight must be considered. The **safely tolerated dose** (STD) is the amount of fluoride that can be ingested without causing any serious reaction for the client. This can be about one-quarter of the **certainly lethal dose** (CLD). The CLD will result in death for the client if emergency care is not rendered. In order to calculate the STD or the CLD, the practitioner must know the percentage of fluoride in the compound, the amount ingested, and the weight of the client.

The CLD of a 70 kg (154 lb) adult is about 5–10 grams of NaF or 32–64 mg of fluoride per kilogram (kg). The CLD for a child depending on weight is 0.5–1.0 grams of sodium fluoride taken at once. The STD for an adult of 70 kg is about 1.25–2.5 grams of NaF or 8–16 mg of fluoride per kilogram (f/kg). For a child the STD is 0.5 grams of sodium fluoride taken at once. In order to compute the amount of fluoride released from a solution, gel, or paste, the following formula is to be used. It has been calculated that less than 1 gram (1,000 mg) of fluoride, if ingested in one huge dose, can be fatal for a child 12 years or younger depending on weight and for a child 6 years or younger, it may be as little as 500 mg of fluoride in order to be lethal.

As an example, if a 2% NaF solution is used, a conversion ratio of the fluoride compound is to be multiplied. To calculate this ratio of a compound such as NaF, the combined molecular weight should be assessed (e.g., Na 23 + F 19 = 42). Then the ratio of fluoride to the compound is 19 to 42 = 19/42, or 0.452. Similarly, the ratio of stannous fluoride is 1 divided by 4.1 and APF (Na_2PO_3) is 1 divided by 7.6. It follows that if a 2% solution of NaF is used and 5 ml of solution were ingested, the amount of available fluoride would be 45.5 mg F. It would require about 105 ml of 2% solution to yield a CDL (1,000 mg, or 1 gram) of fluoride for a child.

Dental Hygiene Applications

With any use of fluoride it is suggested that the clinician be aware of the full amount of fluoride used systemically and topically. Also, the amount of topical fluoride should be considered if the child inadvertently ingests during toothbrushing. Certain people and cultures may eat more shellfish or drink more tea than others, and this needs to be considered in determining fluoride applications.

Consuming products containing calcium (dairy) or magnesium may decrease the absorption of fluorides.

The current and future risk of caries depends on given lifestyle changes and drug therapies. These risks impact upon the recommendations made when fluoride is used as a systemic or topical additive. It is the responsibility of the clinician to determine completely the amount of fluoride and the risk of caries for the patient before prescribing fluoride treatments. Here the dental hygienist plays a primary role in documentation and assessment before the delivery of fluoride treatment to the patient.

Key Points

- Fluoride supplement is primarily used for caries prevention.
- Dental fluorosis is seen when there is excessive ingestion of fluoride.
- Before prescribing or advising on fluoride supplementation, many factors must be assessed, including the age of the child and the amount of fluoride ingested in the diet.
- Once in the saliva, fluoride can remain chemically active for up to 3 hours.

Board Review Questions

1. A condition related to hypomineralization due to excessive ingestion of fluoride is known as (pp. 166–167)
   a. fluorosis.
   b. caries.
   c. hypercalcification.
   d. demineralization.

2. The teeth can acquire fluoride during (pp. 166–167)
   a. pre-eruptive mineralization stage.
   b. pre-eruptive maturation stage.
   c. post-eruptive stage.
   d. a and b
   e. All of the above

3. Which is not an effect of fluoride? (pp. 166–167)
   a. Prevents demineralization
   b. Enhances remineralization if incipient lesion
   c. Alters plaque bacteria
   d. Increases enamel solubility and decreases enamel resistance

4. Soduim fluoride is available in (p. 169)
   a. 2% solution.
   b. 2% gel.
   c. 2% foam.
   d. All of the above

5. Which is *not* an indication for acidulated fluoride application? (p. 170)
   a. Primary teeth
   b. Active caries
   c. Teeth supporting an overdenture
   d. Porcelain restorations

Selected References

Bowen WH. 2002. Fluorosis: Is it really a problem? *JADA* 133:1405–1407.

Hays DR, Westphal C. 2006, May. Fluorides' balancing act. *Dimensions of Dental Hygiene* 20–21.

Healthy People 2010. Office of Disease Prevention and Health Promotion, U.S. Department of Health and Human Services.

Oral Health in America: A Report of the Surgeon General. May 2000.

Weinberg MA. 2005. Guide to fluoride use. *U.S. Pharmacist* 30:48–58.

Web Sites

www.ada.org/public/topics/fluoride/fluoride_article01.asp
www.dentistry.com/oralhygienecenter003.asp
www.atsdr.cdc.gov/tfacts11.html
www.healthypeople.gov
www.oralhealthamerica.org

QUICK DRUG GUIDE

Systemic Fluorides

- Community water fluoridation

Dietary Supplements

- Chewable tablets with/without vitamins Luride Lozi-Tabs; generics
- Drops with vitamins

- Poly-Vi-Flor, Tri-Vi-Flor, Vi-Daylin/F
- Luride, Thera-Flur, Pediaflor drops, Poly-Vi-Flor, generics

Topical Fluorides

Self-applied

- Phos-Flur Rinse
- Fluorigard
- ACT
- PreviDent 5000 Plus
- PreviDent 5000 Booster
- PreviDent Brush-on Gel
- PreviDent Dental Rinse
- Oral-B NeutraCare Rinse
- Gel-Kam Oral Care Rinse ⎫
- Gel-Kam Treatment Gel   ⎬ for dentinal hypersensitivity
- PreviDent 5000 Sensitive ⎭

Office-applied

- Oral-B Minute Foam, Gel
- Oral-B Neutra Foam
- Fluoro-Foam
- Duraphat varnish ⎫ for dentinal hypersensitivity
- Duraflor varnish ⎭

Cardiovascular Drugs

GOAL

To gain knowledge of common drug therapy and dental management of heart-related diseases.

EDUCATIONAL OBJECTIVES

After reading this chapter, the reader should be able to:

1. Describe the different types of heart diseases.

2. List the different categories of drugs used in the treatment of heart conditions.

3. Discuss the adverse side effects of these drugs that are important in the dental office.

4. Describe steps used to monitor a cardiac patient who is being administered a local anesthetic with a vasoconstrictor in the dental office.

KEY TERMS

Cardiovascular system
Hypertension
Angina pectoris
Arrhythmia
Hypercholestolemia

Hyperlipidemia
Anticoagulant drugs
Warfarin
Antiplatelet drugs

Introduction

The **cardiovascular system,** which comprises the heart and blood vessels, functions to supply blood and oxygen to the body through contractions of the heart and the vasculature. As the body's demand for oxygen increases, the vasculature contracts or dilates to direct blood flow to the areas of the body requiring more oxygen. The cardiovascular system can fail either when the heart does not contract sufficiently or there is blockage of a blood vessel, referred to as atherosclerosis. Cardiovascular disorders are classified as hypertension, angina pectoris, heart failure, and arrhythmias.

Hypertension

Pathogenesis

Hypertension is defined as a sustained elevation in arterial pressure due to the amount of blood in the vessel being greater than the space available. In 2003, the Joint National Committee on Prevention, Detection, Evaluation, and Treatment of High Blood Pressure released its seventh report (*JNC-VII*). More current guidelines that have been published include ACCOMPLISH, ON-TARGET, TRANSCEND, HYVET, the Cochrane Collaboration analysis of beta-blockers, ACCORD-BP for hypertension, and JUPITER, SPARCL, ENHANCE, ARBITER 6, and ACCORD-Lipid for dyslipidemia. These trials should be considered as temporary guidelines until existing guidelines are updated. The most current classification of blood pressure is summarized in Table 11-1. According to *JNC-VII,* normal blood pressure is less than 120/80 mm Hg, whereas prehypertension indicates a patient is at risk of developing hypertension. Additionally, there is new emphasis on elevated systolic pressure (SBP) being an important risk factor for cardiovascular disease, rather than elevated diastolic blood pressure, which has been emphasized for many years.

Hypertension affects as many as 50 million Americans. It is listed as the principal cause of death in approximately 40,000 people per year and as a contributory cause of death in more than 200,000 others. Generally, hypertension is an asymptomatic condition in its initial stages.

Blood pressure is regulated by the sympathetic nervous system and the kidneys. Hypertension having no identifiable cause is termed primary or essential and accounts for 90% of all cases. It results in an increase in systolic and diastolic pressure due to alterations in the mechanisms regulating cardiac output and total peripheral vascular resistance. Secondary hypertension is the term given to elevated blood pressure due to a known physical abnormality.

Although the etiology of essential hypertension is relatively unknown, certain genetic and environmental risk factors are listed in Table 11-2. Risk factors for secondary hypertension include renal disease, hyperthyroidism, medication-induced (estrogen), Cushing's disease (glucocorticoid excess), diabetes mellitus, and pheochromocytoma (rare malignant neoplasm). Complications arising from hypertension include stroke and renal failure, which leads to congestive heart failure.

Three factors are responsible for creating blood pressure and controlling cardiac function: cardiac output, peripheral resistance, and blood volume (Figure 11-1).

- *Cardiac output* is the volume or amount of blood pumped out per minute by the ventricle of the heart and is determined by the heart rate and stroke volume, which is the amount of blood pumped by a ventricle in one contraction.
- *Peripheral resistance* (afterload) refers to the resistance of blood vessels to blood flow.
- *Blood volume* is the total amount of blood in the circulatory system, which is approximately 5 liters.

Other factors include:

- *Preload,* the volume of blood returned to the heart before it beats.
- *Contractility,* the forcefulness with which the heart contracts.

The main function of the heart is to receive blood from the body at low pressure and pump it back out to the body at a high enough pressure so that it will be pumped back to the heart. Systolic pressure is the pumping or contraction of the left ventricle, forcing blood out; the diastolic pressure is the relaxation of the left ventricle, allowing for refill with blood.

Treatment

Treatment of essential hypertension is aimed at restoration of the balance between cardiac output and total peripheral vascular

---

TABLE 11-1 JNC-VII Classification of Blood Pressure for Adults

CATEGORY	SYSTOLIC (MM HG)		DIASTOLIC (MM HG)	FOLLOW-UP
Normal	Less than 120	*and*	Less than 80	Check again in 2 years
Prehypertension	120–139	*or*	85–89	Check again in 1 year
Hypertension				
Stage 1	140–159	*or*	90–99	Confirm within 2 months
Stage 2	160 or higher	*or*	110 or higher	Evaluate in < 1 week

When blood pressures fall into different categories, the higher category should be selected to classify the individual's blood pressure status.

Source: Chobanian AV, Black HR, Cushman WC, et al. 2003. The seventh report of the Joint National Committee on Prevention, Detection, Evaluation, and Treatment of High Blood Pressure. *JAMA* 289:2560–2571.

TABLE 11-2 Major Risk Factors for Hypertension

- Smoking
- Obesity
- Sedentary lifestyle
- Alcohol
- Stress
- Male
- Family history of cardiovascular disease
- Postmenopausal woman
- Sodium intake

resistance, so the blood pressure (cardiac output times total peripheral vascular resistance) falls to acceptable levels before irreversible damage occurs to organ systems such as the eyes, the kidneys, or the cardiovascular system. Secondary hypertension is treated by removing the causative agent, re-evaluating the cardiovascular system for damage, and initiating treatment, if necessary.

DID YOU KNOW?

In about 400 B.C. in Greece, Hippocrates knew about arteries and veins, but believed veins carried air.

It is important to realize that treatment of hypertension not only involves pharmacotherapy but major lifestyle modifications, including weight reduction, limiting alcohol consumption, increasing aerobic physical activity, restricting sodium intake, and smoking cessation.

There are over 100 drugs that have been approved by the U.S. Food and Drug Administration (FDA) for the treatment of hypertension. It is important that a drug be selected that is most appropriate for the specific needs of the patient. Many patients with hypertension will have a cormorbidity (another

coexisting disease), which makes choosing the correct medication more challenging to prevent any drug–drug or drug–disease interactions. For instance, patients with hypertension and arthritis may be taking a nonsteroidal anti-inflammatory drug (e.g., ibuprofen) that could lower the effects of some antihypertensive drugs. The desired target blood pressure goal is lower than 140/90 in patients without compelling indicators, and lower than 130/80 on patients with compelling indicators such as diabetes mellitus.

DID YOU KNOW?

Dark chocolate, which is rich in flavonols, can reduce high blood pressure. White chocolate is not rich in flavonols and has no benefit (*Hypertension,* July 18, 2005).

Initial drug therapy of *uncomplicated stage 1 hypertension* [e.g., without another complicating disease (e.g., diabetes)], the following drugs either alone or in combination are recommended:

Thiazide diuretics

Angiotensin-converting enzyme (ACE) inhibitors

Angiotensin II receptor blocker (ARB)

Calcium channel blockers

Patients with *uncomplicated stage 2 hypertension* will require two or more medications to achieve blood pressure goals. Several major classes of antihypertensive agents have been recommended for use as initial therapy (Table 11-3). An outline for the treatment of hypertension is given in Figure 11-2 (page 181). If a patient has concurrent diabetes mellitus (type 1), an ACE inhibitor or ARB is recommended; if the patient has concurrent congestive heart failure, an ACE inhibitor or diuretic is recommended; if the patient had a previous heart attack a beta-blocker is recommended and, in the older adult, a diuretic is preferred.

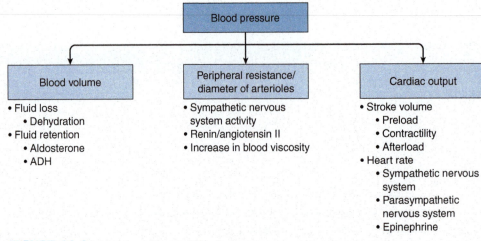

FIGURE 11-1 Major three factors of blood pressure.

TABLE 11-3   Classification of Antihypertensive Agents

DRUG NAME	DENTAL HYGIENE MANAGEMENT
Thiazide Diuretics Chlorothiazide (Diuril) Hydroclorothiazide (Hydrodiuril)	NSAIDs (nonsteroidal anti-inflammatory drugs) such as naproxen sodium and ibuprofen can decrease the effectiveness of the antihypertensive action of the thiazide diuretic, resulting in rapid elevation of blood pressure. Not recommended to use NSAIDs for more than 5 days. Orthostatic hypotension: Monitor blood pressure. To avoid dizziness/fainting when a patient goes from the supine position have the patient sit in an upright position for a few minutes before dismissing him or her. Patients may need to use the restroom facilities (increased urination from the diuretic) more frequently during the dental visit. Adjust your time accordingly. Xerostomia: monitor for dental caries and candidiasis No special precautions with the use of epinephrine.
Loop Diuretics Furosemide (Lasix) Blumetanide (Bumex)	NSAIDs (nonsteroidal anti-inflammatory drugs) such as naproxen sodium and ibuprofen can decrease the effectiveness of the antihypertensive action of the thiazide diuretic, resulting in rapid elevation of blood pressure, Orthostatic hypotension: Monitor blood pressure. To avoid dizziness/fainting when a patient goes from the supine position have the patient sit in an upright position for a few minutes before dismissing him or her. Patients may need to use the restroom facilities (increased urination from the diuretic) more frequently during the dental visit. Adjust your time accordingly. Xerostomia: monitor for dental caries and candidiasis No special precautions with the use of epinephrine.
Potassium-Sparing Diuretics Amiloride (Midamor) Spironolactone (Aldactone) Triamterene (Dyrenium)	NSAIDs (nonsteroidal anti-inflammatory drugs) such as naproxen sodium and ibuprofen can decrease the effectiveness of the antihypertensive action of the thiazide diuretic, resulting in rapid elevation of blood pressure. Orthostatic hypotension: Monitor blood pressure. To avoid dizziness/fainting when a patient goes from the supine position have the patient sit in an upright position for a few minutes before dismissing him or her. Patients may need to use the restroom facilities (increased urination from the diuretic) more frequently during the dental visit. Adjust your time accordingly. Xerostomia: monitor for dental caries and candidiasis No special precautions with the use of epinephrine.
Potassium-Sparing/Thiazide	NSAIDs (nonsteroidal anti-inflammatory drugs) such as naproxen sodium and ibuprofen can decrease the effectiveness of the antihypertensive action of the thiazide diuretic, resulting in rapid elevation of blood pressure. Orthostatic hypotension: Monitor blood pressure. To avoid dizziness/fainting when a patient goes from the supine position have the patient sit in an upright position for a few minutes before dismissing him or her. Patients may need to use the restroom facilities (increased urination from the diuretic) more frequently during the dental visit. Adjust your time accordingly. Xerostomia: monitor for dental caries and candidiasis No special precautions with the use of epinephrine.

(continued)

TABLE 11-3 *(continued)*

DRUG NAME	DENTAL HYGIENE MANAGEMENT
Amiloride/hydrochlorothiazide (HCTZ) (Moduretic)	
Spironolactone/HCTZ (Aldactazide)	
Triamterene/HCTZ (Dyazide)	
ACE (Angiotensin-Converting Enzyme) Inhibitors	NSAIDs (nonsteroidal anti-inflammatory drugs) such as naproxen sodium and ibuprofen can decrease the effectiveness of the antihypertensive action of the ACE inhibitor, resulting in rapid elevation of blood pressure. Orthostatic hypotension: Monitor blood pressure. To avoid dizziness/fainting when a patient goes from the supine position have the patient sit in an upright position for a few minutes before dismissing him or her. Xerostomia: monitor for dental caries and candidiasis No special precautions with the use of epinephrine.
Captopril (Capoten)	
Lisinopril (Prinivil)	
Enalapril (Vasotec)	
Ramipril (Altase)	
Benazepril (Lotensin)	
Fosinopril (Monopril)	
Quinapril (Accupril)	
Moexipril (Univasc)	
Trandolapril (Mavik)	
Angiotensin II Receptor Blockers (ARBs)	NSAIDs (nonsteroidal anti-inflammatory drugs) such as naproxen sodium and ibuprofen can decrease the effectiveness of the antihypertensive action of the antihypertensive, resulting in rapid elevation of blood pressure. Orthostatic hypotension: Monitor blood pressure. To avoid dizziness/fainting when a patient goes from the supine position have the patient sit in an upright position for a few minutes before dismissing them. Xerostomia: monitor for dental caries and candidiasis No special precautions with the use of epinephrine.
Candesartan cilexetil (Atacand)	
Eprosartan (Teveten)	
Irbesartan (Avapro)	
Losartan (Cozar)	
Telmisartan (Micardis)	
Valsartan (Diovan)	
Central Presynaptic α_2-Adrenergic Release Inhibitors	Least affect by combining with NSAIDs. Orthostatic hypotension: Monitor blood pressure. To avoid dizziness/fainting when a patient goes from the supine position have the patient sit in an upright position for a few minutes before dismissing him or her. Xerostomia: monitor for dental caries and candidiasis No special precautions with the use of epinephrine.
Clonidine (Catapres)	
Methyldopa (Aldomet)	
Peripheral Presynaptic Adrenergic Release Inhibitors	NSAIDs (nonsteroidal anti-inflammatory drugs) such as naproxen sodium and ibuprofen can decrease the effectiveness of the antihypertensive action of the antihypertensive, resulting in rapid elevation of blood pressure.

DRUG NAME	DENTAL HYGIENE MANAGEMENT
	Orthostatic hypotension: Monitor blood pressure. To avoid dizziness/fainting when a patient goes from the supine position have the patient sit in an upright position for a few minutes before dismissing him or her.
	Xerostomia: monitor for dental caries and candidiasis
	No special precautions with the use of epinephrine.
Reserpine (Serpasil)	
Guanethidine	
α_1-Adrenergic Blockers (also Vasodilators)	NSAIDs (nonsteroidal anti-inflammatory drugs) such as naproxen sodium and ibuprofen can decrease the effectiveness of the antihypertensive action of the antihypertensive, resulting in rapid elevation of blood pressure.
	Orthostatic hypotension: Monitor blood pressure. To avoid dizziness/fainting when a patient goes from the supine position have the patient sit in an upright position for a few minutes before dismissing him or her.
	Xerostomia: monitor for dental caries and candidiasis
	No special precautions with the use of epinephrine.
Doxazosin (Cardura)	
Prazosin (Minipress)	
Terazosin (Hytrin)	
β-Adrenergic Blockers	NSAIDs (nonsteroidal anti-inflammatory drugs) such as naproxen sodium and ibuprofen can decrease the effectiveness of the antihypertensive action of the antihypertensive, resulting in rapid elevation of blood pressure.
	Orthostatic hypotension: Monitor blood pressure. To avoid dizziness/fainting when a patient goes from the supine position have the patient sit in an upright position for a few minutes before dismissing him or her.
	Xerostomia: monitor for dental caries and candidiasis
Atenolol (Tenormin)	No precautions regarding use of EPI in local anesthetic
Acebutolol (Sectral)	No precautions regarding use of EPI in local anesthetic
Betaxolol (Kerlone)	No precautions regarding use of EPI in local anesthetic
Bisoprolol (Zebeta)	No precautions regarding use of EPI in local anesthetic
Carteolol (Cartrol)	No precautions regarding use of EPI in local anesthetic
Metoprolol (Lopressor)	No precautions regarding use of EPI in local anesthetic
Labetalol (Normodyne)	Use minimal amount of EPI (two cartridges 1:100,000)
Nadolol (Corgard)	Use minimal amount of EPI (two cartridges 1:100,000)
Propranolol (Inderal)	Use minimal amount of EPI (two cartridges 1:100,000)
Calcium Channel Blockers (CCBs)	There is no drug interaction with NSAIDs.
	Orthostatic hypotension: Monitor blood pressure. To avoid dizziness/fainting when a patient goes from the supine position have the patient sit in an upright position for a few minutes before dismissing him or her.
	Gingival enlargement occurs most frequently with nifedipine and amlodipine. Management: meticulous oral home care and maintenance care. Referral to periodontist.
	Xerostomia: monitor for dental caries and candidiasis
Diltiazem (Cardizem)	See above
Verapamil (Calan, Isoptin)	See above
Amlodipine (Norvasc)	See above
Felodipine (Plendil)	See above
Isradipine (Dynacirc)	See above

(continued)

TABLE 11-3 *(continued)*

DRUG NAME	DENTAL HYGIENE MANAGEMENT
Nicardipine (Cardene)	See above
Nifedipine (Adalat, Procardia)	See above
Nisoldipine (Sular)	See above
Direct Vasodilators	NSAIDs (nonsteroidal anti-inflammatory drugs) such as naproxen sodium and ibuprofen can decrease the effectiveness of the antihypertensive action of the antihypertensive, resulting in rapid elevation of blood pressure.
	Orthostatic hypotension: Monitor blood pressure. To avoid dizziness/fainting when a patient goes from the supine position have the patient sit in an upright position for a few minutes before dismissing him or her.
	Xerostomia: monitor for dental caries and candidiasis
	No special precautions with the use of epinephrine.
Hydralazine (Apresoline)	
Minoxidil (Loniten)	
Nitroprusside (Nitropress)	

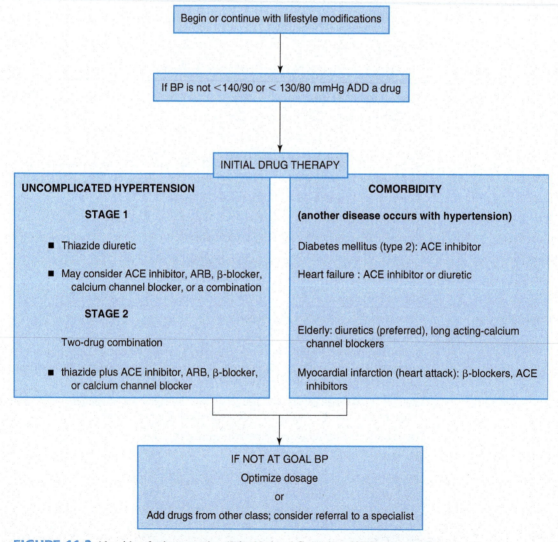

FIGURE 11-2 Algorithm for hypertension (Joint National Committee VII Recommendations).
(Adapted from The seventh report of the Joint National Committee on Prevention, Detection, Evaluation, and Treatment of High Blood Pressure. 2003. JAMA 289:2560–2571.)

Pharmacotherapy

Figure 11-3 illustrates the sites of action of drugs that reduce blood pressure.

DIURETICS Diuretics were the first drugs used in the treatment of hypertension in the 1950s. They are still considered to be the drug of choice because they produce few adverse effects and are very effective for treating mild to moderate hypertension.

There are three classes of diuretics: thiazides, loop, and potassium-sparing, which act in different parts of the kidney (Figure 11-4). Diuretics act by increasing the volume of urine production by excretion of excess fluid in the body (Table 11-3).

Because of increased loss of fluids, electrolyte disturbance with loss of sodium, potassium, and magnesium; dehydration; orthostatic hypotension (due to reduced blood volume); and xerostomia are common adverse effects.

Thiazide Diuretics Thiazide diuretics act in the distal tubule of the kidney to inhibit sodium chloride (NaCl) reabsorption back into the blood allowing an increased level of sodium in the tubule, which holds water, resulting in increased urination (Figure 11-4). Because of the increased sodium load in the tubule, excretion of potassium is usually increased, resulting in hypokalemia. Hydrochlorothiazide is the prototype thiazide.

Over months the diuretic effect of thiazides decreases, with kidney function returning to normal in regard to sodium (sodium reabsorbs back into the blood and is not excreted), but the antihypertensive effect remains. Thiazides are effective in lowering blood pressure 10–15 mm Hg in patients with *mild essential hypertension.* Thiazides may increase total cholesterol and loss of electrolytes, which may predispose the patient with heart disease to arrhythmias. Potassium supplements (e.g., food or drugs) may be necessary to replenish lost potassium. Thiazides are contraindicated in diabetics because they increase blood glucose and may decrease the effectiveness of antidiabetic drugs.

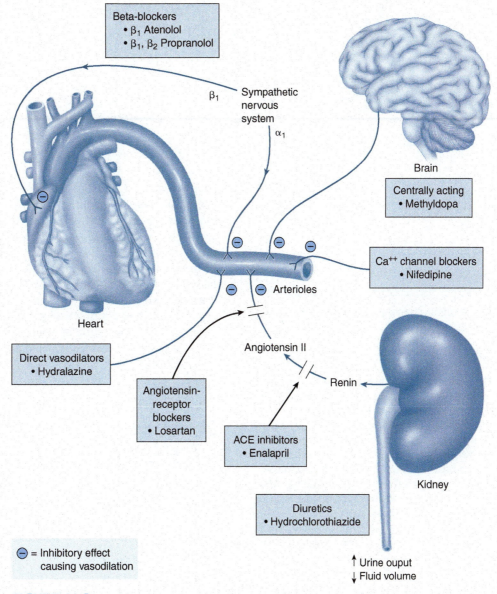

FIGURE 11-3 Diagram showing the sites of action of different antihypertensive drugs.

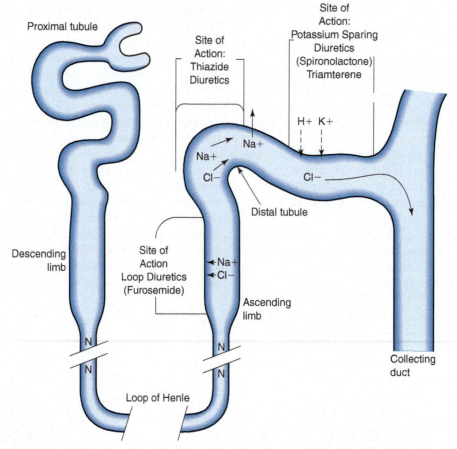

FIGURE 11-4 Site of action of diuretics.

Monitoring of blood electrolytes including K^+, N^+, Mg^+, Cl^- and serum lipids and cholesterol is essential.

Rapid Dental Hint

Patients taking a diuretic such as hydrochlorothiazide or furosemide:

- Drug–drug interaction occurs when an NSAID (nonsteroidal anti-inflammatory drug) such as naproxen sodium or ibuprofen is taken with a diuretic for more than 5 days. This combination of drugs reduces the antihypertensive effect of the thiazide diuretic, which may result in elevated blood pressure.
- Orthostatic hypotension: monitor blood pressure. To prevent dizziness/light-headedness let patient remain in upright position for a few minutes before dismissal.
- Xerostomia: monitor salivary flow/consistency. May have thick/ropey saliva. Recommend adequate fluid intake, fluoride rinses, salivary substitutes.
- Patients may require using restroom facilities more frequently because diuretics increase urination. Adjust your procedure time for this.
- No special precautions with the use of epinephrine.

Loop Diuretics   Loop diuretics are the most effective diuretics and are more potent than thiazides, resulting in greater and more rapid diuresis with loss of fluids through kidney excretion and severe potassium loss and orthostatic hypotension. These drugs inhibit reabsorption of sodium chloride in another part of the kidney called the Loop of Henle but also in the distal tubules (Figure 11-3). Furosemide (Lasix) is the prototype drug, has an onset of about 1 hour after oral administration, and causes significant electrolyte loss because it produces a more dilute urine and excretion of electrolytes. Potassium supplements are usually necessary. Loop diuretics may also increase glucose levels.

Rapid Dental Hint

Patients taking diuretics may develop orthostatic hypotension. Signs: dizziness, light-headedness, pale skin, nausea. Management: monitor blood pressure. After moving the dental chair from a supine position, have patient remain in an upright position for a few minutes before dismissing him or her.

Rapid Dental Hint

Patients taking diuretics may need to use the restroom facilities (increased urination from the diuretic) more frequently during the dental visit. Adjust your time accordingly.

Potassium-Sparing Diuretics   Potassium-sparing diuretics act in the distal tubule, where inhibition of sodium reabsorption results in a corresponding *reduction* in potassium excretion (Figure 11-4), so potassium supplements are not necessary. In order to equalize the potassium effects, these drugs are usually prescribed with a potassium-wasting diuretic such as hydrochlorothiazide. These diuretics work differently than thiazide and loop diuretics.

Spironolactone (Aldactone), a type of potassium-sparing diuretic, is an antagonist of a hormone called aldosterone. Aldosterone prevents the reabsorption of sodium in exchange for potassium.

Triamterene (Dyrenium) promotes sodium excretion in the collecting tubules of the kidneys. Potassium is not exchanged for sodium; sodium is not reabsorbed and stays in the tubules along with water.

Since there is less potassium loss, hyperkalemia can occur, and monitoring of serum potassium levels is necessary.

Rapid Dental Hint

NSAIDs (nonsteroidal anti-inflammatory drugs) such as naproxen sodium and ibuprofen can decrease the effectiveness of the antihypertensive action of the thiazide diuretics and other antihypertensive medications, resulting in rapid elevation of blood pressure. Advise only 5 days of NSAID use.

ADRENERGIC BLOCKERS (ANTAGONISTS) AND ADRENERGIC AGONISTS   Elevated sympathetic nervous system activity may result in transient or sustained hypertension by:

1. Directly stimulating the heart via β_1-receptors
2. The release of NE
3. Constricting peripheral blood vessels via stimulating α_1-receptors

Since hypertension stimulates adrenergic/sympathetic effects, drugs are selected to:

1. Block β_1-adrenergic postsynaptic receptors, preventing stimulation of the heart
2. Stimulate α_2-receptors, which inhibit the release of catecholamines, causing vasoconstriction
3. Block α_1-receptors, which inhibits vasoconstriction

Adrenergic Agents   Presynaptic α_2-adrenergic agonists are divided into *central and peripheral* anti-adrenergics. Centrally acting drugs such as clonidine (Catapres) work in the central nervous system to reduce norepinephrine release by stimulating areas of the brain that inhibit sympathetic outflow. These drugs are not routinely used because of their adverse effects. Peripherally acting drugs such as reserpine deplete the neurons of their catecholamine stores and prevent norepinephrine release from nerves that terminate on the heart.

Selective α_1-adrenergic blockers (vasodilators) decrease blood pressure by causing vasodilatation of peripheral blood vessels. Prototype drugs include prazosin (Minipress) and doxazosin (Cardura). Terazocin (Hytrin) is also used to treat benign prostatic hypertrophy (BPH).

Beta-blockers reduce the heart rate and contractility and decrease CNS sympathetic output. Binding to β-receptors results in decreased norepinephrine release, which is responsible for increased blood pressure.

Rapid Dental Hint

The suffix *–olol* is common to generic beta-blockers.

When selecting a β-blocker for the treatment of hypertension, it is best to use a cardioselective β_1-blocker such as atenolol (Tenormin), so it can be given to patients with diabetes and asthma with fewer undesirable side effects.

ANGIOTENSIN-CONVERTING ENZYME (ACE) INHIBITORS   As mentioned earlier in the chapter, the kidney plays a major role in controlling blood pressure by regulating blood volume. When blood pressure increases in the blood vessels, the kidney can excrete more sodium, which will lower blood volume, resulting in a decrease in cardiac output and the blood pressure returning to normal.

Renin is produced and secreted in the kidney in response to a decrease in renal blood flow. Renin converts angiotensinogen, which is produced in the liver, into angiotensin I. Angiotensin-converting enzyme (ACE), made in the lung, cleaves angiotensin I into angiotensin II, which is a potent vasoconstrictor and causes an increase in blood pressure (Figure 11-5).

ACE inhibitors block the conversion of angiotensin I to the active angiotensin II by inhibiting the converting enzyme. These drugs do not have a substantial effect on cardiac output and heart rate (Table 11-3), but reduce peripheral vascular resistance, resulting in lower blood pressure. ACE inhibitors are ideal in hypertensive patients with diabetes.

While monotherapy with ACE inhibitors in mild-to-moderate hypertension will significantly lower blood pressure, it is usually combined with another antihypertensive agent, such as a diuretic or calcium channel blocker. Precautions must be taken, especially in older adults, because both

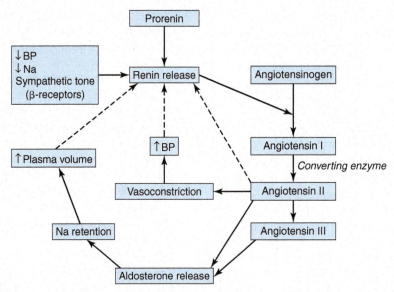

FIGURE 11-5 Renin–angiotensin system.

drugs can cause excessive volume depletion. ACE inhibitors have not been shown to reduce associated cardiovascular outcomes, such as stroke, heart failure, or coronary artery disease.

A common adverse effect of all ACE inhibitors is a nonproductive, persistent cough, which can develop immediately or after months of therapy. It is not dose dependent, which means that it may develop no matter how much of the drug is taken. Other adverse side effects include dizziness, headache, fatigue, angioedema (fluid leakage into the skin), orthostatic hypotension, and xerostomia.

An important drug–drug interaction occurs when an NSAID such as naproxen sodium or ibuprofen is taken with an ACE inhibitor. This combination of drugs reduces the antihypertensive effect of the ACE inhibitor, which may result in elevated blood pressure.

ANGIOTENSIN-II RECEPTOR BLOCKERS (ARBs)   Angiotensin-II receptors are found in a variety of tissues throughout the body. Angiotensin-II receptor blockers (ARBs) block the receptors from receiving angiotensin II, limiting angiotensin II–mediated vasoconstriction and reducing aldosterone secretion. Aldosterone is a mineralocorticoid that acts on kidney cells to increase reabsorption of sodium and water in exchange for the excretion of potassium. These drugs are well tolerated and have a low incidence of cough.

Combination of an ARB and NSAID reduces the antihypertensive effect of the ARBs, which results in elevated blood pressure.

CALCIUM CHANNEL BLOCKERS (CCBs)   Calcium channel blockers were first approved in the treatment of angina in the 1980s. A side effect was lowering of blood pressure in hypertensive patients. As previously discussed, peripheral blood vessels are constricted in hypertension; thus, vasodilation is one of the goals of treatment.

Calcium channel blockers cause vasodilation by inhibiting the influx of calcium into cardiac and smooth muscle by blocking calcium channels. This reduces peripheral vascular resistance, with little effect on cardiac output. Verapamil (Nifedipine) has the most inhibitory effect on cardiac conduction and the greatest effect on decreasing blood pressure, while diltiazem (Cardizem) has a moderate effect on decreasing blood pressure and on cardiac conduction.

Common adverse effects include orthostatic hypotension, reflex tachycardia (increased heart rate due to a rapid fall in BP caused by the drug), hypotension, and gingival enlargement.

There are two classes of calcium channel blockers:

1. Dihydropyridines [e.g., amlodipine (Norvasc), nifedipine (Procardia), felodipine (Plendil)]
2. Nondihydropyridines [e.g., verapamil (Calan) and diltiazem (Cardizem)]. Of the entire class of calcium channel blockers, verapamil and diltiazem have the greatest effect on reducing blood pressure. Calcium channel blockers are the most frequently used because they are good for the treatment of all types of hypertension and can be used in asthmatics. Gingival enlargement is a common adverse side effect.

Rapid Dental Hint

Gingival enlargement occurs most frequently with nifedipine and amlodipine. Management involves meticulous oral home care and maintenance care. Refer to a periodontist.

OTHER VASODILATORS   Direct-acting vasodilators relax smooth muscle cells surrounding blood vessels by an unclear mechanism. These drugs include hydralazine (Apresoline), diazoxide (Hyperstat), minoxidil (Loniten), and nitroprusside (Nitropress). These drugs are usually used in combination with other antihypertensive agents for the treatment of moderate to severe hypertension. Used alone, they cause fluid retention and angina. Minoxidil is used in the management of refractory hypertension where the patient has not responded with other types of drugs. A side effect of minoxidil is hair growth, making it useful treatment for hair loss. This drug is topically applied and is sold under the trade name Rogaine. Nitroprusside and diazoxide are administered intravenously in hypertensive emergencies. These are usually not the drug of choice because of many adverse side effects.

Rapid Dental Hint

Monitor vital signs when administering a local anesthetic with a vasoconstrictor to cardiac patients.

Dental Hygiene Applications

The patient should be asked what medications he or she is currently taking for blood pressure, and if these medications are being taken as prescribed. These medications are usually taken in the morning or at night. Vital signs should be monitored at every dental visit. Since some drugs are used to treat different types of cardiovascular disorders, the clinician should ask the patient for what condition the drug(s) is (are) being taken.

Any hypertensive drug has the ability to cause orthostatic hypotension, a fall in blood pressure of 20/10 mm Hg or more within 5 minutes of standing from a supine position, which can result in syncope. Care must be taken to allow the patient to remain sitting upright for a few minutes after being in a supine position to this.

Using vasoconstrictors in the hypertensive patient is not contraindicated. In the hypertensive patient, high doses (about three to four or more cartridges) of epinephrine may cause excessive cardiac stimulation, resulting in angina or cardiac arrhythmias, which can lead to increased blood pressure and stroke. Patients taking a *nonselective β*-blocker such as propranolol (Inderal), nadolol (Corgard), or timolol (Blocarden) may have an increased vasopressor response to epinephrine. Blood pressure should be monitored before and during dental treatment for any changes. The initial dose should be minimal (1/2 cartridge), injected slowly using aspiration to avoid intravascular injection. After waiting and monitoring for toxicity for a few minutes, more of the anesthetic may be injected. The maximum dose of epinephrine to be used in a patient with controlled hypertension or cardiovascular disease is 0.04 mg, which is equivalent to two cartridges (0.018 mg EPI per cartridge 1:100,000; note that the volume in a cartridge is now 1.7–1.8 ml). The benefits for maintaining adequate anesthesia outweigh the risks for toxicity. Careful monitoring for toxicity (e.g., increased blood pressure, cardiac arrhythmias including tachycardia) is important. Epinephrine 1:50,000 should be avoided, as well as retraction cord containing epinephrine.

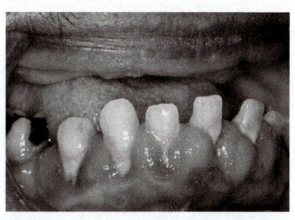

FIGURE 11-6 Gingival enlargement in a patient taking nifedipine.

Levonordefrin, a vasoconstrictor contained in mepivicaine, stimulates primarily α-adrenergic receptors. This will increase blood pressure, and the drug should not be used in the hypertensive patient.

Xerostomia including a dry, sore mouth caused by diuretics and central-acting adrenergic inhibitors are dealt with by educating the patient to increase fluid intake, avoid alcohol and alcohol-containing mouthrinses, and use of artificial salivary drugs.

Gingival enlargement is a common adverse effect of calcium channel blockers (e.g., nifedipine) (Figure 11-6). Discontinuation of the drug usually results in a disappearance of the enlargement. Treatment involves meticulous oral home care and possible surgical removal of excess gingiva.

Rapid Dental Hint

In patients with drug-induced gingival enlargement, consultation with the patients' physician may be necessary to change the calcium channel blocker to another drug category.

Angina Pectoris

Pathogenesis

Angina pectoris (AP) occurs when the metabolic demands of the heart exceed the ability of the coronary arteries to supply adequate blood flow and oxygen to the heart. Although the typical symptom of angina is severe chest pain upon exertion, angina may develop unexpectedly with minimal or no exertion.

The majority of myocardial ischemia (reduced blood flow) represents a manifestation of atherosclerosis (Figure 11-7). Other risk factors for AP include smoking, elevated serum lipids, family history, obesity, male gender, sedentary lifestyle, hypertension, and a type A personality.

Stable angina occurs when chest pain is intermittent on exertion but relieved by rest. Each attack generally resembles the previous attack, to such an extent that the patient can predict

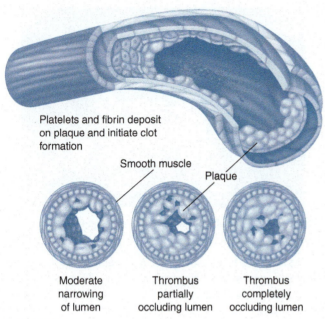

Platelets and fibrin deposit on plaque and initiate clot formation

Smooth muscle

Plaque

| Moderate narrowing of lumen | Thrombus partially occluding lumen | Thrombus completely occluding lumen |

FIGURE 11-7 Atherosclerosis in the coronary arteries.

the attack and change his way of life to avoid the precipitating cause. The classical symptoms are squeezing chest pain that radiates to the left arm, right arm, or both and to the jaw. There may be shortness of breath, nausea, vomiting, and sweating. Acute coronary syndromes (ACS) or myocardial ischemia include unstable angina and myocardial infarction. *Unstable angina* occurs when oxygen demand exceeds oxygen supply at rest and the frequency and severity of attacks increase. *Variant angina* (Prinzmetal's angina) is due to a heart vasospasm, often occurring during sleep. About 90% of patients present with stable angina and 10% have unstable angina that progresses to myocardical infarction and requires antiplatelet drugs and/or surgery.

Pharmacotherapy/Treatment

The goals of treatment are to reduce morbidity and mortality and to control the angina. Risk factors must be controlled, including smoking and alcohol cessation.

The goal of drug therapy is to reduce angina by restoring the balance between heart oxygen supply and demand, either by increasing oxygen supply or decreasing oxygen demand.

The following are drugs/modifications used in the treatment of angina (Table 11-4; Figure 11-8):

- Nitrates
- β_1-blockers
- Calcium channel blockers
- Aspirin: platelet inhibition
- Lifestyle modifications
- Cholesterol reduction
- Homocysteine reduction

NITRATES Nitrates work by relaxing vascular smooth muscle, resulting in vasodilation. This reduces ventricular filling and heart tension and thus oxygen requirements. In addition, nitrates dilate the large coronary arteries. It is recommended for long-term use to do interval dosing with a several-hour "nitrate-free" time, since tolerance can develop. The prototype drug is nitroglycerin, a short-acting nitrate available as a patch (transdermal), topical ointment, or oral formulation.

TABLE 11-4 Anti-Anginal Drugs

DRUG	MECHANISM OF ACTION	DENTAL MANAGEMENT
Nitrates Nitroglycerin (NitroBid, Nitrostat, Nitro-Dur) Isosorbide dinitrate (Isordil)	Dilates and relaxes coronary blood vessels	Headache, dizziness, and/or flushing, orthostatic hypotension. Monitor blood pressure. Allow patient to sit in an upright position in dental chair for a few minutes before dismissing him or her. Epinephrine can be used but limit to 2 cartridges of 1:100,000 because of increased risk of developing tachycardia.
Calcium Channel Blockers Amlodipine (Norvasc) Bedpridil (Vasocor) Diltiazem (Cardizem) Nifedipine (Procardia, Adalat) Verapamil (Calan, Isoptin)	Slows heart rate and dilates coronary arteries	Orthostatic hypotension: Allow patient to sit in an upright position in dental chair for a few minutes before dismissing him or her. Gingival enlargement (especially with nifedipine) No special precautions with epinephrine; however the dosage should still be limited to 2 cartridges of 1:100,000.
Cardioselective Beta-Blockers Atenolol (Tenormin)-β_1 Metoprolol (Lopressor)-β_1 Nadolol (Corgard) Propranolol (Inderal)	Reduces cardiac load and thus oxygen demand	NSAIDs (nonsteroidal anti-inflammatory drugs) such as naproxen sodium and ibuprofen can decrease the effectiveness of the action of the antihypertensive, resulting in rapid elevation of blood pressure. Orthostatic hypotension: Monitor blood pressure. To avoid dizziness/fainting when a patient goes from the supine position have the patient sit in an upright position for a few minutes before dismissing him or her. No special precautions with epinephrine; however since this is a cardiac patient vital signs must be monitored.

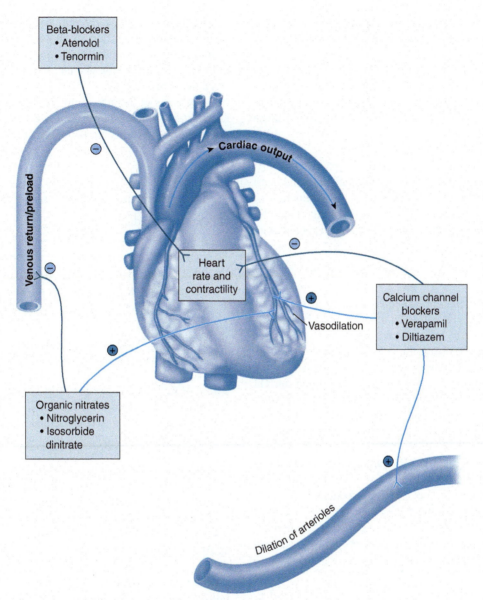

FIGURE 11-8 Mechanisms of action of drugs used to treat angina.

Sublingual nitroglycerin should be given initially at the onset of acute chest pain and continue for prevention of attacks with the patch or ointment form (2%). The sublingual form is used initially because of its fast onset, within seconds. The patch releases 5–10 mg of nitroglycerin over 24 hours. Adverse side effects due to vasodilation include orthostatic hypotension, dizziness, hot flashes, and reflex tachycardia. Nitroglycerin given in sustained-release capsules is used to prevent angina attacks.

Due to the first-pass effect, orally administered nitrates such as isosorbide dinitrate are only effective when given in high doses (30–40 mg qid) but is effective sublingually in a 5 mg dose. Isosorbide dinitrate is used for acute angina attacks and for prophylactic management to prevent angina attacks. It is given sublingually, with an onset of about 5 minutes, or orally, with an onset of 30 minutes and duration of action of about 5 hours.

BETA-BLOCKERS Beta-blockers have been proven to reduce mortality and are used in patients with stable angina who require long-term treatment or in patients who also have hypertension. These drugs decrease myocardial oxygen demand by decreasing heart rate, contractility, and tension. Cardioselective β-blockers are preferred, so only the β_1-receptors are stimulated. These drugs are *cardioselective* because they do not cause bronchoconstriction and the hypoglycemic effects of nonselective beta-blockers. The noncardioselective beta-blockers will block both β_1 and β_2 receptors; these drugs should be used with extreme caution in patients with asthma and diabetes.

CALCIUM CHANNEL BLOCKERS Calcium channel blockers (CCBS) reduce anginal symptoms but do not reduce mortality. Calcium channel blockers are the drug of choice in Prinzmetal's angina but can also be used in chronic stable angina, hypertension, and arrhythmias. CCBs reduce peripheral resistance, decrease in force of heart contraction, and decrease contractility.

NONNITRATES Dipyridamole (Perstantine) is used only for prophylaxis and not for an acute attack, and may decrease platelet aggregation. This drug acts primarily on small-resistance blood vessels in the heart.

ASPIRIN Aspirin or acetylsalicylic acid is a type of antiplatelet drug and is effective in a wide range of atherosclerotic heart diseases, exerting its effect by inhibiting the production of thromboxane A_2 (platelet aggregation), preventing blood clot formation. It has been shown to reduce mortality in patients with unstable angina and prevention of strokes.

Dental Hygiene Applications

Upon review of the patient's medical history, it should be determined when the patient's last attack was and what was the precipitating factor. Patients taking any form of nitrates must be careful when sitting up and getting out of the dental chair. Orthostatic hypotension may develop whereby the patient will get dizzy. Have the patient remain in an upright position in the chair for a few minutes before attempting to get out. Otherwise, there are no contraindications or complications to dental treatment. No special precautions are needed with epinephrine.

It is usually not necessary to discontinue aspirin for routine periodontal debridement.

The use of vasoconstrictors in local anesthetics in stable angina patients is recommended to reduce stress. However, it is suggested to use a maximum of two cartridges containing 1:100,000 epinephrine. Elective dentistry should be postponed in patients with unstable angina.

Heart Failure

Heart failure occurs when decreases in contractility prevent the heart from pumping forcefully enough to deliver blood to meet the body's demands. Decreases in cardiac output activate reflex responses in the sympathetic nervous system, which attempt to compensate for the reduced cardiac output. These reflex responses include increase in heart rate; increased preload, which causes edema; and increased afterload. Ultimately, the heart fails.

Heart failure (or congestive heart failure [CHF]) can be classified into systolic dysfunction (left ventricular) and diastolic dysfunction (right ventricular). Causes of left ventricular heart failure (decreased emptying of the left ventricle) include hypertension, coronary artery disease, mitral regurgitation, anemia (decreased number of red blood cells or hemoglobin), and Paget's disease. These conditions impair the ability of the heart muscle to contract. Symptoms of left heart failure include cough, dyspnea (shortness of breath) during exercise or when lying flat, and pulmonary edema (fluid in lung).

Right ventricular heart failure occurs with a decreased emptying of the right ventricle. Symptoms include pitting edema (fluid accumulation in the interstitial spaces is especially seen in the ankles), liver enlargement, nausea, vomiting, anorexia, and abdominal distention.

The goals of therapy are to relieve the symptoms of heart failure and to prolong the survival rate. Exercise, dietary restrictions, and medications are part of the management guidelines (Table 11-5; Figure 11-9).

Pharmacotherapy

The impaired function of the failing heart can be improved by:

1. Indirectly reducing cardiac workload (decrease preload) and reduction of edematous fluid (preload) with diuretics
2. Increasing heart contractions with cardiac glycosides
3. Using vasodilators to increase cardiac output and blood pressure (ACE inhibitors, angiotensin-II receptor blockers, calcium channel blockers, and direct vasodilators) and/or
4. Reducing sympathetic stimulation to the heart with β_1-blockers (e.g., carvedilol)

DIURETICS Diuretics are the most commonly used drugs for the initial treatment of heart failure. Generally, furosemide or other loop diuretics are used, and a thiazide diuretic can be added if necessary. Loop diuretics are most effective in the treatment of severe CHF because they are effective in reducing systemic, peripheral, or pulmonary edema. Urinary loss of potassium and magnesium is a major problem and must be monitored, as well as dehydration and xerostomia. Although highly effective in the management of acute congestion, diuretics do not prevent disease progression. Once the patient is stabilized with a diuretic, an ACE inhibitor is added.

CARDIAC GLYCOSIDES Since the primary cause of heart failure is a weak myocardium, it is ideal to have a drug that causes the muscle to beat more forcefully (increase heart contractions). The ability to increase the strength of contraction is called a positive inotropic effect. Digitalis (cardiac) glycosides have a positive inotropic effect, negative chronotropic effect (decrease heart rate), and decrease heart size. They cause the heart to beat more forcefully and more slowly, improving cardiac output. The primary cardiac glycoside is digoxin (Lanoxin), which originates from the leaves of the purple foxglove plant (*Digitalis purpurea*). Until the discovery of ACE inhibitors, cardiac glycosides were the mainstay of HF treatment.

Cardiac glycosides have a narrow therapeutic index and can cause fatal adverse effects. At therapeutic doses, these drugs cause an increase in the force of contraction of the cardiac muscle due to an increase in calcium in the cells and decrease heart rate. At slightly higher doses, there is an increased excitability of the heart, seen as tachycardia and arrhythmias. One of the more common adverse effects is hypokalemia, which increases the risk of digitalis cardiotoxicity when combined with diuretics. Treatment with potassium may be indicated in digitalis-induced

TABLE 11-5 Drugs in the Treatment of Heart Failure	
DRUG	**DENTAL HYGIENE MANAGEMENT**
Diuretics *Thiazides* *Loop diuretics* Furosemide (Lasix)	NSAIDs (nonsteroidal anti-inflammatory drugs) such as naproxen sodium (Aleve) and ibuprofen (Advil, Motrin) can decrease the effectiveness of the antihypertensive action of the thiazide diuretic, resulting in rapid elevation of blood pressure. Monitor blood pressure. Orthostatic hypotension: Monitor blood pressure. To avoid dizziness/fainting when a patient goes from the supine position have the patient sit in an upright position for a few minutes before dismissing him or her. Monitor blood pressure. Patients may need to use the restroom facilities (increased urination from the diuretic) more frequently during the dental visit. Adjust your time accordingly. Xerostomia: monitor for dental caries and candidiasis; monitor salivary consistency No special precautions with the use of epinephrine.
Positive Inotropics: *Cardiac Glycosides* Digoxin (Lanoxin)	No interactions with NSAIDs No xerostomia Limit use of local anesthetic to 2 cartridges of 1:100,000 epinephrine
Adrenergic Receptor Agonist Dobutamine (Dobutrex) dopamine	Orthostatic hypotension: Monitor blood pressure. To avoid dizziness/fainting when a patient goes from the supine position have the patient sit in an upright position for a few minutes before dismissing him or her. Monitor blood pressure. Xerostomia: monitor for dental caries and candidiasis; monitor salivary consistency No special precautions with the use of epinephrine.
Vasodilators Hydralazine (Apresoline)	NSAIDs (nonsteroidal anti-inflammatory drugs) such as naproxen sodium (Aleve) and ibuprofen (Advil, Motrin) can decrease the effectiveness of the antihypertensive action of the ACE inhibitor, resulting in rapid elevation of blood pressure. Monitor blood pressure. Orthostatic hypotension: Monitor blood pressure. To avoid dizziness/fainting when a patient goes from the supine position have the patient sit in an upright position for a few minutes before dismissing him or her. Monitor blood pressure. Xerostomia: monitor for dental caries and candidiasis; monitor salivary consistency No special precautions with the use of epinephrine.
ACE Inhibitors Captopril (Capoten) Enalapril (Vasotec) Lisinopril (Prinivil, Zestril) Quinapril (Accupril) Fosinopril (Monopril)	NSAIDs (nonsteroidal anti-inflammatory drugs) such as naproxen sodium (Aleve) and ibuprofen (Advil, Motrin) can decrease the effectiveness of the antihypertensive action of the ACE inhibitor, resulting in rapid elevation of blood pressure. Monitor blood pressure. Orthostatic hypotension: Monitor blood pressure. To avoid dizziness/fainting when a patient goes from the supine position have the patient sit in an upright position for a few minutes before dismissing them. Monitor blood pressure. Xerostomia: monitor for dental caries and candidiasis; monitor salivary consistency No special precautions with the use of epinephrine.
Calcium Channel Blockers Diltiazem (Cardizem) Verapamil (Calan, Isoptin) Amlodipine (Norvasc) Felodipine (Plendil) Isradipine (Dynacirc) Nicardipine (Cardene) Nifedipine (Adalat, Procardia) Nisoldipine (Sular)	Orthostatic hypotension: Monitor blood pressure. To avoid dizziness/fainting when a patient goes from the supine position have the patient sit in an upright position for a few minutes before dismissing him or her. Monitor blood pressure. Xerostomia: monitor for dental caries and candidiasis; monitor salivary consistency No special precautions with the use of epinephrine.

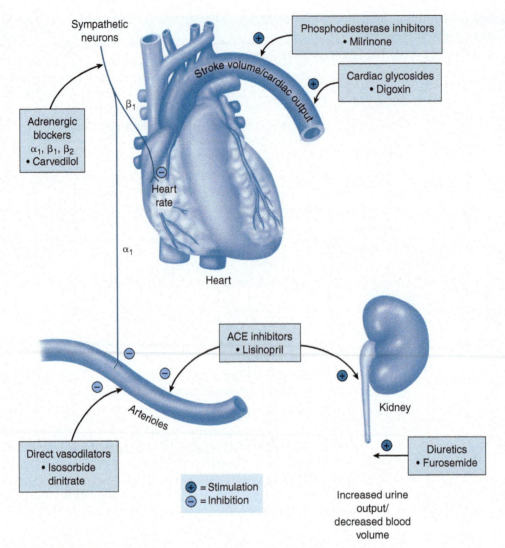

FIGURE 11-9 Mechanisms of action of drugs used for heart failure.

tachycardia. The most common visual disturbances of digitalis toxicity are blurring and change in color vision (yellow, green, red, and white). Digitalis toxicity is managed by discontinuing the drug, treating the electrolyte imbalance, and monitoring arrhythmias.

RDH

Rapid Dental Hint

Patients taking calcium channel blocker for a heart condition:

- No interaction with NSAIDs
- No special precautions with epinephrine
- Monitor for gingival enlargement: meticulous oral hygiene, referral to periodontist for surgical removal of gingiva
- Monitor for orthostatic hypotension: let patient sit in upright position for a few minutes before dismissal

---

RDH

Rapid Dental Hint

Patients taking diuretics and other antihypertensive drugs may develop xerostomia.

Signs and Symptoms: Changes in taste, speaking, swallowing. The gingival/mucosa may appear red and shiny. Examine the oral tissues to see if the dental mirror "sticks" to the buccal mucosa. Examine the tissue for possible fungal infections (candidiasis) in the mouth and dental caries.

Management: Ask the patient if the dry mouth is a problem. Recommend to the patient to use OTC saliva substitutes such as Salivart, Biotène products, Oasis mouthrinse, fluoride rinse. The patient should drink water more frequently. A prescription drug such as pilocarpine or cevimeline may be necessary. It may be necessary to discuss with the patient's physician to change the dose or the medication. Chewing gum with xylitol will help stimulate salivary flow. Schedule more frequent maintenance appointments.

VASODILATORS   Vasodilators are useful in the treatment of HF because of their ability to reduce blood pressure, which decreases edema, and dilate arteries, which increases cardiac output.

ACE INHIBITORS   The primary function of ACE inhibitors is to lower peripheral resistance (reduces load on the heart/afterload) and reduce blood volume by increasing sodium and water excretion. The diminished afterload required of the heart allows for increased cardiac output. A reduction in vascular tone decreases the work and oxygen demand of the failing heart.

In patients who cannot tolerate ACE inhibitors because of cough, either combination therapy with hydralzazine (Apresoline) or a nitrate, or with an angiotensin receptor antagonist such as losartan, valsartan or irbesartan is indicated.

BETA–BLOCKERS β_1-blockers reduce excessive sympathetic stimulation of the heart and circulation in patients with CHF. These drugs should only be used after standard treatment has been tried, never during acute heart failure. One of the newer drugs, carvedilol (Coreg), has considerable vasodilative properties and is the best to use of all β-blockers.

SYMPATHOMIMETICS   Sympathomimetic drugs (β_1-receptor adrenergic agonist) increase contractility with a minimal effect on blood vessels. Dobutamine (Dobutrex) stimulates β_1 receptors on the heart, resulting in an increase in the force of contraction of the heart. Adverse effects include increasing heart rate and hypertension. This drug is also used in the treatment of shock.

Dental Hygiene Applications

Patients with heart failure may be taking similar drugs (e.g., duiretics, ACE inhibitors, beta-blockers) as a hypertensive patient. Thus, when recording the type of medication, it is also important to record the indication for usage.

Administration of a vasoconstrictor (1:100,000 epinephrine) in a local anesthetic should be limited to two cartridges.

Arrhythmias

In an unstimulated neuron, potassium ions (K^+) are present in higher concentration inside the cell than outside, and sodium ions (Na^+) are found in higher concentration outside the cell than inside. In this situation the neuron is polarized. If the cell membrane becomes depolarized, allowing the rapid movement of K^+ ions outside the cell and Na^+ inside the cell, a stimulation or action potential results, which causes the cell to contract. This action potential is the stimulus that normally initiates the contraction of the heart. During the depolarization phase the cell cannot be reactivated by an electrical impulse, and is considered refractory to further stimulation. For the cell to return to a resting state, Na^+ ions must be pumped out of the cell and K^+ ions back into the cell, known as repolarization. This action potential process is spontaneous or automatic.

In the normal heart, an electrical impulse or contraction originates from the sinoatrial (SA) node, a small mass of tissue in the right atria, and travels through the internodal tracts in the atrium to the atrioventricular (AV) node (Figure 11-10). At the AV node, a momentary delay of the impulse allows for atrial contraction and ventricular filling. The impulse then travels through the bundle of His, bundle branches, and Purkinje fibers to stimulate the ventricles to contract and pump blood into the systemic circulation.

An **arrhythmia** occurs when either the impulse rhythm does not start in the SA node, or the rate of heartbeats is abnormal (normally the heart beats about 70–80 times per minute), or it is not under automatic control.

Classification of arrhythmias is based on the anatomical site of the abnormal rhythm: atrial (atrium), ventricular (ventricle), or supraventricular (atrium or above the ventricles).

When the heart is beating too slowly but at a regular rate, it is called sinus bradycardia. There is an increased parasympathetic stimulation that causes the heart to beat slowly. If the heart is beating too fast, it is called sinus or ventricular tachycardia or atrial flutter. Of the different arrhythmias seen in clinical

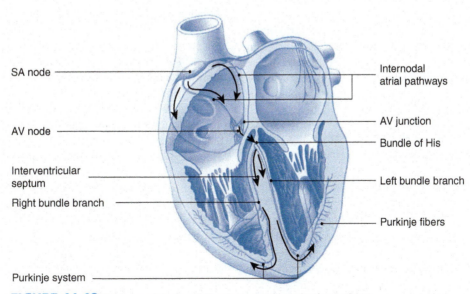

FIGURE 11-10 Diagram of the heart showing normal conduction pathway.

TABLE 11-6　Anti-Arrhythmic Drugs

DRUG

Class I: Sodium Channel Blockers

Class I-A

Quinidine (Quinidine)

Procainamide (Pronestyl)

Disopyramide (Norpace)

Class I-B

Lidocaine (Xylocaine)

Tocainide (Tonocard)

Mexiletine (Mexitil)

Class I-C

Flecainide (Tambocor)

Propafenone (Rythmol)

Class II β-Adrenergic Blockers

Esmolol (Brevibloc)

Metoprolol (Lopressor)

Propranolol (Inderal)

Class III Potassium Channel Blockers

Amiodarone (Cordarone)

Bretylium (injectable)

Sotalol (Betapace)

Class IV Calcium Channel Blockers

Diltiazem (Cardizem)

Nifedipine (Adalat, Procardia)

Verapamil (Calan)

Class I-B: Includes lidocaine (Xylocaine), tocainide (Tonocard), and mexiletine (Mexitil). These drugs shorten the action potential and are used in ventricular arrhythmias.

Class I-C: Includes flecainide (Tambocor) and propafenone (Rythmol). These drugs slow cardiac conduction without affecting the action potential; for supraventricular and ventricular arrhythmias.

- Class II anti-arrhythmics: Include esmolol (Brevibloc), metoprolol (Lopressor), and propranolol (Inderal). These drugs are beta-blockers used for the prevention and treatment of supraventricular arrhythmias. They function to slow the heart rate, decrease the AV node conduction rate, and increase the AV node refractory period.

- Class III drugs: Include amiodarone (Cordarone, Pacerone), bretylium, and sotalol (Betapace). These drugs are potassium channel blockers and prolong the action potential duration and refractory period. Indications for usage are to suppress ventricular arrhythmias.

- Class IV anti-arrhythmics: Include diltiazem (Cardizem, Dilacor) and verapamil (Calan). These drugs are calcium channel blockers that have significant effects on cardiac tissue. They act to decrease the AV node conduction velocity and increase the AV node refractory period. They are used to treat supraventricular tachycardia and suppress AV node conduction.

Other anti-arrhythmics include adenosine (Adenocard), digoxin (Lanoxin) for supraventricular arrhythmias, and magnesium sulfate.

Dental Hygiene Applications

Determine which drugs the patient is taking for a specific cardiovascular condition. There are no special precautions when treating a patient with controlled arrhythmias. The patient's pulse should be taken to determine normal rate and rhythm.

Epinephrine in Cardiac Patients

Although epinephrine stimulates both α- and β-receptors, used in dental anesthesia at low doses (one to two cartridges: 0.17 mg) epinephrine does not stimulate alpha receptors very much but does stimulate the β_2-receptors, which will be occupied because these receptors have a higher affinity for epinephrine. Thus, epinephrine selectively stimulates β_2-receptors, resulting in vasodilation of blood vessels in skeletal muscle. This vasodilation reduces diastolic blood pressure. With an increase in systolic blood pressure and a decrease in diastolic blood pressure, there is no real change in mean blood pressure. It is important to inject slowly and aspirate. The primary effect at high doses (e.g., used in emergency anaphalaxis and cardiac arrest: 0.5 to 1 mg) is vascular smooth muscle contraction through stimulation of α_1-receptors followed by a β_1-adrenergic effect, resulting in increased systolic and diastolic blood pressure.

The following table summarizes the types of cardiovascular diseases, goal of treatment, and medications used to treat the disease.

practice, the most common is atrial fibrillation, where the heart is beating without regard for impulses originating from the SA node. Other types of arrhythmias are ventricular tachycardia, ventricular fibrillation, and premature ventricular contractions (PVCs).

Anti-arrhythmics (Table 11-6) suppress the arrhythmia by blocking either autonomic function or calcium, potassium or sodium channels, which slows conduction of the cardiac impulse. Anti-arrhythmics should only be used to treat symptomatic arrhythmias. Based on these mechanisms, there are four Vaughan Williams classifications of anti-arrhythmics:

- Class I drugs, the largest group of anti-arrhythmics, have a mechanism of action similar to local anesthetics. These drugs block sodium entry into the cell, preventing transmission of the nerve impulse and reducing the rate of depolarization. Class I drugs are further divided into:

  Class I-A: Includes quinidine (Quinidine, Quinaglute), procainamide (Pronestyl, Procan SR), and disopyramide (Norpace). These drugs prolong the action potential in supraventricular and ventricular arrhythmias.

DISEASE	GOAL OF TREATMENT	COMMON DRUGS
Hypertension	1. To decrease blood volume (preload)	Diuretics (thiazides, loop, potassium sparing): increase Na and water excretion
	2. To reduce peripheral resistance	ACE inhibitors: inhibit angiotensin II
	3. To reduce sympthathetic stimulation causing vasodilation (afterload)	α_2-adrenergics (clondine): inhibit NE release
	4. Vasodilation (afterload)	α_1-blockers (Prazocin), calcium channel blockers (nifedipine)
	5. Block β_1-receptors on the heart (reduces cardiac output)	β-blockers (atenolol, metroprolol, etc.)
Angina Pectoris	1. To reduce cardiac output (workload of heart); dilates arteries (decrease afterload)	Nitroglycerin
	2. Smooth muscle relaxation and suppress cardiac activity (decrease afterload)	Calcium channel blockers (diltiazem)
	3. Reduce the frequency of angina; decrease heart rate and contractility	β_1-blockers (atenolol)
Heart Failure	1. Decrease workload (decreasing blood volume)	Diuretics (flurosemide); in mild CHF, use thiazide
	2. Increasing cardiac contractility	Digitalis
	3. Vasodilation	ACE inhibitors, angiotensin II receptor blockers, calcium channel blockers, and direct vasodilators
Arrhythmias	1. Restore heart rate and convert the rhythm	Class I–IV (sodium channel blockers, beta-blockers, potassium channel blockers, calcium channel blockers)

Lipid-Lowering Drugs

It is estimated that nearly 97 million American adults have total serum cholesterol levels of 200 mg/dL or higher. Almost half of deaths occurring from coronary heart disease are due to high cholesterol and lipid plasma levels.

Hypercholesterolemia and **hyperlipidemia** is characterized by an increase in both cholesterol and triglycerides (lipids), respectfully. Cholesterol is an important part of cell membranes and is a precursor to steroid production in the body. Triglycerides are the main storage form of fuel to support the generation of high-energy compounds in the body.

Because lipids are insoluble in plasma, they must be transported in the circulation in the form of lipoproteins (Figure 11-11). There are different types of lipoproteins, including chylomicrons, very low density lipoproteins (VLDL-C), low-density lipoproteins (LDL-C), intermediate-density lipoproteins (IDL-C), high-density lipoproteins (HDL-C), and lipoprotein; the C refers to cholesterol. Each lipoprotein contains various amounts of triglyceride, protein, cholesterol, and phospholipids (Figure 11-12).

In 2001, the National Cholesterol Education Program (NCEP) Expert Panel on Detection, Evaluation, and Treatment of High Cholesterol in Adults (known as the Adult Treatment Panel III, ATP III) made recommendations for cholesterol management. *This panel agreed that elevated LDL cholesterol is the primary target of cholesterol-lowering therapy.* Drug therapy is generally reserved for patients who fail to respond to diet or other measures such as weight reduction, or treatment

of an underlying disease. Cholesterol intake should be under 200 mg a day.

Treatment of hyperlipidemia may consist of implementing dietary restrictions with or without drug therapy. Blood levels of all types of lipids including triglycerides, total cholesterol, and the LDL:HDL ratio must be addressed. Drugs for hyperlipidemia are primarily used to treat hypercholesterolemia and hypertriglyceridemia or both. These drugs include (Table 11-7; Figure 11-13 [page 197]):

- HMG-CoA reductase inhibitors (or "statin" drugs) and bile acid sequestrant drugs used to treat hypercholesterolemia (lowers LDL)
- Niacin and other drugs, used to treat hypertriglyceridemia or marked HDL deficiency
- Fibric acid drugs, used to lower triglycerides
- Combination drugs

HMG-CoA Reductase Inhibitors (Statin Drugs)

These drugs primarily reduce LDL-C and have been shown to slow the progression of coronary artery disease. The mechanism of action is inhibiting the enzyme 3-hydroxy-3-methyl-glutaryl-coenzyme A (HMG-CoA), which results in less cholesterol formation by the liver. The primary adverse effects of the statin drugs include liver toxicity (hepatotoxicity), as seen by elevated

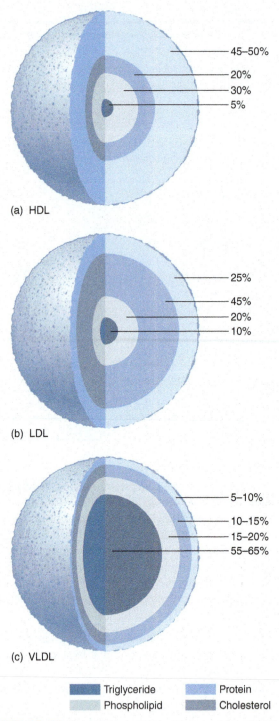

(a) HDL
— 45–50%
— 20%
— 30%
— 5%

(b) LDL
— 25%
— 45%
— 20%
— 10%

(c) VLDL
— 5–10%
— 10–15%
— 15–20%
— 55–65%

Triglyceride   Protein
Phospholipid   Cholesterol

FIGURE 11-11 Composition of lipoproteins: (a) HDL; (b) LDL; (c) VLDL.

serum liver enzymes, and muscle weakness (myopathy). Atorvastatin (Lipitor) is the prototype drug. It has a pregnancy category of X.

Statin drugs are metabolized by CYP3A4. Erythromycin and clarithromycin inhibit this enzyme, resulting in elevated blood levels of the statin drugs; grapefruit juice has the same mechanism of action. Erythromycin or clarithromycin should not be given at the same time as the statin drugs.

Most of the statin drugs, except atorvastatin (Lipitor), should be taken at night because cholesterol synthesis is highest at this time of the day.

DID YOU KNOW?

Grapefruit juice inhibits the breakdown of statin drugs, increasing their blood levels.

RDH

Rapid Dental Hint

Patients taking atovastatin or simvastatin should not take erythromycin or clarithromycin at the same time.

Bile Acid Sequestrants

The bile acid sequestrants bind bile acids (a greenish liquid secreted by the liver, aiding in absorption and digestion) and prevent reabsorption. These drugs (e.g., cholestyramine) are especially valuable in patients with moderately elevated LDL-C, but there is either no change or an increase in triglyceride levels. These drugs may cause constipation and a rash, and interfere with the absorption of digitalis and warfarin.

Fibric Acid Drugs

High triglyceride levels appear to be positively correlated with risk for coronary heart disease. Fibric acid derivatives primarily reduce triglyceride levels and are used in combination with statins. There are many adverse side effects, including allergic reactions, blood disorders, and myopathy. The prototype drug is gemifibrozil (Lopid). Fibric acid analogs can displace other highly protein-bound drugs (e.g., warfarin) from their receptors, causing elevated plasma levels.

Natural Products

Nicotinic Acid

Nicotinic acid (Niacin), a B-complex vitamin, reduces LDL cholesterol, increases HDL cholesterol, and is preferred for lowering triglyceride levels because bile acid sequestrants may raise triglyceride levels. Nicotinic acid is available with a prescription or as an over-the-counter dietary supplement, which is not FDA approved. One form of OTC niacin called nicotinamide has no lipid-lowering effects; patients should be under medical supervision and not self-medicate.

Nicotinic acid causes flushing and an itching or burning feeling of the skin, which may reduce compliance. To help prevent flushing, a nonsteroidal anti-inflammatory drug or aspirin

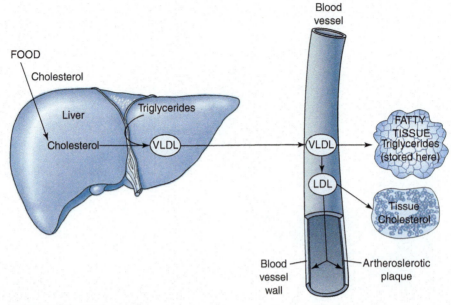

FIGURE 11-12 Lipid metabolism.

can be taken 30 minutes before. Nicotinic acid also causes liver toxicity, gastrointestinal disturbances, glucose intolerance, and peptic ulcers. It is contraindicated in people with diabetes and peptic ulcer disease.

Vitamin E

Vitamin E, a naturally occurring antioxidant and fat-soluble vitamin, may have a protective role against atherosclerosis and coronary artery disease by preventing the oxidation of LDL

TABLE 11-7 Drugs Used in the Treatment of Hyperlipidemia	
DRUG	**ADVERSE EFFECTS**
HMG CoA Reductase Inhibitors ("Statin" Drugs)	Increased liver enzymes, myopathy (muscle weakness)
Pitavastatin (Livalo)	
Lovastatin (Mevacor)	
Simvastatin (Zocor)	
Pravastatin (Pravachol)	
Fluvastatin (Lescol)	
Atorvastatin (Lipitor)	
Bile Acid–Binding Resin (Sequestrants)	GI distress, constipation
Cholestyramine (Quesytran)	
Colestipol (Colestid)	
Fibric Acid Derivatives	Gallstones, myopathy, dyspepsia (indigestion)
Gemfibrozil (Lopid)	
Natural Products	
Niacin	Flushing, hyperglycemia (elevated blood sugar)
Combination Drugs	Back pain, abdominal pain (from the cholesterol absorption inhbitors amlodipine and ezetimibe)
Amlodipine/atorvastatin (Caduet)	
Ezetimibe/simvastatin (Vytorin)	
Other Drugs	Fatigue, headache, coughing, back pain, myalgia
Ezetimibe (Zetia)	

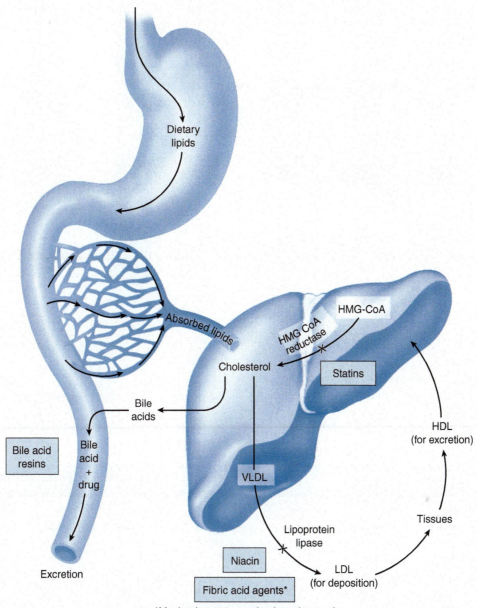

FIGURE 11-13 Mechanisms of action of lipid-lowering drugs.

cholesterol. Adverse effects include muscle weakness, blurred vision, and, in large doses, iron deficiency anemia.

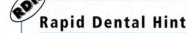

Rapid Dental Hint

Patients taking vitamin E for heart problems may have a tendency to bleeding more during periodontal debridement procedures. Either tell the patient to stop the vitamin E while being treated or it can be easily managed with using pressure.

Coenzyme Q10

Coenzyme Q10 (CoQ10) is a vitamin-like substance found in most animal cells, important in producing energy or ATP. Because the heart requires high levels of ATP, a sufficient level of CoQ10 is essential to that organ. CoQ10 and cholesterol share the same metabolic pathways. CoQ10 has been used to reduce the adverse effects of "statin" drugs. However, this is controversial.

Other Drugs

Ezetimibe (Zetia) inhibits absorption of cholesterol by the small intestine. It is usually administered alone or with HMG-CoA reductase inhibitors as an adjunctive therapy to diet for reduction of elevated total cholesterol and LDL.

Combination Drugs

The newest drugs for LDL reduction are combination drugs, which have less adverse effects and may be more superior to the statins. *These new drugs not only block absorption of cholesterol (cholesterol-absorption inhibitors) from food but reduce the cholesterol that the body makes in the liver.* All of the other drugs, including the statins, affect only dietary cholesterol. Examples of these drugs include amlodipine/atorvastatin (Caduet) and ezetimibe/simvastatin (Vytorin). Ezetimibe and amlodipine are cholesterol absorption inhibitors; atorvastatin and simvastatin are statin drugs. Combination therapy achieves a greater LDL-C reduction than statin monotherapy.

Dental Hygiene Applications

There are no contraindications or precautions to follow for patients on hypolipidemia drugs. Erythromycin should not be prescribed to a patient taking statin drugs. There are no special precautions to follow for these patients regarding the administration of local anesthetics/vasoconstrictors.

Thrombolytic Drugs

Normally, when a blood vessel is injured, a constriction occurs in the vessel that prevents hemorrhage (bleeding). The constriction brings the inner walls of the vessel together and the internal cells become "sticky" and adhere to one another. Normally, within an undamaged vessel, platelets circulate freely and do not stick to the vessel walls; in an injured blood vessel, platelets adhere to the underlying tissues and a platelet plug or clump forms and, finally, a fibrin clot. The clot is then removed by the process of fibrinolysis. Platelets or thrombocytes are small fragments found in the blood that promote blood clotting. This coagulation process prevents blood loss after injury or damage to a blood vessel.

This process occurs as part of the normal hemostasis mechanism. In pathological conditions (e.g., atherosclerosis) of the blood vessels, increased clotting may occur in the presence of thrombus (a fibrinous clot formed in a blood vessel). Formation occurs where a clot forms within a blood vessel that can completely occlude the vessel. Thus, the inhibition of thrombin is essential in preventing and treating thrombo-emoblic disorders.

Anticoagulant drugs retard coagulation and extend the time taken for blood to clot, preventing the occurrence or enlargement of a thrombus (Figure 11-14). These drugs include heparin sodium, given intravenously/subcutaneously, and **warfarin** sodium (Coumadin) in an oral and injectable form. Warfarin is an antagonist of vitamin K. Warfarin is involved in inhibiting:

1. The pathological formation of blood clots within blood vessels by inhibiting the synthesis of clotting factors II, VII, IX, and X, which are made in the liver. It takes about 3 days for an anticoagulant effect to occur.
2. The synthesis of proteins C and S, which are endogenous anticoagulants that inactivate factors V and VII. It takes about 2 days for this to occur.

A period of several days is also required for coagulation factor levels to return to normal after oral anticoagulants are discontinued.

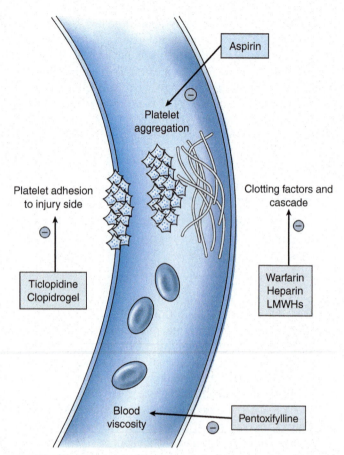

FIGURE 11-14 Mechanisms of action of anticoagulants.

Dicumarol is a coumarin derivative. It is not commonly used because it is not completely absorbed in the GI tract, causing much gastrointestinal upset.

Heparin, one of the oldest drugs currently used, is a naturally occurring anticoagulant produced by basophils and mast cells in the body. Heparin can only be given parenterally because it is degraded when taken orally. It has a short half-life of about one hour, so it must be given frequently or as a continuous infusion. A serious adverse effect is heparin-induced thrombocytopenia whereby platelets aggregate within blood vessels, resulting in clots that can lead to thrombosis.

Indications

Oral anticoagulants are indicated in the long-term management of patients with artificial heart valves and thromboembolic disorder (e.g., deep venous thrombosis, atrial fibrillation). The goal of anticoagulation therapy is to inhibit embolization and prevent the potentially fatal thrombosis. These drugs are also used in conjunction with heparin for the treatment of myocardial infarction.

Dental Management of Patients on Warfarin

The activity of warfarin is expressed using the international normalized ratio (INR). The prothrombin time (PT) test previously was used, but not routinely because of variability among laboratories. Dental patients taking warfarin must be routinely monitored for INR values; the patient's physician should be contacted.

There is much controversy about whether to discontinue warfarin in patients requiring dental treatment: Are they at risk of thromboembolic events if warfarin is stopped? It has been suggested that stopping warfarin can lead to a rebound hypercoagulable state, resulting in a stroke or death. Continuing warfarin therapy does increase the risk of postoperative bleeding, which usually requires intervention.

Rapid Dental Hint

A patient on warfarin (1) must consult from patient's physician and (2) must get INR values not more than 72 hours before periodontal procedures.

INR VALUES AND DENTAL PROCEDURES

Dental Procedures   What dental procedures can be performed while taking warfarin? Ideally, the INR should be measured within 24 hours, but not more than 72 hours, before the dental procedure. For a patient not taking warfarin a normal coagulation profile is an INR of 1.0.

Nonsurgical dental procedures (e.g., periodontal debridement, endodontics, restorative) can be performed without discontinuation of warfarin. In 1992, the American College of Chest Physicians recommended that the therapeutic range of continuous anticoagulant is an INR between 2.0 and 3.0 for all conditions except artificial heart valves, for which the recommended INR is between 2.5 and 3.5. Minor surgical procedures such as a single tooth extraction can be safely performed without altering the warfarin dose with an INR 3. Anticoagulation alterations are required if INR is greater than 4. The target INR differs based on the indication for taking warfarin. For example, if the patient is taking warfarin for atrial fibrillation, deep vein thrombosis or pulmonary embolus, the INR should be 2.5 (range 2.0–3.0). If the patient is taking warfarin for mechanical prosthetic heart valves or recurrence of embolism, then the INR should be 3.5 (range 2.5–3.5) (Table 11-8).

Adverse Effects

The most common adverse effect of oral anticoagulants is bleeding, which may vary in severity from a mild nosebleed to

---

TABLE 11-8   International Normalized Ratio (INR) Guidelines for Dental Treatment

- All patients should have an IHR below 4
- Acceptable INR range 2.0–3.0 in patients with:
  - Pulmonary embolus
  - Deep vein thrombosis (DVT)
  - Atrial fibrillation
  - Bileaflet mitral value
- Acceptable INR range 3.0–4.0 in patients with:
  - Mechanical heart valves
  - Recurrence of embolism while on warfarin

Rapid Dental Hint

Assess your patient's medical history for warfarin use. Contact the patient's physician before any procedures are started. You must know the INR level. In the majority of cases the patient should not discontinue the warfarin.

life-threatening hemorrhage. Patients should report any signs of bleeding and ecchymoses (black-and-blue marks).

Treatment of bleeding may include a decrease in dosage and the administration of phytonadione (vitamin K_1). If bleeding is severe or the INR is markedly elevated (over 20), fresh frozen plasma or factor IX concentrate may be administered to replace clotting factors.

Drug Interactions

Warfarin is completely absorbed after oral administration. Most drug interactions occur because warfarin in about 99% of the drug is bound to plasma proteins, and is almost completely metabolized by CYP1A2, CYP2C9, and CYP3A4 in the liver. The following are common dental drug–drug interactions:

- Erythromycin and clarithromycin (Biaxin) are inhibitors of these enzymes, which will decrease the metabolism of warfarin, thus increasing warfarin blood levels
- Fluconazole (Diflucan) increases warfarin blood levels by inhibiting CYP2C9 enzymes
- Metronidazole inhibits enzymes that metabolize warfarin. These two drugs should be avoided.
- There is an increased risk for bleeding with concomitant administration of aspirin and other nonsteroidal anti-inflammatory drugs such as ibuprofen.

Antiplatelet drugs *inhibit platelet aggregation* and include:

- Aspirin (acetylsalicylic acid or ASA)
- Clopidogrel (Plavix)
- Ticlopidine (Ticlid)

Rapid Dental Hint

A patient is taking warfarin. What should you do before treating the patient? Send the patient to determine the INR value within 72 hours of treatment. Get a medical consult.

DID YOU KNOW?

Tea has tannins, which reduce bleeding. Place a tea bag on the wound if you have slight bleeding after a dental procedure.

- Effient (Prasugrel)
- Abciximab (ReoPro)
- Dipyridamole (Perstantine)
- Aspirin-dipyridamole (Aggrenox)

Aspirin causes gastrointestinal irritation and bleeding due to inhibition of protective prostaglandins. Aspirin is used primarily to prevent arterial thrombosis in patients with ischemic heart disease and stroke, in patients with prosthetic valves, and in patients with unstable angina to prevent myocardial infarction. It is usually given in a low dose of 81 mg daily. Patients who are allergic to aspirin or who cannot tolerate its adverse effects can be prescribed ticlopidine.

Combination therapies that inhibit platelet function by more than one mechanism may be more efficacious than single-agent approaches. Aspirin/extended-release dipyridamole (Aggrenox) is a combination antiplatelet agent with additive antiplatelet effects. Dipyridamole inhibits the uptake of adenosine into the platelets. It is controversial whether to prescribe both aspirin and clopidogrel for additive antiplatelet effect. In 2006, a study by the Cleveland Clinic reported that clopidogrel plus aspirin does not significantly reduce the rate of myocardial infarction, stroke, or cardiovascular death, and thus should not be recommended as a preventative therapy for such diseases.

Low-Dose Heparins

A more recently introduced group of anticoagulants are called low-molecular-weight heparins or LMWHs, such as enoxaparin (Lovenox), ardeparin, and dalteparin (Fragmin). These drugs are used as an anticoagulant in diseases that have thrombosis, and for prophylaxis in situations that lead to a high risk of thrombosis. Low-molecular-weight-heparins were created by breaking apart the heparin molecule to a smaller size, which gets better absorption and has once-daily dosing, rather than a continuous infusion of heparin. There is also a smaller risk of bleeding and thrombocytopenia with LMWHs than heparin. Because LMWHs are administered subcutaneously and does not require coagulation monitoring, outpatient treatment of conditions such as deep vein thrombosis or pulmonary embolism is possible.

Hematopoeitic Drugs

The formation of red blood cells requires iron, vitamin B_{12}, and folic acid. Anemia develops when there is a deficiency in one of these substances. Iron is necessary for hemoglobin production. Iron deficiency anemia caused by chronic blood loss (e.g., pregnancy, menstrual problems) results in small red blood cells with insufficient hemoglobin. As a consequence, iron needs to be replaced by the administration of iron preparations. Oral therapy is continued until the normal range of hemoglobin is attained.

Orally administered iron is in the form of ferrous salts, usually ferrous sulfate, in order for the iron to be absorbed orally. Gastrointestinal upset (nausea, vomiting, and diarrhea) and extrinsic staining of teeth are common adverse side effects. There are no contraindications for dental treatment. Decreased absorption of tetracyclines and ciprofloxacin occurs if taken together.

Dental Hygiene Applications

The international normalized ratio (INR) should be recorded, and is used to monitor the patient's oral anticoagulant therapy. It is a good indicator of bleeding values. The higher the INR the greater the anticoagulant effect.

Oral anticoagulant therapy should not be discontinued; rather, the INR level should be monitored. Dental management of patients on warfarin is dependent upon the INR level. Discontinuing warfarin therapy may result in stroke or death. Dental treatment should be delayed until the INR value is within therapeutic levels of 1.0–4.0. Any dental procedure is contraindicated with INR values greater than 5.0.

Patients also may be taking aspirin prophylactically, either self-medicated or as prescribed by their physician. Aspirin inhibits platelet formation by irreversibly inhibiting cyclooxygenase, an enzyme found in membranes of all cells, including platelets that are responsible for the formation of thromboxane A_2. Thromboxane A_2 causes aggregation of platelets and vasoconstriction. This effect persists for the lifetime of the platelet (about 1 week). If patients are taking aspirin prophylactically, it can be stopped without consequence for dental surgery; however, if taken by order of a physician, it should not be stopped.

Although bleeding may occur if the patient is taking other drugs, such as dipyridamole, it is unlikely to interfere with dental treatment; however, a medical consult is necessary.

Key Points

- Many patients are taking drugs for the heart, including aspirin.
- Take vital signs.
- Confirm that the patient took his or her medication as directed by their physician.
- Most heart drugs cause orthostatic hypotension; have the patient sit upright in the dental chair for a few minutes before arising.
- Patients taking warfarin can receive dental treatment without stopping the drug; get INR levels before any treatment is started.

Board Review Questions

1. Which of the following drugs can cause xerostomia? (p. 189)
   a. Digoxin
   b. Aspirin
   c. Furosemide
   d. Warfarin

2. Which of the following drugs *most* likely causes orthostatic hypotension? (pp. 184, 186)
   a. Diltiazem
   b. Aspirin
   c. Digoxin
   d. Niacin

3. A patient has not discontinued the warfarin he is taking because of heart stents placed last year. This patient will most likely experience (p. 197)
   a. low blood pressure.
   b. elevated blood pressure.
   c. bleeding.
   d. dry mouth.

4. Which of the following drugs needs to be monitored by INR levels? (pp. 197–198)
   a. Warfarin
   b. Acetaminophen
   c. Aspirin regular strength
   d. Low-dose (81 mg) aspirin
   e. Plavix

5. Which of the following drugs is the first-line drug used in the treatment of heart failure in a 50-year-old male? (p. 188)
   a. Hydrochlorothiazide
   b. Aspirin
   c. Digoxin
   d. Nifedipine
   e. Captopril

6. Which of the following drugs should *not* be taken with naproxen (Aleve) for more than 5 days? (p. 177)
   a. Nifedipine (Procardia)
   b. Digoxin (Lanoxin)
   c. Enalapril (Vasotec)
   d. Lidocaine (Xylocaine)

7. Which of the following drugs most likely will cause gingival enlargement? (pp. 179, 184)
   a. Diltiazem (Cardizem)
   b. Verapamil (Calan)
   c. Atenolol (Tenormin)
   d. Amlodipine (Norvasc)

8. Which of the following lab values must be obtained in a patient taking warfarin before periodontal debridement procedures are started? (pp. 188, 198)
   a. International normalized ratio
   b. Partial prothrombin time
   c. Hemoglobin
   d. Hematocrit

9. A patient is taking amlodipine (Norvasc). After periodontal treatment is completed at an office visit and the patient is ready to be dismissed, which one of these procedures should be followed? (p. 186)
   a. Have the patient drink orange juice slowly.
   b. Have the patient sit upright in the dental chair a while.
   c. Administer oxygen.
   d. Administer more local anesthetic.

10. A patient is taking low-dose aspirin to prevent stroke as prescribed by his physician. The patient has no remarkable medical history. Which of the following procedures should be followed before performing oral prophylaxis? (p. 199)
    a. Change the medication to acetaminophen (Tylenol) to prevent bleeding.
    b. Perform the dental procedure without discontinuing the aspirin.
    c. Discontinue aspirin for 5 to 7 days and have the patient come back.
    d. Change the medication to regular strength aspirin.

Selected References

Budenz AW. 2000. Local anesthetics and medically complex patients. *J Cal Dent Assoc* 28:611–619.

Chobanian AV, Black HR, Cushman WC, et al. 2003. The seventh report of the Joint National Committee on Prevention, Detection, Evaluation, and Treatment of High Blood Pressure. *JAMA* 289:2560–2571.

Executive Summary of the third report of the National Cholesterol Education Program (NCEP) Expert Panel on Detection, Evaluation and Treatment of High Blood Cholesterol in Adults (Adult Treatment Panel III). 2001. *JAMA* 285:2486–2497.

Horton JD, Bushwick BM. 1999. Warfarin therapy: Evolving strategies in anticoagulation. *Am Fam Physician* 59:635–645.

Jeske AH, Suchko GD. 2003. Lack of a scientific basis for routine discontinuation of oral anticoagulation therapy before dental treatment. *JADA* 134:1492–1497.

Takahashi Y, Nakano M, Sano K, Kanri T. 2005. The effects of epinephrine in local anesthetics on plasma catecholamine and hemodynamic responses. *Odontology* 93(1):72–79.

Todd DW. 2003. Anticoagulated patients and oral surgery. *Arch Intern Med* 163:1242.

Vlachopoulous C, Aznaouridis K, Alexopoulos N, et al. 2005. Effect of dark chocolate on arterial function in healthy individuals. *American J Hypertension* 18:785–791.

Wahl MJ. 1998. Dental surgery in anticoagulated patients. *Arch Intern Med* 158:1610–1616.

Wahl MJ. 2000. Myths of dental surgery in patients receiving anticoagulant therapy. *J Am Dent Assoc* 131:77–81.

Weir MR. 1996. Angiotensin-II receptor antagonists: A new class of antihypertensive agents. *Am Acad Family Phy* 53:589–594.

QUICK DRUG GUIDE

Antihypertensive Drugs

Diuretics

(Increase elimination of water and salt, which will reduce pressure)

Thiazides

- Chlorothiazide (Diuril)
- Hydrochlorothiazide (Hydrodiuril)

Loop Diuretics

- Furosemide (Lasix)
- Bumetanide (Bumex)

Potassium-Sparing

- Triamterene (Dyrenium)
- Spironolactone (Aldactone)

Angiotensin Inhibitors

(Angiotensin-converting enzyme [ACE] inhibitors: Reduce blood pressure by inhibiting the conversion of angiotensin I to angiotensin II)

- Benazepril (Lotensin)
- Captopril (Capoten)
- Enalapril (Vasotec)
- Fosinopril (Monopril)
- Moexipril (Univasc)
- Quinapril (Accupril)
- Ramipril (Altace)

Angiotensin-II Receptor Blockers (ARBs)

(Block angiotensin II receptor sites)

- Candesartan (Atacand)
- Eprosartan (Teveten)
- Irbesartan (Avapro)
- Losartan (Cozaar)
- Olmesartan (Benicar)
- Telmisartan (Micardis)
- Valsartan (Diovan)

Sympatholytics

(Decrease heart rate and contractility by blocking β-receptors)

β-Receptor Blockers

- Atenolol (Tenormin): cardioselective
- Bisoprolol (Zebeta): cardioselective
- Metoprolol (Lopressor): cardioselective
- Nadolol (Corgard): nonselective
- Propranolol (Inderal): nonselective
- Timolol (Blocadren): nonselective

Centrally/Peripherally α_2-Agonists Acting Drugs

- Clonidine (Catapres)
- Methyldopa (Aldomet)
- Reserpine (generic)

α_1-Adrenergic Blockers

- Prazosin (Minipress)
- Terazosin (Hytrin)

Calcium Channel Blockers

(Prevent calcium from entering the cells of the coronary blood vessels and cause vasodilation)

Nondihydropyridines

- Diltiazem (Cardizem)
- Verapamil (Calan, Isoptin)

Dihyropyridines

- Nifedipine (Procardia)
- Amlodipine (Norvasc)
- Felodipine (Plendil)

Direct Vasodilators

- Hydralazine (Apresoline)
- Minoxidil (Loniten)
- Nitroprusside (Nitropress)

Anti-Angina Drugs

Vasodilators

(Dilate coronary arteries)
- Nitroglycerin (Nitro-Bid, Nitrostat)
- Isosorbide dinitrate (Isordil)
- Isosorbide mononitrate (Imdur)

Calcium Channel Blockers

(Slow heart rate and dilate coronary arteries)
- Amlodipine (Norvasc)
- Bedpridil (Vasocor)
- Diltiazem (Cardizem)
- Nicardipine (Cardene)
- Nifedipine (Procardia, Adalat)
- Verapamil (Calan, Isoptin)

β-blockers

(Reduce cardiac load and thus oxygen demand)
- Atenolol (Tenormin)
- Metoprolol (Lopressor)
- Nadolol (Corgard)
- Propranolol (Inderal)

Heart Failure Drugs

Diuretics

(Increase fluid loss, thus reducing cardiac load)
- Loop diuretics (furosemide)
- Thiazides (hyrochlorothiazide)

Positive Inotropic Drugs

Digitalis Glycosides

(Increase calcium ion concentration, which enhances heart contractility)
- Digoxin (Lanoxin)

Adrenergic Receptor Agonists

(Stimulate β-receptors, which increase cardiac contractility)
- Dobutamine (Dobutrex)
- Dopamine

Vasodilators

- Hyralazine (Apresoline)

Angiotensin-Converting Enzyme Inhibitors

(ACE inhibitors)
- Captopril (Capoten)
- Enalapril (Vasotec)
- Lisinopril (Prinivil, Zestril)
- Quinapril (Accupril)
- Fosinopril (Monopril)

Calcium Channel Blockers

Nondihydropyridines
- Diltiazem (Cardizem)
- Verapamil (Calan, Isoptin)

Dihyropyridines
- Nifedipine (Procardia)
- Amlodipine (Norvasc)
- Felodipine (Plendil)

Antiarrhythmic Drugs

Class I: Sodium Channel Blockers

Class IA
- Disopyrmaide (Norpace)
- Procainamide (Pronestyl)
- Quinidine (Quinidex)

Class IB
- Lidocaine (Xylocaine)
- Mexiletine (Mexitil)

Class IC
- Flecainide (Tambocor)
- Propafenone (Rhythmol)

Class II: β-blockers

- Acebutolol (Sectral)
- Esmolol (Brevibloc)
- Propranolol (Inderal)

Class III: Potassium Channel Blockers

- Amiodarone (Cordarone)
- Bretylium (injectable)
- Sotalol (Betapace)

Class IV: Calcium Channel Blockers

- Diltiazem (Cardizem)
- Verapamil (Calan)

Antihyperlipidemia/Hypertriglyceridemia Drugs

HMG-CoA Reductase Inhibitors ("Statin" Drugs)

- Atorvastatin (Lipitor)
- Fluvastatin (Lescol)
- Lovastatin (Mevacor)

- Pravastatin (Pravacol)
- Rosuvastatin (Crestor)
- Simvastatin (Zocor)

Bile Acid-Binding (Sequestrants) Resins

- Cholestyramine (Questran)
- Colestipol (Colestid)

Other Agents (Natural)

- Nicotinic acid (niacin)
- Vitamin E

Fibric Acids

- Fenofibrate (Lofibra,Tricor)
- Gemfibrozil (Lopid)

Combination Drugs

- Amlodipine/atorvastatin (Caduet)
- Ezetimibe/simvastatin (Vytorin)

Anticoagulants

- Warfarin (Coumadin)
- Dicumarol

- Anisindione (Miradon)
- Heparin

Antiplatelet Drugs

- Aspirin
- Abciximab (ReoPro)
- Clopidogrel (Plavix)

- Dipyridamole (Persantine, Pyridamole)
- Ticlopidine (Ticlid)
- Aspirin/dipyridamole (Aggrenox)

CHAPTER 12

Gastrointestinal Drugs

GOAL

To introduce the fundamentals of drug therapy for common abdominal conditions.

EDUCATIONAL OBJECTIVES

After reading this chapter, the reader should be able to:

1. Describe the current theory of the etiology of peptic ulcer disease.

2. Explain the differences in treatment between peptic ulcer disease and gastroesophageal reflux disease (GERD).

3. Discuss any contraindications or precautions in dental patients with gastrointestinal disorders.

4. Discuss the pharmacologic therapy for GERD.

5. Discuss the treatments for constipation and diarrhea.

KEY TERMS

Gastrointestinal (GI) tract

Peptic ulcer disease

Helicobacter pylori

GERD

Introduction

The **gastrointestinal (GI) tract** comprises the stomach and the intestines. The first part of the small intestine closest to the stomach, where most absorption occurs, is called the duodenum and the large intestine is called the colon. This chapter reviews the drugs that act on the gastrointestinal tract. The following conditions will be reviewed: peptic ulcer disease (PUD), gastroesophageal reflux disease (GERD), inflammatory bowel disease, constipation, diarrhea, and emesis (vomiting).

The GI tract is an interesting part of the body as far as drug intake is concerned. The GI tract is the major route for absorption into the systemic circulation of drugs taken orally. Many drugs affect the GI tract or its mucosal lining; for instance, salicylates (e.g., aspirin) and other nonsteroidal anti-inflammatory drugs directly affect the mucosal lining of the stomach and may cause bleeding. On the other hand, some drugs act locally and affect the GI tract beneficially. Antacids, for example, act locally in the stomach and duodenum to neutralize gastric acid.

Peptic Ulcer Disorders

Peptic-Ulcer Disease

Peptic ulcer disease (PUD) is a general term describing a group of acid-peptic disorders of the upper GI tract, primarily the esophagus, stomach, and duodenum. A peptic ulcer is defined as a circumscribed loss of tissue or break that occurs in the GI mucosa extending through the smooth muscle that lines the GI tract. It occurs when there is an imbalance between gastric acid and pepsin and mucosal defense factors, including prostaglandins, which increases the production of gastric mucus and reduces the formation of gastric acid. An ulcer in the stomach is called a gastric ulcer (GU), a duodenal ulcer (DU) occurs in the duodenum, and an ulcer in the esophagus is called an esophageal ulcer (Figure 12-1). An ulcer can occur anywhere along the GI tract where parts of the mucosa from the tract are exposed to gastric acid and pepsin from the stomach.

A duodenal ulcer is 5–10 times more common than a gastric ulcer. The most common symptom of PUD is epigastric pain, which is more frequent at night, not in the morning when gastric secretion is the lowest, which will usually awaken the individual. Epigastric pain is usually what brings a patient to the physician. Food or antacids usually relieve the pain and the individual has a feeling of being hungry. These ulcers tend to recur many times a year. Heartburn, belching, and bloating are also common symptoms. A differential diagnosis must be made between DU and indigestion, which has similar symptoms. A thorough patient history will determine this. Nausea, vomiting, and weight loss is more commonly seen in gastric ulcers than duodenal ulcers. Eating usually causes pain, so the individual does not eat and loses weight.

DID YOU KNOW?

On average, the stomach produces two liters of hydrochloric acid daily.

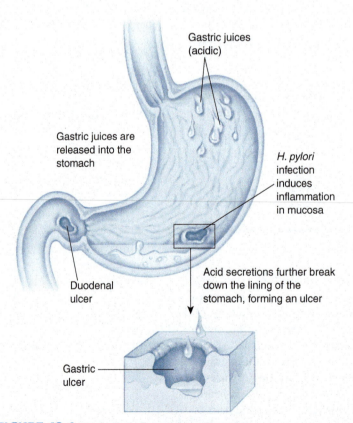

Gastric juices (acidic)

Gastric juices are released into the stomach

H. pylori infection induces inflammation in mucosa

Duodenal ulcer

Acid secretions further break down the lining of the stomach, forming an ulcer

Gastric ulcer

FIGURE 12-1 Mechanism of peptic ulcer formation.

The original theory of the etiology of ulcers involved excessive production and secretion of gastric juice (hydrochloric acid + pepsin) to which the deeper muscle layers of the GI tract are exposed. Gastric juices in the stomach are produced by either physiological means (e.g., smell, sight, and taste of food) or through the central nervous system, where the vagus nerve is stimulated. Histamine, a substance found in highest concentrations in skin, lungs, and GI mucosa, is found inside mast cells in the tissue and is responsible for stimulating the production of gastric juices in the stomach. It is the acidic gastric juices that cause the ulcer in the mucosa and breakdown of the protective barrier lining of the duodenum.

Duodenal ulcers are due to the hypersecretion of acid, and gastric ulcers are due to a decrease in the protective lining of the stomach with a decrease in mucosal resistance and not associated with increased acid secretion.

Currently, however, excessive acid production is thought to be a secondary cause while the primary cause is due to a bacterial infection. Research has found that *Helicobacter pylori (H. pylori) is the bacterium that causes approximately 90% of duodenal and 80% of gastric ulcers.* A blood test can tell if an individual is positive for *H. pylori*. This gram-negative microorganism resides in the mucus layer overlying the gastric epithelium of infected individuals, where it damages the GI mucosa via releasing enzymes that degrade gastric cells and alter the inflammatory response, which may interfere with healing.

Additionally, patients on long-term therapy with aspirin, nonsteroidal anti-inflammatory drugs (NSAIDs), or corticosteroids can develop gastric ulcers. Nonsteroidal anti-inflammatory drugs inhibit both forms of cyclooxygenase enzymes, resulting in a nonselective inhibition of COX-1, which is responsible for protecting the GI mucosa. Other risk factors are environment, cigarette smoking, alcohol consumption, caffeine, and genetics.

> ## DID YOU KNOW?
>
> In 1983, Dr. J. Robin Warren and Dr. Barry Marshall reported finding a new kind of bacteria in the stomachs of people with gastritis. They hypothesized that peptic ulcers are generally caused not by excess acidity or stress but a bacterial infection. In 2005 they won the Nobel Prize for this work.

Gastroesophageal Reflux Disease (GERD)

Gastroesophageal reflux disease, commonly referred to as **GERD**, is one of the most common chronic conditions of the upper gastrointestinal tract. In GERD there is a reflux or "backing up" of gastric contents from the stomach into the esophagus, which generally occurs in many individuals without causing any complications and damage to the mucosal lining of the esophagus. The most common complaint or symptom is heartburn but the individual may also complain of epigastric pain. Most individuals with heartburn will seek therapy on their own with antacids; however, if the acidic gastric contents stay in contact for prolonged periods of time with the mucosal tissue of the esophagus, a form of GERD called reflux esophagitis will develop, which is characterized by inflammation of the esophagus due to excessive acid reflux. Acid reflux into the oral cavity may cause the development of tooth erosion, particularly on the palatal surfaces of the maxillary incisors, which have the greatest contact with the acid. Esophagitis results from excessive reflux of gastric juices rather than excessive acid secretion in the stomach as seen in peptic ulcer disease. Other complications from GERD are dysphagia (difficulty in swallowing) and esophageal ulcers.

Risk factors for GERD include alcohol, smoking, spicy foods, duodenal ulcers, and some medications such as aspirin and NSAIDs, calcium channel blockers (reduce lower esophageal sphincter tone, allowing the reflux of acids), alendronate (Fosamax; for treatment of osteoporosis), and tetracycline. *Helicobacter pylori* infection does not increase the risk of GERD or reflux esophagitis, and is actually associated with a lower severity of symptoms.

PHARMACOTHERAPY FOR PEPTIC ULCER DISEASE AND GERD Since it has been found that PUD is primarily caused by a bacterium, therapy has changed over the years to now include antibiotics in the overall drug regimen. Lowering acid production with medications is the key outcome. Additionally, the patient should, if possible, stop smoking, alcohol consumption (or reduce the amount), caffeine, and use of nonsteroidal anti-inflammatory drugs.

Patients with GERD should also try to lose weight, stop smoking and alcohol consumption, and avoid eating 2–3 hours before bedtime to reduce the amount of acid in the stomach available to reflux.

There are five main types of medications used to treat PUD: antacids, antihistamines, proton pump inhibitors, mucosal defense drugs, and antibiotics (Figure 12-2; Table 12-1).

- *Antacids* are used primarily for symptomatic relief of gastric pain, especially heartburn, and will not really promote healing of the ulcer.
- *Antihistamines* (*Histamine₂-receptor antagonists*; H₂RAs) will provide symptomatic relief of pain and promote healing of the ulcer.
- *Proton pump inhibitors* will provide quick pain relief and accelerated healing of the ulcer.
- *Mucosal defense drugs* have no effect on gastric acid secretion.
- *Prostaglandin*
- *Protective barrier*
- *Antibiotics* are needed to eradicate the *H. pylori* infection.

Drugs used to treat GERD include:

- *Antacids*
- *H₂-receptor antagonists*
- *Proton pump inhibitors*
- *Gastrointestinal stimulant*

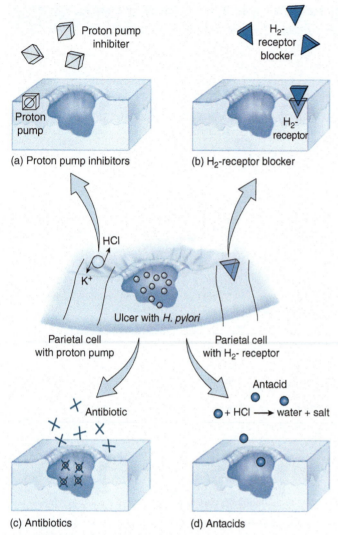

FIGURE 12-2 Mechanism of action of anti-ulcer drugs.

Rapid Dental Hint

In patients taking antacids, H_2RAs, or proton pump inhibitors there are no precautions or contraindications with epinephrine. Also, no special dental management is required.

The only antacid that is used in the treatment of PUD is bismuth subsalicylate (BSS) (Pepto-Bismol), which functions to suppress *H. pylori* infection by inhibiting bacterial adherence to mucosal cells and damages bacterial cell walls. It is recommended that it be used in conjunction with antibiotics. Thus, bismuth is the antacid of choice in the treatment and maintenance of PUD.

DID YOU KNOW?

Patients taking antacids containing calcium, aluminum, or magnesium should not take tetracycline or doxycycline at the same time. Space the dosing apart a few hours.

The duration of action of antacids is short—only about 30 minutes—but if taken 1 to 3 hours after meals and at bedtime, which corresponds to the greatest gastric acid secretion that occurs during a day, the duration of action increases. Antacids are usually used in conjunction with other anti-ulcer medications. If patients with ulcers do not respond to antacids, then other drugs (e.g., antihistamines) should be used.

Adherence is low because:

1. Antacids must be taken frequently, every 2–4 hours, because of the short duration of action, to have a beneficial effect.
2. Antacids generally have a bad taste. Many products have various flavoring agents to mask the bad taste, and refrigeration of the product may improve the taste.
3. Antacids have many adverse effects, such as diarrhea, constipation, belching and flatulence (gas), and have many drug interactions.

Antacids with or without alginic acid and nonprescription histamine$_2$-receptor antagonists are appropriate first-line pharmacological therapy and may provide sufficient acid neutralization/suppression for patients with mild, infrequent GERD symptoms. Because of their rapid onset of action, antacids are useful for quick relief of symptoms.

Alginic acid (which is present in Gaviscon) is not in the true sense an antacid because it does not neutralize acids in the stomach; however, it does form a thick solution of sodium alginate when in contact with gastric acids that floats on the surface of the gastric contents, minimizing the contact of acid

Conventional doses of H$_2$RAs, antacids, or mucosal defense drugs heal approximately 90% of duodenal ulcers (DU) within 8 weeks, while increasing acid suppression with higher H$_2$RA doses or proton pump inhibitors achieves healing rates within 4 weeks. Little data has been established for the efficacy of these drugs in the treatment of DU. NSAID-induced ulcers respond to all of the drugs used for PUD, although healing is more rapid when the NSAID is discontinued.

Antacids Antacids are primarily used in the treatment of dyspepsia (indigestion or heartburn). Antacids are basic salts that dissolve in acid gastric secretions and neutralize some but not all gastric hydrochloric acid, and have a greater effect of increasing the pH in the duodenum than in the stomach. Antacids neutralize or reduce the acidity of gastric juices, but they do not affect the rate or amount of gastric acid secretion by the stomach cells and do not prevent ulcer recurrence. Rather, antacids are usually used to relieve occasional duodenal ulcer symptoms on an as-needed basis by the patient and systemic absorption and adverse effects.

TABLE 12-1 Drugs Used in the Treatment of Peptic Ulcer Disease (PUD) and GERD

DRUG NAME	MECHANISM/INDICATION
Antacids	Relief of epigastric (stomach) pain; indigestion; neutralizes gastric acid juices secreted in the stomach by increasing the pH of gastric secretions; primarily used for heartburn; only bismuth is recommended for duodenal ulcers
Calcium carbonate (Tums, Titralac, Maalox chewable tabs, Gaviscon)	Heartburn/indigestion (GERD); rapid onset of action and a prolonged effect
Bismuth subsalicylate (Pepto-Bismol)	Ulcers because shown to effective against *H. pylori*
Magnesium hydroxide (Milk of Magnesia)	GERD
Aluminum/magnesium hydroxide/simethicone (Maalox, Gelusil liquid, Mylanta liquid)	GERD
Calcium carbonate and magnesium hydroxide (Rolaids)	GERD
Sodium bicarbonate/alginic acid combination (Gaviscon extra strength tabs)	Foaming actions are good for relieving symptoms of GERD only—not indicated for PUD
H$_2$-Receptor Antagonists	Selectively blocks histamine at the histamine receptor; all H$_2$-receptor antagonists act equally—cost is the only deciding factor on which drug to use
	Available over-the-counter, but in a lower strength than by prescription
	The OTC product is only approved for treating heartburn
Cimetidine (Tagamet)	For treatment of duodenal or gastric ulcer and esophagitis
	OTC product only approved for heartburn (100 mg tabs)
Famotidine (Pepcid, Mylanta AR, Pepcid AC)	For duodenal ulcer and heartburn; OTC product only for treating heartburn (10 mg tab)
Nizatidine (Axid)	Treatment of duodenal or gastric ulcer and heartburn
	OTC product only approved for heartburn
Ranitidine (Zantac)	Duodenal and gastric ulcer, esophagitis, heartburn (OTC product only approved for heartburn)
Proton Pump Inhibitors	Suppress gastric acid secretion by inhibiting the gastric-ATPase enzyme pump
Omeprazole (Prilosec); omeprazole/sodium bicarbonate (Zegerid)	Healing of duodenal ulcers in 4 weeks—use in combination with antibiotics for eradication of *H. pylori;* also for maintenance of erosive esophagitis (GERD) and gastric ulcer
Lansoprazole (Prevacid); Prevacid 24 HR OTC	Duodenal ulcer treatment (in combination with other drugs to eradicate *H. pylori*) and maintenance, and NSAID-induced gastric ulcer and GERD
Esomeprazole (Nexium)	For *H. pylori* eradication (when used with amoxicillin and clarithromycin); also for erosive esophagitis; gastroesophageal reflux disease (GERD); NSAID-induced ulcers
Rabeprazole (AcipHex)	Short-term (up to 4) weeks) treatment of the healing and symptomatic relief of duodenal ulcers; short-term (4–8 weeks) treatment in the healing and symptomatic relief of GERD (erosive eosphagitis and heartburn)
Prostaglandin Supplements	
Misoprostal (Cytotec)	Prevention of gastric and duodenal ulcers due to NSAIDs
Protective Barrier Drug	
Sucralfate (Carfate)	For healing of duodenal ulcers, not gastric ulcers
Gastrointestinal Stimulant Drug	
Metoclopramide (Reglan)	GERD; increases muscle contractions in the upper digestive tract, which speeds up the rate at which the stomach empties into the intestines

Note: Lansoprazole, amoxicillin, and clarithromycin are available in a daily administration combination pack (Prevpac).

Source: Antibiotic regimen: American College of Gastroenterology Guidelines. 1998. *American Journal of Gastroenterology* 93:2330.

with the esophagus. When gastroesophageal reflux occurs, it is the sodium alginate—not the acid—that is refluxed from the stomach to the esophagus, resulting in less esophageal irritation.

Sodium bicarbonate is available as baking soda and is combined in many OTC products (e.g., Alka-Seltzer). When taken orally it reacts with acid in the stomach to raise the pH rapidly by

forming sodium chloride, carbon dioxide, and water. In patients on a sodium-restricted diet or decreased renal function, sodium bicarbonate should be taken only on a short-term basis because it is systemically absorbed into the bloodstream. Chronic use can cause alkalosis (increase in bicarbonate and pH) or the "milk-alkali syndrome," which is difficult to diagnose because of its nondescriptive symptoms such as nausea, vomiting, and headache. This syndrome is more likely to occur in individuals who have a high intake of calcium, like pregnant women. It should be used with caution in patients with benign prostatic hypertrophy.

Magnesium hydroxide and aluminum hydroxide (Maalox) are not systemically absorbed and can be used on a long-term basis. The combination minimizes the diarrhea effect produced by the magnesium and the constipating effect produced by the aluminum.

Calcium carbonate (Tums) is a nonsystemic antacid that, when taken on a long-term basis, may cause acid rebound, with more acid being produced. It may also cause kidney stone formation and constipation.

Drug–Drug Interactions   Di- or trivalent ions (Mg^{2+}, Ca^{2+}, Al^{3+}) containing antacids bind to and form an insoluble complex with tetracyclines (tetracycline HCl, minocycline HCl, and doxycycline hyclate) and fluoroquinolone (e.g., Cipro), which will decrease the absorption rate of these antibiotics. Thus, antacids should not be given concurrently with these antibiotics but 1–2 hours before or after taking the antibiotics.

Antihistamines (histamine-receptor antagonist or blocker)   These agents are indicated for the symptomatic relief and healing of ulcers and in alleviating symptoms of duodenal ulcers, gastric ulcers, and GERD. H_2-receptor blockers reduce histamine-stimulated gastric acid secretion by competitively inhibiting H_2-receptors on the parietal cells in the stomach. These agents have a limited effect on gastric acid secretion after food ingestion and are effective in healing ulcers in 6–12 weeks. In contrast to antacids, H_2-receptor antagonists have a similar onset of action to antacids but a much longer duration of action, up to 12 hours, and may provide nighttime relief. Four H_2-receptor antagonists are currently available by prescription and over the counter (the OTC drugs simply have lower doses): cimetidine (Tagamet), famotidine (Pepcid), ranitidine (Zantac), and nizatidine (Axid).

Rapid Dental Hint

The suffix *–tidine* is common to generic H_2-blockers.

All four agents are equally effective and are used in conjunction with antibiotics to eradicate *H. pylori* in PUD. H_2-receptor inhibitors should be taken on an as-needed basis to avoid the development of tolerance. Adverse effects are usually mild and include thrombocytopenia (low blood platelets), headache, diarrhea, and confusion.

Cimetidine (Tagamet) was the first H_2-receptor blocker introduced and has since become available OTC. Cimetidine is involved with many drug–drug interactions because it inhibits CYP_1A_2 enzymes in the liver (Table 12-1). Cimetidine will increase gastric pH for 6 hours. It is not the drug of choice for treatment of longer than 6 weeks because of the development of diarrhea, agranulocytosis [also called neutropenia, where there is a reduction in the blood neutrophil (granulocyte—white blood cell) count], which can lead to increased susceptibility to bacterial and fungal infections and a rebound phenomenon, where new ulcers form.

Proton Pump Inhibitors   Proton pump inhibitors (PPI) provide rapid symptomatic relief with accelerating healing of duodenal ulcers and provide the most rapid symptom relief and highest percentage of esophageal healing of all agents used in GERD management. They are the drug of choice for patients with frequent daily symptoms, moderate to severe GERD symptoms, patients not responding to H_2RAs, and those with complicated disease, including Barrett's esophagus and esophagitis. In most patients, PPIs relieve symptoms within several days of treatment.

Rapid Dental Hint

PPIs can cause xerostomia. Monitor salivary flow and signs of xerostomia and manage accordingly.

Unlike H_2-receptor antagonists, PPIs reduce peak acid output (e.g., food-stimulated acid output) without regard to administration time, although the best time to dose is 30 minutes before breakfast. PPIs achieve almost total suppression of acid secretion because they bind irreversibly to the proton pump in the membrane of the acid-producing cells in the stomach. To restore acid secretion it is necessary either to synthesize new pumps or activate resting pumps, which takes about 3–5 days. The following drugs are PPIs:

- esomeprazole (Nexium)
- lansoprazole (Prevacid)
- omeprazole (Prilosec)
- pantoprazole (Protonix)
- rabeprazole (AcipHex)

Rapid Dental Hint

The suffix *-prazole* is common to generic proton pump inhibitors.

These agents provide long-term and enhanced acid suppression and show high healing rates for PUD. They have been shown to achieve nearly total suppression of acid secretion. The most common adverse effects are headache, skin alterations, diarrhea, xerostomia, and nausea.

All PPIs are highly bound to plasma proteins, so there will be displacement of other highly protein-bound drugs including phenytoin, diazepam, and warfarin, causing elevated plasma levels. All of the PPIs are metabolized by the cytochrome P450 isoenzyme system. Drug interactions are listed in Table 12-1.

Prostaglandin Supplementation Misoprostal (Cytotec) is a synthetic prostaglandin E_2 agent that inhibits gastric acid secretion and increases gastric mucosal defense. It is indicated for the prevention of NSAID-induced gastric and duodenal ulcers. This drug should not be used in pregnant women because it causes uterine contractions.

Protective Barrier Drugs Sucralfate (Carafate) is an aluminum hydroxide–sucrose complex that functions to form a protective barrier or bandage over the GI mucosal lining. It does not alter the pH of gastric juices or inhibit gastric acid secretion, but binds to the gastric mucosa and forms a gel that protects the ulcer from gastric acids. It is indicated for the short-term treatment of duodenal ulcers and for maintenance of healing of a DU. Its efficacy for symptomatic relief of GERD and gastric ulcers has not been established.

Prokinetic Drugs Prokinetic drugs are an alternative to standard doses of H_2RAs. The pathogenesis of GERD can be related to defects in esophagogastric motility, poor esophageal clearance, and delayed gastric emptying time. Therefore, it may be possible to promote healing with the use of a prokinetic drug. A prokinetic drug is used to increase the force of the contraction of the lower esophageal sphincter, thus decreasing reflux of gastric juices and accelerating gastric emptying. Prokinetic drugs are not indicated for the treatment of PUD. Metoclopramide (Reglan) is a dopamine antagonist that blocks dopamine receptors, lowering esophageal sphincter pressure and increasing gastric emptying. It is indicated in the symptomatic relief of GERD, but not for esophageal healing.

PHARMACOTHERAPY FOR *H. PYLORI* INFECTION: ANTIBIOTICS
The use of at least two antibiotics combined with an H_2-receptor antagonist or proton pump inhibitor and/or bismuth comprise the recommended regimen for *H. pylori* infection in PUD (Table 12-1). Using antisecretory drugs without antibiotics is not recommended because there is a high rate of ulcer recurrence and complications. Combination therapy provides better outcomes. Remember to instruct the patient to take yogurt or acidophilus gel caps when taking broad-spectrum antibiotics.

A three-drug regimen is recommended (Table 12-1) versus a two-drug regimen because it is more effective in eradicating *H. pylori*. However, there are more adverse effects, drug–drug

> ### Guidelines for Patients Taking Antacids
>
> - Patients should not take tetracyclines (doxycycline, minocycline) at the same time; they should take antacids at least 2 hours before other medications.
> - Patients with hypertension should avoid sodium-based antacids.

interaction possibilities, and a lower compliance rate. Antibiotic resistance and incomplete treatment are major reasons for treatment failure. Continued therapy for 14 days has been found to be the most reliable and effective regimen.

After the acute disease is under control using antibiotics, antisecretory drugs, and/or bismuth, maintenance therapy is needed. Treatment consists of taking an H_2-receptor antagonist at a lower dosage at bedtime. Even with all of the different therapies, ulcer recurrence is up to 90%.

Treatment of PUD is to relieve ulcer pain, aid in ulcer healing, preventing ulcer recurrence, and eliminating complications. Use of H_2-receptor antagonists, antacids, or sucralfate will heal the ulcer by 8 weeks. PPIs may be more effective and heal ulcers within 4 weeks. Patients positive for *H. pylori* need to take an antibiotic in addition to an antisecretory drug.

Summary of Treatment Guidelines for PUD and GERD

Peptic ulcers: Recommended therapy for duodenal ulcers is: two antibiotics + H_2 antagonist + antacids PRN (as needed)

GERD: The first-line drug therapy for GERD is antacids and a nonprescription H_2RA such as famotidine (Pepcid) or a PPI such as omeprazole (Prilosec). Given the chronic nature of GERD and the high recurrence rates if acid suppressive therapy is discontinued, long-term maintenance therapy is appropriate and indicated for most patients.

Irritable Bowel Syndrome

Irritable bowel syndrome (IBS) is a nonspecific disease with symptoms lasting at least 12 weeks consisting of diarrhea, constipation, and abdominal pain, which is the most common symptom. Diseases that are associated with IBS include fibromyalgia or chronic fatigue syndrome, sleep disturbance, migraines, and chronic stress.

> ### Guidelines for Patients Taking Omeprazole (Prilosec)
>
> - There are interactions with several drugs including diazepam (Valium) and phenytoin (Dilantin).
> - Patients should avoid aspirin and aspirin-containing medications.
> - Dry mouth is an adverse effect.

> ### Guidelines for Patients Taking Ranitidine (Zantac)
>
> - Avoid prescribing aspirin and aspirin-containing medications.
> - Patients with gastroesophageal reflux may present with oral symptoms, including burning mouth and tooth erosion.
> - Recommend reducing acid content in the mouth with sodium bicarbonate mouthrinse.

Irritable bowel syndrome, according to the Rome Criteria, is diagnosed when there are at least 12 weeks of abdominal pain or discomfort that is relieved by defecation and/or onset is associated with change in the form of stool. Onset of IBS is usually in adolescence or early adulthood.

Since the etiology is not fully understood and the symptoms can be vague at times, treatment of IBS is a challenge. A physical examination must be performed to rule out other conditions. Constipation is a side effect of certain medications including antacids, nonsteroidal anti-inflammatory agents, calcium channel blockers (verapamil), iron, and antipsychotics and antidepressants. Diarrhea is a side effect of certain medications, including antacids, antibiotics (e.g., tetracyclines, clindamycin, ampicillin, amoxicillin), and antilipemic agents (gemfibrozil). Psychological issues must be addressed. Dietary modifications should be made to avoid fatty foods, gas-producing foods such as beans, alcohol, and caffeine.

Pharmacotherapy

Pharmacological treatment utilizes any of the following drugs:

1. Antidiarrheal agents: loperamide (Imodium) and cholestyramine (use in patients with high cholesterol levels)
2. Antispasmodic agents: An anticholinergic drug is used to treat the pain and bloating (abdominal distention) caused by IBS. These drugs work by suppressing intestinal contractions after meals or during stressful periods. The following are anticholinergics/antispasmodics: dicyclomine (Bentyl), hyoscyamine (Levsin), donnatal tablets or elixir (phenobarbital, hyoscyamine, atropine, and scopolamine), chlordiazepoxide/clidinium bromide (Librax).
3. Anticonstipation agents: osmotic laxative (lactulose, polyethylene glycol) or other laxatives and increase dietary fiber intake either with foods or supplements, which will act as bulk-forming agents.

Nausea and Vomiting

Emesis (vomiting) is defined as the expulsion of gastric contents through the mouth, whereas nausea is the feeling in the throat that vomiting may happen. Numerous causes of nausea and vomiting include gastrointestinal, cardiovascular (heart failure, myocardial infarction, or heart attack; psychogenic causes (self-induced as seen in bulimia); drug-induced (opiates, antibiotics, chemotherapy, and radiation therapy); pregnancy; changes in position; and many other causes.

Chronic vomiting may cause the enamel on the palatal surfaces of the maxillary incisors to erode, creating a "shiny, smooth" surface (Figure 12-3). A sodium bicarbonate mouthrinse may be recommended to reduce acid content.

Most cases of nausea and vomiting are self-limiting. Treatment is aimed at preventing or eliminating the nausea and vomiting to prevent dehydration. There are many OTC and prescription anti-emetic drugs. Some preparations are listed in Table 12-2.

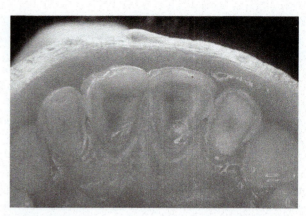

FIGURE 12-3 Erosion of palatal surfaces of maxillary teeth due to chronic vomiting.

Constipation

Constipation is defined as a reduced number of bowel movements and frequently occurs with straining without effect. The patient may complain of abdominal distention or pain. Several risk factors associated with constipation include narcotics (opiates), anticholinergics, calcium channel blockers (especially verapamil), aluminum-containing antacids, and iron products.

Pharmacotherapy

The causative drug can be discontinued, changed to another drug without constipating side effects or, if possible, the dose may be reduced. Chronic constipation can be managed with increasing dietary fiber intake to 20–30 grams/day with an increase in fluid intake. Prune juice contains a substance that helps with constipation.

There are different types of laxatives available:

1. Bulk-forming agents that soften the stool: methylcellulose, polycarbophil, psyllium
2. Emollients that soften the stool: docusate (sodium, calcium, potassium), lactulose, sorbitol, and mineral oil
3. Drugs that cause soft or semisoft stool: disacodyl, senna, magnesium sulfate
4. Drugs that cause watery evacuation: magnesium (citrate, hydroxide, sulfate)

Diarrhea

Diarrhea is a term used to describe watery or loose stools, or excessive stool frequency or amount. Loose or watery stools may be a sign of pathology. Causes may be contaminated food or

TABLE 12-2 Common Anti-Emetics
• Meclizine (Antivert)
• Promethazine (Phenergan)
• Metoclopramide (Reglan)
• Trimethobenzamide (Tigan)
• Prochlorperazine (Compazine)
• Ondansetron (Zofran)

TABLE 12-3 Common Antibiotics Causing Antibiotic-Associated Diarrhea
• Clindamycin
• Amoxicillin
• Ampicillin
• Cephalosporins
• Tetracyclines

TABLE 12-4 Therapy for Nonspecific Diarrhea
• Ioperamide (Imodium)
• Diphenoxylate hydrochloride and atropine sulfate (Lomotil)
• Tincture of opium (Paregoric - Rx)
• Bismuth subsalicylate (Pepto-Bismol; Kaopectate)
• Yogurt or acidophilus tablets
• Octreotide acetate (Sandostatin)

water, infection (bacterial, viral, protozoa), disease (malabsorption syndrome, inflammatory bowel disease such as ulcerative colitis or Crohn's disease), immunocompromised individuals (HIV/AIDS), drugs, irritable bowel syndrome, colon carcinoma, or traveler's diarrhea.

Acute diarrhea lasting less than 3 weeks is most often due to bacterial or viral infection, food poisoning, or drugs. The most common bacteria involved in food poisoning are *Salmonella* and *Escherichia coli* (*E. coli*). Chronic diarrhea lasting more than 4 weeks can lead to dehydration and loss of important minerals and electrolytes.

Antibiotic-Associated Diarrhea

Diarrhea due to antibiotic use, especially broad-spectrum antibiotics (e.g., tetracyclines, amoxicillin) (Table 12-3) is usually caused either by a direct irritant of the drug on the gastrointestinal mucosa (such as tetracycline) or the disruption of normal bowel flora (bacteria that normally live in the gut) leading to the overgrowth of a bacterium called *Clostridium difficle,* which releases toxins that cause inflammation and damage to the intestinal mucosa, resulting in diarrhea.

If diarrhea that results from taking antibiotics is very severe and is watery with exudative mucosal plaque, then it is called pseudomembranous colitis. Pseudomembranous colitis usually is the major cause of hospitalized (noscomial) diarrhea.

The offending drug should be discontinued, if possible, even if diarrhea is a common adverse side effect. Antidiarrhea medication should not be given because it is necessary for the bacterial toxins to be eliminated from the body and giving antidiarrhea medications will not allow this. Yogurt, which has *Lactobacillus acidophilus* culture or acidophilus, is given to replace bowel flora.

Besides antibiotics, other drugs that can cause diarrhea include diuretics, histamine$_2$-receptor inhibitors, digoxin, and nonsteroidal anti-inflammatory drugs.

Treatment of Acute Diarrhea (Other than Antibiotic-Associated Diarrhea)

Once infection, carcinoma, or antibiotic-induced diarrhea is ruled out, acute diarrhea can be treated with many different types of medications (Table 12-4), keeping in mind to prevent dehydration:

1. Loperamide (Imodium), which is available without a prescription, slows down GI motility with few side effects. If diarrhea does not stop within 2 days, then further medical evaluation is needed.

2. Diphenoxylate hydrochloride and atropine sulfate (Lomotil) are available without a prescription. Diphenoxylate is a synthetic opiate, and atropine is an anticholinergic drug that slows down GI motility. This drug can cause dry mouth, blurred vision, urinary retention, tachycardia, and drowsiness. Alcohol and other CNS depressants should be avoided when taking this drug.

3. Tincture of opium (Paregoric) is a liquid narcotic that is used when other antimotility drugs have failed. This drug is also used in AIDS-associated diarrhea.

4. Bismuth subsalicylate (Pepto-Bismol, Kaopectate) is available without a prescription. It has an antisecretory effect on the colon. Antidiarrheal properties make it good in preventing traveler's diarrhea.

5. Yogurt or acidophilus tablets can be taken before the antibiotic is given to reestablish the normal bacterial flora of the intestinal tract. However, with tetracycline HCl, yogurt (a dairy product) should be taken 2 hours before the antibiotic because insoluble complexes are formed that would decrease the absorption of tetracycline. Yogurt can be taken concurrently with doxycycline and minocycline.

6. Octreotide acetate (Sandostatin) is used for refractory diarrhea when all other medications have failed to relieve it. It is administered subcutaneously or intravenously, and is very expensive.

Inflammatory Bowel Disease: Ulcerative Colitis

Ulcerative colitis is a chronic, long-lasting disease resulting in inflammation of the mucosa of the colon and rectum with an unknown etiology. Common symptoms of ulcerative colitis include bloody diarrhea and abdominal pain. Differential diagnoses are irritable bowel syndrome, colon polyps, and colon cancer.

Pharmacological treatment of ulcerative colitis is to reduce the inflammation of the tissues of the colon by using anti-inflammatory drugs, which inhibit leukotriene and prostaglandin synthesis (Table 12-5). The type of drug used depends on the severity of the condition and where in the GI tract the drug is released (e.g., colon, distal ileum, or jejunum). For a mild form of the disease, topical therapy using suppositories, enema, or foam results in a more rapid response, fewer adverse side effects, and less frequent dosing than oral therapy. For mild-to-moderate active disease, or for maintenance of remission, oral drugs are used that include aminosalicylates (e.g., sulfasalazine and mesalamine)

TABLE 12-5 Drugs Used in the Treatment of Ulcerative Colitis

DRUG NAME	DENTAL MANAGEMENT
5-Aminosalicylates (5-ASA)	
Sulfasalzine (Azulfidine)	Avoid antibiotics that could aggravate colitis
Mesalamine (Asacol—tabs, Rowasa—enema, Pentasa—caps)	Monitor for oral ulcerations, xerostomia, and candidiasis; avoid antibiotics that could aggravate colitis
Olsalzine (Dipentum)	Avoid antibiotics that could aggravate colitis
Glucocorticoids	
Prednisone	Consult with patient's physician to determine the need to change dosage. Routine dental procedures including periodontal scaling and root planing does not need to have increased dosage.
Immunosuppressives	
Cyclosporine (Neoral, Sandimmune)	Gingival overgrowth occurs; maintain periodontal health

and corticosteroids (prednisone). Mesalamine (Asacol) does not contain the sulfa component of sulfasalzine and thus has fewer adverse effects. Immunosuppressive drugs (e.g., cyclosporine) have fewer adverse side effects than glucocorticosteroids and are used in refractory (resistant to other drugs) cases.

Rapid Dental Hint

Cyclosporine can cause gingival overgrowth. Monitor patients. Keep meticulous oral home care. If necessary, refer to a periodontist for surgical removal of tissue.

An antibiotic such as metronidazole has been used as an alternative treatment of ulcerative colitis. Supplemental therapy includes the use of antidiarrheal agents and, for those patients in remission, a change in dietary habits to include low-roughage foods.

Rapid Dental Hint

Patients with ulcerative colitis cannot take clindaymcin (Cleocin), an antibiotic frequently prescribed for dental infections.

Dental Hygiene Applications

There are no contraindications or precautions to follow for dental treatment of patients with peptic ulcer disease or gastroesophageal reflux disease. Some gastrointestinal drugs such as cimetidine have many drug interactions about which the dental hygienist should be aware, whether related to dental drugs or not. Since H_2-receptor antagonists are available over the counter without a prescription, many patients will be taking them for heartburn or indigestion.

Patients with GERD may experience symptoms when lying down in the dental chair. The patient may prefer to be lying halfway up and not in a totally supine position.

Since antacids are also available over the counter, many patients may be taking them. When reviewing the medical history with the patient, ask if they are taking antacids. Antacids (aluminum, calcium, and magnesium) interact with certain antibiotics such as tetracyclines and fluroquinolones. These antibiotics should be taken either 1 hour before or 2 hours after taking the antacid.

Xerostomia may be an adverse effect of anticholinergics, anti-emetics, and proton pump inhibitors (PPIs); the patient must be counseled on prevention, including maintenance of optimum oral hygiene.

H_2-receptor inhibitors can inhibit the metabolism of some drugs metabolized by the P450 cytochrome enzyme system, which will increase plasma levels of diazepam, theophylline, warfarin, phenytoin, carbamazepine, lidocaine, propranolol, and tricyclic antidepressants.

Key Points

- *Helicobacter pylori* (*H. pylori*) is a bacterium that causes approximately 90% of gastric and duodenal ulcers.
- Xerostomia may be an adverse effect of anticholinergics, anti-emetics, and proton pump inhibitors (PPIs); the patient must be counseled on prevention, including having optimum oral hygiene.
- Many drug–drug interactions occur with medications for ulcers.
- Diarrhea associated with antibiotic use is caused by *Clostridium difficile.*

Board Review Questions

1. Which of the following gastrointestinal drugs should not be given concurrently with doxycycline? (pp. 207, 209)
   a. Omeprazole
   b. Cimetidine
   c. Antacids
   d. Lansoprazole
2. Which of the following risk factors are primarily involved in causing peptic ulcer disease? (p. 206)
   a. Smoking and alcohol consumption
   b. Caffeine and smoking
   c. *Helicobacter pylori* and NSAIDs
   d. *Streptococcus mutans* and alcohol consumption

3. Which of the following drugs is best for starting initial treatment of mild, intermittent heartburn? (p. 206)
   a. Sodium bicarbonate/alginic combination
   b. Cimetidine
   c. Omeprazole
   d. Lansoprazole

4. Which of the following drugs can cause xerostomia? (p. 209)
   a. Omeprazole
   b. Cimetidine
   c. Ranitidine
   d. Maalox

5. Which of the following drugs has the potential to cause severe diarrhea? (pp. 211–212)
   a. Clindamycin
   b. Ciaspride
   c. Diazepam
   d. Metronidazole
   e. Vancomycin

Selected References

Engstrom PF, Goosenberg EB. 1999. *Diagnosis and management of bowel diseases.* Philadephia: Professional Communications Inc., pp. 15–58, 63–90.

Henderson RP. 2004. In *Handbook of nonprescription drugs,* 14th ed., edited by J. V. Allen et al. Washington, DC: American Pharmaceutical Association, pp. 243–272.

Mears JM, Kaplan B. 1996. Proton pump inhibitors: New drugs and indications. *Am Family Phy* 53:285–292.

Meurer LN, Bower DJ. 2002. Management of *Helicobacter pylori* infection. *Am Fam Phy* 65:1327–1336, 1339.

Pham CQD, Sadowski-Hayes LM, Regal RE. 2006. Prevalent prescribing of proton pump inhibitors: Prudent or pernicious? *Pharmacy and Therapeutics* 31(3):159–167.

Smith C. 1999. Gastroesophageal reflux disease. *U.S. Pharmacist* 24:77–88.

Weart CW. 2002. Opportunities for pharmacist in managing GERD and peptic-ulcer disease. *U.S. Pharmacist* Supplement.

Wells BG, Dipiro JT, Schwinghammer TL, Hamilton CW. 2000. *Pharmacotherapy handbook,* 2nd ed. New York: McGraw-Hill, pp. 251–261, 314–312.

Web Sites

www.cdc.gov/ulcer/
www.medscape.com
www.uspharmacist.com

PEARSON
myhealthprofessionskit™

Use this address to access the Companion Website created for this textbook. Simply select "Dental Hygiene" from the choice of disciplines. Find this book and log in using your username and password to access video clips of selected tests.

QUICK DRUG GUIDE

Antacids

Bismuth Subsalicylate

- Pepto-Bismol

Magnesium Hydroxide

- Milk of Magnesia

Aluminum Hydroxide/Magnesium Hydroxide/ Simethicone

- Maalox liquid
- Gelusil liquid
- Mylanta liquid

Sodium Bicarbonate/Alginic Acid Combination

- Gaviscon

Calcium Carbonate/Magnesium Hydroxide

- Rolaids

Calcium Carbonate

- Tums
- Titralac
- Gaviscon

Anti-Ulcer/GERD Drugs

H_2-Receptor Antagonists

- Cimetidine (Tagamet)
- Famotidine (Pepcid)
- Nizatidine (Axid)
- Ranitidine (Zantac)

Proton Pump Inhibitors

- Omeprazole (Prilosec)
- Lansoprazole (Prevacid)
- Esomeprazole (Nexium)
- Pantoprazole (Protonix)
- Rabeprazole (Aciphex)

Combination

- Omeprazole/sodium bicarbonate (Zegerid)

Prostaglandin Supplements

- Misoprostal (Cytotec)

Protective Barrier Drug

- Sucralfate (Carfate)

Prokinetic Drugs

- Metoclopramide (Reglan)

Antibiotic Combination Treatments

H. pylori *Treatment Regimen (including antibiotics, antihistamines, and antacids)*

- Lansoprazole + clarithormycin + amoxicillin (PrevPac) *or*
- Omeprazole + clarithromycin + amoxicillin *or*
- Lansoprazole *or* omeprazole + clarithromycin + metronidazole *or*

- Lansoprazole *or* omeprazole + bismuth + metronidazole + tetracycline *or*
- Famotidine *or* ranitidine *or* nizatidine + bismuth +metronidazole + tetracycline (Helidac)

Source: Antibiotic regimen: American College of Gastroenterology Guidelines. 1998. *American Journal of Gastroenterology* 93:2330.

GOALS

- To provide an understanding of the various drugs used in the management of lung diseases and of asthma in the dental office.
- To gain knowledge of the various drugs for coughs and colds.

EDUCATIONAL OBJECTIVES

After reading this chapter, the reader should be able to:

1. Classify asthma into different categories.
2. Explain the management of asthma in relation to dental treatment.
3. List and describe current medications used in asthma.
4. Discuss the management of COPD.
5. Describe the management of rhinitis.
6. Discuss the therapy for cough.
7. Discuss adverse effects of antihistamines as they relate to dentistry.

KEY TERMS

Asthma
Bronchospasm
Corticosteroids
Chronic obstructive pulmonary disease

Rhinitis
Antihistamines
Antitussives

Introduction

Disorders of the respiratory tract include asthma, chronic obstructive pulmonary disease (COPD; which encompasses bronchitis and emphysema), and other diseases of the upper and lower respiratory tract, such as allergic rhinitis. Anti-asthmatic medications, antihistamines, decongestants, and antitussives are reviewed in this chapter.

Lung Anatomy

Anatomy of the lungs is as follows:

- Air entering the respiratory system travels through the nose, the pharynx, and the trachea into the bronchi, which divide into smaller passages called bronchioles (Figure 13-1).
- After roughly 23 generations of these airways, the tracheo-bronchial tree ends in sacs called alveoli.
- Airways are surrounded by smooth muscles.
- When the muscles are stimulated, they contract, narrowing the lumen (diameter; opening) of the airway.
- The smooth muscle is controlled by the autonomic nervous system. When the sympathetic nervous system is activated during a stressful situation (e.g., fight-or-flight response) the bronchiolar smooth muscle relaxes and bronchodilation results.
- This allows more air to enter the alveoli, potentially increasing the oxygen supply to the body during stress or exercise (Figure 13-2).

Pathogenesis/Diagnosis: Asthma

Asthma is a chronic lung disease characterized by inflammation of the airways and bronchoconstriction, which improves either spontaneously or with treatment. Asthma affects approximately 15 million Americans. It often begins in childhood, although it can occur at any age. More than 5% of all children younger than age 18 reported having asthma attacks. Asthma is responsible for approximately 2 million emergency department visits and 5,000 deaths per year.

Many cells and cellular elements play major roles in the pathogenesis of asthma.

- T-lymphocytes (white blood cells involved in inflammatory reactions), eosinophils (white blood cells involved in allergic and inflammatory reactions), and mast cells (which make and release histamine, a substance released during allergic reaction in response to an allergen) all contribute to this response.
- These mediators narrow the airway by causing edema and inflammation, and cause bronchoconstriction by stimulating the airway smooth muscles to contract.

The three most common processes that result in airway obstruction are bronchoconstriction, inflammation, and loss of lung elasticity.

Airway obstruction increases airway resistance, resulting in increased work and difficulty of breathing and wheeze and cough. Eventually the obstruction can lead to reduced blood oxygen levels. The first event that occurs is airway inflammation, which is due to the release of inflammatory mediators

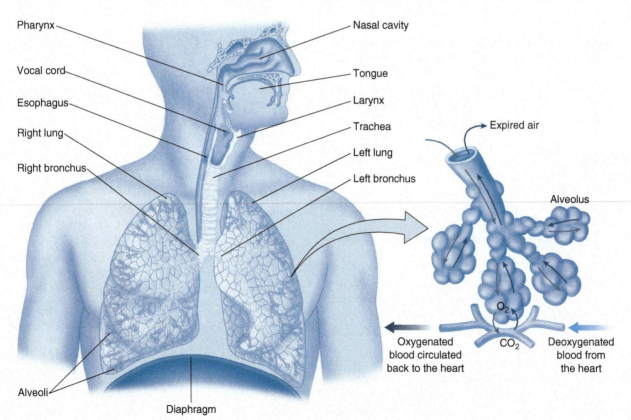

Pharynx — Nasal cavity
Vocal cord — Tongue
Esophagus — Larynx
Right lung — Trachea
Right bronchus — Left lung
— Left bronchus
Expired air
Alveolus
Oxygenated blood circulated back to the heart
O_2
CO_2
Deoxygenated blood from the heart
Alveoli
Diaphragm

FIGURE 13-1 The respiratory system.

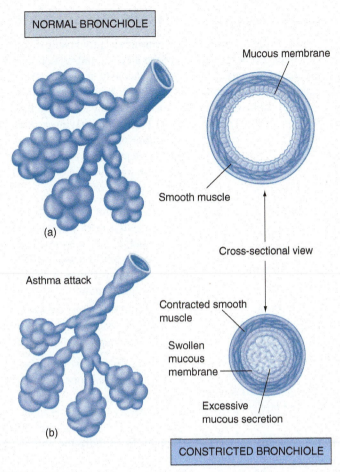

NORMAL BRONCHIOLE

Mucous membrane

Smooth muscle

(a)

Cross-sectional view

Asthma attack

Contracted smooth muscle

Swollen mucous membrane

Excessive mucous secretion

(b)

CONSTRICTED BRONCHIOLE

FIGURE 13-2 Changes in bronchioles during an asthma attack: (a) normal bronchiole; (b) asthmatic bronchiole.

(e.g., histamine, prostaglandins, leukotrienes, and other cytokines) triggered by exposure to allergens such as dust, plant pollen, smoke, and animal dander; exercise; stress; changes in weather; and most frequently upper respiratory viral infection. These inflammatory mediators cause swelling of the airways and provoke contraction of the airway smooth muscle.

Asthma in children is often associated with atopy, which is a genetic susceptibility to produce IgE (antibodies produced in the presence of an antigen or foreign body or allergen) toward allergens. This IgE antibody production is associated with the development of allergies.

When people with asthma are exposed to their triggers (the triggers vary from patient to patient) airway inflammation (mucosal edema and mucous secretions) occurs. *This inflammation may be controlled with anti-inflammatory (cortico-steroids) agents, but not completely eradicated.* The airways

become obstructed by the excess mucous and swelling of airway linings (Figure 13-2). A resulting contraction of the airway smooth muscle, **bronchospasm,** leads to further airway obstruction and limitation of airflow. Airway hyperresponsiveness and subsequent airway obstruction leads to cough, shortness of breath, and wheezing. Effective treatment of asthma should be geared to the reaction of airway inflammation and hyperresponsiveness.

- Bronchospasm is mediated through the β_2-receptors, located on the bronchioles, and may be rapidly relieved by inhaled bronchodilators. Bronchospasm occurs within minutes, while inflammation (mucous secretions) is slower in onset, taking hours. An acute exposure, such as allergy or exercise, causes acute bronchospasm, referred to as the early asthmatic response. Airway inflammation comes on more slowly, known as the late asthmatic response.

- Loss of lung elasticity results from air sac enlargement (distention). Treatment to reverse this condition is more difficult and requires long-term, high-dose drug therapy.

A clinical diagnosis of asthma may be confirmed by pulmonary function testing showing reversible airflow obstruction. The diagnosis is suggested by the following signs or symptoms, which may worsen at night, upon wakening in

BRONCHODILATORS (RESCUE INHALERS)	ANTI-INFLAMMATORY DRUGS (LONG-TERM CONTROL)
Short-acting β_2-agonist (SABA)	Inhaled corticosteroid (ICS)
Anticholinergic	Selective long-acting β_2-agonist (LABA)
Systemic corticosteroid	Mast cell stabilizer
	Leukotriene modifier
	Immunomodulator

the morning, during exercise, with colds, or upon exposure to allergens:

- Wheezing
- Prolonged or troublesome cough
- Difficulty breathing
- Breathlessness (dyspnea)
- Chest tightness

Pharmacotherapy: Controlling Asthma

Drug therapy is targeted toward the inflammation and relieving the bronchospasm (Figure 13-3).

Classification of Medications

- *Quick-relief medications* (also referred to as reliever or acute rescue medications) provide quick reversal of acute airflow obstruction and relief of bronchospasm.

- *Long-term control medications* (also referred to as long-term preventive, controller, or maintenance medications) are taken daily on a long-term basis in order to achieve and maintain control of persistent asthma. Most of these have anti-inflammatory effects.

Severity and Control: Basis of Drug Therapy

In 2007, the *National Institutes of Health (NIH) Expert Panel Report 3* recommend a stepwise approach to the management of asthma that is based on asthma severity and control. Asthma is classified by *severity* depending on the frequency of symptoms:

- *Intermittent* (2 days a week or less; awakenings less than twice a month)
- *Mild persistent* (more than 2 days a week but less than one time a day; awakenings twice a month or more)

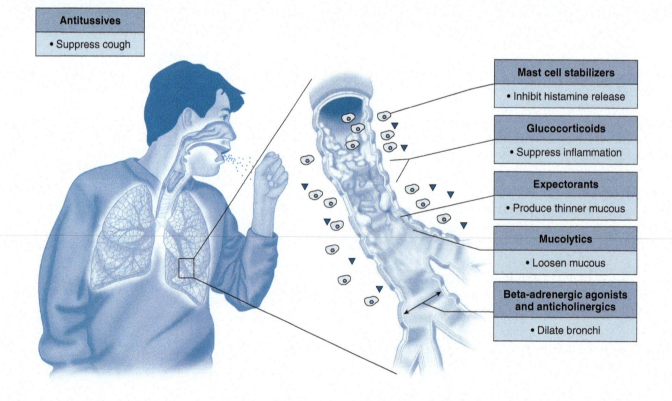

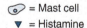

FIGURE 13-3 Drugs used to treat respiratory disorders.

- *Moderate persistent* (every day)
- *Severe persistent* (most of the time)

Asthma *control* is defined as the use of quick-relief medications no more than twice a week and no interference with regular activities. Determining the degree of control is used to monitor and adjust therapy.

STEP-BY-STEP TREATMENT In 2007, the publication *Expert Panel Report 3: Guidelines for the Diagnosis and Management of Asthma* was developed. Table 13-1 summarizes the step-by-step treatment of asthma developed by this panel. Initially different medications are used depending on the severity of the disease. This table helps to determine which type of asthma the patient has and what medication is appropriate.

The number and frequency of medications increase (step up) as the severity of asthma increases, and decreases (step down) when asthma is under control. When beginning therapy, recommendations are to start with the highest appropriate therapy and step down as the patient improves. *Inhaled medications are preferred because of their high therapeutic ratio, with high concentrations of the drug being delivered directly to the airways with few systemic adverse effects.*

Severe asthma attacks are life-threatening and require immediate treatment. An inhaled short-acting β_2-agonist in adequate, frequent doses is essential. Corticosteroid tablets or syrup introduced early in the course of a moderate or severe attack help to reverse the inflammation and speed recovery. Oxygen may be necessary. Theophylline or aminophylline is not recommended if it is used in addition to high doses of β_2-agonist because it provides little additional benefit and increases the likelihood of adverse effects. Epinephrine (adrenaline) is indicated for acute treatment of anaphylaxis.

ROUTES OF DRUG ADMINISTRATION Medications for the management of asthma are administered either by inhaled or systemic routes. Systemic routes are oral or parenteral (intravenous, intramuscular, or subcutaneous). Medications delivered by inhalation directly to the airways have minimal adverse effects and are more effective with a shorter onset of action than when administered orally.

Inhaled drugs are delivered to the lungs by an aerosol, which is a suspension of minute liquid droplets or fine solid particles in a gas. Different devices are used to deliver the aerosol:

- Nebulizer (small machine that vaporizes a liquid medication into a fine mist that is inhaled with a facemask or handheld device) (Figure 13-4)
- Dry powder inhaler (small device that is activated by the process of inhalation to deliver a fine powder to the bronchioles)

TABLE 13-1 Step-Wise Treatment of Asthma in Children ≥ 12 Years of Age and Adults

CLASSIFICATION	LONG-TERM PREVENTION (PREFERRED TREATMENT)	(ALTERNATIVE TREATMENT)	RESCUE INHALERS
Step 1 *Intermittent* asthma	• No medications needed	• No medications needed	• Short-acting bronchodilator: inhaled β_2-agonist (e.g., albuterol) when needed
Step 2 *Mild persistent* asthma (daily medication required)	• Low-dose inhaled corticosteroid (ICS)	• Cromolyn, leukotriene modifier, nedocromil, or theophylline	_____
Step 3 *Moderate persistent* asthma (daily medication)	• Low-dose ICS + Long-acting inhaled β_2-agonist (LABA) or medium-dose ICS	• Low-dose ICS + either a leukotriene modifier or theophylline	_____
Step 4 *moderate persistent* asthma (daily medication)	• Medium-dose ICS + LABA	• Medium-dose ICS + either LABA, theophylline, or zileuton	_____
Step 5 *Severe persistent* asthma (daily medication)	• High-dose ICS + LABA	_____	_____
Step 6 *Severe persistent* asthma (daily medication)	• High-dose ICS + LABA + oral corticosteroid	_____	_____

SABA, short-acting beta$_2$-agonist; ICS, inhaled corticosteroid; LABA, long-acting beta$_2$-agonist.

Source: Expert Panel Report: Guidelines for the Diagnosis and Management of Asthma, National Asthma Education and Prevention Program, 2007.

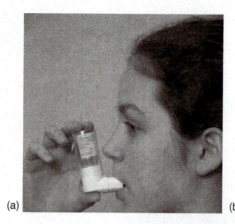
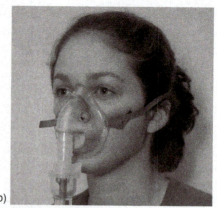
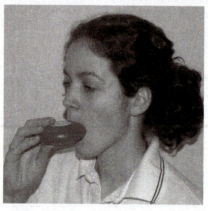

FIGURE 13-4 Inhalers used to deliver asthmatic drugs: (a) Metered-dose inhaler. The patient times the inhalation to the puffs of drug emitted from the MDI. (b) Nebulizer with a face mask. It vaporizes a liquid drug into a fine mist that is then inhaled (c) Metered dose inhaler.

- Metered-dose inhalers (use a propellant to deliver a measured dose of drugs to the lungs during each breath). Most patients who use the metered-dose inhalers, the most common delivery system used, also require a valved holding chamber for optimal drug delivery.

Rescue Medications
- Rescue medications are used for prompt relief of bronchospasm and associated symptoms including cough, chest tightness, and wheezing.
- These medications include (Table 13-2):
  - Selective short-acting β_2-agonists (SABAs): preferred drug
  - Anticholinergics
  - Inhalers, systemic corticosteroids

Bronchodilators: Short-Acting β_2-Agonists (SABAs)
- Provide the quickest onset (5–15 minutes) and relief of symptoms by *bronchodilation* (relaxation of bronchial smooth muscle).
- Prototype short-acting β_2-agonist is albuterol (Ventolin, Proventil).
- Administered either by inhalation (with a metered-dose inhaler or nebulizer) through the mouth, tablets, liquid (syrup), or by injection.
- These drugs should be used in all patients to treat acute symptoms.

- Regular daily use is not generally recommended because tachyphylaxis, due to overstimulation of the receptors, may reduce their effectiveness. When they are needed frequently, this is an indication that more controller therapy

TABLE 13-2   Rescue Inhalers (Bronchodilators) for Bronchospasm

DRUG NAME	ROUTE OF ADMINSTRATION
β_2-Adrenergic (Short-Acting)	
Albuterol (Proventil, Ventolin)	Aerosol inhalation (by mouth), oral (tablet)
Pirbuterol (Maxair)	Inhalation
Terbutaline (Brethine, Brethaire)	Inhalation, oral (tablet), SQ injection
Metaproterenol (Alupent)	Inhalation, oral (tablet)
Levalbuterol (Xopenex)	Inhalation
Anticholinergics	
Ipratropium bromide HFA (Atrovent)	Aerosol inhalation (by mouth)
Ipratropium bromide and albuterol sulfate (Combivent)	Aerosol inhalation (by mouth)
Tiotropium bromide (Spiriva)	Aerosol inhalation (by mouth)

is needed. Inhaled β-adrenergic agonists produce little systemic toxicity because only small amounts of the drug are absorbed. When given orally, a longer duration of action is achieved, but systemic adverse effects such as tachycardia (increased heart rate) and tremor are more frequently experienced. Overuse of inhalation products may reduce the effectiveness of the drug and increase the adverse effects.

Although epinephrine is found in numerous OTC inhalation products (e.g., Primatene Mist, Bronkaid Mist), it is rarely prescribed. It causes bronchodilation by stimulation of the β_2-receptors and vasoconstriction, and decreases secretion by stimulation of the α_1-receptors. It is primarily used in emergency situations for severe bronchoconstriction, or in some cases of croup (condition of the larynx, particularly in children and infants, characterized by respiratory difficulty and brassy cough). Epinephrine is contraindicated in patients with uncontrolled hypertension, hyperthyroidism, and narrow-angle glaucoma.

The oldest oral sympathomimetic is ephedrine, which causes vasoconstriction. Over-the-counter preparations with ephedrine include Broncolate and Primatene tablets. Although still available in many OTC products, newer selective β_2-agonists have replaced it because of possible links to stroke and heart attack because of its β_1-receptor activity.

Adrenergic agonist agents relax airway smooth muscle that results in bronchodilation. Because epinephrine and isoproterenol (Isuprel) are not β_2-receptor selective and also stimulate β_1-receptors, they cause more cardiac stimulation and are rarely used in the treatment of asthma.

Anticholinergic Agents   Cholinergic innervation is an important factor in the regulation of airway smooth muscle tone. Anticholinergic agents are usually used when patients cannot tolerate β_2-agonists or as an adjunct to β_2-agonists for additional relief of bronchoconstriction. These drugs reduce the symptoms of cough, wheezing, and chest tightness. Inhaled anticholinergic drugs are generally not sufficiently effective when used alone, but are beneficial when combined with β-agonists or corticosteroids. Anticholinergics are not used for allergen or exercise-induced asthma.

Ipratropium bromide (Atrovent) is the prototype anticholinergic. The mechanism of action of ipratropium is to inhibit acetylcholine receptors on smooth muscle, resulting in bronchodilation. Adverse side effects are xerostomia and taste alteration (bitter

---

Dental Guidelines for Patients Taking Ipratropium (Atrovent)

- Monitor salivary flow.
- Patients may need daily fluoride treatments at home if dry mouth is persistent.
- Patients should use salivary substitutes if dry mouth is persistent.

---

taste). The patient should rinse the mouth after each inhalation dose to prevent dryness. Anticholinergics should be used with caution in patients with narrow-angle glaucoma, prostatic hypertrophy, or bladder-neck obstruction because they may increase pressure within the eye and cause urinary retention, respectively.

Systemic Corticosteroids   Systemic **corticosteroids** are used when asthma cannot be controlled by bronchodilators alone. Corticosteroids taken orally take more than 4 hours to have a therapeutic effect by reducing inflammation. Systemic steroids are used for acute asthma, while for chronic, long-term maintenance therapy (prevention of attacks), inhaled steroids are used. Since the adverse effects of orally administered steroids include gastric irritation (ulcers), hypokalemia (low blood potassium levels), fluid retention, hyperglycemia (high blood glucose), increased appetite, acne, behavioral changes, growth suppression and, with long-term use, decreased immune function, they should be discontinued as quickly as possible.

LONG-TERM PREVENTIVE MEDICATIONS
Inhaled Corticosteroids (ICSs)   Inhaled corticosteroids are the drug of choice for persistent asthma. Safety and efficacy of these drugs has been shown down to age 1. Regular use of inhaled corticosteroids in adults can reduce hospitalizations and complications (e.g., death) from asthma and improve lung function and quality of life, including decreasing days of work or school missed.

Corticosteroids are the most potent and effective *anti-inflammatory* agents and should be first-line therapy for long-term management of mild, moderate, and severe persistent asthma (Table 13-3). In moderate to severe asthma the addition of a long-acting β_2-agonist may improve control (Table 13-3), although the leukotriene modifiers may serve this role as well.

Dental Guidelines for Patients Taking Albuterol (Proventil)

- May leave patients in a semisupine chair position.
- After each inhalation, patients should rinse their mouth with water to prevent dryness.
- May need daily fluoride treatments at home if dry mouth is persistent.
- Use salivary substitutes if dry mouth is persistent.
- Patients should have the inhalant available during dental treatment.

Dental Guidelines for Patients Taking Systemic Corticosteroids

- Monitor patients for oral candidiasis (thrush; white areas that do not rub off).
- Monitor the patients' salivary flow.
- Patients taking steroids for more than 2 weeks may require additional doses for stressful dental procedures; consult with their physician.
- Patients should avoid aspirin because of gastrointestinal problems.
- Frequent oral prophylaxis.

TABLE 13-3 Long-Term Control Medications

DRUG NAME	ROUTE OF ADMINSTRATION
Corticosteroids (anti-inflammatory)	Inhalation (meter-dose inhalers)
Beclomethasone dipropionate (Beclovent, Vanceril)	
Budesonide (Pulmicort)	
Flunisolide (Aerobid)	
Fluticasone (Flovent, Advir)	
Mometasone (Asmanex)	
Triamcinolone (Azmacort)	
Selective β_2-Agonists (Long-Acting) (bronchodilator)	Inhalation
Salmeterol (Serevent)	Inhalation
Formoterol (Foradil)	Inhalation
Methylxanthines (bronchodilator)	Systemic
Theophylline (Slo-Phyllin, TheoDur, Theo-24)	Oral (tablets, capsules, syrup)
Mast Cell Stabilizers (anti-inflammatory)	
Cromolyn sodium (Intal)	Inhalation
Nedocromil (Tilade)	Inhalation
Leukotriene Modifiers (anti-inflammatory)	
Zafirlukast (Accolate)	Tablets
Montelukast (Singulair)	Tablets
Zileuton (Zyflo)	Tablets
Immunomodulators (anti-inflammatory)	
Omalizumab (Xolair)	Subcutaneous injection

Combination therapy with an inhaled corticosteroid and a long-acting β_2-agonist is the recommended treatment for adults and children over 5 years of age with *moderate to severe asthma*. The GOAL (Gaining Optimal Asthma controL) study (2004) reported that when taking a combination of inhaled corticosteroids and long-acting β-agonists, most patients achieved control of their asthma.

Adverse effects from inhaled corticosteroids may include:

* Cough
* Oral candidiasis (thrush)
* With very high doses, growth suppression

Patients should brush the teeth and rinse the mouth with water after every inhalation dose to prevent fungal infections. When a patient uses the inhaler with a valved holding chamber, the incidence of oral candidiasis drops markedly.

Dental Guidelines for Patients Taking Inhaled Corticosteroids

Beclomethasone: Qvar, Beclovent
Fluticasone: Flovent, Advair
Budesonide: Pulmicort
Flunisolide: Aerobid
Mometasone: Asmenex
Triamcinolone: Azmacort

* Monitor for fungal infection in oral cavity.
* Patients should brush their teeth and rinse mouth with water after inhalation dose.
* May require fluoride treatments at home for dry mouth.
* Hoarseness may develop.

Selective Long-Acting β_2-Agonists (LABA) (bronchodilators)

* Salmeterol (Serevent) and formoterol (Foradil) (Table 13-3)
  * *Bronchodilators,* causing the airway smooth muscle to relax
  * Used with a low or medium dosage of an inhaled corticosteroid to improve asthma control *but should not* be used alone
  * May allow a reduction of the dosage of corticosteroid used
  * Salmeterol is available in a fixed combination Diskus with Flovent, called Advair
  * Adverse effects of the long-acting β-agonists include:
    * Xerostomia
    * Black-Box Warning: Increased risk of asthma-related deaths. Only use as additional therapy if patient not controlled with other medications such as ICS.
    * Tachycardia (increased heart rate)
    * Headache
    * When used alone, overstimulation of the β-agonist receptors, which makes the short-acting agonists less effective

Methylxanthines

* Theophylline and aminophylline
* Bronchodilators that relax the airway smooth muscle to control asthmatic symptoms
* These drugs are no longer recommended for acute exacerbations or as a drug of choice for asthma. Decades ago, they

Dental Guidelines for Patients Taking Salmeterol (Serevent)

* Assess salivary flow; assess need for fluoride rinse.
* Stress importance of good oral hygiene.
* Monitor vital signs, especially patients with heart disease.
* Keep patients in a semisupine position.

were the mainstay of chronic therapy and when used intravenously served as the main emergent treatment of acute asthma. They have been supplanted by the drugs discussed above. Serum levels must be monitored to avoid toxicity.

• Many drug interactions occur with theophylline; for example, concomitant erythromycin or clarithromycin (Biaxin) may elevate the blood level of theophylline.

• Caffeine is a type of methylxanthine drug. About 100 mg of caffeine is present in a cup of coffee (only about 65 mg in instant coffee), sufficient to cause mild bronchodilation in patients with asthma.

Mast Cell Stabilizers

• Cromolyn sodium and nedocromil sodium

• Have anti-inflammatory actions that inhibit the release of histamine and other mediators of allergic reactions leading to airway inflammation

• Both medications are administered by inhalation and may be an alternative treatment in mild persistent asthma.

DID YOU KNOW?

Moses Maimonides recognized the beneficial effects of strong tea in people with asthma.

DID YOU KNOW?

Cola drinks contain about 35 mg caffeine; a cup of hot chocolate contains about 4 mg.

Leukotriene Modifiers

• Orally administered agents

• Alternative first-line treatment for mild persistent asthma, and may serve as adjuncts to inhaled corticosteroids for more severe disease.

• Block the activity of arachidonic acid derivatives (e.g., leukotrienes), which are involved in the inflammatory pathway.

• Montelukast (Singulair) is the most prescribed because of its once-a-day dosing and its approval for young children. These drugs reduce the need for short-acting, inhaled β_2-agonists.

Immunomodulators Omalizumab is indicated as adjunctive therapy in patients with severe allergic asthma who cannot be controlled with ICSs.

Other Agents Combination therapy of ipratropium bromide (anticholinergic) and albuterol sulfate (Duoneb) can be helpful for COPD; and, as above, fluticasone/salmeterol (Advair) is beneficial for patients with moderate or severe asthma who benefit from the addition of a bronchodilator, rather than increasing the anti-inflammatory therapy.

COPD (Bronchitis/Emphysema) Treatment

Chronic obstructive pulmonary disease (COPD) encompasses diseases that cause *chronic* (long-term) obstruction of air flow. Chronic bronchitis, an inflammation characterized by excessive mucous in the bronchi causing a productive (mucous-producing) cough, and emphysema, an irreversible destruction of alveolar walls with dilation of air spaces, are the major components of COPD.

There is no cure for COPD. Its medication management involves a variety of step-by-step treatment regimens similar to those for asthma. The goals of treatment are to improve chronic obstruction and to treat and prevent acute episodes. Treatment starts with smoking cessation. Pharmacotherapy begins with short-acting bronchodilators for mild disease and long-acting drugs as the disease becomes more chronic and severe (Table 13-4). The most commonly used initial drug is a β_2-agonist inhaler. Inhalation is preferred over the oral route because of increased efficacy and reduced toxicity. If chronic, mild symptoms continue then ipratropium bromide inhaler is started. Long-term oxygen therapy is occasionally required.

Rapid Dental Hint

Remind your patients who use a steroid inhaler to rinse the mouth with water after use.

TABLE 13-4	Step-by-Step Approach for Managing COPD (Bronchitis and Emphysema)		
SEVERITY OF DISEASE	CLINICAL SYMPTOMS	TREATMENT	OTHER
At risk	Productive cough	No bronchodilator needed	Smoking cessation
I	Productive cough	Short-acting bronchodilator as needed	Smoking cessation
II	Productive cough	Tiotropium with or without short-acting β_2-agonist	Smoking cessation, exercise
III	Productive cough, out of breath on mild exertion	Tiotropium, long-acting β_2-agonist	Smoking cessation, exercise, oxygen therapy
IV	Productive cough, out of breath on mild exertion	Tiotropium, long-acting β_2-agonist, inhaled corticosteroids	Smoking cessation, exercise, oxygen therapy

Drugs for Cold

Rhinitis, inflammation of the nasal mucosa (mucous membranes in the nasal cavities), is most frequently caused by allergic reactions to pollen, mold spores, dust, and other allergens or by viruses, such as rhinoviruses and other agents related to the common cold (Figure 13-5). Rhinitis may be seasonal in the case of allergic rhinitis or may be an acute, self-limiting condition in the case of viral rhinitis. Characteristics of both types of rhinitis are nasal congestion, rhinorrhea (runny nose), itching, sneezing, mucus production, vasodilation, and airway narrowing. Conjunctivitis (inflammation of the conjunctiva of the eye) is usually seen more in allergic rhinitis, but accompanies some viral infections.

Viral rhinitis or—as it is more often called—the common cold is a self-limiting condition and is best treated conservatively. Aches and pain are best relieved with a nonsteroidal anti-inflammatory drug (ibuprofen) or acetaminophen. Nasal decongestants (e.g., psuedoephedrine, phenylephedrine) may be helpful.

A distinction must be made between allergic rhinitis and the common cold. The common cold is a self-limiting condition that is caused by viruses and is infectious and communicable. Viruses can be spread through the air by droplets from a sneeze or cough and by touching the nose, eyes, or mouth after contact. Allergic rhinitis is a risk factor for the development of asthma and nasal polyps. Cold symptoms usually last for 1–2 weeks.

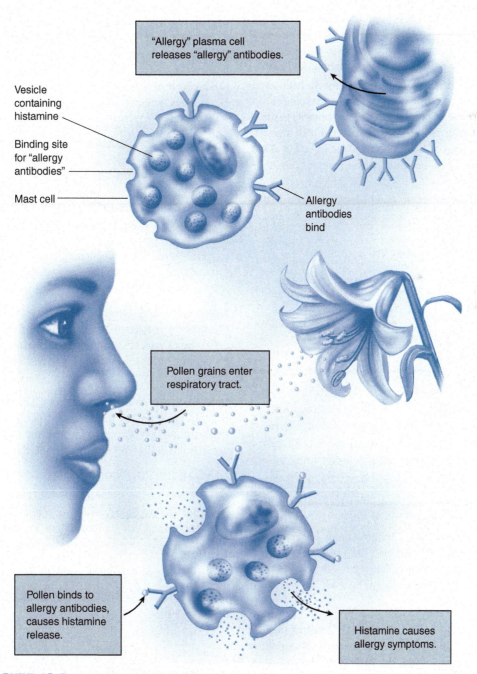

FIGURE 13-5 Development of allergic rhinitis.

Most of the symptoms associated with rhinitis are due to the release of histamine from mast cells and basophils (type of white blood cell). Three types of histamine receptors are found in the body: H_1, H_2, and H_3.

DID YOU KNOW?

Several clinical studies show an association between asthma and rhinitis. People with asthma have some nasal component to their disease.

- H_1-receptors are located on the smooth muscle of the bronchi, veins, capillaries, heart, and gastrointestinal tract and are involved in allergic reactions that cause rhinitis. Activation of H_1-receptors causes bronchoconstriction, vasodilation, constriction of the intestinal smooth muscle, itching, and pain.
- H_2-receptors are located on the brain, stomach, heart, and blood vessels. Activation of these receptors causes an increase in gastric acid production in the stomach, vasodilation (lowers blood pressure), and relaxation of smooth muscle. These receptors are not primarily involved in allergic reactions, and drugs that bind to these receptors are used for the treatment of ulcers.
- H_3-receptors are presynaptic receptors located on histamine-releasing cells, which upon stimulation inhibit histamine release.

Drugs used to treat rhinitis are classified into:

1. Antihistamines
2. α-Adrenergic agonists
3. Topical corticosteroids
4. Mast cell stabilizers

DID YOU KNOW?

In 2005, the *Journal of Allergy and Clinical Immunology* found that 54% of people in the United States are allergic to at least one of 10 common allergens. The most common allergic reactions were to dust mites, rye grass, ragweed, and cockroaches. Men are more likely than women to have allergies.

Antibiotics are not useful for treating colds because they kill bacteria, not viruses. Inappropriate use of antibiotics for the common cold is a major factor in allowing bacteria to become resistant to antibiotics that previously killed them.

Antihistamines

Histamine by itself has no known clinical use. **Antihistamines** are drugs that block the histamine (H_1)-receptors, eliminating the symptoms (sneezing, itching, rhinorrhea) associated with rhinitis but are ineffective in treating the common cold.

TABLE 13-5 First-Generation Antihistamines
DRUG NAME
Diphenhydramine (Benadryl) 25 mg tabs OTC
Chlorpheniramine (Chlor-Trimeton) 4 mg, 8 mg ext-rel, 12 mg tabs OTC
Promethazine (Phenergan)
Hydroxyzine (Atarax, Vistaril) OTC
Clemastine (Tavist) OTC
Cyproheptadine (Periactin)

Antihistamines are contraindicated in narrow-angle glaucoma, prostatic hypertrophy, stenosing peptic ulcer disease, and bladder obstruction because they have anticholinergic properties.

H_1-receptor blockers are used to treat allergic reactions (allergic rhinitis) and motion sickness. Since they are not selective to the bronchioles, these drugs will bind to the receptors on other organs, producing many adverse side effects. There are two types of H_1-receptor antihistamines: first generation and second generation.

SEDATING (FIRST-GENERATION) ANTIHISTAMINES Some first-generation H_1-receptor blockers (Table 13-5) are diphenhydramine (Benadryl), chlorpheniramine (Chlor-Trimeton), hydroxyzine (Atarax, Vistaril), dexchlorpheniramine (Prolarmine), promethazine (Phenergan), and clemastine (Tavist). Dimenhydrinate (Dramamine) and meclizine (Antivert) are used to treat motion sickness or vertigo. Most adverse effects are due to anticholinergic activity. As a result, the drugs may cause dry mouth, blurred vision, tachycardia, and urinary retention. Common adverse effects include drowsiness and/or sedation, xerostomia, and urinary retention.

NONSEDATING ANTIHISTAMINES Second-generation H_1-receptor blockers (Table 13-6) are fexofenadine (Allegra), cetirizine (Zyrtec), and loratadine (Claritin). Second-generation H_1-receptor blockers cause less sedation than first-generation agents.

INTRANASAL ANTIHISTAMINES The antihistamines mentioned above are all given orally. Azelastine (Astelin) is an antihistmine that is applied intranasally (sprays in the nose) for the treatment of symptoms of allergic rhinitis.

α-Adrenoceptor Agonists (Nasal Decongestants)

- Alpha$_1$-adrenoceptor agonists act as *nasal decongestants by constricting blood vessels in the nasal mucosa,* as well as other blood vessels throughout the body. Vasoconstriction reduces the blood supply to the nose and decreases edema.

TABLE 13-6 Second-Generation Antihistamines
DRUG NAME
Cetirizine (Zyrtec)
Fexofenadine (Allegra)
Loratadine (Claritin)

- OTC drugs include oxymetazoline (Afrin) and phenylephrine (Neo-Synephrine, Sinex). These drugs have a rapid onset of action. However, after 3–5 days of these drugs a rebound congestion occurs and may be worse than before with damage to the mucosa and severe nasal obstruction.
- Since they stimulate α-adrenergic receptors causing vasoconstriction, they should not be used or used with caution in patients with hypertension, hyperthyroidism, diabetes mellitus, cardiovascular disease, glaucoma, urinary obstruction, or if taking a beta-blocker drug or monoamine oxidase inhibitor (MAOI) for depression.
- Other adverse effects include nervousness, tremor, insomnia, dizziness, and chronic mucosal inflammation (after prolonged use).
- Pseudoephedrine (Sudafed) is a systemic nasal decongestion available in either tablets or in a syrup form. It is also found in anticough syrup mixtures. Since it is a sympathomimetic, caution should be used in hypertensive patients.

Topical (Intranasal) Corticosteroids

Topical (intranasal) corticosteroids—which include beclomethasone (Beconase, Vancenase), mometasone (Nasonex), fluticasone (Flonase), budesonide (Rhinocort), and flunisolide (Nasalide)—reduce the inflammation. Intranasal corticosteroids are the most effective drugs for relieving symptoms of sneezing, itching, congestion, and rhinorrhea. They are administered as nasal sprays to reduce systemic absorption and adverse side effects; however, there are concerns related to diminished growth in children. Some adverse side effects include nasal irritation, burning, sneezing, sore throat, and headache. Oral antihistamines are an alternative in patients who cannot tolerate or do not want to use corticosteroids.

CROMOLYN AND NEDOCROMIL Cromolyn (Nasalcrom), available over the counter as a nasal spray, and nedocromil (Tiladle) have anti-inflammatory activity and are also used to treat asthma and allergic rhinitis. They are relatively safe drugs that are administered using a spinhaler or nasalmatic device.

Anticholinergic Agents

Ipratropium (Atrovent) is a bronchodilator applied as a nasal spray. It is approved for asthma and for rhinitis, but does not relieve nasal congestion.

Drugs for Cough

Cough is produced by the cough reflex. The initial stimulus for cough most likely starts in the mucosa from the nose through the branching points in the tracheobronchial tree, where irritation results in bronchoconstriction. Cough receptors in the trachea and bronchioles send nerve information to the cough center in the brain, and the cough reflex is triggered. Stimuli that start a cough include dust, pollen, and other irritants.

Antitussives are used to suppress the cough. Centrally acting drugs suppress cough by depressing the cough center in the brain. This group of medications includes codeine, hydrocodone, hydromorphone, and dextromethorphan.

Codeine, a narcotic, is the gold standard to which other antitussive agents are compared. Due to the risk of respiratory depression, codeine should be used with caution in patients with pulmonary diseases such as asthma.

Dextromethorphan is a nonnarcotic agent that does not possess the same adverse effects as codeine, including low respiratory depression. Many OTC drugs contain dextromethorphan (e.g., Robitussin, Vicks).

These drugs are available in various liquid cough preparations that include other agents. In the United States, cough syrups that contain codeine and hydrocodone are classified as Schedule V controlled substances and require a prescription.

Benzonatate (Tessalon), a nonnarcotic agent, is an orally administered drug that reduces the activity of peripheral cough receptors. Respiratory depression is not inhibited at recommended doses.

Expectorants

Expectorants stimulate the production of a watery, less viscous mucous. Guaifenesin is added to most oral nonprescription preparations (e.g., Mucinex) and works by irritating the gastric mucosa, which stimulates respiratory secretions. It is a safe medication with few adverse effects. Water can also be used as an effective expectorant.

Dental Hygiene Applications

Once it is determined that a patient has asthma, it is important to know if the patient has had recent symptoms, what therapy he or she is taking, and the date of the last severe attack. Consultation with the patient's physician may be necessary for severe asthma. If the patient is using an inhaler, it should be used just before the appointment, and it must be available throughout.

When systemic corticosteroids (e.g., prednisone) are taken, endogenous (within the body) production and secretion decrease. The patient's physician should be contacted to determine if any additional therapy is necessary. More than 20 mg a day or 2 mg/kg/d for at least 14 days may alter the patient's immunity. This should be taken into account when scheduling invasive procedures. Most routine dental procedures do not require supplemental steroids. However, patients undergoing extensive dental treatment (e.g., extraction, surgery) may need to increase the steroid dose the morning of the appointment. Consult with the patient's physician.

Aspirin and other nonsteroidal anti-inflammatory drugs [e.g., naproxen (Aleve), ibuprofen (Advil, Motrin, Nuprin)] may be contraindicated in patients, especially children, with asthma and nasal polyps since these drugs can precipitate or exacerbate an aspirin-induced bronchospasm that can be life-threatening.

The anticholinergic side effects (e.g., xerostomia) of first-generation antihistamines have implications in dentistry. The dental clinician should educate the patient on how to reduce the symptoms of dry mouth. The patient should be informed to drink plenty of water and avoid alcohol, including alcohol-containing mouthrinses. The majority of patients may be on antihistamines frequently during the year, if a seasonal allergic rhinitis is involved.

Many preparations for rhinitis and cough are over the counter. The dental clinician should interview the patient concerning *all* medications, including over-the-counter drugs.

Key Points

- Asthma has both a bronchospasm component and an inflammatory component; drug therapy focuses on both of these processes. In most patients, chronic anti-inflammatory therapy is absolutely necessary.
- Bronchospasm is mediated through the β_2-receptors, located on the bronchioles, and is rapidly relieved by inhaled bronchodilators.
- Asthma-related deaths are significantly lower in patients taking inhaled corticosteroids.
- According to the NAEPP (National Asthma Education and Prevention Program) Expert Panel Report Update, 2007, chronic inhaled corticosteroid use is safe in adults and children, and is recommended as the first-line therapy in adults and children with *persistent* asthma (mild, moderate, or severe).
- For quick relief of a bronchospasm and its accompanying acute symptoms, including cough and wheezing, a short-acting β_2-selective agonist (e.g., albuterol) is the drug of choice.
- The addition of a long-acting β_2-agonist [e.g., salmeterol (Serevent), fluticasone propionate/salmeterol xinafoate (Advair Diskus)] to an inhaled corticosteroid is superior to all other combinations, as well as to higher doses of inhaled corticosteroids alone. However, in 2006 the FDA added a black-box warning to long-acting β_2-agonists (LABA); these drugs may increase the risk of asthma-related deaths. The FDA states that patients with asthma should not stop taking their LABA medications and should consult their physician with concerns regarding the new labeling changes. The new labels recommend Serevent and Advair not be the first medicine used to

treat asthma, and should only be added to the treatment plan for patients whose symptoms are not controlled on other asthma drugs such as low-to-medium inhaled corticosteroids.

- Aspirin and nonsteroidal anti-inflammatory agents (NSAIDs) may be contraindicated in patients with asthma.
- Brush teeth and rinse mouth after each use of a corticosteroid inhaler to help prevent fungal infection.
- Smoking cessation is a critical step in the management of COPD, and is to be encouraged by the dental office.
- Many dental patients are taking OTC antihistamines, which may cause xerostomia due to its anticholinergic effects.
- Second-generation antihistamines are reported to cause less xerostomia.
- Antitussives and expectorants are used to control coughs.

Board Review Questions

1. After which of the following drugs used to treat asthma should the dental hygienist instruct the patient to rinse the mouth? (p. 222)
   a. Ipratropium
   b. Cromolyn sodium
   c. Beclomethasone
   d. Theophylline
2. Which of the following drugs *may be* contraindicated in asthmatics? (p. 228)
   a. Aspirin
   b. Acetaminophen
   c. Vitamin C
   d. Folic acid
3. Which of the following drugs is the drug of choice for the *quick relief* of bronchospasm? (pp. 219, 221, 228)
   a. Albuterol
   b. Ipratropium
   c. Hydrocortisone
   d. Salmeterol
4. Which of the following drugs is classified as a β_2-agonist bronchodilator? (p. 221)
   a. Albuterol
   b. Ipratropium
   c. Hydrocortisone
   d. Montelukast
5. Which of the following drugs is used to control mild persistent asthma? (p. 223)
   a. Albuterol
   b. Ipratropium
   c. Inhaled beclomethasone
   d. Salmeterol
6. Which of the following antihistamines has anticholinergic effects? (p. 226)
   a. Loratadine
   b. Fexofenadine
   c. Diphenhydramine
   d. Azelastine

7. Which of the following drugs is preferred for long-term control of asthma? (pp. 219, 222)
   a. β_1-receptor agonists
   b. β_2-receptor agonists
   c. Inhaled corticosteroids
   d. Oral corticosteroids

8. Which of the following adverse effects occurs with antihistamines? (p. 226)
   a. Dry mouth
   b. Increased salivation
   c. Dry skin
   d. Moist skin

9. Which of the following terms defines "suppressing a cough"? (p. 227)
   a. Expectorant
   b. Antitussive
   c. Antihistamine
   d. Antiasthma

10. Which of the following types of agents are nasal decongestants? (p. 227)
    a. β_1-receptor agonists
    b. β_2-receptor blockers
    c. α_1-receptor agonists
    d. α_2-receptor blockers

Selected References

Bateman ED, Boushey HA, Bousquet J, et al. 2004. GOAL Investigators (Group Gaining Optimal Asthma ControL) study. *Am J Respir Crit Care Med* 170:836–844.

Casserly JE. Breathe easy: An update on asthma. *Pharmacy Times*. Assessed online January 20, 2011, at www.pharmacytimes.com.

Diagnosis and management of allergic rhinitis. 2001. *American Family Physician,* Monograph No. 3.

Mintz, M. 2004. Asthma Update: Part II, Medical Management. *Am Fam Physician* 70:1061–1066.

National Guideline Clearinghouse (NGC). Agency for Healthcare Research and Quality. www.guideline.gov.

National Institutes of Health, National Heart, Lung, and Blood Institute. National Asthma Education and Prevention Program Expert Panel Report 3. Guidelines for the Diagnosis and Management of Asthma, Expert Panel Report 3. 2007. NIH Publication. No. 08–5846. Bethesda, MD: National Institutes of Health.

Ostrom NK. 2001. Asthma management: Proper uses of pharmacotherapy. *U.S. Pharmacist* 26(12):53–64.

Wheeler PW, Wheeler SF. 2005. Vasomotor rhinitis. *Am Fam Physician* 72:1057–1062.

Web Sites

www.nhlbi.nih.gov/guidelines/asthma/asthgdln.pdf
www.niaid.nih.gov/factsheets/cold.htm
www.medicalnewstoday.com/info/asthma/useful-links.php
www.lungusa.org/finding-cures/grantopportunities/trend reports/asthma-trendreport.pdf
www.ncbi.nlm.nih.gov/pubmed/12572181

PEARSON
myhealthprofessionskit™

Use this address to access the Companion Website created for this textbook. Simply select "Dental Hygiene" from the choice of disciplines. Find this book and log in using your username and password to access video clips of selected tests.

QUICK DRUG GUIDE

Long-Term Control of Asthma

Corticosteroids (Inhaled) for Inflammation

- Beclomethasone (QVAR)
- Budesonide (Pulmicort)
- Flunisolide (Aerobid)
- Fluticasone (Flovent, Advir)
- Mometasone (Asmanex)
- Triamcinolone (Azmacort)

Selective β_2-Agonists (Long-Acting): Bronchodilator

- Salmeterol (Serevent)
- Formoterol (Foradil)

Methylxanthines

- Theophylline (TheoDur)

Mast Cell Stabilizers

- Cromolyn sodium (Intal)
- Nedocromil (Tilade)

Leukotriene Modifiers

- Zafirlukast (Accolate)
- Montelukast (Singulair)
- Zileuton (Zyflo)

Quick-Relief Medications

Selective β_2-Adrenergic (Short-Acting): Bronchodilators (for Bronchospasm)

- Albuterol (Ventolin, Proventil): Drug of choice
- Pirbuterol (Maxair)
- Terbutaline (Brethine)
- Metaproterenol (Alupent)
- Levalbuterol tartrate (Xopenex)

Anticholinergics: Bronchodilators

- Ipratropium bromide (Atrovent)
- Ipratropium bromide and albuterol
- Sulfate (Combivent)
- Tiotropium bromide (Spiriva)

Corticosteroids (Oral) (Anti-Inflammatory)

- Dexamethasone
- Hydrocortisone
- Methylprednisolone
- Prednisolone
- Prednisone

Drugs for Cough and Colds

First-Generation Antihistamines (H$_1$-Receptor Antagonists) (relief of allergy symptoms, motion sickness)

- Diphenhydramine (Benadryl)
- Azatadine (Optimine)
- Chlorpheniramine (Chlor-Trimeton)
- Clemastine (Tavist)
- Cyproheptadine (Periactin)
- Dexbrompheniramine (Drixoral)
- Dexchlorpheniramine (Polaramine)
- Hydroxyzine (Atarax)
- Promethazine (Phenergan)
- Triprolidine (Actifed)

Second-Generation/Nonsedating Antihistamines

- Cetrizine (Zyrtec)
- Fexofenadine (Allegra)
- Loratadine (Claritin)

Intranasal Corticosteroids (Treating Allergic Rhinitis)

- Beclomethasone (Vancenase, Beconase)
- Budesonide (Rhinocort)
- Flunisolide (Nasalide)
- Fluticasone (Flonase)
- Mometasone (Nasonex)
- Triamcinolone (Nasacort)

Sympathomimetics (Treating Nasal Congestion Due to Allergic Rhinitis and the Common Cold)

- Epinephrine (Primatene)
- Oxymetazoline (Afrin)
- Phenylephrine (Neo-Synephrine)
- Pseudoephedrine (Sudafed)

Antitussives (Cough)

- Codeine
- Dextromethorphan (many OTC products)
- Hydrocodone

Expectorants

- Guaifenesin (many OTC products)

Neurological Drugs

GOAL

To gain knowledge of the various drugs used to control seizures, Parkinson's disease, and migraine headaches.

EDUCATIONAL OBJECTIVES

After reading this chapter, the reader should be able to:

1. List the different types of epilepsy.

2. Describe the management of a patient undergoing an epileptic seizure in the dental chair.

3. List and discuss drug–drug interactions with anti-epileptic drugs.

4. List and discuss drugs used in the treatment of Parkinson's disease.

5. Discuss the drug management of headaches.

KEY TERMS

Seizures

Anti-epileptic drugs

Parkinson's disease

Extrapyramidal

Migraine

Epilepsy

Pathophysiology

Epilepsy is a relatively common central nervous system disorder affecting about one in 200 individuals. This disorder is characterized by the repeated occurrence of **seizures,** defined as the abnormal, excessive discharges of brain neurons and changes in the electrical activity in the brain (Table 14-1). Convulsions or violent, involuntary contractions of the voluntary muscles may or may not occur with a seizure. If a seizure occurs, it is often intermittent and brief. Drooling and tongue biting are common symptoms.

Seizures may result from hypoxia (lack of oxygen), birth injury to the brain, fever, alcohol intoxication/withdrawal, brain tumors, head trauma, or stroke. In some patients, epilepsy may be genetic.

A partial seizure originates in one cerebral hemisphere in the brain; the patient does not lose consciousness during the seizure. A generalized seizure originates in both cerebral hemispheres, with a loss of consciousness. Seizures are accompanied by characteristic changes in the electroencephalogram (EEG). Most seizures last for about 10 seconds to 5 minutes. Seizures may be preceded by an aura, a warning similar to a light, noise, or feeling to the individual that a seizure is going to occur.

The two main types of generalized seizure are tonic-clonic seizures and absence seizures. Absence seizures (formerly known as petit mal seizures) most often occur in children and last less than 20 seconds.

Tonic-clonic seizures (formerly known as grand mal) are the most common type of seizure in all age groups. During these seizures tongue biting may occur. A tonic-clonic seizure usually lasts 1–2 minutes, after which the patient becomes confused, drowsy, and sleepy. Seizures may be preceded by an aura; intense muscle contractions indicate the tonic phase. A cry may occur after the onset of the seizure due to air being forced out of the lungs. The clonic phase is characterized by alternating contraction and relaxation of muscles.

Status epilepticus is a medical emergency that occurs when a seizure is repeated continuously. It could occur with any type of seizure, but usually generalized tonic-clonic seizures are seen.

Anti-Epileptic Drug Therapy

Treatment or control of seizures depends on the type of seizure. There are specific first-line drugs for each type. Drugs that control generalized tonic-clonic seizures are not effective for absence seizures.

Rapid Dental Hint

Ask your patient the last time he or she had an attack and what provoked it.

FIRST-GENERATION/TRADITIONAL DRUGS

Phenobarbital (Luminal) In 1912, phenobarbital, a type of barbiturate that was then used to induce sleep, was found to have antiseizure activity and was the first **anti-epileptic drug.** Although it is among the oldest and safest anti-epileptic drugs, its use has declined in favor of newer drugs. It is a second-line drug in adults with partial and generalized seizures except absence seizures. The mechanism of action is to enhance the effects of gamma-amino-buyteric acid (GABA), prolonging the chloride channel opening, and blocking the sodium channel. The half-life of phenobarbital is long, between 72 and 125 hours, so it takes

---

TABLE 14-1   Classification of Seizures (Commission of Classification and Terminology of the International League Against Epilepsy)

Partial (focal) Seizures

- Simple partial seizure (no loss of consciousness)
- Complex partial seizure (impairment of consciousness)
- Secondarily generalized seizure

Generalized Seizures

- Tonic-clonic seizures (formerly called grand mal; an aura or symptoms may appear before the seizure occurs; jerking of the extremities with loss of consciousness)
- Absence seizures (formerly called petit mal; in young children and adolescents ages 2–12; many seizures a day with a momentary loss of consciousness with eye blinking and muscle jerks)
- Myoclonic seizures (sudden, short jerks or muscle contractions of the extremities that can occur at any age; associated with hereditary disorders)
- Clonic seizures (contraction and relaxation of muscles of the entire body)
- Tonic seizures (increased muscle tone; loss of bladder and bowel control)
- Atonic seizures (sudden loss of muscle tone similar to slumping to the ground)
- Febrile seizures (in children, and last for just a few minutes; the child has a fever)

Unclassified Epileptic Seizures

- Status epilepticus (emergency situation characterized by continuous, prolonged seizures longer than 20 minutes)

a long time (about 3 weeks) to get to steady state levels. Phenobarbital is rapidly and completely absorbed following oral doses.

Its high incidence of adverse effects has precluded its use as a primary drug: sedation, high abuse potential, dizziness, and respiratory depression.

Phenytoin Phenytoin (Dilantin) was first introduced in 1938 for the treatment of seizures and is still widely used. It was the first nonsedating anti-epileptic drug. Phenytoin decreases passive sodium influx across brain cell membranes by blocking sodium channels, decreasing excessive abnormal discharge of neurons.

Phenytoin is the first-line therapy for partial (both simple and complex) seizures, generalized tonic-clonic seizures, and status epilepticus, but is ineffective in absence seizures. Phenytoin combined with diazepam (Valium), a benzodiazepine, are the drugs of choice in the maintenance of patients with status epilepticus.

Phenytoin has a narrow therapeutic index, so even small fluctuations in plasma levels can cause toxicity. Missed doses will result in a marked change in plasma concentration. Since

Guidelines for Dental Patients Taking Phenytoin (Dilantin)

- Monitor for gingival enlargement.
- Monitor and emphasize oral hygiene; difficult for patients to adequately maintain oral hygiene because of tissue overgrowth.
- Place patients on frequent recall appointments to monitor gingival condition.

different drug formulations from various manufacturers can affect absorption, it is best to use the same drug manufacturer and not to change brands because severe changes in the serum levels can occur. Frequent blood level monitoring is best for optimal dosing.

Many adverse effects can occur, which are concentration dependent, including gingival enlargement (Figure 14-1), nausea, vomiting, and slurred speech. There is some evidence that phenytoin is teratogenic causing fetal hydantoin syndrome, where there is a deficiency in prenatal growth, mental retardation, cleft palate, and heart deformities; it has a pregnancy category of D.

The patient should be informed that if gingival enlargement occurs it will remain as long as the patient is taking phenytoin. Surgical removal of the excessive gingival tissue may be necessary but the enlargement most likely will recur. Meticulous oral home care is important for these patients.

RDH

Rapid Dental Hint

There is a drug–drug interaction between doxycycline and phenytoin. Do not administer both together.

Carbamazepine Carbamazepine is the drug of choice for controlling partial and generalized tonic-clonic seizures. It was originally developed for the treatment of trigeminal neuralgia, a painful inflammation of the trigeminal nerve (fifth cranial nerve), and it is also effective for bipolar disorder.

The mechanism of action is similar to phenytoin—blocking sodium channels and prolonging the inactivation state of these channels, allowing the drug to inhibit the development of an action potential or firing of the neurons involved in the seizure.

RDH

Rapid Dental Hint

Remember to assess patients taking phenytoin for gingival enlargement. It is difficult for patients to maintain effective oral hygiene. Gingivectomy/gingivoplasty may be indicated.

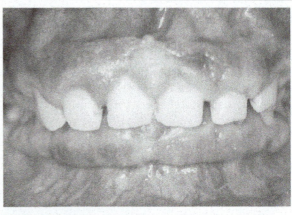

FIGURE 14-1 Gingival enlargement in a patient taking phenytoin.

Severe blood disorders may develop with carbamazepine, such as aplastic anemia, the failure of the bone marrow to produce red blood cells, white blood cells, and platelets. This can result in bleeding gingiva and agranulocytosis (decreased number of circulating neutrophils or white blood cells). A medical consult from the patient's physician is needed for dental treatment; lab tests are necessary when taking carbamazepine.

Carbamazepine is metabolized by the P450 liver cytochromes (CYP3A4) and can reduce effectiveness of oral contraceptives. When taken with erythromycin and clarithromycin, carbamazepine levels become elevated. Carbamazepine induces the metabolism of doxycycline, resulting in lower blood levels of the antibiotics.

Oxcarbazepine Oxcarbazepine (Trileptal) is similar to carbazepine, but has fewer adverse effects. Like carbamazepine, oxcarbazepine blocks the neuronal sodium channel during sustained rapid repetitive firing. It is used as monotherapy for partial-mixed epilepsy and as monotherapy in patients with refractory partial seizures. It does not increase the metabolism of warfarin, cimetidine, or erythromycin.

Valproic Acid Valproic acid is used for controlling all types of generalized seizures (including absence, myoclonic, and partial seizures). It blocks sodium channels and increases GABA synthesis, inhibits GABA degradation in the brain, and is metabolized in the gut to valproic acid.

There are many adverse effects, including xerostomia, inhibition of platelet aggregation (which may be reflected in altered bleeding time and frank hemorrhage), GI complaints, nausea, vomiting, weight gain, hair loss, drowsiness, behavior changes, and tremor. There are three black-box warnings: (1) severe, fatal hepatotoxic reactions may occur, especially in infants under 2 years; (2) it can produce teratogenic effects such as neural tube defects, and has a pregnancy category of D; and (3) cases of life-threatening pancreatitis have been reported in both children and adults.

Guidelines for Dental Patients Taking Carbamazepine

- Patients should avoid erythromycin, clarithromycin (Biaxin), and doxycycline.
- Monitor for xerostomia.
- Monitor for blood disorders: infections, spontaneous bleeding (not provoked with an instrument), and poor healing.
- Monitor blood lab values.
- Look for oral ulcerations and glossitis.
- Tell patients to maintain good oral hygiene.

Rapid Dental Hint

Valproic acid can cause xerostomia. Monitor your patient.

Ethosuximide Ethosuximide (Zarotin) is the drug of choice in controlling absence (petit mal) seizures. Its mechanism of action is inhibiting calcium influx into the brain cell by blocking the T-type calcium channels.

Common adverse effects include nausea, vomiting, anorexia, dizziness, confusion, and leukopenia (low white blood cell count).

Benzodiazepines Lorazepam, administered intravenously (IV), is the drug of choice in status epilepticus and in alcoholic-related seizures. Clonazepam (Klonopin) can be used for controlling myoclonic seizures in children.

SECOND-GENERATION DRUGS Newer anti-epileptic drugs are called second-generation drugs and tend to have more specific sites of action and fewer adverse effects (Table 14-2). These include:

TABLE 14-2 Drugs Used in the Treatment of Epileptic Seizures

TYPE OF SEIZURE	DRUG OF CHOICE	ALTERNATIVE DRUG
Complex/partial seizures	Carbamazepine (Tegretol)	Phenobarbital (Luminal)
	Valproic acid (Depakene, Depakote)	Primidone (Mysoline)
	Phenytoin (Dilantin)	Gabapentin (Neurontin)
		Lamotrigine (Lamictal)
Generalized tonic-clonic (grand mal) seizures	Carbamazepine (Tegretol)	Phenobarbital (Luminal)
	Phenytoin (Dilatin)	Gabapentin (Neurontin)
	Topiramate (Topamax)	Lamotrigine (Lamictal)
	Levetiracetam (Keppa)	
Absence (petit mal) seizures	Ethosuximide (Zarontin)	Clonazepam (Clonopin)
		Valproic acid (Depakene, Depakote)
Febrile seizures in children	Phenobarbital (Luminal)	
Myoclonic seizures	Clonazepam (Klonopin)	
Status epilepticus	Lorazepam (Ativan) (IV)	

- Levetiracetam (Keppra)
- Tiagabine (Gabitril)
- Lamotrigine (Lamictal)
- Gabapentin (Neurontin)
- Pregabalin (Lyrica)
- Felbamate (Felbatol)
- Topiramate (Topamax)
- Zonisamide (Zonegran)

Rapid Dental Hint

Remember that one of the most important complications of anti-epileptic drugs is to increase congenital malformations.

OTHER INDICATIONS FOR ANTI-EPILEPTIC DRUGS Besides being used in the management of seizures, anti-epileptic drugs are also used in the treatment of:

1. Anxiety disorders
2. Bipolar disorder
3. Migraine
4. Neuropathic pain (e.g., diabetic peripheral neuropathy, postherpetic neuralgia)

Table 14-2 summarizes the drugs of choice and alternative drugs for the treatment/control of epileptic seizures.

Dental Hygiene Applications

Reviewing the patient's medical history and interviewing the patient allows the dental hygienist to determine the type of seizure the patient has, cause of seizures, the age of onset, medications used, and degree of control. It is important to determine the patient's adherence in taking the drug. If the patient is not routinely taking his or her medication, a consult with the physician may be needed. The patient should be asked when his or her last epileptic episode was and if there was a loss of consciousness.

Parkinson's Disease

Parkinson's disease is a chronic, progressive, degenerative central nervous system disorder first described by Dr. James Parkinson in 1817. It affects about 1 million people in the United States and occurs in men more often than in women, with an

Guidelines for Dental Patients Taking Valproic Acid (Depakote)

- Emphasize good oral hygiene.
- Evaluate for blood-clotting ability during periodontal debridement, since inhibition of platelet aggregation may occur.
- Monitor for xerostomia.

average age of onset at 65 years. It is characterized by a reduction in the neurotransmitter *dopamine* in a specific area of the brain called the basal ganglia, a collection of cell bodies in the central nervous system.

Clinical Presentation

Symptoms of Parkinsonism develop due to depletion of dopamine. The classic four symptoms of Parkinsonism are a resting tremor, muscle rigidity, bradykinesia, and postural instability.

RESTING TREMOR In 75% of patients, a resting tremor is the first notable symptom. The tremor begins as a fine "pin rolling" of one hand at rest where the patient rubs the thumb and forefinger together in a circular motion. With purposeful movement, the tremor may disappear. This is different from an essential tremor, which is seen during muscle movement.

MUSCULAR RIGIDITY Stiffness may resemble symptoms of arthritis. Some patients have difficulty in bending over or moving extremities. A stiff "poker face" may develop later on in the disease.

BRADYKINESIA Bradykinesia, which is the most noticeable of all symptoms, is displayed as difficulty initiating movement (slowness of movements) and controlling fine muscle movements. Patient may have difficulty in chewing, swallowing, and speaking. Walking often becomes difficult and the patient has a slow-moving shuffle or "short-step" gait.

POSTURAL INSTABILITY Poor posture and imbalance may result in falls.

Rapid Dental Hint

Parkinson's tremor may begin in the jaw; monitor elderly dental patients.

The diagnosis of Parkinson's disease is made clinically because there are no diagnostic laboratory tests.

Pathophysiology

Functionally in the brain, the initiation of muscle movement is through the pyramidal system, and the control of muscle movement is through the **extrapyramidal** system. Manifestations of Parkinson's disease are seen as an increase in extrapyramidal adverse effects due to a decreased synthesis and release in *dopamine (DA),* which is responsible for "turning off the extrapyramidal system." Low production of dopamine is due to the degeneration and destruction of dopamine-producing neurons found within an area of the brain known as the substantia nigra. Loss of dopaminergic cells in the *substantia nigra* is the hallmark of Parkinson's disease. When dopamine is not being produced it cannot reach other areas of the brain that require it. The most important area in the brain for dopamine contact is the *corpus striatum,* which is responsible for controlling unconscious muscle movement. Additionally, there is an elevated level of *acetylcholine (ACh),* which causes an excitatory action that is associated with muscle movement. Thus, Parkinson's disease is associated with an imbalance between the dopaminergic and cholinergic systems in the brain. Balance, posture, and involuntary muscle movement depends on an equilibrium between dopamine (inhibitory) and acetylcholine (stimulatory) in the *corpus striatum.* If dopamine is absent, ACh can stimulate this area of the brain.

Drug-Induced Parkinsonism

Drug-induced Parkinsonism may have identical clinical signs to Parkinson's disease. Drugs most commonly implicated in inducing Parkinsonian symptoms are antagonistic to dopaminergic response. These drugs include some antipsychotics and metoclopramide (Reglan; for gastroesophageal reflux disease).

Drug-induced Parkinsonism is reversible, but it may take up to a few months after discontinuing the drug before symptoms disappear completely.

Pharmacological Treatment

Unfortunately, there is no cure for Parkinson's disease; however, drugs focus on reducing symptoms in some patients by restoring the balance between dopamine and ACh. This is accomplished by *increasing the activity of DA or decreasing the activity of ACh.* Dopamine activity is increased either by giving dopamine (dopamine agonists) or increasing the endogenous (within the body) levels of dopamine. Anticholinergic drugs will block the effect of ACh within the corpus striatum (Table 14-3).

DOPAMINERGIC DRUGS   Dopaminergic drugs are used to increase dopamine levels in the corpus striatum. The drug of choice is levodopa/carbidopa (Sinemet) and is most effective in relieving muscle rigidity and bradykinesia. Since dopamine cannot get through the blood–brain barrier and get into the brain, it must be given in the form of levodopa, which, once past the blood–brain barrier, converts into dopamine. Thus, levodopa or L-dopa is changed into dopamine in the brain, replacing the missing dopamine (Figure 14-2).

Common adverse effects include orthostatic hypotension, psychiatric disturbances (e.g., hallucinations, nightmares, depression), and involuntary orofacial movements and "swings." Dark color may appear in the saliva, urine, or sweat.

Rapid Dental Hint

Patients taking levodopa/carbidopa for Parkinson's disease may experience orthostatic hypotension. Let the patient sit in an upright position for a few minutes before dismissing him or her. Monitor blood pressure.

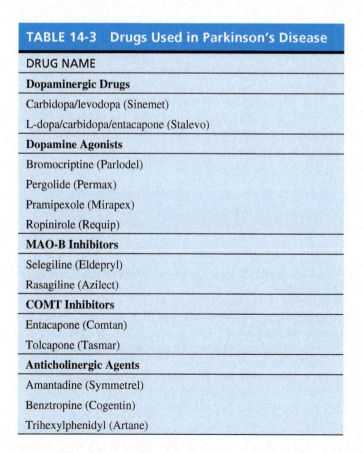

TABLE 14-3   Drugs Used in Parkinson's Disease
DRUG NAME
Dopaminergic Drugs
Carbidopa/levodopa (Sinemet)
L-dopa/carbidopa/entacapone (Stalevo)
Dopamine Agonists
Bromocriptine (Parlodel)
Pergolide (Permax)
Pramipexole (Mirapex)
Ropinirole (Requip)
MAO-B Inhibitors
Selegiline (Eldepryl)
Rasagiline (Azilect)
COMT Inhibitors
Entacapone (Comtan)
Tolcapone (Tasmar)
Anticholinergic Agents
Amantadine (Symmetrel)
Benztropine (Cogentin)
Trihexyphenidyl (Artane)

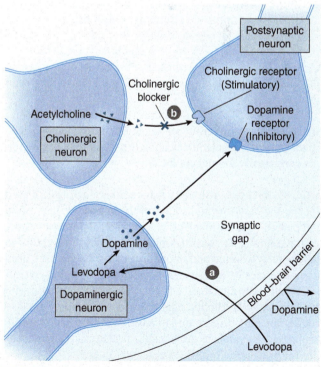

FIGURE 14-2 Mechanism of action of anti-Parkinson drugs. (a) Levodopa therapy increases dopamine production; (b) cholinergic blocker decreases acetylcholine reaching the receptor.

To decrease the amount of L-dopa used and reduce the incidence of adverse effects and to maximize levodopa in the brain, another drug, carbidopa, is added. Carbidopa, which is given in a combined formulation with L-dopa, increases the CNS penetration of L-dopa, so an effective dose is attained more rapidly while reducing adverse effects. Carbidopa does not cross the blood–brain barrier and does not affect the metabolism of L-dopa. The combination of L-dopa and carbidopa is the foundation and the drug of choice for moderate to severe disease.

L-dopa therapy is most effective during the first year of the disease, with a marked decrease in effectiveness by 3 years; by 5 years the signs and symptoms are back to the predrug level. This phenomenon, where the patient experiences fluctuations in their response to L-dopa with an increase in involuntary muscle movement of the orofacial and limb muscles, is referred to as the "on–off effect."

DID YOU KNOW?

Amantidine was originally used as an antiviral drug to prevent the Asian flu. When it was given to a Harvard Medical School patient who also had Parkinson's disease, the condition improved. Today, amatadine is still given to high-risk patients to prevent influenza A virus respiratory infections.

Rapid Dental Hint

Remember to assess your patients with Parkinson's disease for xerostomia.

Rapid Dental Hint

Patients taking drugs for Parkinson's disease may experience xerostomia. Monitor patients' salivary consistency. No special precautions are needed with epinephrine.

Rapid Dental Hint

The main symptoms of Parkinson's disease are usually stiffness, tremor (shaking), and slowness of movement. Your patients may have difficulty getting in and out of the dental chair.

DOPAMINE AGONISTS   The dopamine agonist agents act directly to stimulate dopamine receptors. There are four dopamine agonists used to treat Parkinson's disease: bromocriptine (Parlodel), Pergolide (Permax), pramipexole (Mirapex), and ropinirole (Requip). These drugs are commonly used with levodopa to delay the onset of levodopa-motor complications. The most frequent adverse effects are orthostatic hypotension, daytime sleepiness, mental confusion, hallucinations, and nightmares, which are greater than seen with L-dopa.

The newest FDA-approved drug, ropinirole (Requip), significantly reduces "wearing-off" time. Requip should be added into the patient's regular medication if it is not reducing symptoms consistently throughout the day.

ANTICHOLINERGIC AGENTS   Anticholinergic drugs are used either in the early or mild stages of the disease or later on in combination with levodopa/carbidopa, and are primarily effective for tremors. These drugs block cholinergic receptors to balance acetylcholine and dopamine levels. Commonly used anticholinergics include benztropine (Cogentin), trihexyphenidyl (Artane), and amantadine (Symmetral), which is used with levodopa. Anticholinergic agents are not commonly used to treat Parkinson's disease due to adverse effects and inability to improve bradykinesia. Amantadine is also used prophylactically for prevention of influenza A viral infection.

As with all types of anticholinergic drugs, common adverse effects include xerostomia, urinary retention, constipation, blurred vision, dry skin, and drowsiness.

MONOAMINE OXIDASE B (MAO-B) INHIBITOR AND COMT (CATECHOL-O-METHYLTRANSFERASE) INHIBITOR   Selegiline (Eldepryl) and rasagiline (Azilect) are MAO-B inhibitors that block the enzyme MAO-B, which metabolizes dopamine and increases levels in the brain. Rasagiline is used alone or in combination with L-dopa. The main advantage of rasagiline is that it does not have the toxic metabolic breakdown products of selegiline.

The newest class of anti-Parkinson drugs is COMT (catechol-O-methyltransferase) inhibitors. These drugs are used as an adjunct to carbidopa/levodopa to help with motor complications due to levodopa.

Guidelines of Dental Patients Taking Anti-Parkinson Drugs

- Anti-Parkinson drugs have a high incidence of causing dry mouth and other anticholinergic side effects.
- Monitor dental patient for caries, periodontal disease, and oral candidiasis.
- Optimum oral hygiene.
- Supplemental topical fluoride and drinking water is recommended.
- Avoid alcohol, smoking, and depressants, which could aggravate the dry mouth.
- For orthostatic hypotension, have patient remain upright in the dental chair a few minutes before rising. Monitor vital signs.
- Since these drugs also cause dizziness and confusion, monitor the patient.

Dental Hygiene Applications

Most anti-Parkinson drugs cause anticholinergic adverse effects and orthostatic (postural) hypotension. The patient must be counseled by the dental clinician about xerostomia.

The vital signs of the patient should be monitored. After supine positioning to avoid orthostatic hypotension, have the patient remain in an upright position in the dental chair for a few minutes before arising.

Aggregated mouth and tongue movements and xerostomia may be a sign of a serious adverse effect of the medication or the disease process. A physician's consult may be needed.

There are no specific precautions needed with regard to the use of vasoconstrictors in local anesthetics.

Alzheimer's Disease

Like Parkinson's disease, Alzheimer's is a neurodegenerative disease characterized by the destruction of cholinergic and other neurons in the central nervous system. As the disease progresses less acetylcholine is produced. The etiology is unknown and there is no cure. In the United States, Alzheimer's accounts for about 60% of all cases of dementia in people over 65 years of age, and is associated with about 100,000 deaths per year. This disease has overwhelming effects on the individual's emotional, memory, and physical function.

There are currently four prescription drugs approved by the FDA to treat people with Alzheimer's disease. Treating the symptoms can provide patients with comfort, dignity, and independence for a longer period of time. These medications do not stop the progress of the disease.

Cholinesterase inhibitors function to prevent the breakdown of acetylcholine, important for memory and thinking: galantamine (Razadyne), rivastigmine (Exelon), and donepezil (Aricept).

An N-methyl D-aspartate (NMDA) antagonist, memantine (Namenda), is indicated for moderate to severe Alzheimer's disease. This drug works by regulating glutamate, which is produced in excessive amounts and may cause brain cell death.

Headache

The International Classification of Headache Disorders identifies 165 headache types, divided into primary and secondary headaches depending on the underlying risk factors. Primary headache disorders, which account for 97–98% of all headaches, are characterized by the lack of an identifiable and treatable underlying cause. Examples of primary headache disorders include migraine, tension-type, and cluster headaches. Secondary headache disorders are associated with an identifiable cause such as headache or facial pain attributed to disorders of the neck, eyes, ears, nose, sinuses, teeth, mouth, or other facial or cranial structures; head or neck trauma; drug substance or its withdrawal; infection; cranial neuralgias; brain tumors; meningitis; temporal arteritis; intracranial lesions; and primary angle closure glaucoma.

Migraine

In the United States, approximately 29 million people (18% of women, 6% of men) suffer from **migraine.** Migraine is a recurring, episodic, and often severe headache disorder, with attacks lasting 4–72 hours. Migraine is further divided into several subtypes including, among others, migraine without aura and migraine with aura.

To establish a diagnosis of *migraine without aura,* five attacks lasting 4–72 hours must have occurred. It is usually associated with photophobia (sensitivity to or intolerance of light) and phonophobia (fear of sounds, including your own voice), nausea and vomiting, and cutaneous allodynia, a nonpainful stimulus on the skin that is perceived as painful, and is experienced by some patients during an attack.

Migraine with aura, experienced by about 20% of patients, is characterized by episodes of headache with features similar to those of migraine without aura in addition to aura symptoms that precede or occur with the onset of pain. Most aura symptoms develop gradually over 5–20 minutes and last less than 60 minutes. Aura represents a transient episode of focal neurological dysfunction caused by an imbalance between excitatory and inhibitory neuronal activity at different levels in the central nervous system. A visual aura may be bright flashing lights and a sensory aura may take the form of a paresthesia that involves the arm, face, hands, and body. About 25% of people experience a postdrome, which involves changes in mood and behavior after the migraine attack. Precipitating factors include caffeine (and caffeine withdrawal), menstruation, stress, smoking, lack of sleep, certain foods, and strenuous exercise. Attacks are commonly unilateral.

> **DID YOU KNOW?**
>
> Some scenes in *Alice in Wonderland* are based on visual aura of migraine.

A migraine attack develops over four phases:

- Prodrome (hours to days before the attack)
- Aura
- Headache
- Postdrome (recovery)

Pain during the headache phase is due to vasodilation of cerebral blood vessels, which is caused by the neurons in the trigeminal nerve releasing substance P (a chemical messenger that signals the brain to feel pain when it is released). Additionally, low levels of serotonin, a neurotransmitter in the brain, may result in dilation of cerebral blood vessels, initiating the manifestation of head pain. At this stage in the migraine process, activation of specific subtypes of 5-HT_1 receptors has proven clinically effective in relieving migraine pain.

Rapid Dental Hint

Pain from migraine is due to vasodilation of blood vessels in the brain and low levels of serotonin.

Medication-Overuse Headaches

Medication-overuse headache (MOH) is a syndrome/cycle that starts when a patient takes too much headache medication, which contributes to the headache rather than easing it. Anyone with a history of migraine headache is at risk for developing a MOH. Unfortunately, drug companies and advertisements contribute to the development of medication-overuse headaches. Many over-the-counter pain relievers that contain caffeine are the culprits (e.g., Excedrin Migraine and Excedrin Tension Headache). Caffeine present in coffee and sodas and pain relievers may all contribute to medication-overuse headaches. To stop rebound headaches, the amount of pain medication should be reduced or stopped. Signs and symptoms of rebound headache include nausea, anxiety, insomnia, and restlessness.

Drug Therapy

Drug therapy is aimed at aborting a migraine at the time it occurs, symptomatic pain relief, and preventing a migraine from occurring. The use of any symptomatic therapy, either prescription or OTC, should not be more than twice a week. Beyond that, the patient should be taking preventative medications. Therapy should start by eliminating all products containing caffeine, which causes vasoconstriction. Table 14-4 lists the classifications of drugs used in the treatment of acute migraine attacks and for prophylaxis (chronic therapy).

DID YOU KNOW?

The medicinal use of coffee by Islamic physicians probably began before the second millennium A.D. The first documented use of coffee as a beverage was by the Sufis of Yemen, who were using the drink to stay awake during prayers in the 1400s. By 1510 there were coffeehouses in Mecca and Cairo.

TREATMENT OF ACUTE MIGRAINES (ABORTIVE)

Triptans   Triptans, the newest drugs for migraine management, are effective and well tolerated drugs for the *treatment of acute migraine* to abort the attack, but are not used prophylactically. Triptans bind with high affinity to the 5-HT_1 (serotonin) receptors and are referred to as selective serotonin agonists. Activation of these receptors results in cranial vessel constriction and reduction transmission in trigeminal pain pathways. They have a rapid onset of action. Formulations

available include oral, suppositories, injections, nasal sprays and a needle-free, subcutaneous delivery (sumatriptan). Orally

TABLE 14-4   Drugs Used in the Treatment of Migraine
DRUG NAME
Acute Treatment (Abort Migraine)
Triptans
• Almotriptan (Axert)
• Eletriptan (Relpax)
• Frovatriptan (Frova)
• Naratriptan (Amerge)
• Rizatriptan (MAXALT, MAXALT-MLT)
• Sumatriptan (Imitrex)
• Zolmitriptan (Zomig)
Nonnarcotic Analgesics
• Acetaminophen (Tylenol)
• Aspirin, acetaminophen, and caffeine (Excedrin Migraine)
• Nonsteroidal anti-inflammatory drugs (NSAIDs)
• Ibuprofen (Advil, Motrin, Nuprin); naproxen (Aleve)
Combination NSAID/Triptan
• Sumatriptan and naproxen sodium (Treximet)
Analgesics Combination
• Codeine, acetaminophen, caffeine, butalbital (Fioricet)
Ergot
• Ergotamine (Ergomar), caffeine (Carfergot)
Anticonvulsants
• Topiramate (Topamax)
• Valproic acid (Depakote)
Prophylaxis
Calcium Channel Blockers
• Diltiazem (Cardizem)
• Nifedipeine (Procardia)
• Verapamil (Calan, Isoptin)
Beta-Blockers
• Atenolol (Tenormin)
• Metoprolol (Lopressor)
• Propranolol (Inderal)
• Timolol (Blocadren)
Tricyclic Antidepressants
• Amitriptyline (Elavil)
• Imipramine (Tofranil)
• Nortipytyline (Pamelor)
• Protriptyline (Vivactil)
Botulinum Toxin
• Botulinum toxin Type A (Botox)

administered triptans provide pain relief within 30 minutes. Injected sumatriptan has an onset of action of less than 15 minutes.

Triptans are contraindicated in patients with ischemic heart disease (e.g., angina pectoris, history of myocardial infarction, or silent ischemia) or in patients who have symptoms of ischemic heart disease and coronary artery vasospasm. Triptans may increase blood pressure and should not be given to patients with uncontrolled hypertension. Caution should be used when using local anesthetics containing epinephrine. The patient's blood pressure should be monitored.

The combined use of triptans and antidepressants, including selective serotonin reuptake inhibitors (SSRIs) such as Prozac or Zoloft or selective serotonin/norepinephrine reuptake inhibitors (SNRIs) such as Cymbalta or Effexor, *may* result in a serotonin syndrome resulting from excessive blood levels of serotonin. Symptoms include restlessness, hallucinations, fast heartbeat, diarrhea, nausea and vomiting, and rapid changes in blood pressure. Serotonin syndrome *may* be more likely to occur when starting or increasing the dose of a triptan, SSRI, or SNRI. This combination is not contraindicated, but care should be taken when the two drugs are taken concurrently.

Common adverse reactions include head and jaw discomfort, flushing, dizziness, sleepiness, and tiredness.

Ergot Derivatives   Drugs such as ergotamine (Ergomar) and dihydroergotamine nasal spray (Migranal) are α-adrenergic blockers and vasoconstrictors of cranial smooth muscle.

Elevated blood levels occur when taken with erythromycin and clarithromycin. Many adverse effects, including nausea, localized edema and itching, and numbness and tingling in fingers and toes, preclude its long-term use and for prevention.

Analgesics   For mild migraine attacks, analgesics alone or in combination with caffeine have been used. Overuse of analgesics and caffeine can aggravate the migraine. Most of the pain relievers that patients use are over the counter. Excedrin Migraine (which is the same as regular Excedrin) contains acetaminophen, aspirin, and caffeine. Caffeine, a vasoconstrictor, is added to pain relievers to make them more effective in relieving headaches. Two tablets contain the same amount of caffeine as a cup of coffee. Long-term use of analgesics is discouraged, as this may lead to headaches on withdrawal. Adverse effects include gastrointestinal upset and bleeding and nausea. Nonsteroidal anti-inflammatory drugs include ibuprofen and naproxen; these reduce the release of serotonin and can be used in combination with triptans.

Narcotic analgesics containing codeine are used for more severe pain. These prescription products include Fiorinal (a combination of codeine, aspirin, butalbital, and caffeine) and Fioricet (acetaminophen, butalbital, and caffeine). These drugs are also available without codeine. There are many adverse effects including dependency, constipation, sedation, and drowsiness that preclude long-term use.

MIGRAINE PROPHYLAXIS   Choosing a drug for prevention is based on the adverse effect profile of the drug and on the medical status of the patient.

Anticonvulsants   Topiramate (Topamax) is approved for migraine prevention in adults and not for acute treatment. It is a sulfamate-substituted monosaccharide with a broad spectrum of anticonvulsant activity. Its precise mechanism of action is unknown. Common adverse effects include lowered bicarbonate levels in the blood, resulting in an increase in the acidity of the blood (metabolic acidosis) and hyperventilation (rapid, deep breathing) or fatigue. Maintenance of adequate fluid intake is important to minimize the risk of renal stone formation. Other side effects are tingling in arms and legs, loss of appetite, nausea, diarrhea, taste change, and weight loss. There are no contraindications with epinephrine.

Valproic acid (Depakene) is approved for migraine prophylaxis and can take up to 2–3 weeks to be effective. Common adverse effects, including weight gain, sedation, and xerostomia, may preclude its use in certain patients.

Beta-Blockers   The use of beta-blockers for the treatment of migraines started in the 1960s when people being treated for heart problems found that their migraines lessened. The mechanism of action may be due to limiting the tendency for cranial blood vessels to overdilate. It may take up to 4-6 weeks to see a reduction in migraine frequency. Timolol and propranolol are FDA approved.

Nonselective beta-blockers are contraindicated in patients with asthma. The amount of epinephrine should be limited to 0.04 mg (two cartridges of 1:100,000) when taking a nonselective beta-blocker.

Calcium Channel Blockers   Similar to beta-blockers, calcium channel blockers were originally used to treat cardiovascular conditions. These drugs may also work by stabilizing blood vessel membranes by preventing them from overdilating. It can take up to 2 months to see effects.

Tricyclic Antidepressants   Antimigraine action is separate from antidepressant effect. For migraine prevention, a lower dose is prescribed than would be used for the treatment of depression and it can take up to 3–4 weeks before the drug is effective. The dose of epinephrine should be limited to 0.04 mg.

Botulinum Toxin Type A   Injection of botulinum toxin type A (Botox), derived from the exotoxin of bacteria, besides being used cosmetically and for dystonia (sustained contraction of muscles), has been used in the prevention of migraines for up to 6 months. Although the exact mechanism is unclear, it has been hypothesized that it works by inhibiting the release of transmitters from pain-sensitive nerve endings.

Alternative Treatments

Some alternative medications used in the prophylaxis of migraine include feverfew, petasites, magnesium, riboflavin, coenzyme Q10, and melatonin. There are no randomized, controlled studies using melatonin. There is concern with the lack of standardization regarding the contents and purity of herbal supplements.

A number of alternative treatments have been recommended in the treatment and prevention of migraine including hypnosis, biofeedback, meditation, acupuncture, massage, transcutaneous electrical nerve stimulation, and magnesium supplements.

Dental Hygiene Applications

Migraine is the most common headache disorder, affecting approximately 29 million people in the United States, and is present in one in four households. During a migraine, stimulation of the trigeminal nerve (the fifth cranial nerve, carrying sensory information from the face) may cause referral of pain to any of the nerve's three branches, resulting in facial pain.

Many dental patients will be taking one type of headache medication. There are no precautions for using local anesthetics with epinephrine in patients taking migraine drugs, except for nonselective beta-blockers and triptans.

Key Points

- Take a complete medical history.
- Determine when the patient's last epileptic seizure was and what brought it on.
- Monotherapy is the preferred treatment option for epilepsy.
- What medication does the patient take, and is it taken regularly?
- Be prepared if the patient has a seizure in the dental chair.
- Get a medical consultation and lab blood tests.
- Patient management in the dental chair is an important part of treatment.
- Monitor the patient for xerostomia.
- There are no special precautions for using vasoconstrictors in local anesthetics.

Board Review Questions

1. Which of the following anti-epileptic drugs decreases doxycycline serum levels? (p. 234)
   a. Phenytoin
   b. Valproic acid
   d. Primidone
   e. Levetiracetam
2. Which of the following antiseizure drugs increases the incidence of gingival enlargement? (p. 234)
   a. Phenobarbital
   b. Lamotrigine
   c. Carbamazepine
   d. Phenytoin
   e. Ethosuximide

3. Which of the following drugs is used to treat trigeminal neuralgia? (p. 234)
   a. Phenytoin
   b. Carbamazepine
   c. Phenobarbital
   d. Valproic acid
   e. Primidone
4. Which of the following drugs are used to treat migraines? (pp. 236, 239)
   a. Triptans
   b. Anticonvulsants
   c. Beta-blockers
   d. All of the above
5. Which of the following are two common adverse effects of drugs used to treat Parkinson's disease? (pp. 237, 238)
   a. Hypertension and diarrhea
   b. Xerostomia and orthostatic hypotension
   c. Orthostatic hypotension and nasal congestion
   d. Hypertension and constipation

Selected References

American Academy of Neurology and the American Epilepsy Society. 2004, April. AAN Guideline Summary for Clinicians. Efficacy and Tolerability of the New Antiepileptic Drugs, I: Treatment of New Onset Epilepsy.

American Academy of Neurology and the American Epilepsy Society. 2004, April. AAN Guideline Summary for Clinicians. Efficacy and Tolerability of the New Antiepileptic Drugs, II: Treatment of Refractory Epilepsy.

American Academy of Neurology and the American Epilepsy Society. 2004, April. AAN Guideline Summary for Clinicians. Treatments for Refractory Epilepsy.

DeVane CL. 2001. Substance P: A new era, a new role. *Pharmacotherapy* 21(9):1061–1069.

Dodick DW, Mauskop A, Elkind AH, et al. 2005. Botulinum toxin type A for the prophylaxis of chronic daily headache: Subgroup analysis of patients not receiving other prophylactic medications: A randomized double-blind, placebo-controlled study. *Headache* 45:315–324.

Evans RW, Taylor FR. 2006. "Natural" or alternative medications for migraine prevention. *Headache* 46:1012–1018.

Faulkner MA. 2006. The role of the pharmacist in the management of Parkinson's disease: Its symptoms and comorbidities. *U.S. Pharmacist,* Continuing Education Series.

French JA, Kanner, AM, Bautista J, Abou-Khalil B, Browne T, Harden CL, et al. 2004. Efficacy and tolerability of the new antiepileptic drugs. I. Treatment of new onset epilepsy: Report of the Therapeutics and Technology Assessment Subcommittee and Quality Standards Subcommittee of the American Academy of Neurology and the American Epilepsy Society. *Neurology* 62:1252–1260.

Hamel E. 1999. The biology of serotonin receptors: Focus on migraine pathophysiology and treatment. *Can J Neurol Sci* 26:S2–6.

Hargreaves RJ, Shepheard SL. 1999. Pathophysiology of migraine-new insights. *Can J Neurol Sce* 26(Suppl. 3):S12–S19.

Headache Classification Subcommittee of the International Headache Society. 2003. The International Classification of Headache Disorders, 2nd ed. *Cephalalgia* Supplement 1:1–150.

LaRoche SM. 2004. The new antiepileptic drugs. *JAMA* 291:605–614.

Lipton RB, Stewart WR, Celentano DD, et al. 1992. Undiagnosed migraine headaches—a comparison of symptom-based and reported physician diagnosis. *Arch Intern Med* 152:1273–1278.

Merck. 2005. *Monographs in medicine: A study of migraine.* Whitehouse Station, NJ: Merck & Co., Inc.

Ochoa JG. 2006. *Antiepileptic drugs: An overview.* www.emedicine.com.

Padmanabhan R, Abdulrazzaq YM, Bastaki SM, Shafiullah M, Chandranath SI. 2003. Experimental studies on reproductive toxicologic effects of lamotrigine in mice. *Birth Defects Res B Dev Reprod Toxicol* 68(5):428–438.

Parks Jr BR, Dostrow VG, Noble SL. 1994. Drug therapy for epilepsy. *American Fam Physician* 50:639–648.

Parmet S, Lynm C, Glass RM. 2004. Epilepsy. *JAMA* 291:654.

Schapira AV, Olanow CW. 2004. Neuroprotection in Parkinson's disease. *JAMA* 291:358–364.

Schuurmans A, van Weels C. 2005. Pharmacologic treatment of migraine: comparison of guidelines. *Can Fam Physician* 51(6):838–843.

Serge J, Pierre-Louis C. 2000. New drugs: Which should be included in the formulary? All new drugs should be included. *Arch Neurol* 57:272–273.

Silberstein SD, Olesen J, Bousser M-G, Diener H-C, et al., 2005. The International Classification of Headache Disorders, 2nd edition (ICHD-II)—revision of criteria for 8.2, *Medication-overuse* headache. *Cephalalgia* 25:460–465.

Tea CP, Williams BR, Atkinson R, Gill MA. 2003. Management and treatment of Parkinson's disease. *U.S. Pharmacist* 28:93–100.

Wenzel RG, Sarvis CA, Krause, ML. 2003. Over-the-counter-drugs for acute migraine attacks: Literature review and recommendations. *Pharmacotherapy* 23(4):294–505.

Web Sites

www.Parkinsons.org

www.nia.nih.gov/Alzheimers/Publications/medicationsfs.htm

PEARSON
myhealthprofessionskit™

Use this address to access the Companion Website created for this textbook. Simply select "Dental Hygiene" from the choice of disciplines. Find this book and log in using your username and password to access video clips of selected tests.

QUICK DRUG GUIDE

Drugs for Epilepsy

- Carbamazepine (Tegretol, Carbiarol): first-line therapy—oxcarbazepine; partial/mixed and refractory partial (Trileptal); partial/tonic-clonic/mixed seizures
- Ethosuximide (Zarontin): petit mal seizures only
- Gabapentin (Neurontin): partial seizures
- Lamotrigine (Lamictal): partial seizures and refractory partial
- Levetiracetam (Keppra): partial seizures and primary generalized tonic-clonic seizures in patients 6 years of age and older
- Phenytoin (Dilantin): first-line therapy; tonic-clonic and complex partial seizures
- Phenobarbital (Luminal): tonic-clonic seizures, partial seizures

- Pregabalin (Lyrica): partial seizures
- Primidone (Mysoline): grand mal seizures
- Tiagabine (Gabitril): partial mixed and refractory partial seizures
- Topiramate (Topamax): partial/tonic-clonic seizures and refractory partial seizures
- Valproic acid (Depakene): first-line therapy; complex and simple partial seizures
- Zonisamide (Zonegran): partial seizures
- Benzodiazepines: lorazepam (Ativan)—only used for status epilepticus

Drugs for Parkinson's Disease

Dopamine Replacement
- Carbidopa/levodopa (Parcopa)
- Carbidopa/levodopa/entacapone (Stalevo)

Monoamine Oxidase Inhibitor
- Rasagiline (Azilect)
- Selegiline (Eldepryl)

COMT (Catechol-O-Methyltransferase) Inhibitor
- Entacapone (Comtan)
- Tolcapone (Tasmar)

Dopamine Agonists
- Bromocriptine (Parlodel)
- Pergolide (Permax)
- Pramipexole (Mirapex)
- Ropinirole (Requip)

Anticholinergic Agents
- Amantadine (Symmetrel)
- Benztropine (Cogentin)
- Trihexylphenidyl (Artane)

Drugs for Alzheimer's Disease

- Donepezil (Aricept)
- Galantamine (Razadyne)

- Memantine (Namenda)
- Rivastigmine (Exelon)

Drugs for Migraine

Triptans (Serotonin Receptor Agonists)
- Almotriptan (Axert)
- Eletriptan (Relpax)
- Frovatriptan (Frova)
- Naratriptan (Amerge)
- Rizatriptan (MAXALT, MAXALT-MLT)
- Sumatriptan (Imitrex)
- Zolmitriptan (Zomig)
- Sumatriptan and naproxen (Treximet)

Anti-epileptics
- Levetiracetam (Keppra)
- Topiramate (Topamax)
- Valproic acid (Depakene)
- Zonisamide (Zonegran)

Ergot Derivatives

- Ergotamine (Ergomar)
- Ergotamine, caffeine (Carfergot)
- Dihydroergotamine (migranal nasal spray)

Calcium Channel Blockers

- Diltiazem (Cardizem)
- Nifedipeine (Procardia)
- Verapamil (Calan, Isoptin)

Beta-Blockers

- Propranolol (Inderal)
- Timolol (Blocadren)

Tricyclic Antidepressants

- Amitriptyline (Elavil)
- Imipramine (Tofranil)
- Nortipytyline (Pamelor)
- Protriptyline (Vivactil)

Analgesics

- Acetaminophen (Tylenol)
- Aspirin, acetaminophen, and caffeine (Excedrin Migraine)
- Ibuprofen (Advil, Motrin, Nuprin)
- Naproxen (Aleve)

Narcotic Analgesics

- Codeine, acetaminophen, caffeine, butalbital (Fioricet)

Botulinum Toxin

- Botulinum toxin Type A (Botox)

15

Psychiatric Drugs

GOAL

To provide an understanding of psychiatric medications used to treat psychiatric and dental disorders and how to manage these patients in the dental office.

EDUCATIONAL OBJECTIVES

After reading this chapter, the reader should be able to:

1. Discuss the biochemical etiology of the various psychiatric disorders.

2. Describe the major classes of psychotherapeutic medications.

3. Discuss the adverse effects of psychiatric medications.

4. Discuss the impact of these adverse effects during dental treatment.

KEY TERMS

Antipsychotics

Antidepressants

Anxiolytic agents

Sedative/hypnotics

Psychopharmacology

Extrapyramidal side effects

Mood disorders

Introduction

Psychopharmacology is one of the most rapidly growing areas of clinical pharmacology. There are three major symptoms of psychiatric/emotional disorders: anxiety, depression (mood disorders), and psychosis. Psychiatric medications are classified according to therapeutic applications including:

- **Antipsychotics** for the treatment of psychoses such as schizophrenia
- **Antidepressants** (mood-elevating agents) for the treatment of depression and mood-stabilizing agents for the treatment of manic or bipolar disorders (formerly known as manic-depressive disorder)
- **Anxiolytic agents** for the treatment of anxiety disorders
- **Sedative/hypnotics** (e.g., barbiturates) for the induction of sleep

Many dental patients may be taking one or more of these medications either for a psychiatric disorder, alleviating anxiety before a dental procedure, nocturnal bruxism, or chronic orofacial pain. The majority of these drugs cause xerostomia, which may lead to the development of caries and periodontal disease. Thus it is important for the dental hygienist to be familiar with psychiatric medications, to monitor patients taking these medications, and to instruct patients on proper oral home care.

A publication from the American Psychiatric Association entitled the *Diagnostic and Statistical Manual of Mental Disorders,* Fourth Edition (DSM-IV; 1994), allows the physician to diagnose a wide range of psychiatric disorders. Essentially, the DSM-IV is organized by symptoms that are related to specific diagnoses.

Psychopharmacology deals with drugs used to treat psychosomatic disorders, which have a biochemical origin in the brain. In psychiatric disorders of the central nervous system, many CNS neurotransmitters are involved in causing signs and symptoms of the disease.

Basic Pharmacology

For a drug to be effective there must be equilibrium among absorption, distribution, metabolism, and excretion. Especially for psychiatric drugs to reach the brain, the drug must also effectively cross the blood–brain barrier. Since most psychiatric drugs are weak bases, they are readily absorbed from the intestine and best absorbed on an empty stomach. Psychiatric drugs have numerous adverse oral side effects that may interfere with adequate management of the dental patient.

Rapid Dental Hint

Patients taking any type of psychiatric drug should be monitored for xerostomia, which may lead to caries and periodontal diseases.

Antipsychotic Drugs

Psychosis is a mental disorder characterized by gross impairment of thought and behavior, in which a person cannot differentiate between real and unreal thoughts. *Positive symptoms* add on to normal behavior and consist of hallucinations, delusions, paranoia, and suspiciousness. *Negative symptoms* consist of emotional and social withdrawal and lack of interest. *Schizophrenia,* the most common type of psychosis, affects only approximately 1% of the American population. It usually occurs in males and begins in adolescence or early adult life.

The etiology of schizophrenia is essentially unknown; however, there are several hypotheses, including a strong genetic predisposition and a chemical imbalance in the brain. It is a chronic disease for which there is no cure.

Dopamine Receptors

Dopamine receptors play a role in the etiology of schizophrenia and in the mechanism of action and adverse effects of antipsychotics. Controlling dopamine and dopamine receptors is essential for the treatment of schizophrenia (Figure 15-1).

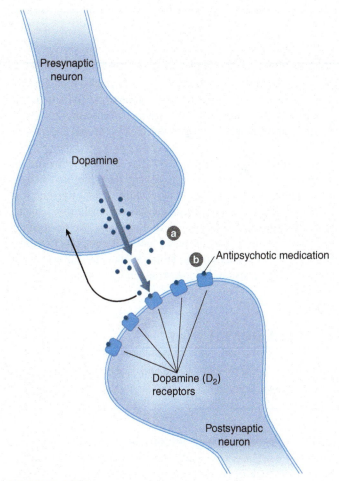

FIGURE 15-1 Mechanism of action of antipsychotic drugs. (a) Overproduction of dopamine; (b) antipsychotic medication occupies D_2 receptors, preventing dopamine from stimulating the postsynaptic neuron.

Medications

All antipsychotic drugs act by binding to the dopamine (D_2) receptor, preventing dopamine from attaching. This results in decreased dopamine activity in the neuronal synapse. Antipsychotics are often referred to as *dopamine antagonists*. When about 65% of the D_2 receptor is blocked by the drug, psychotic behavior is reduced. The older theory of the pharmacodynamics of antipsychotics stated that the stronger an antipsychotic was in binding and blocking the D_2 receptor, the more potent it was as an antipsychotic. However, the current theory is that the *strength (affinity) to the receptor is not correlated with efficacy*. For example, clozapine is the weakest binding antipsychotic, but it has the most efficacy on positive symptoms.

DID YOU KNOW?

Fifty years ago antipsychotics were discovered accidentally, while being used for other indications. The discovery of chlorpromazine's antipsychotic action started during the 1930s, based on the mood-altering side effects of its antihistamines such as diphenhydramine (Benadryl).

Adverse Effects

Besides binding to dopamine receptors, which are responsible for their antipsychotic action, antipsychotics also bind nonspecifically to muscarinic receptors (anticholinergic), α_1-adrenergic receptors, and histamine (H_1) receptors (antihistaminic), resulting in a variety of adverse effects that are also related to dentistry.

BINDING TO MUSCARINIC RECEPTORS Binding to muscarinic receptors causes *anticholinergic effects,* including xerostomia, constipation, blurred vision, tachycardia, sexual dysfunction, and urine retention. The mouth can be extremely dry, causing the dental mirror to stick to the oral mucosa. The decrease in salivary flow may lead to dental and root caries, periodontal disease, and oral candidiasis. Drugs to increase salivary flow, salivary substitutes, and moisturizers may be required.

Rapid Dental Hint

Monitor patients who are taking psychiatric drugs for xerostomia, periodontal diseases, and root caries.

BINDING TO DOPAMINE RECEPTORS Binding to the D_2 receptors correlates not only to antipsychotic effects but also to movement disorders called **extrapyramidal side effects** (EPS). It has been estimated that between 50 and 75% of patients on antipsychotics eventually develop some form of EPS, which can interfere with management of the dental patient. This can be permanent, even when the drug is discontinued.

The extrapyramidal side effects that can occur within days from starting the medication include:

- Dystonia (abnormal muscle contraction)
- Acute akathisia (the most common EPS; sense that the patient must keep moving; swaying from foot to foot)
- Parkinsonism (tremors, impaired gait); benztropine (Cogentin) may help relieve early-onset adverse effects
- Tardive dyskinesia, an EPS that is not always reversible and is characterized by involuntary, persistent movements of the tongue (rolling) and lips (lip smacking), lateral jaw movements, chewing movements, blinking, rocking back and forth, and facial muscle movement. Oral dyskinesias may result in bruxism, broken teeth, tongue trauma, and ulcerations. Since the patient cannot remain "still" and is always moving, dental management of these patients is difficult. Approximately 20% of patients and 50% of older adults on long-term neuroleptics experience tardive dyskinesia. There is no recognized treatment.

Rapid Dental Hint

Dental patients with extrapyramidal side effects (e.g., constant jaw and lip movement, facial muscle movement) may be difficult to manage.

BINDING TO HISTAMINE RECEPTORS Binding to H_1 receptors results in antihistamine adverse effects including sedation, drowsiness, and weight gain (and serotonin receptor blockade).

BINDING TO α_1-ADRENERGIC RECEPTORS Another concern of neuroleptics is cardiac safety. Binding to the α_1-adrenergic receptors causes orthostatic hypotension, dizziness, syncope, palpitations, and reflex tachycardia.

Rapid Dental Hint

Dental patients taking antipsychotic drugs may experience orthostatic hypotension. Monitor blood pressure. Have the patient remain in an upright position in the dental chair for a few minutes before getting up.

Most neuroleptics cause a prolongation of the QT interval, which can lead to a potentially fatal ventricular tachycardia. The highest incidence occurs with thioridazine, followed by ziprasidone, quetiapine, risperidone, olanzapine, and haloperidol. It also occurs in atypical antipsychotics, but to a lesser extent. Because of this, it is important to question the patient about all medications, prescription as well as OTC, to avoid cardiac problems. Precautions should be taken when using local anesthetics containing epinephrine, which could increase the cardiac adverse effects.

Rapid Dental Hint

Adverse effects of antipsychotics that could interfere with dental treatment include sedation, extrapyramidal effects (e.g., oral dyskinesia—movement of tongue, jaw, and lips), xerostomia, and orthostatic hypotension. Extra time may be needed for an appointment.

Types of Antipsychotics

Antipsychotics (also called *neuroleptics*) are classified as *typical antipsychotics* and *atypical antipsychotics*. Typical antipsychotics are the older drugs and have been the treatment of choice for psychoses for 50 years (Table 15-1).

With the limitations of the traditional antipsychotic agents (e.g., adverse effects, treatment failure, adherence problems, and limitation in treating negative symptoms), the introduction of newer, atypical antipsychotics has broadened the therapeutic spectrum to include negative symptoms and fewer serious adverse effects (e.g., orthostatic hypotension, xerostomia), although there are still many adverse effects (Table 15-2).

Rapid Dental Hint

Patients taking atypical antipsychotics are at increased risk for diabetes. Monitor periodontal disease status.

Clozapine (Clozaril) was the first atypical antipsychotic available in the United States. Clozapine causes seizures and blood disorders such as agranulocytosis (white blood cell count decreases to under 1,000 mm³), which is a FDA black box warning. Clozapine is usually used for refractory cases where other treatments have failed. It is necessary to take a blood test weekly to check on white blood cell levels.

TABLE 15-1 Common Typical "Older" Antipsychotics

Typical Antipsychotics

Low Potency
- Chlorpromazine (Thorazine)
- Thioridazine (Mellaril)

High Potency
- Trifluoperazine (Stelazine)
- Fluphenazine (Prolixin)
- Thiothixene (Navene)
- Haloperidol (Haldol)
- Loxapine (Loxitane)
- Molindone (Moban)

TABLE 15-2 Atypical Antipsychotics

- Risperidone (Risperdal); considered to be first-line therapy
- Olanzapine (Zyprexa)
- Ziprasidone (Geodon)
- Quetiapine (Seroquel)
- Clozapine (Clozaril)
- Iloperidone (Fanapt)
- Lurasidone (Latuda)
- Asenapine (Saphris)

Because psychosis involves the expression of multiple symptoms and many patients respond only partially to antipsychotics, combination pharmacotherapy may be necessary. Thus, antipsychotics can be used with other drugs such as valproate, an anticonvulsant drug.

Rapid Dental Hint

For patients taking a phenothiazine type of antipsychotic such as risperidone (Risperdal), a change in blood pressure is common. Monitor the patient's blood pressure. Limit the amount of epinephrine to avoid hypotension problems. Avoid possible intravascular injection of the local anesthetic solution.

Drug Interactions of Dental Significance

1. Since all antipsychotics are metabolized in the liver, the P450 cytochrome enzymes (CYP2D6, CYP1A2, CYP3A4) will affect their metabolism either by increasing or decreasing blood levels.
   - Clozapine, quetiapine (Seroquel), and ziprasidone (Geodon) inhibit the metabolism of erythromycin and clarithromycin; avoid concurrent use. Consult with the patient's physician.

Guidelines for Dental Patients Taking Antipsychotics

- Anticholinergic adverse effects; monitor patients for xerostomia, root caries, and oral candidiasis.
- Monitor patients for orthostatic hypotension: Patients should remain in an upright position in the dental chair before standing.
- Greater incidence of hyperglycemia (diabetes mellitus) in patients with schizophrenia; monitor patient for periodontal disease.
- Tardive dyskinesia: Dental management may be difficult due to abnormal muscle movement.
- Limit the use of epinephrine; avoid use of epinephrine-impregnated retraction cord.

2. Most antipsychotics can cause α-adrenergic receptor blockade. Thus, epinephrine-containing local anesthetics may cause hypotension and reflex tachycardia. Epinephrine should be administered cautiously to prevent intravascular injection. The dental hygienist should monitor vital signs in patients taking antipsychotics. The maximum number of cartridges that should be used is two of 1:100,000 epinephrine. Levonordefrin should be avoided because of high toxicity.

Rapid Dental Hint

The Food and Drug Administration (FDA) has requested that manufacturers of atypical antipsychotic drugs include a warning on the label of these drugs describing the risk of off-label use (using the drug for a condition that is not FDA indicated) to older patients with dementia. These patients who have dementia and take an atypical antipsychotic show a greater mortality (death) rate.

Drugs for Mood Disorders

Mood disorders are characterized by marked mood swings and include major depressive episode (depression), dysthymia, and bipolar disorder. Mood disorders can be treated by nonpharmacological methods (e.g., psychotherapy, hypnosis, electroconvulsive therapy), pharmacotherapy, or a combination of both.

Depression

ANTIDEPRESSANTS: ETIOLOGY/DIAGNOSIS OF MAJOR DEPRESSION **Major depression** is a common illness, affecting approximately 5–10% of the population. In order to diagnose depression, a certain number of symptoms (at least five) must be present every day for at least 2 weeks. These symptoms include depressed mood, markedly diminished interest or pleasure in activities, weight gain, sleep changes, feelings of worthlessness or guilt, poor concentration, thoughts of death, and fatigue or loss of energy. Dysthymia is a milder type of depression, causing less impairment.

Mechanism of Action   There are many theories about how antidepressant drugs work. It is known that a biochemical imbalance occurs in depression. It is believed that depression causes decreased levels of norepinephrine and/or serotonin in the brain, which occurs either because of an increased breakdown of these neurotransmitters by enzymes, a decrease in their synthesis in the presynaptic neuron, or reuptake of the neurotransmitter back into the presynaptic axon terminal that released it. In any case, there are reduced levels of norepinephrine and serotonin (regulates mood) in the neuronal synapse junction. There is usually a delay of onset of action of antidepressants, taking at least 2–3 weeks until therapeutic effects are seen. Full recovery from depression may take several months.

Thus, the purpose of some antidepressant medication, such as the tricyclics and selective serotonin reuptake inhibitors, is to increase the concentration of norepinephrine and/or serotonin by inhibiting or blocking the reuptake into synaptic terminals on the neuron. The subsequent increase in the amounts of these neurotransmitters available at the synapse may compensate for their deficit seen in depressed individuals. The other type of antidepressant, MAOIs, acts by inhibiting monoamine oxidase (MAO), an enzyme responsible for the breakdown of catecholamine neurotransmitters such as epinephrine and norepinephrine.

TABLE 15-3   Classification of Antidepressants: Treatment of Major Depressive Disorder
DRUG NAME
Tricylic Antidepressants (TCAs)
Amitriptyline (Elavil)
Comipramine (Anafranil)
Desipramine (Norpramin)
Doxepin (Adapin, Sinequan)
Imipramine (Tofranil)
Nortriptyline (Pamelor)
Protriptyline (Vivactil)
Trimipramine (Surmontil)
Selective Serontonin Reuptake Inhibitors (SSRIs)
Citalopram (Celexa)
Escitalopram (Lexapro)
Fluoxetine (Prozac)
Fluvoxamine (Luvox)
Paroxetine (Paxil)
Sertraline (Zoloft)
Atypical Antidepressants
Amoxapine (Asendin)
Bupropion (Wellbutrin)
Maprotiline (Ludiomil)
Mirtazapine (Remeron)
Nefazodone (Serzone)
Trazodone (Desyrel)
Selective Serotonin Norepineprhine Reuptake Inhibitors (SNRIs)
Duloxetine (Cymbalta)
Venlafaxine (Effexor)
Desvenlafaxine (Pristiq)
Monoamine Oxidase Inhibitors (MAOIs)
Isocarboxazid (Marplan)
Phenelzine (Nardil)
Tranylcypromine (Parnate)
Herbal Supplement
St. John's wort

Classification of Antidepressants   There are different classifications of antidepressant drugs, each with a specific mechanism of action (Table 15-3):

- Tricyclic antidepressants (TCAs)
- Selective serotonin reuptake inhibitors (SSRIs)
- Monoamine oxidase inhibitors (MAOIs)

TRICYCLIC ANTIDEPRESSANTS   The *tricyclic antidepressants (TCAs)* were first introduced in 1957 and are used in the treatment of depression (Table 15-3). The TCAs work by inhibiting the reuptake or inactivation of norepinephrine and/or serotonin from the synapse, resulting in elevated levels of these neurotransmitters, which would improve the depression (Figure 15-2). Thus, TCAs act like norepinephrine/serotonin reuptake inhibitors. Besides depression, TCAs are indicated for the dental management of nocturnal bruxism and chronic orofacial pain.

Adverse Effects   The biggest problem when deciding which antidepressant to use is its adverse effect profile. Adverse effects of TCAs are due to the *nonselective* affinity and blockade of other receptors, including muscarinic (cholinergic), histaminic, and α-adrenergic receptors (Table 15-4).

Rapid Dental Hint

There are many dental adverse effects in patients taking TCAs, including xerostomia and orthostatic hypotension. Do xerostomia counseling (e.g., drink plenty of water; use salivary substitutes or moisturizers; avoid alcohol and fluoride supplements). For orthostatic hypotension: monitor blood pressure and allow patient to sit in an upright position before getting up from the dental chair.

These adverse effects can best be managed either by changing the medication or reducing the dosage. Xerostomia may be severe enough that it causes difficulty in swallowing or speech and can lead to the development of dental/root caries and periodontal disease.

Because TCAs increase heart rate, they should not be used in patients with heart conduction disorders or those recovering from a heart attack. TCAs may precipitate arrhythmias in patients with preexisting conditions.

TCAs must be discontinued slowly to avoid withdrawal symptoms. Since the advent of newer antidepressants, TCAs

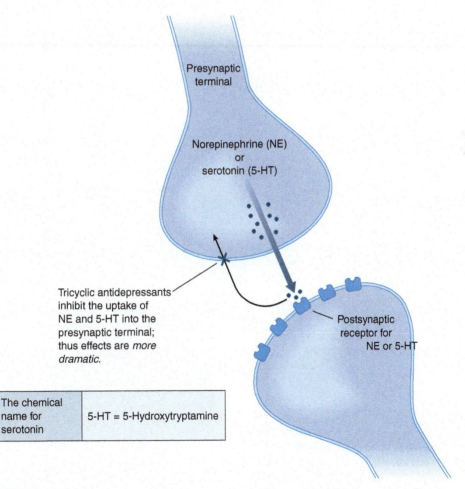

FIGURE 15-2 Tricyclic antidepressants produce their effects by inhibiting the reuptake of neurotransmitters into the nerve terminal. The neurotransmitters particularly affected are norepinephrine and serotonin.

TABLE 15-4 Major Adverse Effects of TCAs

MUSCARINIC BLOCKADE	HISTAMINE BLOCKADE	α-ADRENERGIC BLOCKADE
Xerostomia	Drowsiness, sedation	Orthostatic hypotension, dizziness
Blurred vision		
Urinary retention	Weight gain	Reflex tachycardia
	Hypotension	Sexual dysfunction
Constipation		
Increased heart rate		
Memory dysfunction		

have been used less frequently, primarily because of their low margin of safety in overdose and numerous adverse drug effects.

Drug Interactions of Dental Significance It is not necessary to avoid using epinephrine-containing local anesthetics, but to limit the amount to 0.04 mg, which is present in about two cartridges of lidocaine 2% with 1:100,000 epinephrine. Epinephrine (EPI) is inactivated by either the enzyme catechol-O-methyl transferase (COMT) or by reuptake into the nerve terminal. TCAs block the reuptake of both NE and EPI, allowing accumulating levels (Figure 15-3).

Levonordefrin-containing local anesthetic (carbocaine) is *contraindicated* in patients taking a tricyclic antidepressant because accidental intravascular (into the arteries) can result in acute hypertension and cardiac arrhythmias.

SELECTIVE SEROTONIN REUPTAKE INHIBITORS (SSRIs) The neurotransmitter serotonin (5-hydroxytryptamine; 5-HT) was discovered in 1954 to be present in the brain and that the synthesis or function was reduced in depressed individuals. In order to improve the profile of antidepressants, research started in the late 1960s aimed at developing more potent and more *selective*

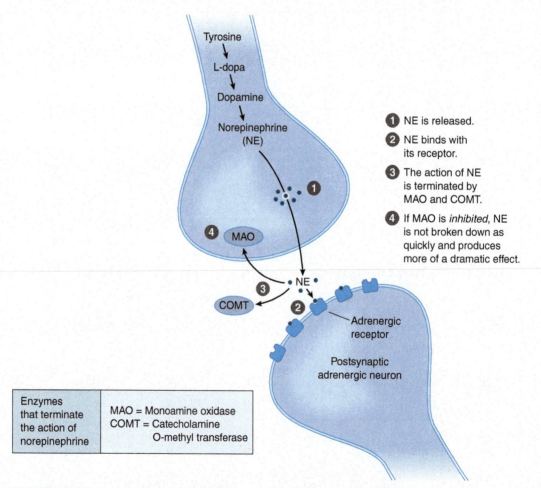

FIGURE 15-3 Termination of norepinephrine activity through enzyme activity in the synapse.

drugs for the *inhibition of serotonin reuptake.* This was desirable, since many of the adverse effects of tricyclic antidepressants are thought to be due to their nonselective binding to and blocking of receptors for acetylcholine and histamine.

Rapid Dental Hint

In patients taking an SSRI, there may be less complaints of xerostomia.

SSRIs are a type of antidepressant drug first introduced in 1988 (Table 15-3). The prototype SSRI is fluoxentine (Prozac). Development of SSRIs was intended to focus more on the increasing serotonin levels in the brain while producing fewer adverse effects. These drugs selectively inhibit serotonin reuptake into the neuron vesicles by blocking the reuptake serotonin receptor site on the presynaptic neuron, without affinity for the uptake inhibition of norepinephrine and other neurotransmitter amines (Figure 15-4). Besides depression, some SSRIs are used to treat anxiety disorders, eating disorders (anorexia nervosa or bulimia), fibromyalgia, premenstrual syndrome, obsessive–compulsive disorder, and panic disorder.

Rapid Dental Hint

In patients taking an SSRI, there are no special concerns regarding the use of epinephrine in a local anesthetic.

Adverse Effects   SSRIs do not have the same affinity to other receptors, so they do not exert the same anticholinergic, antihistaminic, anti-adrenergic effects. In general, these drugs do not cause drowsiness or sedation because they do not bind to the histamine receptors. Thus, the SSRIs have a different adverse effect profile that includes gastrointestinal discomfort (nausea, diarrhea), nervousness, headache, reduced appetite, sexual dysfunction, and weight loss. Additionally, SSRIs can induce bruxism. There is an increased risk of gastrointestinal bleeding, especially if the patient has preexisting risk factors or is taking other drugs (ibuprofen, aspirin, warfarin) that increase risk. SSRI use increases risk of bleeding by 3.6

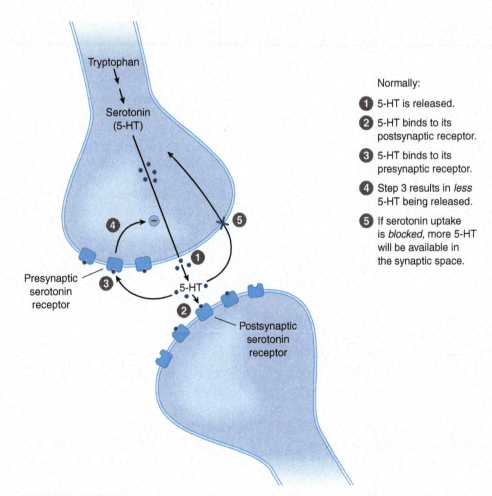

FIGURE 15-4 SSRIs block the reuptake of serotonin into nerve terminals, resulting in increased serotonin levels.

times, compared with the risk in the general population for those who don't use SSRIs, but there is a 12-fold risk increase when nonsteroidal anti-inflammatories (NSAIDs) and SSRIs are combined.

Rapid Dental Hint

In patients taking an SSRI the use of NSAIDs (e.g., ibuprofen, naproxen) is not recommended. Recommend acetaminophen.

Drug–Drug–Food Interactions   In January 2006, the FDA-approved safety labeling revisions for venlafaxine (Effexor and Effexor XR) to warn of the risk for sustained hypertension associated with their use in some patients. Monitor blood pressure in these patients.

A "serotonin syndrome" can occur due to elevated serotonin blood levels that are potentially very dangerous and fatal. This usually is caused by a combination of two or more drugs, one of which is an SSRI and the other a MAOI. Symptoms include severe hypertension, rapid eye movement, rapid muscle contraction, feeling drunk, dizziness, confusion, diarrhea, and eventually cardiovascular collapse and death.

Since serotonin reuptake blockade has no effect on the disposition of EPI because EPI uses the NE reuptake pump, there are no precautions or concerns for using EPI in patients taking SSRIs.

SEROTONIN-NOREPINEPHRINE REUPTAKE INHIBITORS (SNRIs)   Serotonin-norepinephrine reuptake inhibitors (SNRIs) work by inhibiting the reuptake of the neurotransmitters serotonin and norepinephrine. This results in an increase in the concentrations of serotonin and norepinephrine.

ATYPICAL ANTIDEPRESSANTS   There are other types of antidepressants that have action similar to the TCAs but are classified as atypical. These drugs include nefazodone (Serzone), bupropion (Wellbutrin), maprotiline (Ludiomil), and trazodone (Desyrel) (Table 15-3).

Guidelines for Dental Patients Taking Antidepressants

- Limit use of epinephrine to two cartridges of 2% lidocaine with 1:100,000 epinephrine if patient is taking a TCA.
- No concerns with the use of EPI in a patient taking a SSRI.
- Monitor for xerostomia: caries, periodontal disease (SSRIs produce less xerostomia than TCAs).
- Use caution with orthostatic hypotension (usually with TCAs). Monitor blood pressure.

Rapid Dental Hint

Bupropion (Wellbutrin), an antidepressant, is also used as a smoking cessation drug and is marketed as Zyban.

MONOAMINE OXIDASE INHIBITORS (MAOIs)

Drug–Drug–Food Interactions of Dental Significance   MAOIs may increase action of sympathominmetics (e.g., epinephrine in lidocaine, phenylephrine, pseudoephedrine); it is not necessary to avoid using epinephrine (EPI), but limit its use to 0.04 mg, the amount present in two cartridges of lidocaine 2% with 1:100,000 epinephrine; avoid levonordefrin. While the patient is taking an MAOI, they must not eat any foods containing tyramine, including aged cheeses, bananas, raisins, avocados, aged meat, soy sauce, yeast, beer, wines, yogurt, sour cream, bologna, salami, hot dogs, green figs, sauerkraut, and pickled herring.

DID YOU KNOW?

Antidepressants were originally developed as antihistamines. They were discovered in the 1950s. The first modern antidepressant, iproniazid, was originally developed to treat tuberculosis, but it was found that it was mood elevating and stimulated activity in patients. The first tricyclic antidepressant was imipramine.

HERBAL REMEDIES   Herbal remedies for the treatment of depression are not approved by the U.S. Food and Drug Administration. There are concerns over the "purity" of the ingredients in the formulations as well as their efficacy. An example of an herbal supplement that is not FDA approved for the management of depression is St. John's wort, which comes from the flowering plant *Hypericum perforatum*. There are many adverse side effects, including xerostomia, GI disturbances, restlessness, headache, dizziness, and confusion.

Rapid Dental Hint

Antidepressants increase the risk of suicidal thinking and behavior (suicidality) in short-term studies in children and adolescents with major depressive disorder (MDD) and other psychiatric disorders. Children and adolescents taking antidepressant medication must be aware and observed closely for suicidality. In 2004, this warning was added to the beginning of the package insert in bolded font and enclosed in a black box. Additionally, there is a warning for clinical worsening and suicide risk in adult patients with MDD.

Bipolar Disorders (BPD)

Bipolar disorder (BPD) is a common chronic, serious psychiatric condition characterized by an irregular course of episodes of mania and depression. An individual can experience manic, hypomanic, depressive, and mixed episodes. Bipolar disorder is most commonly misdiagnosed as unipolar (major) depression because patients often present while at the depressive rather than the manic stage, and thus are incorrectly treated. The older term for this condition is manic depression. Patients with undiagnosed bipolar disorder are at increased risk for suicide. To be diagnosed with BPD the individual must have the following episodes for a specific duration of time:

- *Manic episodes* (or mania) are characterized by an abnormally elevated or irritable mood; aggressive, happy, euphoric, grandiose (exaggerated sense of self-importance), impulsive behavior; decreased sleep; and increased activity. Must have symptoms for at least 1 week.
- *Hypomanic episodes* are not full-blown mania but a milder form that does not interfere with an individual's daily functioning. At least 4 days with three or more symptoms.
- *Depressive episodes* are characterized by feeling sad, decreased interest (low mood), low self-esteem, sleep disturbance, and appetite disturbance. At least 2 weeks with five or more symptoms most of the day/nearly every day.

Mixed episodes are characterized by both mania and depression (both high and low mood) over a 1-week period.

DSM-IV classifies bipolar disorders as:

- *Bipolar I disorder:* Considered the classic form of manic depression, in which manic, depressive, hypomanic, or mixed states can occur. There must be a full manic episode for a diagnosis of bipolar I.
- *Bipolar II disorder:* Patients never experienced a full manic episode, but have experienced at least one hypomanic episode and at least one episode of major depression.
- *Cyclothymic disorder:* Chronic (more than 2 years), fluctuating mood disturbances involving many periods of mild

hypomanic and depressive symptoms that do not meet the criteria for either mania or major depression.

In most cases, patients with major depression/mood disorder have shown a tendency toward certain comorbid conditions in which there is another illness associated with the depression/mania, such as substance abuse or anxiety.

PHASES OF TREATMENT Standard pharmacological treatment of symptoms of bipolar disorder involves (Table 15-5):

- Acute therapy: treatment of the acute episode of the manic and depressed stage
- Maintenance therapy: prevention of the relapse of these episodes

Many types of drugs are used to treat BPD, including mood stabilizers, antidepressants, and antipsychotics. *Mood stabilizers* to treat the mania exert their effects by "stabilizing from above," and *antidepressants* to treat the depression exert their effects by "stabilizing mood from below." In 2002, the American Psychiatric Association (APA) updated its guidelines for the treatment of patients with bipolar disorder. The main changes reflected the shifts in the evidence for use of treatment other than lithium.

> ### DID YOU KNOW?
>
> Napoleon and Beethoven are just a few of the famous people diagnosed with bipolar disorder.

Treatment of the Manic/Mixed (Acute) Episode Although most of the data of the effectiveness of mood stabilizers in bipolar illness come from studies using monotherapy (one drug), in clinical practice most bipolar patients are treated with more than one drug. Combination therapy also has the potential to improve the therapeutic:side effect ratio and for long-term stabilization.

TABLE 15-5 Common Bipolar Disorder Medications	
DRUG NAME	**DENTAL MANAGEMENT**
Lithium carbonate (Eskalith)	• Medical consult with the patient's physician may be necessary. • Have patient sit in upright position in dental chair before getting up. • Dry mouth: Advise patient to drink water, avoid alcohol-containing mouthrinses, use artificial saliva (if needed), and brush frequently. • Lithium can cause orthostatic hypotension: monitor BP and patient should sit in upright position in dental chair before standing.
Carbamazepine (Equetro)	• Monitor for a decrease in WBC counts. • Monitor cardiovascular signs at each visit.
Gabapentin (Neurontin)	• Monitor for xerostomia.
Lamotrigine (Lamictal)	• Lamotrigine can cause orthostatic hypotension: monitor BP and patient should sit in upright position in dental chair before standing.
Valproic acid (Depakene),	• Monitor the patient's clotting.

APA recommends as stage 1 primary agents:

- For *mild* acute manic (agitated) episode (monotherapy): lithium, divalproex (valproate/valproic acid), or an atypical antipsychotic such as risperidone (Risperdal), ziprasidone (Geodon), aripiprazole (Abilify), olanzapine (Zyprexa), or quetiapine (Seroquel)
- For *mixed* episode: divalproex, aripiprazole, risperidone, or ziprasidone
- For *severe* manic or mixed episodes (two-drug combination): lithium + atypical antipsychotic *or* valproate plus an atypical antipsychotic

Lithium (Lithobid)   Discovered in 1949, lithium is the gold standard mood stabilizer. The specific mechanism of action in mania is relatively unknown. By decreasing or preventing manic episodes, subsequent depression episodes may be avoided. Lithium may also help to reduce rapid cycling (four or more episodes of mania, hypomania, or depression in the preceding 12 months) experienced by some patients. Patients taking lithium alone had significantly fewer suicide attempts.

Since lithium has an FDA black-box warning for a *narrow therapeutic index,* blood tests must be taken to find the optimal therapeutic dosage and to avoid toxicity even at doses close to therapeutic levels. Chronic lithium toxicity generally occurs after long-term therapy with high dosages.

DID YOU KNOW?

When the soda 7-Up was originally introduced in the 1930s, it contained lithium.

Since lithium is widely distributed throughout the body, there are numerous adverse effects, involving the central nervous system, gastrointestinal tract, cardiovascular system, kidneys (renal), blood system (hematological), urinary tract, and skin. Some of these adverse effects include cardiac arrhythmias, fine hand tremor, polydipsia (increase in thirst), polyuria (increase in urination), dizziness, drowsiness, tongue movements, xerostomia, metallic taste, dry skin, hypothyroidism, diarrhea, and an increase in white blood cell count (neutrophilia).

There are multiple drug–drug interactions with lithium. Since lithium is 100% orally absorbed from the gastrointestinal tract and excreted unchanged in the urine there are many drugs that alter its clearance. Metronidazole taken with lithium may increase lithium toxicity. Since lithium is not metabolized in the liver, the cytochrome P450 enzymes are not involved in these drug interactions.

Nonsteroidal anti-inflammatory drugs (e.g., ibuprofen) increase lithium blood levels by decreasing its clearance in the urine.

Rapid Dental Hint

In patients taking lithium *do not* recommend NSAIDs (e.g., ibuprofen, naproxen sodium). There is a drug–drug interaction that increases lithium levels. Consult with patient's physician.

In patients taking lithium do not prescribe metronidazole (an antibiotic). Use another antibiotic or consult with the patient's physician.

Since lithium can decrease salivary flow, it is important to assess the patient for caries, periodontal diseases, and oral candidiasis. A lichenoid drug reaction can occur with lithium. Since lithium can cause orthostatic hypotension, the dental hygienist should monitor vital signs and have the patient remain in the dental chair in an upright position for a few minutes before standing up.

Divalproex Sodium (Depakote)   In 1995, divalproex sodium (Depakote) was the first anticonvulsant approved as a mood stabilizer, and is most effective in treating mixed episodes. Often it is combined with lithium in lower doses to reduce adverse effects and improve therapeutic response.

Divalproex sodium is a compound comprised of sodium valproate and valproic acid, and dissociates to the valproate ion in the gastrointestinal tract. Divalproex acts by increasing levels of Γ (gamma)-aminobutyric acid (GABA), a neurotransmitter in the brain, either by inhibiting its metabolism or by enhancing postsynaptic GABA activity.

The most commonly reported gastrointestinal adverse effects reported at the beginning of therapy are nausea and vomiting and indigestion. Inhibition of platelet aggregation may cause altered bleeding times. It is recommended that valproate blood concentration and platelet counts be monitored once weekly during acute treatment with maintenance monitoring as clinically indicated. Valproate can produce teratogenic effects

Rapid Dental Hint

Dental management of patients taking lithium:

1. Do xerostomia counseling and assess patient for caries, candidiasis, and periodontal disease
2. Patients complaining of a dry mouth may be suffering from dehydration due to lithium-induced polyuria (increased thirst). Refer patient to their physician.
3. Tongue movements: try using the mouth mirror for tongue control.
4. Monitor for orthostatic hypotension: take blood pressure and allow patient to remain in an upright position before dismissing.

such as neural tube defects. Divalproex is available as enteric-coated tablets and extended-release tablets, which allow for absorption in the small intestine and not the stomach, where GI adverse effects occur. Additional adverse effects include weight gain and hair loss.

Rapid Dental Hint

Patients taking valproate may have increased bleeding during periodontal procedures because it impairs platelet aggregation. It is important to see blood values before treatment. Send for a medical consultation.

It is well absorbed orally from the gastrointestinal tract and is about 90% bound to plasma proteins, so it displaces and is displaced by other drugs highly protein bound, such as warfarin, aspirin, and phenytoin.

The FDA has a black-box warning for hepatic failure, which may result in death. The drug is extensively metabolized in the liver by the cytochrome P450 system.

Rapid Dental Hint

Patients taking lithium, valproate, and carbamazepine should have blood values monitored and reported. Ask your patient about his or her blood values.

There is increased chance of bleeding if taken with aspirin or a nonsteroidal anti-inflammatory drug.

Atypical Antipsychotics   The APA recommends the use of an atypical antipsychotic as monotherapy for less ill patients or in combination with lithium for more severely ill patients.

Olanzapine   Olanzapine (Zyprexa), the first atypical antipsychotic drug approved as a mood-stabilizing drug, has been FDA approved since 2000. It is used either as monotherapy for manic episodes or as an add-on agent for mania partially responsive to conventional mood-stabilizing drugs. Olanzapine and aripiprazole (Abilify) are the only drugs FDA approved for relapse prevention of manic episodes. There are no established blood levels associated with antimanic response, so there is no need for blood level monitoring.

Quetiapine   Quetiapine (Seroquel) is an antipsychotic agent that is FDA approved for acute manic episodes. Since it may cause orthostatic hypotension, use caution with dental patients when uprighting from the dental chair.

Anti-epileptic Mood Stabilizers: Carbamazepine   Carbamazepine (Equetro) is an anticonvulsant drug used to treat acute bipolar I mania and mixed episodes, and is better for long-term use. Fatigue is a common and annoying adverse effect, which makes adherence a problem. Because of its similarity in chemical structure to tricyclic antidepressants, MAOIs should not be given concurrently. Carbamazepine is metabolized by the CYP3A4 isoenzymes in the liver. Many dental drugs such as erythromycin, clarithromycin, and ciprofloxacin inhibit the metabolism of carbamazepine, causing increased blood levels (Table 15-5).

Other Anti-epileptic Drugs for Treatment of Bipolar Disorder   If the patient does not respond to these drugs, several newer anticonvulsants such as lamotrigine (Lamictal) and gabapentin (Neurontin) may be effective. Lamotrigine is indicated in the depressed phase of bipolar disorder or as adjunctive add-on in acute mania. It has been associated with development of a severe systemic rash. On September 29, 2006, the FDA announced that first-trimester exposure to lamotrigine may increase the risk for cleft lip or palate in newborns.

Rapid Dental Hint

Patients taking carbamazepine: erythromycin and clarithromycin increase blood levels of carbamazepine by inhibiting the metabolism of carbamazepine. Management: Choose a different antibiotic like azithromycin or consult with patient's physician.

TREATMENT OF THE DEPRESSIVE EPISODES OF BIPOLAR DISORDER   As mentioned earlier, bipolar depression can be difficult to recognize and distinguish from generalized depression. Currently, lithium is the only proven agent for treatment of bipolar depression, but lamotrignine is also shown good results. Other drugs include a combination of olanzapine and fluoxetine (Prozac). Antidepressant monotherapy is not recommended due to the chance of starting a manic episode or inducing a pattern of rapid cycling; the evidence of long-term effectiveness of antidepressant therapy is also weak.

If the acute depressive episode does not respond to these medications, the next step would be to add on bupropion (Wellbutrin) or paroxetine (Paxil). Alternative secondary steps include adding an SSRI or venlafaxine (Effexor). For patients who are severely depressed, electroconvulsive therapy should be considered.

MAINTENANCE PHASE FOR BIPOLAR I DISORDER   Once the acute crisis is over, patients may remain at particularly high risk of relapse for up to 6 months. This phase of treatment, also referred to as continuation treatment, is aimed at preventing recurrences of mood episodes (depression, mania, hypomania, mixed episodes) and maximizing the patient's quality of life.

APA Guidelines for Treating Manic and Depressive Episodes in Bipolar Disorder	
EPISODES	**DRUGS**
Manic/Mixed	
Severe	*Two-drug combination:* Lithium or valproate + atypical antipsychotic (such as olanzapine or risperidone) (Alternative: carbamazepine)
Moderate (less severe)	*Monotherapy:* Lithium, valproate, or an atypical antipsychotic (olanzapine)
Depressive	
First-line pharmacological treatment	Lithium *or* lamotrigine
Alternative, especially for severely ill	Lithium + antidepressant
Depressive episode that does not respond to first-line treatment	Add: lamotrigine, bupropion, *or* paroxetine (Alternative step: Add an SSRI)
Maintenance	Lithium, valproate
	(Alternatives: lamotrigine, olanzapine, carbamazepine)

Drugs approved for maintenance therapy in bipolar illness (American Psychiatric Association, 2005) include lamotrigine (Lamictal), lithium, or valproate. Lamotrigine is especially effective in preventing relapse into depression; lithium is more effective in preventing relapse of mania. The addition of an antidepressant to lithium maintenance therapy has failed to prevent bipolar depression.

Anxiolytics (Anti-Anxiety Agents)

Anxiety disorders are the most common type of psychiatric disorder, but less than 30% of people will seek treatment. Anxiety is an emotion experienced by almost everyone. It is important to distinguish normal fears from abnormal anxiety. Usually, if an individual is in a situation that may be conceived as threatening or dangerous, a state of anxiety is produced; however, if anxiety occurs without sufficient reason and interferes with an individual's health, then it is referred to as pathological anxiety. Only pathological anxiety needs to be treated.

Anxiety has an effect on the body (somatic) as well as psychological changes. Symptoms of anxiety include chest pain, tachycardia, trembling, tremors, restlessness, abdominal pain, diarrhea, fatigue, palpitations, insomnia, irritability, headache, dizziness, shortness of breath, profuse sweating, apprehension, and nausea. Chronic stress and anxiety may contribute to increased acid production and development of ulcers. The individual appears to be nervous, frightened, and has a feeling of impending doom. The individual actually enhances his or her somatic symptoms into a serious medical condition.

The DSM-IV-TR™ divides clinical anxiety into the following components:

- Generalized anxiety disorder (GAD)
- Panic disorder
- Phobias
- Posttraumatic stress disorder (PTSD)
- Obsessive–compulsive disorder (OCD)
- Other anxiety disorders (e.g., alcohol-induced anxiety disorder, substance-induced anxiety disorder, or separation anxiety)

To be diagnosed as generalized anxiety disorder, the anxiety must be present continuously for at least 6 months. Obsessive–compulsive disorder is characterized by the presence of persistent thoughts and impulses that need to be carried out purposively. Panic disorder is characterized by unexpected, recurrent periods of intense fear that last several minutes. Posttraumatic stress disorder occurs after exposure to a psychologically distressing event where physical harm is anticipated.

There are many theories as to the etiology of anxiety. Normal arousal occurs with antagonism of the inhibitory neurotransmitter called GABA (gamma-aminobutyric acid), resulting in elevated GABA levels in the brain. If this arousal is consistent and GABA is continuously fired, a clinically apparent anxiety state develops. Serotonin is also involved in the pathogenesis of anxiety.

Pharmacology

BENZODIAZEPINES Benzodiazepines are the drug of choice in the pharmacological treatment of generalized anxiety disorder because they are the most rapidly acting and effective anxiolytic agent (Table 15-6). But they do have side effects, including sedation and physical dependency. Some states (including New York) require that benzodiazepines be a Schedule II controlled drug just like narcotics because of its abuse potential.

Benzodiazepines are used for short-term treatment for the acutely anxious patient experiencing functional disability, and should not be used for the treatment of mild anxiety or depression. Duration of therapy is usually 2–6 months. For long-term treatment, an antidepressant such as an SSRI (selective serotonin reuptake inhibitor) or SMRI (selective mixed reuptake inhibitor) should be considered.

Mechanism of Action Benzodiazepines bind to receptors on GABA and stimulate or activate them by increasing membrane permeability to chloride ions. This results in an increased effect of GABA, which is an inhibitory neurotransmitter. Decreased GABA levels in the brain are supposed to reduce/eliminate anxiety symptoms.

Indications Benzodiazepines have a wide range of indications due to their different dose levels, onset, and duration of actions. Benzodiazepines are classified as anxiolytics (relief of anxiety), sedatives (tranquilizing), hypnotics (sleep-inducing drugs), muscle relaxants, and anticonvulsants. The anti-anxiety effect is caused by sedation, while the hypnotic effect produces insomnia. The short-acting, rapid-onset benzodiazepines, e.g., lorazepam (Ativan), alprazolam (Xanax) at low doses relieve dental anxiety with little sedation, which is unique with these drugs. But at higher doses, lorazepam is a sedative/hypnotic taken at bedtime. A benzodiazepine that has an onset of 15–45 minutes and is intermediate/long acting is best to induce sleep in insomniacs. These drugs are classified as hypnotics. Benzodiazepines are also used in the treatment of alcohol withdrawal. Thus deciding which drug to use depends on the condition being treated and the pharmacokinetics of the drug.

Drugs with a long elimination half-life such as diazepam (Valium) should not be given to elderly patients because they have a reduced metabolism and may not be able to metabolize the drug efficiently, resulting in elevated blood levels and toxicity. However, an advantage of benzodiazepines is the wide margin of safety between therapeutic and toxic doses, so there is a less likely chance of overdosing.

Adverse Effects   All of the benzodiazepines are similar in effects, with the most common side effect being central nervous system (CNS) depression, including sedation, drowsiness, and respiratory depression. Sedation is dose related: The higher the dose, the more sedation occurs. Xerostomia is a dental-related side effect that should be monitored in patients.

Tolerance does occur within 3–14 days; more and more of the drug is needed to get a therapeutic response. Because of this, overdosing is also less likely to occur. Dependence is most likely to occur in patients with a past history of alcoholism or substance abuse if taken for prolonged periods of time (even with normal doses, dependence may occur as soon as within 4–6 weeks of starting the drug). Excessive ingestion (overdose) is not likely to result in respiratory depression.

Withdrawal symptoms occur if benzodiazepines are taken for long periods. When discontinuing the drug, the dose should be decreased slowly over time. Benzodiazepines with short half-lives such as alprazolam have the greatest tendency for dependency and withdrawal symptoms. Thus the lowest possible dose for the shortest period of time is the best regimen, which may be difficult since many patients with anxiety or panic disorder may be in treatment for months to years. Intravenous flumazenil (Mazicon, Romazicon) antagonizes the effects of benzodiazepines on the CNS, including sedation and psychomotor impairment.

The benzodiazepines should not be given to women in the first trimester of pregnancy, or in patients with alcohol intoxication, acute angle glaucoma, or a history of substance abuse.

Drug–Drug Interactions of Dental Significance   Alcohol and other CNS depressants should be avoided to prevent additional drowsiness and sedation. Benzodiazepines are metabolized by the liver P450 enzymes (CYP3A4). They are either transformed by oxidative pathways in the liver or metabolized by conjugation into water-soluble products in the liver, whereby the metabolite products formed are inactive. Epinephrine is not contraindicated with benzodiazepines (Table 15-6).

Rapid Dental Hint

Dental management of patients taking benzodiazepines [e.g., alprazolam (Xanax)]:

1. Do xerostomia counseling and assess patient for caries, candidiasis, and periodontal disease. More frequent maintenance appointments for fluoride application. Recommend salivary substitutes/artificial saliva, chewing gum with xylitol, avoid alcohol (even alcohol-containing mouthrinses), and more frequent sipping of water.

2. Consider the patient's stress level; may have shorter appointments

3. No special limitations in using epinephrine

4. Do not give erythromycin or clarithromycin with any benzodiazepine. Use azithromycin.

OTHER DRUGS: GAD   Drugs other than benzodiazepines have been used to treat anxiety. All drugs with serotonin reuptake inhibiting properties are effective in treating general anxiety disorder (GAD). Buspirone (Buspar) is a nonbenzodiazepine that is an agonist at serotonin type 1A receptors and is effective in the treatment of some anxiety disorders. It is very well tolerated by patients. Buspirone should not be given to patients also taking MAOIs.

Propranolol, a β-blocker, has also been used to relieve anxiety. Propranolol does not act centrally in the brain to relieve symptoms of anxiety, but reduces the autonomic symptoms of anxiety (e.g., the tachycardia that results from anxiety).

Sedative/Hypnotic Drugs

A sedative/hypnotic drug is a sedative that depresses activity of the central nervous system and reduces anxiety and tension and induces sleep.

Barbiturates

Barbiturates at one time were used in the treatment of anxiety, but are no longer because of their ability to cause overdosing, tolerance (more of the drug is needed to produce the same therapeutic effect), and dependence (increased need to want a psychoactive drug), and have been replaced by the benzodiazepines. Barbiturates are used mainly as:

• Hypnotics (tranquilizing, sleep inducing) in the short-term (2-week) treatment of insomnia (sleep disturbance)

• Anticonvulsants in the treatment of seizures

• Preoperatively to relieve anxiety and provide sedation

The benzodiazepines are also used as sedatives/hypnotics and anticonvulsants and have fewer adverse effects than

TABLE 15-6 Commonly Used Anxiolytics: Drugs for Treatment of Generalized Anxiety Disorders

DRUG NAME	MECHANISM/INDICATION
Benzodiazepines	Stimulates the inhibitory neurotransmitter GABA
Alprazolam (Xanax; Niravam—orally dissolving)	Panic disorder; dental anxiety
Lorazepam (Ativan)	Dental anxiety
Chlordiazepoxide HCl (Librium, Libritabs)	Anti-anxiety; alcohol withdrawal; preoperative sedation; sedative/hypnotic
Clonazepam (Klonopin)	Panic disorder
Diazepam (Valium)	Dental anxiety, alcohol withdrawal; anticonvulsant (IV), skeletal muscle relaxant; very rapid onset
Halazepam (Paxipam)	Anti-anxiety; treat phobias
Clorazepate (Tranxene)	Dental anxiety; very rapid onset
Buspirone (Buspar)	Selective serotonin receptor agonists; only has anxiolytic properties
Hydroxyzine (Atarax)	Antihistamine; pruritus; preoperative and postoperative sedation

barbiturates. When taken for insomnia (difficulty in sleeping), barbiturates can cause hangover and daytime sedation and if used longer than 2 weeks, the drugs lose their effectiveness in producing sleep. Today, it is preferred to use the benzodiazepines as sedative-hypnotics and anxiolytics because benzodiazepines have a higher therapeutic index, making them a safer drug.

When taken orally, barbiturates pass the blood–brain barrier into the brain and produce changes in CNS moods, ranging from excitation, to mild sedation, to hypnosis (altered state of awareness) and to anesthesia in high doses. Barbiturates produce respiratory and brain depression. Death can occur in an overdose.

PHARMACOLOGY These drugs work similarly to the benzodiazepines by enhancing the binding of GABA to GABA receptors, increasing GABA activity, and allowing chloride ion channels to open.

In usual dosages, barbiturates also suppress respiratory activity, such as seen in sleep.

Barbiturates are classified according to their lipid solubility and duration of action (Table 15-7). Ultrashort-acting barbiturates are highly lipid-soluble and have a very short duration of action. They are used as IV anesthetics, and are not given orally.

Short- and intermediate-acting barbiturates [pentobarbital (Nembutal)] are less lipid-soluble and their effects last longer than the ultrashort-acting barbiturates. These drugs are used for sleep induction (sleeping pills).

Long-acting barbiturates are the least lipid-soluble, with much longer duration of action. These drugs are used as sedatives for a tranquilizing or anti-anxiety effect.

Barbiturates are slowly metabolized in the liver by the liver P450 microsomal enzymes.

ADVERSE EFFECTS Adverse effects include drowsiness, headache, nausea, and vomiting, impaired consciousness, excitement, and CNS depression. In toxic doses, death occurs by respiratory depression. With continued use, development of tolerance and dependency are likely, which makes the ultrashort-acting barbiturates, such as pentobarbital, a frequently intentionally abused drug. Dependency presents a clinical picture similar to alcoholism. Ingestion of excessive quantities of barbiturates usually results in respiratory depression and coma.

These drugs are addicting. Abrupt discontinuation of barbiturates can cause withdrawal symptoms consisting of tremors, nausea, vomiting, seizures, and cardiac arrest.

Barbiturates used for insomnia are only given for short-term usage because chronic use can cause rebound insomnia.

DRUG–DRUG INTERACTIONS OF DENTAL SIGNIFICANCE Barbiturates induce P450 enzymes in the liver, which increases the metabolism of many drugs.

OTHER SEDATIVE/HYPNOTIC MEDICATIONS

Chloral Hydrate Chloral hydrate (Noctec) is a prodrug; it must be metabolized in the liver to its active form. It is used primarily for sedation in children and is frequently used in the dental office as pre-anesthetic sedation before a dental procedure. It has an unpleasant taste and has a low therapeutic index, indicating it has a high incidence of toxicity.

Zolpidem Zolpidem (Ambien) is used as a hypnotic in patients with problems with early morning awakening. It is used only for short-term treatment of insomnia.

Zaleplon Zaleplon (Sonata) is used on a short-term basis in patients who have difficulty with falling asleep or morning grogginess. Possible drug interactions occur with rifampin, phenytoin, carbamazepine, and phenobarbital.

Attention-Deficit/Hyperactivity Disorder (ADHD)

Many children seen in the dental office may be diagnosed with attention-deficit/hyperactivity disorder (ADHD). It affects 3–5% of all children, and approximately 2 million American

TABLE 15-7 Sedative/Hypnotics: Induction of Sleep	
DRUG NAME	**USES**
Benzodiazepines	
Short-acting hypnotics	To induce sleep (conscious/preoperative sedation) Used for sedation in dental offices
Midazolam (Versed)	Intravenous
Triazolam (Halcion)	Very rapid onset
Intermediate-acting hypnotics	To induce sleep
Estazolam (Prosom)	Rapid onset
Temazepam (Restoril)	Rapid onset
Long-acting hypnotics	To induce sleep
Flurazepam (Dalmane)	Very rapid onset
Quazepam (Doral)	Rapid onset
Zaleplon (Sonata)	Rapid onset, very short duration; short-term treatment of insomnia—must dose during the night
Zolpidem (Ambien)	Selectively binds to serotonin-1 receptor; short-term treatment of insomnia (2–3 weeks); rapid onset
Others Chloral hydrate (Noctec)	Rapid onset; short-term sedative/hypnotic to allay anxiety or induce sedation preoperatively; reduce anxiety; associated with drug withdrawal
Barbiturates	All barbiturates increase GABA activity and are sedative/hypnotics
Phenobarbital (Luminal)	Sedative/hypnotic; epilepsy (anticonvulsant)
Intermediate/Short-Acting	Insomnia (sleep disorder)
Amobarbital (Amytal)	Sedation (insomnia), anxiety, preanesthetic medication (for hypnotic effects)
Butabarbital (Butisol)	Sedative
Pentobarbital (Nembutal)	Sedative/hypnotic (insomnia) (short-term use only)
Secobarbital (Seconal)	Sedative/hypnotic (insomnia) (short-term use only)

children. Children with ADHD have difficulty concentrating on certain tasks, do not have a wide attention span, and are easily distracted. Adults are now being diagnosed with ADHD. Signs and symptoms include forgetting appointments, difficulty staying seated, and constantly losing things.

The goal of treatment is to improve behavior and academic performance in children. If diagnosed properly, these children are taking a CNS stimulant (Schedule II drugs) such as an amphetamine (Adderall XR). These drugs have sympathomimetic effects, and the amount of epinephrine-containing local anesthetics should be kept to a minimum. Vital signs should be monitored. Methylphenidate (Concerta) and atomoxetine (Strattera) are other drugs used in the management of ADHD.

Use of Anti-Anxiety Drugs in the Dental Office

Dental clinicians can prescribe anti-anxiety drugs for sedation of the apprehensive dental patient, treatment for bruxism, and orofacial pain (Table 15-8).

Anxious Dental Patient

Benzodiazepines are considered the drug of choice for relieving anxiety associated with dental procedures. Benzodiazepines are anti-anxiety drugs. The most commonly used oral benzodiazepines are diazepam (Valium), triazolam (Halcion), clorazepate (Tranxene), and lorazepam (Ativan). Generally, these drugs are given in a single dose either the night before or one hour before the dental procedure. An adverse side effect of benzodiazepines is sedation. Triazolam, which has a more rapid onset of action and shorter half-life, shows less postoperative sedation. The patient should have a designated driver taking them to and from the dental office.

Intravenous benzodiazepines such as diazepam (Valium) and midazolam (Versed) are used in the dental office for conscious sedation. Complications may arise during intravenous administration of these drugs, and must be recognized for early and appropriate treatment. Venipuncture complications include hematoma, fluid extravasation, and intra-arterial drug injection. Drug-related side effects such as nausea and vomiting can occur. Practitioners must have emergency drugs and equipment available in the dental office at all times.

Bruxism

Many patients who have nocturnal bruxism also have anxiety problems. The management of bruxism is using appliances and in some cases medications. A benzodiazepine such as diazepam (Valium) 5–10 mg or clorazepate (Tranxene) taken at bedtime can be effective in these patients. Benzodiazepines should not be used for more than 2 weeks because of the potential for abuse

TABLE 15-8 Anti-Anxiety Drugs Used in the Dental Office

CONDITION	DRUG	DOSE	DENTAL MANAGEMENT
Apprehensive patient	*Benzodiazepines:*		Postoperative sedation; abuse/dependence issues
	Diazepam (Valium)	5–10 mg one hour before dental treatment	Do not give to patients who are also taking phenytoin (Dilantin) and cimetidine (Tagamet)
	Lorazepam (Ativan)	1–2mg one hour before dental procedure	Avoid with alcohol and other CNS depressants
	Triazolam (Halcion)	0.25–0.5 mg one hour before dental treatment	Diazepam and triazolam decreased metabolism with erythromycin
Bruxism	*Benzodiazepines:*		
	Diazepam (Valium)	5–10 mg at bedtime (limited therapy to 2 weeks)	Abuse/dependence issues
			Do not give to patients who are also taking phenytoin (Dilantin) and cimetidine (Tagamet)
			Avoid with alcohol and other CNS depressants
	Antidepressants:		
	Amitriptyline (Elavil)	Starting dose: 10 mg at bedtime, then gradually increase	Anticholinergic side effects, including xerostomia
	Doxepin (Sinequan)		
Chronic Orofacial Pain	*Antidepressants:*		
	Amitriptyline (Elavil)	Initial dosing 10–25 mg at bedtime with weekly increments to a target dose of 25–150 mg	

and dependency. Tricyclic antidepressants such as amitriptyline (Elavil) can also be used when appliance therapy has failed. The starting dose is 10 mg at bedtime and gradually increases every few days.

Dental Hygiene Applications

Drugs used in psychiatry have many adverse effects that are implicated in dental treatment. There is a high incidence of dry mouth, which can be so severe that a mouth mirror can stick to the oral mucosa. Instruct the patient to drink plenty of water and use a saliva substitute available at the pharmacy. Examples of saliva substitutes are Optimoist Liquid and Salivart Synthetic Saliva Solution. Reduction in salivary flow can also cause candidiasis. The patient should be instructed to avoid alcohol, smoking, and antihistamines, which also reduce salivation.

Since patients with dry mouth are prone to caries, regular in-office fluoride treatment and/or self-applied fluorides may be indicated. A 0.05% sodium fluoride over-the-counter rinse (e.g., PreviDent) or 0.4% stannous fluoride over-the-counter gel (e.g., GelKam) may be useful for home use.

To prevent dental/root caries, foods that are high in sugar and acid should be avoided; sugar promotes bacterial growth and acid causes demineralization. Instruct the patient to use a soft or extra-soft toothbrush.

The **extrapyramidal side effects** seen with antipsychotics may pose a patient management problem. The patient may be in constant motion, moving the lips, tongue, and head. Unfortunately, nothing can be done to eliminate this; the dental clinician has to be aware of it so injuries can be avoided.

Many antipsychotics block α-adrenergic receptors, resulting in hypotension (postural), angina, and diarrhea. Patients should remain sitting upright in the dental chair for a few minutes before rising.

There is no compelling evidence that antipsychotic drugs cause diabetes, but there is a greater prevalence of hyperglycemia in patients with serious mental illness. Patients with schizophrenia have an eightfold to tenfold higher risk of diabetes than the general population. It has been documented that diabetes is an established risk factor of periodontal diseases. Thus patients taking antipsychotic medications for schizophrenia should be monitored for the periodontal diseases.

There is much controversy regarding the use of local anesthetics containing vasoconstrictors. The question arises as to whether the use of EPI in cardiac patients and in patients taking antidepressants (other than SSRIs and drugs that do not affect the levels of NE/EPI) will increase blood pressure and heart rate. The use of epinephrine in local anesthetics as a vasoconstrictor is *not* contraindicated in patients taking antidepressants, antipsychotics, anxiolytics, or barbiturates. Since some antidepressants (e.g., tricyclic antidepressants) inhibit the reuptake of norepine-phrine, it was presumed that there would be an additive effect with epinephrine (from the local anesthetic) in the synaptic area, which could possibly result in a hypertensive crisis (extremely elevated blood pressure). Epinephrine contained in local anes-thetics functions as a vasoconstrictor to delay systemic absorp-tion, which then increases the duration of anesthesia. Using vasoconstrictors in these types of patients may actually prevent the release of endogenous epinephrine. Thus patients taking tri-cyclic antidepressants that elevate NE levels should be treated like cardiac patients in terms of EPI administration. One to two cartridges of 2% lidocaine with 1:100,000 epinephrine (0.04 mg epinephrine) should be used in a patient taking a TCA. Retrac-tion cords containing epinephrine are contraindicated.

Since MAOIs inhibit the enzyme that breaks down NE and serotonin; use of these drugs with EPI is not of much concern. Some newer antidepressants (e.g., SSRIs) do not affect the lev-els of NE. Levonordefrin, the vasoconstrictor in carbocaine, should be avoided in patients taking tricyclic antidepressants due to enhanced sympathomimetic effects. Also, retraction cord containing epinephrine should be avoided in these patients.

Key Points

- Summary
- Most psychiatric drugs cause xerostomia, which may lead to carious lesions. Monitor patients; advise patients to drink plenty of water, use sugarless gum, and use salivary substi-tutes such as Optimoist, Salivart, or Moi-Stir Swabsticks.
- Xerostomia is due to a decreased salivary flow (anticholin-ergic effects).
- Epinephrine may be given in limited amounts to patients taking TCAs. Retraction cord containing EPI is contraindicated.
- Levonordefrin, a vasoconstrictor in local anesthetics, is contraindicated in patients taking TCAs.
- No contraindications for EPI in patients taking SSRIs.
- Tardive dyskinesia (repetitive involuntary movements of the tongue, lips, and jaw) are adverse side effects of anti-psychotic drugs. These movements make management of dental patients difficult.
- TCAs and SSRIs have cardiac side effects (e.g., tachycar-dia, increased blood pressure, and arrhythmias).
- Most psychiatric drugs cause orthostatic hypotension. The patient should sit in an upright position in the dental chair for a few minutes before getting out of the chair.

- Patients taking divalproex (Depakote) should have a medi-cal consult regarding platelet counts.
- Benzodiazepines are used for sedation of the anxious dental patient and in the management of nocturnal bruxism.
- TCAs are used in the management of nocturnal bruxism when appliance therapy has failed.
- Lithium, used in the treatment of the acute manic phase of mixed bipolar disorder, may cause a metallic taste in the mouth due either to the taste of the lithium tablet or due to the secretion of lithium in the saliva. There are increased lithium blood levels if taken with nonsteroidal anti-inflam-matory drugs [ibuprofen (Advil, Motrin), naproxen (Aleve)].
- Carbamazepine (Tegretol), used in the treatment of sei-zures and non-FDA-approved in the treatment of manic-depressive disorder, may cause sores in the mouth, which may be an early sign of a blood disorder. Do not prescribe erythromycin or clarithromycin.

Board Review Questions

1. Which of the following drugs requires regular blood tests to determine the white blood cell levels? (p. 249)
   a. Thorazine
   b. Resperidone
   c. Clozapine
   d. Ziprasidone

2. Which of the following adverse effects makes treating a patient on a psychiatric drug difficult? (pp. 248, 249)
   a. Dystonia
   b. Akathisia
   c. Drug-induced Parkinsonism
   d. Tardive dyskinesia

3. With which of the following drugs does epinephrine (1:100,000) need to be limited to 2 cartridges? (p. 252)
   a. Amitriptyline (Elavil)
   b. Sertraline (Zoloft)
   c. Fluoxetine (Prozac)
   d. Paroxetine (Paxil)

4. Local anesthetics containing epinephrine are contrai-ndicated in the dental patient taking fluoxetine requiring local anesthesia because epinephrine will cause ortho-static hypotension. (pp. 253, 254)
   a. The first statement is true and the reason is correct.
   b. The first statement is true and the reason is incorrect.
   c. The first statement is not true but the reason is correct.
   d. The statement and the reason are not correct.

DISEASE	THERAPY	TRANSMITTER RECEPTOR ACTIONS
Schizophrenia	Antipsychotics	Dopamine (DA), 5-HT$_{2A}$ receptor antagonism
Depression	Antidepressants	Serotonin and/or norepinephrine reuptake blockade
Anxiety	Anxiolytics	GABA receptor blockade; serotonin reuptake inhibition

5. Which of the following is a common adverse effect of psychiatric drugs and requires patient counseling in the dental office? (pp. 254, 259, 263)
   a. Tardive dyskinesia
   b. Orthostatic hypotension
   c. Weight gain
   d. Xerostomia
   e. Sedation

Selected References

ADA Guide to Dental Therapeutics, 3rd ed. 2003. Chicago: American Dental Association.

American Academy of Family Physicians. 2000. Diagnosis and management of depression. *American Family Physician* Monograph No. 2. Kansas, MO: Author.

American Psychiatric Association. 1994. *Diagnostic and statistical manual of mental disorders,* 4th ed. Washington, DC: Author.

American Psychiatric Association. 2005, May. Bipolar disorder management: A new edition. *Annual Meeting Highlights.* Atlanta, GA.

American Society of Health-System Pharmacists. *AHFS Drug Information 2001,* edited by GK McEvoy. Bethesda, MD: American Society of Health-System Pharmacists,

Citrome L, Goldberg JF. 2005. Bipolar disorder is a potentially fatal disease. *Postgrad Med* 117:9–11.

Gentile S. 2007. Atypical antipsychotics for the treatment of bipolar disorder. *CNS Drugs* 21(5):367–387.

Goldberg JF, Citrome L. 2005. Latest therapies for bipolar disorder: Looking beyond lithium. *Postgrad Med* 117:25–26, 29–32, 35–36.

Gonzales-Pinto A, Gutierrez M, Ezcurra J, et al. 1998. Tobacco smoking and bipolar disorder. *J Clin Psychiatry* 59:225–228.

Hawton K. 2005. Suicide risk and attempted suicide in bipolar disorder: A systematic review of risk factors. *J Clin Psychiatry* 66:693–704.

Henin A, Mick E, Biederman J, et al. 2007. Can bipolar disorder-specific neuropsychological impairments in children be identified? *J Consult Clin Psychol* 75(2):210–220.

Hirschfeld RM, Vornik LA. 2005. Bipolar disorder—Costs and comobidity. *Am J Manag Care* 11 (Suppl.).

Kastrup E. 2005. *Drug facts and comparison.* St. Louis, MO: J.B. Lippincott.

Mattson MP, Kapogiannis D, Greig NH. 2010. Tweaking energy metabolism to prevent and treat neurological disorders. *Clin Pharm Ther* 88(4):437–439.

Muzyka BC, Glick M. 1997. The hypertensive dental patient. *JADA* 128:1109–1120.

Sanger TM, Tohen M, Vieta E, et al. 2003. Olanzapine in the acute treatment of biopolar I disorder with a history of rapid cycling. *J Affect Disord* 73:155–161.

Suppes T, Dennehy EB, Hirschfeld, RM, et al. 2005. The Texas Implementation of Medication Algorithms: Update to the algorithms for treatment of bipolar I disorder. *J Clin Psychiatry* 66:870–886.

Web Sites

medscape.com
psychiatrictimes.com
psych.org
psychiatryonline.org

PEARSON
myhealthprofessionskit™

Use this address to access the Companion Website created for this textbook. Simply select "Dental Hygiene" from the choice of disciplines. Find this book and log in using your username and password to access video clips of selected tests.

QUICK DRUG GUIDE

Antipsychotics

Typical Antipsychotics

Phenothiazines

- Chlorpromazine (Thorazine)
- Mesoridazine (Serentil)
- Thioridazine (Mellaril)
- Fluphenazine (Prolixin)
- Perphenazine (Trilafon)
- Trifluoperazine (Stelazine)

Nonphenothiazines

- Thiothixene (Navane)
- Haloperidol (Haldol)
- Loxapine (Loxitane)
- Molindone (Moban)

Atypical Antipsychotics

- Clozapine (Clozaril)
- Risperidone (Risperdal)
- Olanzapine (Zyprexa)
- Quetiapine (Seroquel)
- Ziprasidone (Geodon)

Drugs for Mood Disorders: Antidepressants

Tricylic Antidepressants (TCAs)

- Amitriptyline (Elavil)
- Imipramine (Tofranil)
- Trimipramine (Surmontil)
- Doxepin (Adapin, Sinequan)
- Desipramine (Norpramin)
- Nortriptyline (Pamelor)
- Protriptyline (Vivactil)
- Comipramine (Anafranil)
- Amoxapine (Asendin)

Monoamine oxidase inhibitors (MAOIs)

- Phenelzine (Nardil)
- Isocarboxazid (Marplan)
- Tranylcypromine (Parnate)

Selective Serontonin Reuptake Inhibitors (SSRIs)

- Fluoxetine (Prozac)

- Paroxetine (Paxil)
- Sertraline (Zoloft)
- Citalopram (Celexa)
- Fluvoxamine (Luvox)

Atypical Antidepressants

- Mirtazapine (Remeron)
- Reboxetine (Edronax)
- Bupropion (Wellbutrin)
- Trazodone (Desyrel)
- Nefazodone (Serzone)

Serotonin-Norepinephrine Reuptake Inhibitors (SNRIs)

- Venlafaxine (Effexor)
- Desvenlafaxine (Pristiq)
- Duloxetine (Cymbalta)

Drugs for Mood Disorders: Mood Stabilizers (Bipolar Disorder)

Mood Stabilizing: Acute Mania

- Lithium carbonate (Eskalith)
- Valproic acid (Depakene), divalproex sodium (Depakote)
- Olanzapine (Zyprexa)
- Carbamazepine (Equetro)

Depressive Disorder

- Lithium carbonate (Eskalith)
- Lamotrigine (Lamictal)
- Nonresponsive: addition of
- Bupropion (Wellbutrin)
- Paroxetine (Paxil)

Anxiolytics/Hypnotics

Benzodiazepines

Short-Acting Anxiolytics

- Alprazolam (Xanax)
- Lorazepam (Ativan)
- Oxazepam (Serax)

Long-Acting Anxiolytics

- Prazepam (Centrax)

Intermediate-Acting Hypnotics

- Estazolam (Prosom)
- Temazepam (Restoril)
- Chlordiazepoxide HCl (Librium, Libritabs)
- Clorazepate (Tranxene)
- Diazepam (Valium)
- Halazepam (Paxipam)

Short-Acting Hypnotics

- Midazolam (Versed)
- Triazolam (Halcion)
- Zolpidem (Ambien)

Long-Acting Hypnotics

- Flurazepam (Dalmane)
- Quazepam (Doral)

Other Anti-Anxiety Drugs

- Buspirone (Buspar)
- Sertraline (Zoloft)
- Venlafaxine extended-release (Effexor XR)
- Paroxetine (Paxil)

Barbiturates

Long-Acting

- Phenobarbital (Luminal)

Intermediate/Short-Acting

- Amobarbital (Amytal)
- Butabarbital (Butisol)
- Pentobarbital (Nembutal)
- Secobarbital (Seconal)

Ultra-Short-Acting

- Thiopental (Pentothal)

Drugs for Attention-Deficit/Hyperactivity Disorder (ADHD)

Amphetamine

- Dextroamphetamine sulfate
- Dextroamphetamine saccharate
- Amphetamine aspartate monohydrate

- Amphetamine sulfate (Adderall XR) CII
- Methylphenidate (Concerta) CII
- Atomoxetine (Strattera)

Endocrine and Hormonal Drugs

After reading this chapter, the reader should be able to:

1. Illustrate the pathogenesis of diabetes mellitus.

2. Compare the indications and effects of the available medications used to treat diabetes mellitus.

3. Explain the dental management of diabetic patients.

4. Describe the various drug–drug interactions of diabetic medications.

5. State the dental management of patients with thyroid disorders.

6. State the management of dental patients taking corticosteroids.

7. Describe the dental indications of topical corticosteroids.

8. Describe important dental concerns of corticosteroids.

9. Summarize the components of oral contraceptives and dental concerns.

10. Describe oral signs and symptoms of ONJ.

11. Discuss the guidelines for dental patients taking bisphosphonates.

12. List dental risk factors for ONJ.

KEY TERMS

Diabetes mellitus
Hyperglycemia
Insulin
Insulin resistance
Thyroid gland
Corticosteroids
Glucocorticoids

Gonadocorticoids
Adrenal crisis
Sex hormones
Anti-inflammatory
Bisphosphonates
Osteonecrosis of the jaw

GOALS

- To provide knowledge of the various medications used in the treatment of diabetes mellitus.
- To provide an understanding of thyroid conditions and how to manage these patients in the dental office.
- To gain knowledge about the dental management of patients taking corticosteroids.
- To provide the dental professional with a basic understanding of the various hormonal drugs, including oral contraceptives, and their relationship to dental treatment.
- To familiarize the student with current information regarding the use of drugs called bisphosphonate derivatives and the development of osteonecrosis of the jaw (ONJ).
- To inform the student about recommendations and guidelines for dental patients taking bisphosphonates.

Diabetes Mellitus

Diabetes mellitus makes up a group of hormonal diseases characterized by alterations in carbohydrate, protein and lipid metabolism resulting in elevated levels of blood glucose. This **hyperglycemia** is due to a lack of insulin secretion by the pancreas, a reduction in insulin action, or a combination of both. Plasma glucose concentrations are usually maintained between 40 and 160 mg/dL. Glucose is a sugar that is taken up into the cells by insulin and is used as energy by the cells. **Insulin** is a hormone made and secreted by the beta cells of the islets of Langerhans in the pancreas. When insulin does not function properly or is not produced in efficient amounts to take up the glucose into the cells, glucose remains in the blood and causes a condition called hyperglycemia or diabetes mellitus, which is characterized by glucose intolerance. The liver, however, continues to make glucose (gluconeogenesis) and additional glucose is secreted into the blood stream (Figure 16-1). The elevated glucose levels affects almost all organs in the body, including the cardiovascular system, eyes, nerves, kidneys, and the periodontum.

Over the years the classification of diabetes mellitus has changed. Diabetes mellitus is no longer referred to as juvenile- or adult-onset diabetes, nor is it referred to as insulin-dependent and non-insulin-dependent. In 1997, new terms used to classify diabetes mellitus were developed. Diabetes mellitus is now classified as type 1 and type 2.

Type 1

Type 1 diabetes mellitus (formerly juvenile-onset or insulin-dependent diabetes) is due to an *absolute* insulin deficiency as a result of destruction of pancreatic islet beta-cells. Without adequate insulin to allow glucose from the blood to enter cells, the cells starve while glucose accumulates in the blood. The cells do not have glucose as a source of energy, so they begin to break down fat. Free fatty acids accumulate in the blood which are converted into ketones, which may result in ketoacidosis, a potentially life-threatening condition. Diabetic ketoacidosis occurs when there is hyperglycemia (more than 250 mg/dL) and urinary ketone bodies, which result in a metabolic acidosis characterized by drowsiness, nausea, sweating, tachycardia, and coma. Type 1 diabetes is primarily an autoimmune process whereby insulin autoantibodies in the body are involved in pancreatic cell destruction. The onset of type 1 diabetic symptoms is usually quick.

Type 2

Type 2 diabetes mellitus (formerly adult-onset diabetes mellitus or non-insulin-dependent diabetes mellitus) is the more prevalent form of diabetes, and its incidence is increasing due to an increased aging population and obesity. Type 2 diabetes mellitus is characterized by insulin resistance with adequate or near adequate and, perhaps even excessive, amounts of insulin. Unlike type 1 diabetes, autoimmune destruction of the beta-cells does not occur in type 2 diabetes mellitus but rather genetics (heredity/family history) play a major role in its development. The typical type 2 diabetic is usually obese and symptoms of the disease are seen gradually. Diabetic ketoacidosis is not usually seen in type 2 diabetics because adequate endogenous insulin is produced to keep ketone formation low.

Insulin Resistance: Type 2 Diabetic

Understanding the concept of insulin resistance is necessary for managing the type 2 diabetic. **Insulin resistance** is defined as decreased insulin effectiveness with a reduced sensitivity of the cells to respond to insulin. After insulin is secreted by the

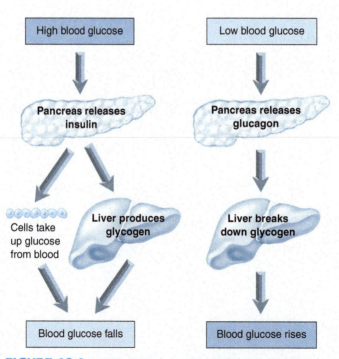

FIGURE 16-1 Insulin, glucagon, and blood glucose.

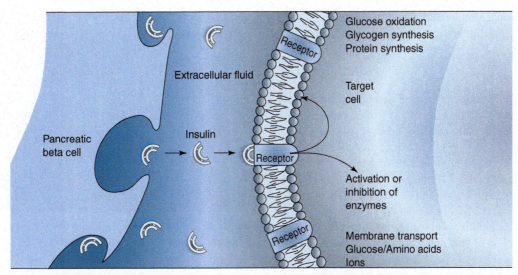

FIGURE 16-2 Plasma insulin binds to receptors on target cells to enter the cells, which starts actions that lead to insulin's biological effects.

beta cells, it binds to insulin receptors on adipose, liver, and muscle cells, as well as other cell types. Insulin must bind with these receptors and become active in bringing glucose into the cell and stimulating glucose metabolism (Figure 16-2). In type 2 diabetes, insulin receptors in the target tissues have become insensitive or resistant to insulin so it can bind to the receptor, but there is a defect in both insulin action and secretion, making the insulin ineffective in glucose uptake into the tissues. When insulin resistance develops, the beta cells are forced to compensate by secreting more insulin (*hyperinsulinemia*). Over time, the beta cells of the pancreas lose their ability to produce insulin in sufficient quantities to overcome insulin resistance. This condition is referred to as *impaired glucose tolerance* or prediabetes. This results in high blood glucose levels, especially after meals, which is called postprandial hyperglycemia. The degree of insulin defects is influenced by many factors, including obesity, smoking, and decreased physical activity. Continued insulin resistance and insulin deficiency ultimately will result in type 2 diabetes.

Diagnosis

Common signs and symptoms of type 1 diabetes include:

1. Polyphagia (increased appetite)
2. Polyuria (increased urination)
3. Polydipsia (increased thirst)
4. Weight loss
5. Weakness
6. Xerostomia
7. Burning tongue/mouth
8. Periodontal disease (also seen in type 2 diabetes)

Symptoms may not be apparent in type 2 diabetics because the disease is slow in development. Most individuals are obese, and most are diagnosed with diabetes because of an abnormal random blood glucose test.

There are other types of diabetes, including gestational diabetes, when pregnant women have hyperglycemia. Diabetes can result from taking drugs such as corticosteroids, or from other diseases such as Cushing's syndrome.

Criteria for diagnosing diabetes mellitus have changed over the years from those previously recommended by the National Diabetes Data Group (NDDG) and the World Health Organization (WHO). The following are different ways to diagnosis diabetes mellitus:

1. *Random (not fasting) plasma glucose.* If ≥200 mgdL, then a fasting plasma glucose (FPG) test should be done.
2. A subsequent (FPG) test should be performed to confirm the results of the random plasma glucose test. Diabetes is characterized by the presence of a fasting hyperglycemia: plasma glucose of 126 mg/dL after fasting (no caloric intake for at least 8 hours) overnight.
3. In patients with an abnormally high FPG value, an *oral glucose tolerance test* (OGTT) may be performed; however, since it is an expensive test and many false positives can occur, patients have to follow strict preparation rules. Patient preparation for an OGTT involves a carbohydrate diet and 10- to 12-hour fasting before the test. Plasma glucose levels are taken at different times after taking a carbohydrate (glucose) solution. A 2-hour postprandial (2 hours after consuming the carbohydrate solution) glucose of 200 mg/dL is diagnostic of diabetes. Many drugs that can produce a false positive (getting positive results when they should be negative) include thiazide diuretics, corticosteroids, propranolol, oral contraceptives, and phenytoin.

DID YOU KNOW?

Diabetes also occurs in animals, including cats.

Impaired glucose tolerance (IGT) is diagnosed by an OGTT, with the 2-hour postprandial (after a meal) value of 140 mg/dL, but >200 mg/dL.

Complications

Individuals with diabetes are at an increased risk for microvascular (the terminal ends of blood vessels: arterioles, capillaries, and venules) complications of the eye (retinopathy), gingiva, kidneys, nerves (neuropathy), and extremities (e.g., foot ulcers). Macrovascular (arteries) complications include coronary artery disease. Diabetics are at increased risk for congestive heart disease (CHD) and peripheral vascular disease and stroke. Coronary artery disease is the major cause of death in both type 1 and type 2 diabetics. All of these conditions are associated with insulin resistance (increased production of insulin by the beta cells). Other diseases associated with insulin resistance and diabetes are hyperlipidemia and hypertension. *Diabetes is a risk factor for developing periodontal diseases, and individuals with periodontal disease are at risk for developing diabetes mellitus* (Figures 16-3 and 16-4).

Rapid Dental Hint

Remember to screen and monitor your diabetic patients for periodontal disease.

Control and Management

The ultimate goal for diabetic control and reduction in complications is glycemic control. Glycosated hemoglobin, or HbA1c, is a test that monitors how the patient is controlling the diabetes. This test measures the percentage of hemoglobin in the red blood cells that is bound to glucose. When hemoglobin becomes glycosated it will stay bound to that red blood cell for the life of that cell. HbA1c levels reflect glycemic control over the preceding 2–3 months and are useful in determining the efficacy of treatment. The goal is to have an HbA1c of 7% or lower (this test

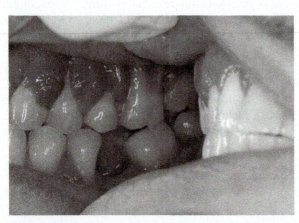

FIGURE 16-3 Patient diagnosed with type 2 diabetes mellitus. Periodontal examination revealed deep periodontal pockets and bleeding. Radiographic bone loss was evident. (Courtesy, Dr. David Lefkowitz)

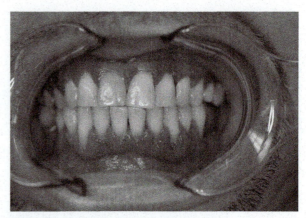

FIGURE 16-4 Severe periodontitis in a patient with uncontrolled diabetes. (Courtesy, Dr. David Lefkowitz)

should be done about every 3 months) and preprandial (before meals) fasting blood glucose of 80–120 mg/dL (Table 16-1).

Rapid Dental Hint

Before starting periodontal treatment you need to know the patient's HbA1c. If unknown, contact the patient's physician. If HbA1c is >7%, treatment should not be started and, a physician's consult is required.

Patients usually self-monitor blood glucose and urinary glucose. Accu-Check™ is one type of monitoring device available.

Diet modification is critical for type 1 diabetics and can be used as monotherapy in type 2 diabetics. Weight loss in type 2 diabetics will improve insulin secretion, which may reduce the risk of microvascular and macrovascular complications. Exercise may improve insulin sensitivity and reduce plasma glucose. The importance of smoking cessation should be reinforced. These patients may need exogenous insulin to help maintain type 2 status.

Rapid Dental Hint

Make sure your patients eat and take diabetic meds prior to dental treatment.

TABLE 16-1 Glycosolated Hemoglobin (HBA1c) Levels

- Normal level: treatment can precede 5.0–6.0%
- Treatment goal: treatment can precede <7.0%
- Alternative diabetic management required >8.0%

(increased risk for complications such as delayed wound healing)

Pharmacology

ORAL HYPOGLYCEMICS Antidiabetic drugs are classified into oral and injectable agents (Tables 16-2 and 16-3). The decision to use a specific drug is based on whether there is an absolute insulin deficiency of insulin (as seen in type 1 diabetes) or a defect in insulin action and secretion (as seen in type 2 diabetes). In type 1 diabetes, insulin is essential because there is no insulin being produced by the beta cells. In type 2 diabetes, rather than an absolute insulin deficiency, insulin is being produced even in excess (hyperinsulinemia), but there is a problem with its action and secretion. If monitoring and lifestyle modifications (e.g., weight loss/exercise, smoking cessation) are not successful in glucose control of type 2 diabetes, oral antidiabetic agents must be used. Proper diet and exercise can sometimes increase the sensitivity of insulin receptors to the point that drug therapy is not needed.

ORAL ANTIDIABETIC AGENTS All oral antihyperglycemic agents reduce blood glucose levels by different methods and/or degrees, but all need insulin in order to be effective. Intact beta cells are needed for these drugs to work. Therapy is

TABLE 16-2 Agents Used in the Treatment of Diabetes Mellitus

DRUG NAME

First-Generation Agents

Chloropropamide (Diabinese)

Tolazamide (Tolinase)

Tolbutamide (Orinase)

Second-Generation Agents

Glipizide (Glucotrol)

Glyburide (DiaBeta, Micronase)

Glyburide, micronized (Glynase)

Glimepiride (Amaryl)

Biguanides

Metformin (Glucophage)

Combination Drugs

Glyburide/metformin (Glucovance)

Metformin/glipizide (Metaglip)

Metformin/rosiglitazone (Avandamet)

Thiazolidinediones

Pioglitazone (Actos)

Rosiglitazone (Avandia)

Alpha-Glucosidase Inhibitors

Acarbose (Precose)

Miglitol (Glyset)

Meglitinides

Repaglinide (Prandin)

Nateglinide (Starlix)

TABLE 16-3 Insulin Preparations

DRUG NAME

Rapid-Acting Insulins

Recombinant Human Insulin Preparations

Insulin regular (human insulin)

(Humulin R, Novolin R, Regular Iletin II)

Insulin Analog Preparations

Insulin human inhalation powder (rDNA origin) (Exubera)

Insulin glulisine (rDNA original) (Apidra)

Insulin aspart (rDNA origin) (NovoLog FlexPen, NovoLog Mix 70/30, Novolog FlexPen)

Insulin lispro (rDNA origin) (Humalog, Humalog Pen)

Intermediate- and Long-Acting Insulins

Recombinant Human Insulin Preparations

NPH Insulin (human insulin) (Humulin N, Novolin N, NPH Iletin I, NPH Iletin II)

Human regular and human NPH mixture

(Humulin 70/30, Humulin 50/50, Novolin 70/30)

Insulin isophane human (NPH) (Humulin N, Novolin N)

Insulin zinc human (Humulin L, Novolin L)

Analog Preparations

Insulin glargine (Lantus)

Insulin determir (Levemir)

PZI—insulin lispro protamine 75%/insulin lispro 25% (Humalog Mix)

usually initiated with a single agent. If therapeutic goals are not achieved, two agents are given. Oral antidiabetic agents are divided into six classifications:

1. *Sulfonylureas* have been around for over 40 years and were the first oral agents used in the treatment of type 2 diabetes mellitus, particularly in patients in whom diet fails to control the hyperglycemia. Sulfonylureas, or insulin secretion stimulators, work by stimulating the release of insulin from the pancreatic beta cells and to increase the binding of insulin to the receptors on target tissues (cells), increasing insulin sensitivity and increasing glucose transport in the tissues. These agents are used by almost 30–40% of all individuals with type 2 diabetes mellitus. Sulfonylureas can cause hypoglycemia because of their ability to increase insulin secretion. First-generation agents are no longer the first-line drugs being replaced by second-generation sulfonylureas and other newly introduced (within the last 12 years) drugs.

   Second-generation sulfonylureas (including glimepride, glipizide, and glyburide) also work by stimulating the release of insulin from the beta cells but are more potent (smaller doses are used) with fewer adverse effects, including less weight gain, less hypoglycemia, and fewer drug–drug interactions. Patients recently diagnosed (less than 5 years) and older than 40 years of age and obese who cannot control their glucose levels with exercise or diet respond well with sulfonlyureas. Dosage adjustment is necessary in patients with liver disease. In patients who do not respond to sulfonylureas alone, another antidiabetic drug is added or used.

2. *Biguanides* work by decreasing glucose production and release by the liver and stimulating glucose uptake into tissues. Metformin is an example of a biguanide. Unlike the sulfonylureas, biguanides alone do not cause weight gain or hypoglycemia. In obese individuals, they increase insulin sensitivity, resulting in weight loss. Since metformin does not affect insulin production or secretion (release), it does not cause hypoglycemia or hyperinsulinemia. It is generally used in combination with insulin or a sulfonylurea. Adverse effects include anorexia, diarrhea, nausea, and abdominal discomfort. Metformin reduces triglyceride and LDL cholesterol. Metformin is contraindicated and should not be used in patients with renal (kidney) disease, respiratory disease, or cardiac insufficiency.

3. *Alpha-glucosidase inhibitors* reduce postprandial (after eating) hyperglycemia by reversibly inhibiting the alpha glucosidase enzymes in the small intestine, delaying carbohydrate absorption, and delaying and reducing a rise in blood glucose after meals. Gastrointestinal discomfort is the most common adverse effect and is contraindicated in patients with inflammatory bowel disease or any obstructive bowel conditions. Acarbose (Precose) and miglitol (Glyset) are in this category. These medications do not cause weight gain or hypoglycemia when used alone. However, when used with a sulfonylurea, side effects may occur.

4. *Thiazolidinediones* (TZDs) are a relatively new class of drugs used to reduce insulin resistance by enhancing the effects of circulating insulin by improving insulin sensitivity in muscle and fat cells. These agents are used only as a second-line therapy and some in combination with other antidiabetic agents such as a sulfonylurea or metformin. Two thiazolidinedoines currently approved in the United States are rosiglitazone (Avandia) and pioglitazone (Actos). Adverse affects include fluid retention (which may exacerbate heart failure), weight gain, and severe liver damage. Since they do not stimulate insulin secretion, hypoglycemia does not occur. Major health risks including heart attack and stroke, and even death, have been associated with Avandia. The FDA issued a black-box warning alert about the potential harm that the drug can cause. The drug will be taken off the market as of November 2011.

5. *Meglitinides* are the newest class of oral hypoglycemics. They increase insulin secretion from beta cells of the pancreas, but from a different site than the sulfonylureas. These drugs are taken before meals to stimulate insulin release and control the rise in postprandial glucose plasma levels. Two drugs in this category are repaglinide (Prandin) and nateglinide (Starlix). Weight gain is a common adverse side effect. Hypoglycemia and effects on blood lipids are not seen.

6. *Combination drugs* combine metformin with glipizide (Metaglip), glyburide (Glucovance), and rosiglitazone (Avandamet). Various oral hypoglycemic drugs have different mechanisms of action. As diabetes progresses, more metabolic disorders arise. Combination therapy is needed to treat the more complex and varied complications. For example, a patient may be taking a sulfonylurea to enhance insulin secretion and a TZD to reduce insulin resistance and hyperglycemia.

Insulin Pharmacology: History

- Insulin is required in type 1 diabetics because there is an absolute or total deficiency of insulin and it needs to be replaced from an exogenous source to prevent ketoacidosis. About 30% of diabetics in the United States are taking insulin.

- Although not used as a first-line treatment in type 2 diabetes, insulin (with oral agents) can be used to supplement deficient levels of insulin in the blood, especially in patients who have had diabetes for a long time and are unable to achieve adequate glycemic control (more than 350 mg/dL) with oral agents alone.

- Diet, exercise, and oral agents are usually tried first in type 2 diabetics.

Guidelines for Dental Patients Taking Oral Hypoglycemics

1. Must have HbA1c levels before dental treatment begins. Get a medical consult from the patient's physician.

2. Ask the patient what their blood glucose (sugar) level was today, and if they took their medication as directed. A random plasma glucose level of ≥200 mg/dL and a FPG (fasting plasma glucose) of ≥126 mg/dL should be consulted with the patient's physician before dental treatment is started.

3. Early morning appointments should be scheduled to avoid stress-induced hypoglycemia.

4. Monitor for periodontal disease in your patient.

Guidelines for Dental Patients Taking Oral Hypoglycemic Agents—Glipizide (Glucotrol)

- Monitor the periodontal condition of diabetic patients.
- Stress meticulous home care.
- Patients should have frequent recall appointments.
- Patients should avoid aspirin and nonsteroidal anti-inflammatory drugs (e.g., ibuprofen).
- Question patients about self-monitoring of their diabetic condition.
- Encourage patients to follow a prescribed diet and regularly take the medication to avoid hypoglycemic episodes.

- Insulin is a hormone (protein) produced by and secreted from the beta cells in the pancreas. When endogenous insulin is not being produced or in ineffective amounts, exogenous insulin must be introduced into the blood to maintain adequate blood levels. Insulin regulates plasma glucose levels by decreasing liver glucose production and increasing glucose uptake into the cells. Insulin is biologically inactive until it is bound by specific receptors located in target cells.

Insulin Secretion and Absorption

- *Endogenous insulin* is normally released from the pancreas when blood glucose levels are elevated.
- *Prandial insulin* is released into the blood sporadically in two phases in response to elevated blood glucose after a meal.
  - In phase 1, insulin is released within seconds of eating and lasts for about 10 minutes.
  - Phase 2 insulin release occurs within 15 minutes of phase 1 and lasts for about 2 hours and is responsible for lowering the postprandial rise in blood glucose.
- *Basal insulin* is released continuously during the day at low levels in response to continuous liver glucose output.

DID YOU KNOW?

In 1921, Dr. Frederick Grant Banting and Charles Best discovered insulin by tying string around the pancreatic ducts of several dogs. When they examined the pancreases of these dogs several weeks later, all of the pancreas cells were gone and only pancreatic islets were left. These islets contained a protein they called insulin.

Goal of Insulin Therapy

The goal of insulin therapy is to mimic prandial and/or basal insulin production so blood glucose can be controlled continuously during the day and night, and limit the potential for hypoglycemic effects.

Insulin Regimen

Insulin preparations (Table 16-3) are classified as rapid, intermediate, or long-acting. The regimen for controlling hyperglycemia is a basal-bolus regimen, which includes an intermediate- or long-acting insulin injected once or twice daily to mimic basal insulin secretion, and a rapid- or short-acting insulin injected at mealtime to mimic prandial insulin secretion. The use of an insulin pump can accomplish this.

Some patients may not like to have multiple injections during the day. An alternative choice includes premixed insulin formulations that contain both a rapid- or short-acting insulin and an intermediate-acting insulin that can be administered in one injection twice daily (see Table 16-3).

Formulations

Recombinant Human Insulin Preparations

SHORT- OR RAPID-ACTING INSULIN In the past, insulin preparations came from animal sources, primarily pork because beef caused allergic reactions in humans. In 1986, *recombinant human insulin* first emerged. Today, recombinant human insulin is produced from either genetically altered bacteria (*Escherichia coli*) or yeast that has the same amino acid chain sequence as human insulin. Recombinant human insulin has fewer impurities, limiting significant allergic reactions, and is more rapid in onset and shorter in duration than pork insulin. Regular human insulin (R) and neutral protamine Hagedorn (NPH) are types of human insulin formulations.

Regular human insulin (R) is FDA approved for the treatment of type 1 and type 2 diabetes and mimics postprandial pancreas insulin release to reduce meal-related glucose levels (Table 16-2). It has a quick onset and short duration, which allows for postprandial glucose control. It should be injected about 30 minutes before meals. Regular insulin can be mixed with another type of insulin. It is available in a vial or a prefilled pen.

INTERMEDIATE-ACTING INSULIN Isophane insulin suspension (NPH; neutral protamine Hagedorn) was developed to reduce the number of injections required to achieve glycemic control. It is formulated as a crystalline suspension (cloudy). It is FDA approved for the treatment of type 1 and type 2 diabetes. It has a longer duration of action than rapid-acting insulin and is injected once or twice daily to mimic endogenous basal insulin release throughout the day.

NPH is available in a vial and a prefilled pen. It can be mixed with other insulin preparations including regular, insulin lispro, insulin aspart, and insulin glulisine, or a premixed formulation (available with regular).

INSULIN ANALOG PREPARATIONS Because of the pharmacological limitations of the human insulin formulations, various insulin analogs have been developed. In 1996, the first *insulin analog,* insulin lispro, was introduced. Insulin analogs are synthetically derived preparations based on the human insulin structure but slightly modified, resulting in altered pharmacokinetics that mirror the pharmacokinetics of endogenous insulin. Insulin aspart (NovoLog), insulin glulisine, and insulin lispro (Humalog) are insulin analog preparations. Today, only recombinant human insulin and insulin analog preparations are available. Beef and pork insulin were discontinued in 2003 and 2005, respectively.

RAPID-ACTING INSULIN ANALOG PREPARATIONS Insulin lispro (Humalog), insulin aspart (NovoLog), and insulin glulisine (Apidra) are rapid-acting insulin analogs. These formulations are being used more frequently because they are absorbed more quickly (10–15 minutes) and have a shorter duration of action (less than 5 hours) than human insulin (onset: 30–60 minutes). They are usually used with insulin infusion pumps.

INTERMEDIATE-ACTING ANALOG PREPARATIONS   There are no intermediate-acting analog preparations.

LONG-ACTING ANALOG PREPARATIONS   Insulin glargine was the first long-acting insulin analog, introduced in the United States in 2003, and requires only one injection during the day, which avoids nocturnal (nighttime) hypoglycemia (low glucose), whereas most other insulins require multiple injections daily. It should not be mixed in the syringe with any other insulin.

Adverse effects include injection site reactions and limitations for mixture with other insulin preparations.

Insulin detemir (Levemir) was FDA approved in 2005. It has a duration of action of up to 24 hours and is injected either once or twice daily.

Mixing Insulin Preparations and Premixed Insulin Preparations

Multiple daily dose insulin (MDI) therapy using a basal-bolus regimen offers tight glycemic control by mimicking endogenous insulin activity. However, it requires frequent blood glucose monitoring and multiple injections during the day. Different insulin preparations can be mixed together in the same syringe to deal with the different onset and duration of action of the insulin. When insulin is mixed, regular insulin, which is clear, must be drawn first into the syringe followed by another type of insulin, which is cloudy.

Many people have difficulty mixing the different insulin preparations or are unable to do multiple injections. Premixed insulin preparations are available that minimize the number of injections while offering both postprandial and basal insulin control. However, if patients require tight glycemic control and have not modified their lifestyle, these premixed preparations should not be used because dose adjustment cannot be done with premixed preparations. Premixed formulations contain both a rapid-acting and an intermediate-acting insulin that can be administered in one injection twice daily. It is administered as a subcutaneous injection in the abdomen, arm, buttocks, or thigh.

Insulin Delivery Devices

Insulin is available in vials as well as in a prefilled pen device. Rapid-acting insulin can also be used in an insulin pump, which delivers intensive insulin therapy with better absorption, decreased risk of nighttime and activity-related hypoglycemia, and allows a more flexible lifestyle. The pump is placed on the abdomen and is programmed to give small doses of insulin subcutaneously into the abdomen at predetermined intervals, with larger doses (boluses) at mealtime.

Newest Insulin Formulation

In 2006, inhaled (nasal spray) insulin (Exubera) was approved by the FDA. The inhaled powder is a form of recombinant human insulin that is used in the treatment of type 1 and type 2 diabetes. Peak levels were achieved in about 30–90 minutes. In type 1 diabetes, inhaled insulin may be added to a longer-acting insulin as a replacement for short-acting insulin taken with meals. In type 2 diabetes, inhaled insulin may be used alone, along with oral hypoglycemics or with longer-acting insulin.

Adverse Effects

The most common adverse effect of insulin is hypoglycemia, due either to too much insulin being injected or improper timing of the injections with meals. Patients and dental offices should have a source of simple sugar (e.g., orange juice) in case of hypoglycemic reactions. Hypoglycemia progresses rapidly, whereas hyperglycemia is slow in progression. Glucagon (GlucaGen Hypokit) given IV, IM, or SC is administered for some diabetic patients when they are in hypoglycemic shock. Patients taking insulin should be advised of the possibility of hypoglycemic attacks at any time, and be prepared to treat them by taking sugar or glucose tablets.

Other adverse effects include:

- Hyperglycemia
- Weight gain
- Pain at injection site
- Lipohypertrophy [proliferation of subcutaneous fat (adipose) tissue] at the injection site
- Allergic reaction

Rapid Dental Hint

To prevent insulin shock (hypoglycemia), make sure patients have taken medication as usual and an adequate intake of food/sugar. Have orange juice or other forms of sugar available in the clinic/dental office.

Guidelines for Dental Patients Taking Insulin

- Patients must be adequately controlled.
- A common adverse effect is hypoglycemia.
- Signs and symptoms of hypoglycemia: sweating, palpitations, pallor, dizziness
- Management of hypoglycemia: raising blood sugar to normal. Have patient drink 4 oz orange juice. Patient should feel better. Dental treatment can continue.
- Determine if patients are self-monitoring blood glucose.
- What is the HbA1c?
- Make early dental appointments.
- Make sure patients took insulin as directed.
- Assess and monitor for periodontal diseases, caries, and candidiasis.
- Aspirin and NSAIDs (e.g., ibuprofen) increase hypoglycemic effects.
- Epinephrine decreases the effect of insulin due to epinephrine-induced hyperglycemia; caution in amount of epinephrine-containing local anesthetic.

Dental Hygiene Applications

Patients in the dental office should be screened and monitored for periodontal disease, since diabetes mellitus is a documented risk factor for periodontal diseases. On the other hand, patients with periodontal disease should be cognizant of the development of diabetes mellitus. Patient education is an integral part of treatment of the periodontal patient with diabetes.

Other oral manifestations of diabetes mellitus include xerostomia, burning tongue/mouth, and *Candida* (fungal) infections. These factors must be monitored in the diabetic patient because xerostomia can lead to increased incidence of caries.

As diabetes progresses, many organs become affected and the patient most likely will be taking many other different types of drugs such as antihypertensives and drugs to lower cholesterol (antihyperlipidemic drugs). A review of all medications a diabetic is taking is important to determine adverse side effects and drug interactions.

Patients should be asked at the beginning of every appointment if they took insulin/oral agents as directed that day, since many diabetic patients (especially those taking insulin) are susceptible to hypoglycemic reactions (profuse sweating, fainting, palpitations, hunger, nervousness, or unconsciousness). The dental clinician should ask patients if they are prone to hypoglycemic reactions. If a patient becomes hypoglycemic, sugar, orange juice, or glucose tablets can be given if a patient is conscious. If a patient becomes unconscious, then additional medical assistance should be called and injection of glucagons administered. Dextrose (glucose) can also be used. Most diabetic patients monitor their blood glucose levels at home with a finger-stick test. Ask patients the results of the test for that day.

Epinephrine decreases the effect of insulin due to epinephrine-induced hyperglycemia. Thus, epinephrine counters the effect of insulin, which may interfere with diabetic control. Precautions should be taken to minimize the amount of epinephrine used in local anesthetics.

Thyroid Drugs

Thyroid Gland Hormones

The **thyroid gland** (Figure 16-5), located on the front side of the neck, produces and releases a hormone (protein) called *thyroxine* (T_4, levothyroxine). At the target tissues, thyroxine is converted to the active form, *triiodothyronine*(T_3), which enters the cells and binds to receptors. About 87% of T_3 is derived from T_4 and the remaining 13 percent is synthesized by the thyroid gland. Iodine is required for the synthesis of T_4 and is provided by dietary intake of iodized salt. For therapeutic purposes (medications for replacement of thyroid hormone), T_4 is used because more constant blood levels can be achieved due to its longer duration of action with a half-life of 7 days than T_3, with a half-life of 1 day.

Thyroid gland hormones regulate the *basal metabolic rate,* which is the baseline speed at which cells perform their functions and are essential for carbohydrate, protein, and lipid metabolism in the body. As cellular metabolism increases, thyroid hormone increases body temperature. The gland also regulates blood pressure and growth and development.

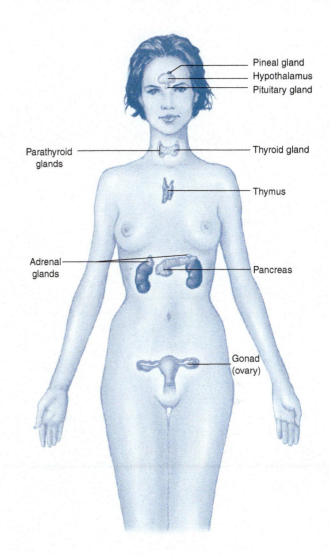

FIGURE 16-5 Location of thyroid gland.

Thyroid-stimulating hormone (TSH), which comes from the hypothalamus, stimulates growth of the thyroid gland and synthesis and secretion of the thyroid hormones (Figure 16-6). The thyroid forms a *negative feedback loop:* Secretion of TSH declines as the blood level of thyroid hormones rises (T_4), and vice versa (e.g., peaks at night and lower levels during the day).

Once released into the bloodstream, thyroid hormones can exist in the bound (to a protein) or unbound form. Thyroid hormones are highly protein bound (99.9% for T_4 and 99.5% for T_3), so only a little of the free unbound form is actually binding to receptors and producing an effect in the body. The conversion to T_3 is critical because T_3 has greater biological activity than T_4.

To determine if an individual has a thyroid disorder, hyperthyroidism, or hypothyroidism, a blood test is taken that measures unbound T_4 and TSH levels.

Pharmacology: Antithyroid Drugs

Hyperthyroidism (thyrotoxicosis) or excessive production of thyroid hormones must be treated by reducing the levels of the thyroid hormones. The most common type of hyperthyroidism is called Graves' disease, an autoimmune disease in which the body

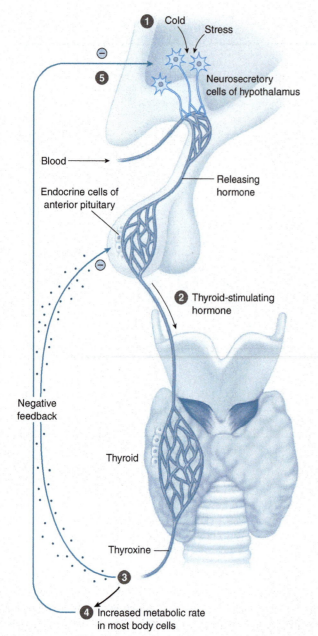

FIGURE 16-6 Mechanism of the thyroid gland showing a stimulus (1) that causes the release of TSH (2) and then the release of thyroid hormone (3). There is an increase in basal metabolic rate (speed by which cells perform their functions (4). This effect creates a negative feedback loop (5) where TSH production is suppressed when T4 levels are high, and vice versa.

develops antibodies against its own thyroid gland. Other causes of overactivity includes multinodular goiter or Plummer's disease (enlargement of thyroid gland) and tumors. Pharmacological treatment options include the following antithyroid drugs (Table 16-4):

1. *Thioamide drugs:* Propylthiouracil (PTU) and methimazole (Tapazole) work by inhibiting thyroid hormone production by interfering with the incorporation of iodine. These drugs are used as short-term treatment of Graves' disease. There is a high incidence of agranulocytosis (blood disorder of the neutrophils; a reduction of the white blood cells).

2. *Radioactive iodine (RAI):* Another first-line treatment for Graves' disease. The patient drinks an oral liquid containing sodium iodide that concentrates and destroys the overactive thyroid gland. After RAI, the patient usually has hypothyroidism and must take thyroid supplements for the rest of his or her life.

3. *Iodine:* Iodine-containing compounds including Lugol's solution (5% iodine (I_2) 10% potassium iodide (KI)). These agents are primarily used for the treatment of thyrotoxic crisis or, as it is sometimes called, thyroid storm, a life-threatening condition featuring acute manifestations of thyrotoxicosis including hypertension, tachycardia, confusion, vomiting, and coma. Surgical removal of the gland is also a recommended treatment for thyroid storm.

   Lugol's solution is available over-the-counter in the United States as of January 2007, although the DEA is considering a public ban on all iodine solutions of greater than 2.2% because iodine is required for the production of methamphetamine. Lugol's solution is available over-the-counter in Canada.

4. Beta-blockers (propranolol, nadolol) are not approved in the United States by the FDA for the treatment of thyrotoxicosis.

5. Other drugs include calcium channel blockers (diltiazem or verapamil), which block the effects of thyroid hormone, but do not have an effect on the underlying disease. Corticosteroids can be used for treating thyroid storm but there are many adverse effects that preclude its use as the first line of treatment.

Pharmacology: Hypothyroidism

Hypothyroidism is a common disorder that results from a deficiency in secretion of T_4 and T_3 from the thyroid gland. It frequently occurs after a patient is treated with radioactive iodine, whereby the thyroid gland becomes inactive (hypothyroid) and requires replacement therapy. It can be caused by thyroid gland failure, autoimmune thyroiditis (Hashimoto's disease), cretinism (congenital hypothyroidism), tumors, or be drug induced (e.g., lithium, iodides, sulfonylureas). Diagnosis is based on elevated levels of TSH. Initially, T_4 levels may be normal, but later on in the disease there are decreased levels. Symptoms of hypothyroidism in adults, also known as myxedema, include slowed body metabolism, slurred speech, depression, bradycardia, weight gain, low body temperature, and intolerance to cold environments. Treatment goals for hypothyroidism are to return thyroid hormone levels to normal with the used of medications. Periodic (monthly) blood tests should be performed while the patient is taking thyroid replacement medications to monitor for TSH and T_4 levels.

1. Thyroid USP (Armour) is manufactured from desiccated (dry) pig, beef, or sheep thyroid gland, and contains iodine. This product has unpredictable hormonal stability.

2. Levothyroxine (Synthroid, Levothroid) is synthetic T_4 hormone that is identical to the T_4 secreted from the thyroid gland and is one of the most commonly prescribed drugs in the United States. This is the drug of choice for thyroid hormone replacement. This product has predictable absorption,

TABLE 16-4   Disorders and Treatment of the Thyroid Gland

DISORDER	SIGNS AND SYMPTOMS	DRUG TREATMENT

Hyperthyroidism	Sweating, weight loss, nervousness, oversensitivity to heat, fatigue, moist skin, tachycardia (in Graves' disease there is exophthalmos, or bulging of the eye); Plummer's disease (toxic multinodular goiter): symptoms of hyperthyroidism but without exophthalmos	Goal: to reduce thyroid levels
		Thiourea drugs:
		  propylthiouracil (PTU)
		  methimazole (Tapazole)
		Radioactive iodine (RAI)
		Beta-blockers: propranolol, nadolol
		Iodine compounds:
		  Lugol's solution
		  Potassium iodide (SSKI)

Hypothyroidism	Cold intolerance, weakness, tiredness, fatigue, hoarseness, constipation, aches, pains, depression	Thyroid USP L-thyroxine (Levoxyl, Synthroid, Levothroid) L-triiodothyronine (Cytomel)

is stable, potent, has a long duration of action, is less expensive than the other products, and can be administered once daily. Although T_3 has greater biological activity than T_4, administration of L-thyroxine results in a concentration of T_4 that is converted to T_3.

3. L-triiodothyronine (Cytomel) is synthetic T_3 hormone. Daily multiple dosing is required. Hard to monitor blood levels.

4. Liotrix (Thyrolar) is synthetic T_4:T_3. This product is not really necessary because T_4 is converted to T_3 in the peripheral tissues and it is expensive.

Rapid Dental Hint

Dental treatment modifications may be necessary for patients with thyroid disorders; assess your patient. In patients taking levothyroxine, epinephrine is all right to use.

ADVERSE EFFECTS Adverse effects occurring in overdosage include irritability, nervousness, insomnia, headache, palpitations, and weight loss. Excessive doses can lead to heart disorders, including congestive heart failure and myocardial infarction.

Liothyronine has a high incidence of cardiac side effects. Thyroid USP may cause allergic reactions, since it is derived from animal sources.

Dental Hygiene Applications

There are no special precautions to follow when treating dental patients who are well controlled with thyroid medication. Most patients presenting to the dental office will be controlled and under the care of a physician; however, patients may be seen with undiagnosed hypothyroidism or hyperthyroidism, where routine dental treatment may result in adverse outcomes. If there is no documentation on the patient's medical history about thyroid disorders but several signs and symptoms point to thyroid disease, it is prudent to get a medical consult from the patient's physician. Epinephrine (1:100,000) is limited to two cartridges in hyperthyroid patients; however, patients with thyroid storm will most likely not be seen in the dental office, since it is a life-threatening disorder and patients are very ill. Monthly blood tests should be done to maintain normal thyroid hormone levels.

Adrenal (Steroid) Hormones

Adrenal Glands

The adrenal glands are located next to the kidneys (Figure 16-5). One part of the adrenal gland, the adrenal medulla, produces and secretes epinephrine and norepinephrine, which stimulate the sympathetic division of the central nervous system. Epinephrine is responsible for converting stored glycogen (carbohydrates) into glucose in the liver. This process is called glycogenolysis.

The other part of the adrenal gland is the adrenal cortex. The adrenal cortex produces and releases steroid hormones into the circulation. When released into the circulation, these natural hormones have many effects on the body and are essential for life. These hormones allow the body to endure stresses put upon it such as injury, disease, and mental strain.

The release of **corticosteroids** by the adrenal cortex is controlled by the hypothalamus and anterior pituitary gland via ACTH (adrenocorticotropic hormone), which stimulates corticosteroid release. All human steroids are synthesized from cholesterol found in the body. Three natural corticosteroids that the body produces and secretes are classified by their actions:

1. *Mineralocorticoids.* The primary mineralocorticoid is aldosterone. Mineralocorticoids have the responsibility of maintaining the levels of sodium and potassium in the body. They conserve or maintain the body's concentration

of water at a near constant level. They exert most of their effect on the kidneys, causing selective excretion of excess potassium in the urine and at the same time retain sodium. The medical use of mineralocorticosteroids is limited.

2. *Glucocorticoids.* Hydrocortisone (cortisol) is the primary glucocorticoid. **Glucocorticoids** or glucocorticosteroids regulate energy metabolism by causing proteins (e.g., muscles) and lipids (e.g., body fats) to be broken down and converted into glucose (glycogenolysis). They cause carbohydrates stored in the form of glycogen to be converted back to glucose and deposited into the blood, where they are available for the tissues in the body. About 15–30 mg of cortisol is secreted in the body daily. Glucocorticoids also suppress inflammatory processes (anti-inflammatory) within the body (e.g., bee sting, arthritis), have anti-allergic properties, and are important to the body's immunological defense reactions.

3. *Gonadocorticoids*, or sex hormones. Male and female sex hormones produced by the adrenal cortex supplement those produced by the testes and ovaries. The female hormones are called estrogen and progesterone, and the male androgens include testosterone; the androgens are referred to as anabolic steroids.

Systemic Adrenocortical Steroids

Naturally occurring cortisol is not used, but is substituted for by others that can be produced more economically for the treatment of specific systemic medical conditions.

MINERALOCORTICOIDS: INDICATIONS Clinically, synthetic mineralocorticoids affect the kidneys by increasing sodium retention and potassium loss. Thus, mineralocorticoids are used primarily in patients with a medical condition called hypoadrenalism to replace and maintain loss of fluids and electrolytes. Fludrocortisone (Florinef) is the drug that is used for mineralocorticoid replacement.

GLUCOCORTICOIDS: INDICATIONS Clinically, synthetic glucocorticosteroids are used primarily as **anti-inflammatory** agents in the treatment of the following medical conditions:

- Asthma
- Rheumatoid arthritis
- Bursitis
- *Pneumocystis jiroveci* pneumonia in HIV-infected patients
- Viral croup (upper airway obstruction with cough in children)
- Systemic lupus erythematosus (SLE)
- Ulcerative colitis
- Antirejection for organ transplant
- Inflammatory conditions of the eye and skin
- Bullous disorders (e.g., pemphigus vulgaris and erythema multiforme)
- Stress-induced shock syndrome
- Severe allergic reactions
- Joint diseases (given as intra-articular injections every 1–6 weeks)

The immunosuppressive action of glucocorticoids allow them to be used in the management of organ transplant patients to prevent organ rejection. Corticosteroids are also used in the treatment of Addison's disease (adrenal insufficiency) and in the treatment of dental-related ulcerative inflammatory lesions such as lichen planus, burning tongue, and aphthous stomatitis (canker sores). Corticosteroids are known to be beneficial in treating herpes zoster infection, but their effectiveness in the treatment of recurrent herpes labialis infection is unknown; however, corticosteroids in combination with an antiviral agent may be safe and beneficial for herpes labialis. Corticosteroids by themselves are not so effective in reducing inflammation in viral lesions, and will mask symptoms of infection.

Steroid hormones act by controlling the rate of protein synthesis inside cells. When taken systemically, glucocorticosteroids are absorbed into the circulation and enter sensitive cells, where they bind to protein receptors and regulate the levels of specific proteins and enzymes, which result in its anti-inflammatory effects. Corticosteroids also exert an anti-inflammatory effect by inhibiting the release of histamine from mast cells.

GLUCOCORTICOIDS: SYSTEMIC PRODUCTS Table 16-5 lists the more commonly used systemic glucocorticosteroids, which are classified according to their duration of action:

1. Short-acting
2. Intermediate-acting
3. Long-acting

Corticosteroids are also classified according to their anti-inflammatory potency. Hydrocortisone has the least anti-inflammatory activity, while betamethasone and dexamethasone are the most potent anti-inflammatory steroids.

Rapid Dental Hint

Patients taking a corticosteroid such as prednisone can develop diabetes from the prednisone and it is called corticosteroid-induced diabetes mellitus. Monitor your patient for periodontal disease. Local anesthetic containing epinephrine can be safely administered.

ADVERSE EFFECTS Short-term, low-dose steroid therapy rarely results in any adverse effects. However, as the dosage and duration of therapy increases, so does the risk of unwanted side effects. Long-term therapy is more related with severe adverse events including:

- Suppressing normal adrenal gland function
- Osteoporosis
- Hyperglycemia
- Hypertension
- Candidiasis (including intraoral)

TABLE 16-5 Systemic Glucocorticosteroids		
DRUG NAME	**MECHANISM OF ACTION**	**DENTAL MANAGEMENT**
Short-acting (8–12 hours) Cortisone (generic, Cortone) Hydrocortisone, Cortisol (generic, Cortef)	After absorption into the bloodstream the drug enters the cell, where it binds to receptors, allowing change in certain proteins and enzymes, resulting in anti-inflammatory effects.	Consult with the patient's physician if taking corticosteroids. Long-term therapy may need to have supplemental steroids to avoid stressful situations. Usually for periodontal debridement there will not be a change in dosage.
Intermediate-acting (12–36 hours) Methylprednisolone (generic, Medrol) Prednisolone (generic, Orapred, Prelone Prednisone (generic, Meticorten, Deltasone) Triamcinolone (generics, Aristocort, Kenacort)	Prednisone is usually the first drug of choice because of low cost and fewer adverse side effects (sodium and water retention).	Consult with the patient's physician if taking corticosteroids. Long-term therapy may need to have supplemental steroids to avoid stressful situations. Usually for periodontal debridement there will not be a change in dosage.
Long-acting (36–54 hours) Betamethasone (generic, Celestone) Dexamethasone (generic, Decadron)	Dexamethasone has the greatest anti-inflammatory activity.	Consult with the patient's physician if taking corticosteroids. Long-term therapy may need to have supplemental steroids to avoid stressful situations. Usually for periodontal debridement there will not be a change in dosage. Oral solution (e.g., syrup) can be used in the management of some oral diseases (e.g., aphthous ulcers, lichen planus)

- Peptic ulcers
- Psychiatric disorders
- Poor/delayed wound healing
- Immune suppression
- With prolonged use there is a reduction in protein production and fat deposition in areas that were previously occupied by muscle, producing the characteristic "moon face" and "buffalo hump." These features simulate the disease called Cushing's syndrome. Corticosteroids also cause water and sodium retention (except for prednisone), calcium excretion, and potassium imbalance (Table 16-6).

Rapid Dental Hint

NSAIDs should not be used in patients taking corticosteroids because there is an increased risk of GI bleeding and ulcers.

In long-term therapy, alternate-day dosing should be used. Doubling the dosage and administering the drug every other day in the morning mimics the endogenous (body's own) corticosteroid circadian rhythm. The goal of steroid therapy should be to maintain the lowest dosage possible while obtaining the desired clinical response.

Rapid Dental Hint

Look for intraoral candidiasis in patients taking systemic corticosteroids.

Corticosteroids should be used with caution or not be given to patients with herpes simplex, glaucoma, diabetes mellitus, peptic ulcer disease, osteoporosis, congestive heart failure, hypertension, infections (fungal, bacterial, viral), and psychiatric disorders.

WITHDRAWAL OF CORTICOSTEROIDS   When corticosteroids are to be withdrawn, there is a "tapering" period so that patients do not experience withdrawal syndrome. This allows the body to recover the normal secretion of endogenous corticosteroids. In most patients the dosage is tapered over 2 months or more. Symptoms of adrenal insufficiency that are seen if the steroid is withdrawn rapidly include headache, fatigue, joint pain, nausea, vomiting, weight loss, fever, and peeling of the skin.

TABLE 16-6 Common Adverse Effects of Corticosteroids

SHORT-TERM THERAPY (1 WEEK OR LESS)	LONG-TERM (CHRONIC) THERAPY
Peptic ulcer (gastrointestinal bleeding)	Cushing's syndrome (moonface, buffalo hump)
Psychosis (psychiatric disorders)	Peptic ulcers
Hypertension	Psychosis
Hyperglycemia (diabetes mellitus)	Potassium imbalance (cardiac problems)
Sodium and water retention	Diabetes mellitus
	Sodium and water retention

Rapid Dental Hint

For certain less stressful procedures (e.g., periodontal debridement, restorative), no dosage adjustment is necessary. When necessary, consult with your patient's physician.

DRUG INTERACTIONS Corticosteroids (e.g., hydrocortisone, methylprednisolone) are metabolized by the CYP3A4 isoenzymes in the liver. Metabolism of corticosteroids is enhanced, decreasing plasma levels, when taken with carbamazepine (Tegretol), phenobarbital, phenytoin (Dilantin), and rifampin. Glucocorticoids may increase the dosage requirement for insulin.

Topical Corticosteroids

Synthetically produced steroid agents are also used topically (e.g., cream, ointment) for skin and oral lesions (e.g., aphthous stomatitis, vesiculo-bullous diseases on the oral mucosa, burning mouth/tongue) as well as ear, nose, and throat conditions. Table 16-7 lists the common topical steroid preparations according to the degree of potency. For example, hydrocortisone is the least potent and best to use in infants and children because of minimal systemic absorption. Local and systemic adverse effects from topical corticosteroids are minimal. Absorption through the skin varies with the different formulations. Some formulations are fluoridated (a fluorine atom is added to the molecule), which prolongs the duration of action and increases the anti-inflammatory action, but unfortunately increases the incidence of adverse effects, including mineralocorticoid activity (e.g., sodium and water retention). Over-the-counter topical corticosteroids are available as hydrocortisone 0.5% and 1%.

For dental application on oral mucosa, a special formulation is available, a type of oral paste made from carboxymethylcellulose, gelatin, and pectin dispersed in a plasticized hydrocarbon gel that is composed of 5% polyethylene in mineral oil. This oral paste or adhesive is available as Orabase (Colgate Oral Hoyt, Canton, MA). Different compounds are added to this adhesive paste including benzocaine (topical anesthetic) and hydrocortisone acetate 5 mg (0.5%), which is available under the name Orabase HCA (hydrocortisone) Oral Paste (Colgate Oral Hoyt). Topical corticosteroids are indicated for any ulcerations or irritations of the oral mucosa [e.g., oral lichen planus, lupus erythematosus, and recurrent aphthous ulcers (canker sores)].

Corticosteroids alone are not effective against viral infections, and they are immunosuppressive, which would further aggravate the lesions or increase the incidence of herpes simplex infections. In addition to using Orabase HCA, formulations of high-potency gels or very high-potency ointments (see Table 16-7) such as fluocinonide gel 0.05% (Lidex, Lidex-E) or clobetasol propionate 0.05% can be used for shorter periods of time. The affected area in the mouth should be dried and then the paste should be "dabbed" on, not rubbed, with a clean finger or cotton swab.

Systemic absorption occurs when topical corticosteroids are applied to oral mucosa. Absorption increases with increased potency of the steroid and with prolonged usage.

Topical corticosteroids are available in different formulations and strengths. Since creams are oil-in-water emulsions, they must be rubbed in well until the cream is not seen. Ointments provide more occlusive covering than creams and are best suited for dry skin. Lotions are made of suspensions of powder or liquid in a water (aqueous) vehicle and are best for inflamed and tender areas because they are "cooling" and lubricate the area.

Dental Hygiene Applications

When exogenous glucocorticosteroids are taken systemically, the internal or endogenous production of these hormones by the adrenal cortex may be "turned off," resulting in adrenal gland suppression. There is concern regarding dental patients who may be at risk of experiencing **adrenal crisis** (acute adrenocortical insufficiency) during or after stressful invasive procedures; however, literature suggests that this is a rare event in dentistry.

Patients' physicians should be contacted for any dental surgical procedures.

The usual recommended dose of predisone is 5–60 mg/d in single or divided doses. Short-term treatment usually does not present with any adverse effects, including adrenal suppression. More than 20 mg a day or 2 mg/kg/d for at least 14 days may alter the patients' immunity. This should be taken into account when scheduling invasive procedures (e.g., extractions, periodontal surgery, implant surgery, incision and drainage of infections). The clinician should confirm that patients took the recommended dose of steroid within 2 hours of the procedure. It may be advantageous to increase the dose so as not to exacerbate the medical condition. The normal dose may need to be increased and tapered back to the normal dosage after the procedure; however, some studies no longer support

TABLE 16-7 Selected Topical Corticosteroids for Dermatological and Oral Lesions

DRUG NAME (GENERIC)

Lowest-potency, Group VII

- Hydrocortisone 2.5% (various brand names—Cortaid, Cortizone—OTC; 0.5% and 1%)
- Hydrocortisone acetate 0.5% (in Orabase: for dental lesions)

Group VI

- Alclometasone (Aclovate)
- Flurandrenolide (Cordran 0.0125%) F
- Dexamethasone (Decadron) F
- Triamcinolone acetonide cream (Aristocort, Kenalog 0.025%) F
- Triamcinolone acetonide dental paste 0.1% (Oralone)

Group V

- Hydrocortisone valerate 0.2% cream (Westcort)

Group IV

- Desoximetasone (Topicort 0.05%) F
- Flucoinolone acetonide (Synalar) F
- Hydrocortisone valerate ointment (Westcort 0.2%) F

Medium-Potency, Group III

- Betamethasone valerate ointment (Valisone)
- Flurandrenolide (Cordran) F
- Halcinonide (Halog 0.025%) F
- Triamcinolone acetonide ointment (generic, Aristocort, Kenalog 0.1%) F

High-potency, Group II

- Amcinonide (Cyclocort) F
- Betamethasone dipropionate F (Diprosone)
- Desoximetsone (Topicort 0.25%) F
- Fluocinolone (Synalar HP 0.2%) F
- Fluocinonide gel (Lidex) F

Highest-potency, Group I

- Clobetasol propionate (generic, Temovate) F
- Diflorasone diacetate (Psorcon) F
- Halobetasol propionate (Ultravate) F

All are available by prescription only except for those listed as OTC.

Hydrocortisone acetate in Orabase is used orally.

High-potency gel or very high-potency ointment can also be used orally.

F denotes fluorinated (increased potency)

routine recommendations for corticosteroid supplementation (Miller CS, Little JW, Falace DA. 2001. Supplemental corticosteroids for dental patients with adrenal insufficiency. *JADA* 132(11):1570–1579). For minor, less stressful procedures such as periodontal probing, scaling and root planing, restorative, and orthodontics, no corticosteroid adjustments are required.

Sex Hormones and Contraceptives

Sex hormones or steroids are specific proteins produced and secreted by male and female organs called gonads (ovaries and testes), the adrenal cortex, and the placenta during pregnancy that affect the growth or function of the reproductive organs and the development of secondary sex characteristics. The female sex hormones are estrogens and progestins, which include progesterone; the major male sex hormone are androgens, which include testosterone.

The gonadotropins, secreted by the anterior pituitary gland, are responsible for controlling the activity of the reproductive organs and controlling the synthesis of the hormones produced by the male and female. The primary gonadotropins are FSH (follicle stimulating hormone), LH (luteinizing hormone), ICSH (interstitial cell stimulating hormone), PL (prolactin), and GH (growth hormone).

Estrogens control contractility of the myometrium and contribute to the development of the primary female sexual characteristics (ovaries and uterus) and secondary characteristics (cervix, vagina, mammary gland). Estrogens also control the menstrual cycle. Sex hormones are used to treat various medical conditions. These hormones can be used alone or in combination with other sex hormones.

Estrogens

INDICATIONS AND MECHANISM OF ACTION Estrogens are available naturally or synthetically with estrogenic activity (Table 16-8). Three natural estrogens the female body produces are estradiol (the main estrogen secreted by the ovary), estrone, and estriol. Estrogen is used as:

1. Hormone replacement therapy (estrogen alone or in combination with progestins) to reduce the symptoms of menopause in postmenopausal women
2. Oral contraceptives in combination with progestins
3. Treatment of uterine bleeding due to a hormone imbalance
4. Amenorrhea (lack of menstruation)
5. Vulvar and vaginal atrophy (postmenopausal symptoms)
6. Prevention and treatment of osteoporosis
7. Treatment of skin lesions (e.g., acne)

Estrogens also increase HDL and triglyceride levels, and decrease LDL cholesterol levels. Estrogen products are available in different formulations including oral tablet, vaginal tablet, vaginal ring, vaginal cream, and transdermal (skin) system.

> ## DID YOU KNOW?
>
> The birth control pill was first patented in 1960.

Estrogen acts by diffusing through the cell membranes and binding to estrogen (protein) receptors to activate it. This activated receptor binds to specific DNA sequences, eliciting a hormone response.

Older formulations of estrogen underwent first-pass metabolism through the liver where they were extensively converted to inactive metabolites. Today, newer formulations using small particles (micronized estradiol) allow estradiol to be absorbed rapidly and undergo little first-pass metabolism. Additionally, the development of nonoral administration (patch, vaginal, implant, and intramuscular injection) of estradiol bypasses the oral route and avoids the first-pass effect, so a smaller dosage can be used. The development of conjugated estrogens allowed the drug to be metabolized in the gastrointestinal tract rather than undergoing extensive first-pass metabolism in the liver. Estradiol is metabolized in the liver to sulfate and glucuronide conjugates by intestinal bacteria. This allows for more rapid reabsorption into the circulation and back into the liver. This process of enterohepatic

circulation prolongs the action of the drug and reduces elimination. It has been suggested that some antibiotics (e.g., amoxicillin, clarithromycin, metronidazole, tetracycline, doxycycline, and ampicillin) that kill bacteria in the intestines may reduce the enterohepatic circulation of estrogen, resulting in a decrease in serum levels and reducing effectiveness of the contraceptive. It is advisable to inform patients of such interaction and discuss with the patient's physician additional or alternative methods of contraception.

Rapid Dental Hint

A female patient is taking an oral contraceptive and amoxicillin is prescribed for an endodontic infection. The patient should be advised to use an alternative birth control method while on the antibiotic.

ADVERSE EFFECTS Estrogens are contraindicated and should never be given to patients with breast cancer (or uterine, cervical, and vaginal cancer), pregnant patients, patients with liver disease, or patients with a vascular thromboembolic (blood clot) condition. There can be an increased risk for blood clots if patients smoke and take oral contraceptives. Many oral contraceptives are being taken off the market due to high mortality.

Estrogens may increase the risk, especially if used long term, of cerebral vascular accident (stroke)—especially in smokers, certain carcinomas (endometrial), endometrial hyperplasia, and gallbladder disease. Increased incidence of breast cancer in patients taking estrogens on a long-term basis is controversial. Additionally, estrogens cause nausea and vomiting, headache, dizziness, and breast tenderness.

Nonsteroidal Estrogens

Nonsteroidal estrogens, such as diethylstilbesterol (DES), were first introduced to prevent miscarriages, but it was found that the fetus was affected and that the children had a high incidence of development of vaginal cancer. Today, they are used only in the treatment of inoperable breast cancer.

Anti-Estrogens

Anti-estrogens are drugs that inhibit the actions of estradiol by binding to the estrogen receptor, preventing estradiol from binding. Tamoxifen (Nolvadex), anastrozole (Arimidex), exemestane (Aromasin), and toremifene (Fareston) are anti-estrogen drugs used in the treatment of breast cancer. Clomiphene (Clomid) is used to treat infertility by stimulating ovulation, causing the release of multiple mature ova.

Progestins

Progestins modify some of the effects of estrogens and may reduce the incidence of endometrial hyperplasia. There are two main groups of progestins: progesterone (naturally occurring; includes

TABLE 16-8 Sex Hormone Products

DRUG NAME	INDICATIONS
Estrogens	Estrogen replacement therapy (ERT)
Estradiol, micronized (Estrace); oral, vaginal cream	ERT; patch may provide more constant levels of estrogen
Estradiol transdermal system (Estraderm, Climara, Vivelle, Esclim, generics); skin patch	ERT
Conjugated estrogens (generics; Premarin); oral, IM, vaginal cream	ERT
Ethinyl estradiol (Estinyl); oral	ERT; oral contraceptives
Estradiol cypionate (Depo-Estradiol, generics)	ERT; oral contraceptives
Quinestrol (Estrovis)	ERT
Progestins	
Hydroxyprogesterone caproate (Duralutin, Pro-Depo, generics); injectable	Abnormal uterine bleeding, amenorrhea (no menstruation), and endometriosis
Medroxyprogesterone acetate (Provera, generics); oral	Abnormal uterine bleeding, amenorrhea (no menstruation), and endometriosis
Medroxyprogesterone acetate (Depo-Provera); injectable	Contraception
Megestrol (Megace); oral	Advanced breast cancer and endometrial cancer
Norethindrone (Norlutin); oral	Abnormal uterine bleeding, amenorrhea (no menstruation), and endometriosis
Norethindrone acetate (Aygestin, Norlutate); oral	Abnormal uterine bleeding, amenorrhea (no menstruation), and endometriosis
Progesterone micronized (Prometrium); oral	Hormone replacement to prevent endometriosis
Hormone Replacement Therapy: Estrogen + Progesterone Products	Replacement of estrogen with progesterone in women with menopause
Activella (estradiol/norethindrone); oral	
CombiPatch (estradiol/norethindrone); patch	
Estratest (esterified estrogens/methyltestosterone); oral	
Estratest H.S. (esterified estrogens/methyltestosterone); oral	
FemHRT 1/5(ethinyl estradiol/norethindrone); oral	
Ortho-Prefest (estradiol/norgestimate); oral	
Premphase (conjugated estrogens/medroxyprogesterone); oral	
Prempro (conjugated estrogens/medroxyprogesterone); oral	
Oral Contraceptives Estrogen + Progestin	To prevent pregnancy (ovulation)
Monophasic	
Loestrin (ethinyl estradiol/norethindrone acetate)	
Lo/Ovral (ethinyl estradiol/norgestrel)	
Demulen (ethinyl estradiol/ethynodiol diacetate)	
Modicon, Brevicon (ethinyl estradiol; norethindrone)	
Ovcon (ethinyl estradiol/norethindrone)	
Norinyl, Ortho-Novum (ethinyl esradiol/norethindrone)	
Norlestrin (ethinyl estradiol; norethindrone acetate)	
Ovral (ethinyl estradiol; norgestrel)	
Ortho Evra (norelgestromin/ethinyl estradiol)	
Norinyl (Mestranol; norethindrone)	
Enovid (Mestranol; norethynodrel)	

(continued)

TABLE 16-8 *(continued)*	
DRUG NAME	**INDICATIONS**
Biphasic	
Ortho-Novum (ethinyl estradiol; norethindrone)	
Triphasic	
Tri-Levlen; Triphasil (ethinyl estradiol; levonorgestrel)	
Ortho-Novum (ethinyl estradiol; norethindrone)	
Tri-Norinyl (ethinyl estradiol; norethindrone)	
Androgens	
Fluoxymesterone (Halostestin, generics); oral	Inoperable breast cancer in women
Methyltestosterone (Android, generic); oral	Inoperable breast cancer in women
Testosterone (Androderm, generic); IM	Treatment for male hypogonadism
Anabolic Steroids	
Nandrolone decanoate (Deca-Durabolin); injectable	Postmenopausal osteoporosis

dydrogesterone, hydroxyprogesterone, and medroxyprogesterone) and testosterone (norethindrone and norethynodrel). Progestins are used as antifertility agents (contraceptives) by decreasing ovulation, treatment of menstrual disorders, treatment of endometriosis (ovarian suppression), and in hormone replacement therapy (HRT) with estrogens (Table 16-8).

Because of the similar structure in progesterone and testosterone, progesterone may cause masculinity in females. Other adverse side effects of progestins include weight gain, hypertension, edema, cervical and breast changes, depression, acne, and thrombophlebitis.

Progestin Inhibitors

Progestin inhibitors inhibit the action of progestin at the progesterone receptors. Mifepristone (RU 486), called the "morning after" pill, is used to abort the embryo.

Estrogen/Hormonal Replacement Therapy

Estrogens are used for estrogen replacement therapy in menopausal and postmenopausal women for the prevention of osteoporosis. Additionally, estrogens may lower the incidence of menopausal symptoms, such as hot flashes, mood changes, and vaginitis, and reduce the incidence of cardiovascular disease. Estradiol, estropipate, and conjugated estrogens are primarily used in ERT. When estrogen only is used it is called estrogen replacement therapy (ERT), when estrogen is used in combination with progestins it is referred to as hormonal replacement therapy (HRT). In women without a hysterectomy (with a uterus), progesterone should be added to the estrogen, which may reduce the incidence of endometrial hyperplasia.

There is controversy concerning the preventive values of using ERT or HRT in menopausal/postmenopausal women. While there may be a reduction in the risk of bone fractures, with long-term therapy there may be an increased risk of breast cancer, stroke, and thromboembolism. HRT is contraindicated in women who are pregnant, or have liver disease, breast cancer, thromboembolic disorders, and vaginal bleeding. Smoking may

decrease the effectiveness of estrogen on bone and may increase the risk of thromboembolic disease.

Table 16-7 lists some estrogen-only ERT products, which include transdermal estradiol, conjugated estrogens, and micronized estradiol and estrogen plus progesterone HRT products.

Phytoestrogens, which are plant-derived products with so-called natural estrogen activity, are available in the health stores and should be used with caution, since the purity of the product as well as its side effects are unknown.

Oral Contraceptives

ESTROGENS + PROGESTINS; PROGESTIN ONLY Estrogens are used in oral contraceptives in combination with progestins to suppress the FSH (follicle-stimulating hormone) and thus inhibit ovulation (Table 16-8). Essentially, contraceptives work by mimicking pregnancy. Oral contraceptives are also used to treat endometriosis. Although most contraceptives are given orally, a few products are administered through a transdermal patch or a long-lasting depot, a long-lasting formulation that requires only weekly or monthly dosing.

ESTROGEN + PROGESTIN Combination oral contraceptives contain estrogen, generally in the form of ethinyl estradiol, and a progestin (Table 16-8). They are taken for 20–21 days and then discontinued for the following 6–7 days when menstruation occurs. The newer generation of oral contraceptives contains newer progestins that have no estrogenic effect and less androgenic (acne, depression, hirsutism, weight gain) effect. Combination oral contraceptives are available as monophasic, biphasic, and triphasic, corresponding to the progestin content.

Adverse effects of combination contraceptives include vaginal yeast infections; depression; headache; nausea; weight gain; leg, chest, or abdominal (stomach) pain; shortness of breath; and breast tenderness.

Oral contraceptives are contraindicated in pregnancy, liver disease, breast cancer, history of myocardial infarction, thromboembolism, and thrombophlebitis (especially in smokers). Oral contraceptives should be used with caution in women with gallbladder disease, and in women over age 35 who are smoking.

The newer progestins, such as norgestimate and desogestrel, cause fewer side effects than the older progestins.

PROGESTIN ONLY   The so-called minipill (norethindrone) is a type of progestin-only contraceptive. Progestin oral contraceptives are given continuously, with no days off. Progestin-only contraceptives are indicated in women who smoke, where estrogen is contraindicated, and in older women. It is indicated in patients at high risk to side effects from estrogen.

Drug Interactions: Sex Hormones

Tobacco smokers taking estrogen alone or in combination with progestins have an increased risk of stroke. Estrogens reduce the effects of oral anticoagulants (e.g., warfarin), resulting in clotting; adjustment of warfarin may be needed. Estrogens may inhibit the metabolism of benzodiazepines (Valium, Xanax), resulting in increased serum levels of benzodiazepines. Broad-spectrum antibiotics (e.g., tetracyclines, ampicillin, amoxicillin) have been stated in medical literature to interact with oral contraceptives (mainly the estrogen part), resulting in a decreased effectiveness of the oral contraceptive. Phenytoin may decrease the estrogen effect by increasing its metabolism.

Male Sex Hormones: Androgens and Anabolic Steroids

Male sex hormones have androgenic and anabolic effects. Androgens (testosterone) are used in the treatment of hypogonadism—which increases development of male puberty and growth when it is delayed—and inoperable breast cancer in women. Most testosterone products undergo extensive first-pass metabolism in the liver, reducing the oral bioavailability. Most products are given parentally (IM) or transdermally (Table 16-8).

Anabolic steroids are testosterone-like compounds with hormonal activity used to hasten weight gain after severe trauma or surgery and alleviate postmenopausal osteoporosis. They are taken (inappropriately) by athletes to increase muscle mass and strength.

> **DID YOU KNOW?**
>
> Women taking oral contraceptives may show signs of gingival inflammation including bleeding on probing.

Bisphosphonates/Osteoporosis

In the mid-1990s **bisphosphonates** were first introduced and prescribed as alternatives to hormone replacement therapies (HRTs) for osteoporosis and to treat osteolytic tumors and possibly slow tumor development. In 1996, Fosamax™ (alendronate) was the first bisphosphonate drug approved for osteoporosis (low bone mass and reduced bone strength that leads to fractures of the spine, wrist, and hip) in postmenopausal women.

Over the past five years there have been major dental concerns regarding a rare adverse reaction of **osteonecrosis of the jaw** (ONJ) induced by bisphosphonates.

Indications

Bisphosphonates are prescribed in the treatment and prevention of:

1. Corticosteroid-induced osteoporosis
2. Postmenopausal osteoporosis
3. Hypercalcemia with metastatic cancer to help decrease bone pain and fracture by reducing blood calcium levels
4. Paget's disease
5. Chronic renal disease in patients undergoing dialysis (precipitates bone fragility)

Classification of Bisphosphonates

Commonly prescribed bisphosphonates are listed in Table 16-9.

General Pharmacology: Osteoporosis

Bisphosphonates act by inhibiting bone resorption by decreasing the action of osteoclasts. The osteoclastic resorption of mineralized bone and cartilage is blocked through its binding to bone which keeps the bone more dense. Also, bisphosphonates inhibit the increased osteoclastic activity and skeletal calcium release

TABLE 16-9	Bisphosphonates			
GENERIC NAME	TRADE NAME	ROUTE OF ADMINISTRATION	INDICATION	POTENCY FACTOR
Etidronate	Didronel	Oral	Paget's disease	1
Tiludronate	Skelid	Oral	Paget's disease	10
Clodronate	Bonefos, Loron, Ostac	Oral	Hypercalcemia (bone metastases)	10
Alendronate	Fosamax	Oral	Osteoporosis	500
Risedronate	Actonel	Oral	Osteoporosis	2,000
Ibandronate	Boniva	Oral/IV	Osteoporosis	1,000
Pamidronate	Aredia	IV	Bone metastases	100
Zoledronate	Zometa	IV	Bone metastases	10,000

into the bloodstream induced by various stimulatory factors released by tumors.

Risk Factors

Risk factors with the development of bisphosphonate-induced ONJ include:

- Current or history of taking bisphosphonates (especially IV formulations but also oral)
- History of cancer (breast, lung, prostate, multiple myeloma, or metastatic disease to the bone), osteoporosis, Paget's disease, chronic renal disease on dialysis

The following are local dental risk factors for ONJ in patients taking intravenous or oral bisphosphonates:

- Periodontal surgery
- Extractions
- Dental implant surgery
- Ill-fitting dentures that are irritating to the tissues
- Less likely with endodontic therapy, orthodontics, scaling and root planing
- Bisphosphonate ONJ can also occur spontaneously without any prior dental procedure

Clinical Presentation

Osteonecrosis is necrosis or death of bone and can cause severe, extensive, and irreversible damage to the jaw bone (occurs more frequently in the mandible than maxilla). Oral lesions appear similar to those of radiation-induced osteonecrosis. There usually is a delayed or completely absent healing of the periodontium after dental extraction or surgery for more than 6 weeks or can occur spontaneously.

The following are signs and symptoms of ONJ (Figures 16-7 and 16-8):

- Irregular mucosal ulcer with exposed bone in the maxillofacial area
- Pain or swelling in the area
- Infection

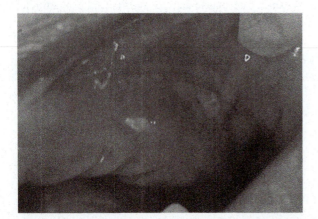

FIGURE 16-7 Edentulous patient with pieces of bone that became necrotic and continued to slough off after tooth extraction. (Courtesy, Jacqueline M. Plemons, DDS, MS, Baylor College of Dentistry; *U.S. Pharmacist.* Reprinted with permission from U.S. Pharmacist, Jobson Medical Information LLC.)

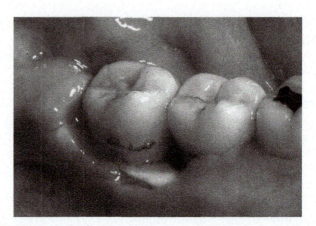

FIGURE 16-8 Case of ONJ that occurred spontaneously. Note the white area, which is exposed necrotic bone. (Courtesy, Jacqueline M. Plemons, DDS, MS, Baylor College of Dentistry; *U.S. Pharmacist.* Reprinted with permission from U.S. Pharmacist, Jobson Medical Information LLC.)

- Pain
- Mobility of teeth
- Numbness or heavy sensation

Novartis (East Hanover, NJ), a drug company that manufactures Aredia and Zometa, developed a staging criteria for ONJ (see Table 16-10).

Management

Treatment of ONJ depends on the severity of the case. Regardless of the severity, any necrotic bone should be removed. Conservative treatment of ONJ is recommended, including antibiotics, oral rinses (chlorhexidine), pain control, and periodontal debridement where needed.

Dental Hygiene Applications: Bisphosphonates

There are concerns regarding the dental management of patients currently taking or with a history of taking bisphosphonates because of the development of ONJ. Although the majority of reports of bisphosphonate-associated ONJ are in patients taking IV bisphosphonates, more reports are being documented in patients taking oral bisphosphonates. Thus, patients undergoing long-term IV or oral bisphosphonate therapy should be treated with caution and close observation after dental procedures. It is important to discuss the patient's dental needs with his or her physician.

The Food and Drug Administration, drug companies, and dental societies/associations (e.g., American Academy of Periodontology, American Association of Endodontists, American Academy of Oral Medicine, and American Association of Oral and Maxillofacial Surgeons) have issued precautions and

TABLE 16-10	Staging Criteria for ONJ
GRADE	SYMPTOM SEVERITY
1	Asymptotic
2	Mild
3	Moderate
4	Severe

recommendations for dentists to follow regarding prevention, diagnosis, and treatment guidelines for ONJ.

It is advised that patients have a dental examination and all dental procedures be completed prior to the start of bisphosphonate therapy; a careful medical history is needed to determine if a patient will require or is currently on bisphosphonates. Patients should go for routine dental maintenance visits at least every 6 months and maintain good oral hygiene. Routine restorative and dental hygiene procedures may be performed. An elective dental procedure is not advised in patients on IV bisphosphonates.

Dental Hygiene Applications

During a medical history interview, it is important to note if patients are taking contraceptives. Ethinyl estradiol, which is the primary drug used in contraceptives, may become ineffective in preventing pregnancy if patients are also taking broad-spectrum antibiotics such as tetracyclines, amoxicillin, or metronidazole (Flagyl). Consultation with the patient's physician may be necessary to change the method of contraception.

It has been stated in older dental literature that estrogens may cause increased gingivitis and gingival bleeding. Most of these studies were done in the 1960s and 1970s. The formulation of oral contraceptives has changed over the years resulting in less estrogen, which causes less gingival tissue change.

Key Points

- Adrenal crisis is rare in dentistry.
- Increases in systemic corticosteroid doses are not usually necessary in dental patients undergoing routine dental care (e.g., oral prophylaxis, scaling/root planing, operative).
- An increase in dose is necessary for patients undergoing stressful dental procedures such as extractions, periodontal surgery, and implant surgery.
- Systemic and topical corticosteroids are used in the treatment of many dental/oral conditions.
- A preparation containing hydrocortisone acetate in a paste (Orabase®) is used in patients with oral mucosa ulceration or irritation.
- Human insulin preparations: Regular insulin (rapid-acting) and NPH (intermediate-acting). All other insulin formulations are insulin analog preparations.
- Diabetics are more prone to the development of periodontal disease, and patients with periodontal disease have an increased incidence of development of diabetes.
- Other oral manifestations of diabetes mellitus include xerostomia, burning tongue/mouth, and *Candida* (fungal) infections.
- Epinephrine increases blood glucose. Patients who are not well controlled, with fluctuating blood glucose levels, or taking high doses of insulin should have the amount of epinephrine limited.
- Interview patients about the type of diabetic medication being taken. Make sure the medication is taken as directed and patients have eaten before dental treatment.

- There are no special precautions to follow regarding the use of epinephrine in patients taking thyroid medication as long as the condition is controlled and not hyperthyroidism.
- Oral manifestations of undiagnosed thyroid disease can be recognized during a dental exam.
- There is a possible drug–drug interaction between broad-spectrum antibiotics (e.g., tetracyclines) and oral contraceptives. Alternative contraceptive methods may have to be used.
- Oral contraceptives usually do not cause gingival inflammation because current formulations contain less estrogen.

Board Review Questions

1. Which of the following medications is most susceptible in causing hypoglycemia? (p. 274)
   a. Micronase
   b. Metformin
   c. Insulin
   d. Pioglitazone
   e. Repaglinide

2. Which of the following medications should *not* be given to a diabetic taking insulin? (p. 274)
   a. Ibuprofen
   b. Penicillin
   c. Acetaminophen
   d. Vitamin C

3. To which of the following classifications does metformin belong? (p. 272)
   a. Alpha-glucosidase inhibitors
   b. Biguanides
   c. Meglitindies
   d. Thiazolidinediones
   e. Insulin

4. Which of the following adverse effects is seen with insulin and should be carefully monitored while seeing a dental patient? (p. 274)
   a. Hypoglycemia
   b. Anorexia
   c. Constipation
   d. Hyperlipidemia
   e. Liver enzyme problems

5. In which of the following organs is insulin produced and secreted? (p. 268)
   a. Heart
   b. Kidney
   c. Liver
   d. Pancreas
   e. Lung

6. Which of the following substances should be given in limited amounts to uncontrolled diabetics? (pp. 274, 275)
   a. Water
   b. Epinephrine
   c. Lidocaine
   d. Benzocaine

7. Which of the following oral conditions occurs more frequently in a diabetic? (p. 275)
   a. Tooth decay
   b. Lip numbness
   c. Periodontal disease
   d. Increased salivation

8. If a conscious patient becomes hypoglycemic in the dental chair, which of the following substances should be administered? (p. 274)
   a. Sugar
   b. Water
   c. Coffee
   d. Tea

9. Which of the following systemic conditions could a diabetic also have? (p. 270)
   a. Hyperlipidemia
   b. Sinusitis
   c. Headaches
   d. Depression

10. Most of the insulin used today is: (p. 273)
    a. Animal
    b. Plant
    c. Recombinant human
    d. Combination plant and animal

11. Which of the following drugs may interact with Ortho-Novum? (pp. 282)
    a. Aspirin
    b. Tetracycline
    c. Chlorhexidine
    d. Ibuprofen
    e. Vitamin C

12. Which of the following statements is true concerning replacement of hormones in postmenopausal women? (p. 275)
    a. When estrogen is used alone, it is referred to as hormonal replacement therapy (HRT).
    b. Progesterone is usually combined with estrogen in women with a uterus.
    c. When estrogen is combined with progesterone, it is referred to as estrogen replacement therapy.
    d. An adverse side effect of estrogen therapy is depression.
    e. Patients taking estrogen may complain of xerostomia.

13. There is a high incidence of gingival overgrowth in patients taking oral contraceptives *because* most products on the market today contain lower concentrations of estrogen. (pp. 284, 285)
    a. Statement is true and the reason is correct.
    b. Statement is true and the reason is incorrect and not related.
    c. Statement is false but the reason is correct.
    d. Both the statement and reason are incorrect.

14. Which of the following hormones consists of the mini-pill? (p. 285)
    a. Estrogen
    b. Progestin

c. Estrogen/progestin
d. Androgen

15. Which of the following is an anti-estrogen drug? (p. 282)
    a. Tamoxifen
    b. Progestin
    c. Estrogen
    d. Metronidazole

16. Which of the following is the most common medication used to treat patients with hypothyroidism? (p. 275)
    a. Levothyroxine
    b. Thyroid USP
    c. Liotrix
    d. Iodide
    e. Propranolol

17. Which of the following blood markers are used to monitor for thyroid function? (pp. 275, 276)
    a. T_3 and T_4
    b. T_4 and TSH
    c. T_4 and pituitary stimulating hormone
    d. Iodine and T_3

18. All of the following are signs and symptoms of hyperthyroidism *except* one; which is the exception? (pp. 275, 276)
    a. Dry skin
    b. Nervousness
    c. Sweating
    d. Heat intolerance
    e. Palpitations

19. Which of the following medications is derived from animals? (p. 276)
    a. Thyroid USP
    b. Levothyroxine
    c. Liotrix
    d. Liothyronine

20. The primary classification of hydrocortisone is (pp. 278, 279)
    a. Anti-inflammatory
    b. Antihypertensive
    c. Antimicrobial
    d. Antifungal
    e. Antiviral

21. Which of the following steroid hormones is naturally occurring? (p. 278)
    a. Prednisone
    b. Prednisolone
    c. Cortisol
    d. Betamethasone
    e. Triamcinolone

22. All of the following are adverse side effects of corticosteroids *except* one. Which one is the exception? (pp. 285, 286)
    a. Hypertension
    b. Psychosis
    c. Peptic ulcers
    d. Water retention
    e. Heat tolerance

23. Which of the following conditions can be seen in patients taking oral bisphosphonates for the management of osteoporosis? (pp. 285, 286)
   a. Herpes labialis
   b. Aphthous ulcer
   c. Burning mouth
   d. Ulcerative lichen planus
   e. Osteonecrosis of the jaw (ONJ)

24. Which of the following is the cause of osteonecrosis of the jaw (ONJ) in patients taking bisphosphonates? (p. 279)
   a. Increase bone deposition
   b. Increase bone resorption
   c. Decrease cementum resorption
   d. Inhibit cementum deposition
   e. Inhibit bone resorption

Selected References

American Association of Endodentists. 2007, Winter. Bisphosphonate-associated osteonecrosis of the jaw. Chicago: Author.

American Association of Oral and Maxillofacial Surgeons. 2006, September 25. Position Paper on Bisphosphonate-related Osteonecrosis of the Jaws. Rosemont, IL: Author.

Corgel JO. 2007. Implants and oral bisphosphonates. *J Periodontol* 78:373–376.

DeRossi SS, Hersh EV. 2002. Antibiotics and oral contraceptives. *Dent Clin North Am* 46(4):653–664.

Evans A, Krentz AJ. 1999. Benefits and risks: of transfer from oral agents to insulin in type 2 diabetes mellitus. *Drug Saf* 21:7–22.

Fletcher SW, Colditz GA. 2002. Failure of estrogen plus progestin therapy for prevention. *JAMA* 288(3):366–367.

Grossi SG, Genco RJ. 1998. Periodontal disease and diabetes mellitus: A two-way relationship. *Ann Periodontol* 3(1):51–61.

Haines ST, Cushenberry LM, LeRoith D, Steil CF. 2001. New approaches to insulin therapy for diabetics. In *Special Report: A continuing education program for pharmacists*. Washington, DC: American Pharmaceutical Association.

Haupt BA. 2000, July. Management of thyroid disorders. *U.S. Pharmacist* (Suppl.).

Koda-Kimble MA, Young LY, Kradjan WA, Guglielmo BJ. 2002. Thyroid disorders. In *Handbook of applied therapeutics*, 7th ed. Baltimore: Lippincott Williams & Wilkins.

Mattson JS, Cerutis DR. 2001. Diabetes mellitus: A review of the literature and dental implications. *Compendium Dent Educ* 22(9):757–773.

Mealy BL. 2008. The interactions between physicians and dentists in managing the care of patients with diabetes mellitus. *JADA* 139:4S–7S.

Miller CS, Little JW, Falace DA. 2001. Supplemental corticosteroids for dental patients with adrenal insufficiency. *JADA* 132(11):1570–1579.

Moritz AJ, Mealey BL. 2006. Periodontal disease, insulin resistance, and diabetes mellitus. *Grand Rounds in Oral-Systemic Medicine* 1(2):13–20.

Muzyka BC. 2000. Revisiting the use of glucocorticosteroids in dentistry. *Practical Perio Aesthetic Dent* 2:814.

Pinto A, Glick R. 2002. Management of patients with thyroid diseases. *JADA* 133:849–858.

Ruggiero S, Gralow JRE, Marx AO, Hoff MM, Shubert J, Huryn M, et al. 2006. Practical guidelines for the prevention, diagnosis, and treatment of osteonecrosis of the jaw in patients with cancer. *J Oncology Practice* 2(1):7–14.

Takiya L, Dougherty T. Pharmacist's guide to insulin preparations: A comprehensive review. *Pharmacy Times*. Continuing education program 290-000-05-016-H01.

Thorstensson H, Kuylensteirna J, Hugoson A. 1996. Medical status and complications in relation to periodontal disease experience in insulin-dependent diabetics. *J Clin Periodontol* 23:194–202.

Webb MR. 2000. Treatment options for type 2 diabetes. *American Family Physician* Monograph no. 1.

Wells BG, DiPiro JT, Schwinghammer TL, Hamilton CW. 2000. Thyroid disorders. In *Pharmacotherapy handbook*, 2nd ed. Norwalk, CT: Appleton & Lange, pp. 213–225.

White Jr. JR, Campbell RK. 2003. Type 2 diabetes and insulin resistance: Counseling patients in the pharmacy. *U.S. Pharmacist* 28:65–87.

Wilson GR, Curry Jr. WR. 2005. Subclinical thyroid disease. *Am Fam Physician* 72:1517–1524.

World Health Organization. 1985. *Diabetes Mellitus: Report of a WHO Study Group*. Technical Report Serial No. 727. Geneva: Author.

Zoorob RJ, Cender D. 1998. A different look at corticosteroids. *Am Fam Physician* 59:443–452.

Web Sites

www.diabetesmonitor.com
www.diabetes.org
www.medscape.com
www.thyroid.org
www.medscape.com
www.novartis.com
www.jop.stateaffiliates.asco.org/JanuaryIssue/Summary-Guidelines.pdf
www.aae.org
www.perio.org

PEARSON
myhealthprofessionskit

Use this address to access the Companion Website created for this textbook. Simply select "Dental Hygiene" from the choice of disciplines. Find this book and log in using your username and password to access video clips of selected tests.

QUICK DRUG GUIDE

Antidiabetic Drugs

Sulfonylureas

First-Generation Agents

- Chlopropamide (Diabinese)
- Tolazamide (Tolinase)
- Tolbutamide (Orinase)

Second-Generation Agents

- Glipizide (Glucotrol)
- Glyburide (DiaBeta, Micronase)
- Glyburide, micronized (Glynase)
- Glimepiride (Amaryl)
- Glipizide ext-rel (Glucotrol XL)

Biguanides and Combinations

- Metformin (Glucophage, Fortamet)
- Metformin/rosiglitazone (Avandamet)
- Metformin/glyburide (Glucovance)
- Metformin/glipizide (Metaglip)
- Rosiglitazone/glimepiride (Avandaryl)

Thiazolidnedoines

- Rosiglitazone (Avandia)
- Pioglitazone (Actos)

Glucosidase Inhibitors

- Acarbose (Precose)
- Miglitol (Glyset)

Insulins

Rapid-Acting

- Insulin human inhalation powder (rDNA origin) (Exubera)
- Insulin glulisine (rDNA original) (Apidra)
- Insulin aspart (rDNA origin) (NovoLog FlexPen, NoVoglog Mix 70/30, NovoLog FlexPen)
- Insulin lispro (rDNA origin) (Humalog, Humalog Pen)
- Insulin regular (human insulin) (Humulin R, Novolin R, Regular Iletin II)

Intermediate- and Long-Acting

- Isophane insulin suspension (human insulin) (NPH, Humulin N; Novolin N, Iletin I, NPH Iletin II)
- Insulin zinc human (human insulin) (Humulin L, Novolin L)
- Human regular and human NPH mixture (Humulin 70/30, Humulin 50/50, Novolin 70/30)
- Insulin Glargine (Lantus) (analog)
- Insulin Determir (Levemir) (analog)
- PZI: Insulin lispro protamine 75%/insulin lispro 25%

Thyroid Drugs

Hyperthyroidism

Thiourea Drugs

- Propylthiouracil (PTU)
- Methimazole (Tapazole)

Radioacative Iodine (RAI)

Iodine Compounds

- Lugol's solution/potassium iodide (SSKI)

Hypothyroidism

- Thyroid USP
- L-thyroxine (Levoxyl, Synthroid, Levothroid)
- L-triiodothyronine (Cytomel)
- Liotrix (Thyrolar)

Systemic Corticosteroids

Short-Acting (8–12 hours)

- Cortisone (generic, Cortone); tabs
- Hydrocortisone, Cortisol (Cortef, various brand names); tabs

Intermediate-Acting (12–36 hours)

- Methylprednisolone (generic, Medrol); tabs
- Prednisolone (generic, Orapred, Prelone); tabs, syrup
- Prednisone (generic, Meticorten, Deltasone)
- Triamcinolone (Aristocort, Kenacort, generics)

Long-Acting (36–54 hours)

- Betamethasone (Celestone); tabs, syrup
- Dexamethasone (Decadron, generic)

Topical Corticosteroids (Drug Name/Generic)

Low-Potency Group IV

- Hydrocortisone (generic, Cortef, Synacort) Rx
- Hydrocortisone (various brand names—Cortaid, Cortizone—OTC; 0.5% and 1%)
- Hydrocortisone acetate (in Orabase®)
- Alclometasone (Aclovate)
- Flurandrenolide (Cordran 0.0125%) F
- Dexamethasone (Decadron) F
- Triamcinolone acetonide (Aristocort Kenalog 0.025%) F
- Triamcinolone acetonide F dental paste

Medium-Potency Group III

- Betamethasone benzoate (Uticort) F
- Desoximetasone (Topicort 0.05%) F
- Flurandrenolide (Cordran) F
- Flucoinolone acetonide (Synlar) F
- Halcinonide (Halog 0.025%) F
- Hydrocortisone valerate (Westcort 0.2%) F
- Mometasone furoate (Elocon) F
- Triamcinolone acetonide (generic, Aristocort, Kenalog 0.1%) F

High-Potency Group II

- Amcinonide (Cyclocort) F
- Betamethasone dipropionate F (diprosone)
- Desoximetsone (Topicort 0.25%) F
- Fluocinolone (Synalar HP 0.2%) F
- Fluocinonide (Lidex) F
- Triamcinolone acetonide (generic, Aristocort, Kenalog 0.5%) F

Very-High-Potency Group I

- Betamethasone dipropionate (Diprolene 0.05%) F
- Clobetasol propionate (generic, Temovate) F
- Diflorasone diacetate (Psorcon) F
- Halobetasol propionate (Ultravate) F

F denotes if the formulation is fluoridated, which prolongs the duration of action.

Estrogens

- Estradiol, micronized (Estrace); oral, vaginal cream
- Estradiol transdermal system (Estraderm, Climara, Vivelle, Esclim, generics); skin patch
- Conjugated estrogens (generics; Premarin); oral, IM, vaginal cream
- Ethinyl estradiol (Estinyl); oral
- Estradiol Cypionate (Depo-Estradiol, generics)
- Quinestrol (Estrovis)

Progestins

- Hydroxyprogesterone caproate (Duralutin, Pro-Depo, generics); injectable
- Medroxyprogesterone acetate (Provera, generics); oral
- Medroxyprogesterone acetate (Depo-Provera); injectable
- Megestrol (Megace); oral
- Norethindrone (Norlutin); oral
- Norethindrone acetate (Aygestin, Norlutate); oral
- Progesterone micronized (Prometrium); oral

Hormone Replacement Therapy

Estrogen + Progesterone Products

- Activella (estradiol/norethindrone); oral
- CombiPatch (estradiol/norethindrone); patch
- Estratest (esterified estrogens/methyltestosterone); oral
- Estratest H.S. (esterified estrogens/methyltestosterone); oral
- FemHRT 1/5 (ethinyl estradiol/norethindrone); oral

- Ortho-Prefest (estradiol/norgestimate); oral
- Premphase (conjugated estrogens/ medroxyprogesterone); oral
- Prempro (conjugated estrogens/medroxyprogesterone); oral

Oral Contraceptives

Estrogen + Progestin Products

Monophasic

- Loestrin (ethinyl estradiol/norethindrone acetate)
- Lo/Ovral (ethinyl estradiol/norgestrel)
- Demulen (ethinyl estradiol/ethynodiol diacetate)
- Modicon, Brevicon (ethinyl estradiol; norethindrone)
- Ovcon (ethinyl estradiol; norethindrone)
- Norinyl, Ortho-Novum (ethinyl estradiol; norethindrone)
- Norlestrin (ethinyl estradiol; norethindrone acetate)
- Ovral (ethinyl estradiol; norgestrel)
- Ortho Evra (Norelgestromin/ethinyl estradiol)
- Norinyl (Mestranol; norethindrone)
- Enovid (Mestranol; norethynodrel)

Biphasic

- Ortho-Novum 10/11 (ethinyl estradiol; norethindrone)

Triphasic

- Tri-Levlen; Triphasil (ethinyl estradiol; levonorgestrel)
- Ortho-novum 7/7/7 (ethinyl estradiol; norethindrone)
- Tri-Norinyl (ethinyl estradiol; norethindrone)

Androgens

- Fluoxymesterone (Halostestin, generic); oral
- Methyltestosterone (Android, generic); oral
- Testosterone (Androderm, generic); IM

Anabolic Steroids

- Nandrolone decanoate (Deca-Durabolin); injectable

Herbal and Natural Remedies

GOAL

To introduce the dental hygienist to the actions, drug interactions, and concerns of common herbal and nutritional supplements seen in the dental practice.

EDUCATIONAL OBJECTIVES

After reading this chapter, the reader should be able to:

1. Discuss the views of complementary and alternative medicine.

2. Describe the actions of various herbal products used in dentistry.

3. List common adverse side effects and drug–herb interactions.

4. Discuss the role of herbal medicine in dentistry.

KEY TERMS

Alternative medicine

Homeopathy

Herbal supplements

Nutritional supplements

Homeopathy and Natural Products

Plants have been used for their medicinal value for thousands of years. Most early medications, and approximately 25% of our current prescriptions, are plant based. An herb is technically a botanical without woody tissue such as stems or bark. In Europe the treatment of diseases using plant-based therapies has achieved the status of an accepted discipline.

Complementary and **alternative medicine** refers to the use of products that are not considered to be part of conventional healthcare. Essentially, these "natural" products focus on the mind and body of the individual as well as emphasizing self-care. The term *pharmacognosy* refers to the study of natural products that are the results of plant and animal metabolism. For example, cannabis (marijuana) consists of the dried flowering tops of the plants of *Cannabis sativa,* and calcium alginate used for dental impressions is extracted from seaweed.

Alternative healthcare deals with **homeopathy,** naturopathy, and chiropractic therapy. Samuel Hahnemann founded the practice of homeopathy. Physicians used homeopathy in the late eighteenth and early nineteenth centuries. Essentially, the basis of homeopathy is that the cause of disease is the disturbance of a spiritual vital force, which manifests as specific symptoms. Today's conventional medicine treatment of symptoms from diseases involves using medicines that oppose the action of the symptoms; for instance, the use of antipyretics such as aspirin or acetaminophen for patients with fever will lower the fever but causes fever in toxic doses. Nitroglycerin treats angina but causes angina in toxic doses. Hahnemann recognized that many natural products produce pharmacological effects, which he called "symptoms." He believed that using these substances in toxic doses in healthy individuals produces symptoms similar to a given disease. Patients' symptoms disappear following a minimal dose of the substance that has a toxicology profile matching the symptoms patients display; homeopathy deals with "like cures like." Hahnemann did recognize that giving these substances could aggravate the condition and present with other side effects. He decided to dilute the substance to the point where the symptoms were no longer present. Dilutions of the substance reduce the concentration of the active substance to very low levels. Homeopathic medicines have official compendial status in the United States. The Homeopathic Pharmacopoeia of the United States/Revision Service (HPRS) is recognized as the official compendium of homeopathy.

The use of **herbal** and **nutritional dietary supplements** to treat diseases is considered to be biologically based therapies. Beginning in the late 1970s and continuing today, herbal medicine has experienced a comeback, with nearly 60 million Americans taking nonprescription herbal medicines every day. These people have the impression that natural substances have more healing power than synthetic medications. Also, these products are readily available at a reasonable cost. The percentage of people aged 45 to 64 who take herbal supplements increased about 50% between 1998 and 2002. Billions of dollars are spent yearly on herbal medicines. Many people take over-the-counter herbal products alone or with prescription medicines without informing their physician.

Safety Concerns

One of the major skepticisms is whether these products are safe and effective. In 1990, the Food and Drug Administration classified herbal medicines as food supplements. The Dietary Supplement and Health Education Act (DSHEA) of 1994 classifies vitamins, minerals, amino acids, and herbs as dietary supplements, which allows the marketing of these "food supplements" without the approval of any government agency for testing for safety, efficacy, or standards of manufacturing. The FDA is only required to prove that these products are unsafe. Dietary supplements do not have to be tested prior to marketing, and the effectiveness of the product does not have to be demonstrated by the manufacturer. The product label must include a disclaimer that the product is not FDA evaluated or approved and it is not intended to diagnose, treat, or prevent any disease. The DSHEA does not regulate the accuracy of the label; the product may or may not contain the product listed in the amounts claimed. Herbal products therefore cannot be marketed for the diagnosis, treatment, cure, or prevention of disease. However, these products can be labeled explaining their proposed effect on the human body (e.g., alleviation of fatigue) or their role in promoting general well-being (e.g, enhancement of mood). Dietary supplement labeling requires the wording "dietary supplement" as part of the product name, and it must include a "supplement facts" panel on the ingredients. Also, products derived from plants must designate the plant part and the Latin binomial.

It must be emphasized that herbal products can be beneficial but also have harmful effects. Patients using herbs should make their physicians aware of this. Herbs should not be used by patients with serious medical conditions, pregnant women, nursing women, or young children unless under the care of a physician. It is recommended to start with the lowest recommended dose and then to increase if needed.

Active Ingredients

There are many herbal products on the market. Some common herbs are listed in Table 17-1.

The two primary formulations of herbal products are solid and liquid. Solid formulations include tablets, capsules, salves, and ointments. Liquid formulations are made by extracting the active chemicals from the plants using solvents such as water, alcohol, or glycerol. The liquids are then concentrated in various strengths. Extracts are concentrated formulations of fluids, powders, solids, and oils. Teas are prepared by drying the herb, which is marketed in its coarse cut form or in tea bags.

Herbal products are made from natural chemicals extracted from a plant and are produced either in the original form or refined, where the essential extract is removed from the plant, concentrated, and then added back into the original form to make it more concentrated. The active ingredients in an herbal product may be present in only one specific part of the plant or in all parts. For example, the active ingredient in ginger is composed of roots found below ground, whereas in St. John's wort it comes from leaves and stems which are above the ground. Every herb contains many active chemicals rather

TABLE 17-1   Nutraceuticals

HERBAL PRODUCT	USES	ADVERSE EFFECTS	DRUG INTERACTIONS
Betel nut (Areca catechu)	Masticatory stimulant	Oral leukoplakia, stained teeth and gingiva bronchoconstriction	May interact with antipsychotics, causing bradykinesia and jaw tremor
Chamomile (different species) (flower of plant)	Reduces flatulence, diarrhea, upset stomach, common cold, mild sedation	Allergic reactions	Aspirin: increased bleeding Benzodizepines: CNS depression
Dong Quai (*Radix Angelicae Sinensis*) (root of plant)	Gynecological conditions, muscle relaxant, high blood pressure, constipation, ulcers, arthritis	Photosensitivity, bleeding	Aspirin: increased bleeding
Echinacea (*Echinacea angustifolia*) (different plant parts)	Strengthens immune system, prevents colds and flu	Fever, nausea, vomiting, hepatoxicity if used longer than 8 weeks	Increased liver toxicity: acetaminophen, ketoconazole
Ephedra (*E. sinica*)	Respiratory conditions, weight loss	Hypertension, cardiac arrhythmias, anxiety	Can increase sympathomimetic actions of drugs
Garlic (*Allium sativum*) (comes from garlic bulbs)	Decreases cholesterol levels, lowers blood pressure, and is an anticoagulant	Bleeding; topical garlic may cause the appearance of a chemical burn	Increased bleeding: aspirin, NSAIDs, warfarin; insulin: additive hypoglycemic effect reduces saquinavir (Fortovase) serum levels
Ginger (comes from the ginger root)	Anti-emetic (nausea), vertigo	Bleeding	Aspirin, NSAIDs, warfarin: additive anticoagulant effects
Ginkgo (*Gingko biloba*) (comes from leaves and seeds)	Improvement of cognitive functioning in Alzheimer's disease (dementia); also used for sexual dysfunction caused by selective serotonin reuptake inhibitors (SSRIs)	Bleeding	Additive bleeding effects: warfarin, NSAIDs/aspirin
Ginseng (*Panax* spp.) (plant root)	Increases vitality, elevates energy levels	Bleeding, hypoglycemia, hypertension	Increased bleeding: aspirin Diuretics: increased diuresis Insulin and oral hypoglycemics: increased hypoglycemic effect Digoxin: may increase toxicity
Glucosamine and chondroitin (glucosamine is derived from chitin from shrimp and crabs and chondroitin is from cow cartilage; glucosamine is also available in synthetic form)	Osteoarthritis	Bleeding	Increased bleeding: Anticoagulants, NSAIDs; contraindicated if allergic to shellfish
Green tea (fresh or dried tea leaves)	Prevents cancer, causes weight loss	Caffeine-related irritability, irregular heartbeat, diarrhea, vomiting, headache	Atropine
Kava kava (*piper methysticum*) (comes from the root of the plant)	Treatment of anxiety, insomnia, and muscle tension Possesses antipyretic (fever reducer) and local anesthetic properties	Interferes with blood clotting, sedation, oral and lingual dyskinesia, rash, painful twisting movement of the trunk, liver problems	May increase the effects of local anesthetics Increased CNS depression with alcohol, opiates, barbiturates, benzodiazepines Levodopa/carbidopa; worsening of Parkinson's symptoms Phenothiazines: Increased risk of tardive dyskinesia

(continued)

TABLE 17-1 *(continued)*

HERBAL PRODUCT	USES	ADVERSE EFFECTS	DRUG INTERACTIONS
			Warfarin/aspirin/NSAIDs: prolonged bleeding
Licorice (*Glycyrrhiza glabra*)	Stomach ulcer	Hypertension	Increased levels of digoxin; increased blood pressure with ACE inhibitors
Melatonin (endogenous hormone secreted by the pineal gland)	Jet lag, insomnia, anticancer	Drowsiness	Unknown
Saw palmetto (*Serenoa repens*) (comes from fruit and berries)	Treatment of symptoms of benign prostate hyperplasia	Bleeding, gastrointestinal upset	Additive effect with oral contraceptives; decreased iron absorption
St. John's wort (*hypericum perforatum*) (comes from flowers, leaves, and stems)	Mild to moderate depression	Xerostomia, gastrointestinal upset, allergic reactions, fatigue, dizziness, confusion, photosensitivity, bleeding	Reduced effectiveness of oral contraceptive; may reduce digoxin serum levels; serotonin syndrome (tremors, seizures, hypertension) in patients taking SSRIs, tricyclic antidepressants, MAOIs for depression
			NSAIDs/aspirin/warfarin: prolonged bleeding
			Cyclosporine: may decrease cyclosporine levels
Valerian root (*Valeriana Officinalis*) (root of the plant)	Insomnia, restless motor syndrome	Headaches, dizziness, GI upset	Antidepressants/anti-anxiety drugs: increased CNS depression

than just one, like in conventional medicines. Most of these chemicals have not been isolated and identified so the strength of the product varies considerably, which makes standardization difficult. Additionally, the chemical composition of herbal supplements is unpredictable. Some standardizations, which are printed on the product label and may differ from one manufacturer to another, have been documented, including:

- *Kava kava,* which contains about 40–45% kavalactones
- *Ginkgo biloba* contains 24% ginkgo flavone glycosides, 60 mg ginkgo biloba extract, and 6% terpene lactones
- *St. John's wort,* which contains 0.3–0.5% hypericins and 3–5% hyperforin

Adverse Effects

Adverse effects can occur with herbal/natural supplements. Most reactions are due to filler substances added to the herbal product but not on the label.

More commonly encountered adverse effects include sedation and bleeding, which manifests either via direct effects on capillaries, by interfering with platelet adhesion, or by increasing fibrinolytic activity. Caution should be used when prescribing aspirin or NSAIDs to patients taking herbs that could increase bleeding, including ginger, garlic, and ginkgo. Another adverse effect is an allergic reaction to the herb, which can manifest in the oral cavity (e.g., gingiva, tongue).

Dental Implications

Various herb or dietary supplements are used to treat various oral conditions/lesions. Table 17-2 lists some supplements commonly used.

Rapid Dental Hint

Prolonged bleeding may occur during periodontal debridement in patients taking ginger, ginkgo, ginseng, St. John's wort, garlic and glucosamine/chondroitin. Bleeding will most like be controlled in healthy patients. If the patient is also taking aspirin or other blood thinner, consult with the patient's physician. These products should be stopped up to 5–7 days before periodontal/implant/extraction surgery.

Dental Hygiene Applications

The increasing popularity of over-the-counter natural and herbal products demands that dental clinicians be more knowledgeable about the effects that these supplements have on oral health and treatment. Patients' medical history should include the use of nutraceuticals, since many have adverse side effects and drug

TABLE 17-2 Oral Conditions and the Appropriate Herbal Supplement

ORAL CONDITION	SUPPLEMENT
Aphthous ulcers (canker sores)	Aloe vera, red raspberry
Oral fungal infections (thrush)	Tea tree oil, cinnamon
Periodontal disease	Coenzyme Q10, sanguinaria, goldseal
Caries	Licorice root (glycyrrhiza glabra)
Oral inflammation (mucositis) in cancer patients	Chamomile, vitamin E

interactions that may affect dental treatment. Most of these effects are associated with sedative, hepatotoxic, and antiplatelet properties of the herbs. Many nutraceuticals can increase the risk of bleeding, especially when taken with anticoagulants or NSAIDs. Products that cause bleeding may have to be discontinued before surgical procedures.

Key Points

- Nutraceuticals are not FDA approved; however, many dental patients take various dietary supplements for different medical/dental conditions.
- Always ask patients, besides prescription and OTC drugs, if they are taking any type of nutraceutical.
- In a reference look up any potential drug–herb interaction.
- Many products cause bleeding, which may interfere with some surgical dental procedures.

Board Review Questions

1. A patient is taking 81 mg of aspirin and garlic for his high cholesterol levels. Which of the following conditions could the hygienist expect to see while treating this patient? (pp. 295, 296)
   a. Bleeding
   b. Xerostomia
   c. Red, shiny tongue
   d. Gingival enlargement

2. Which of the following herbs can be used in the treatment of oral thrush? (p. 297)
   a. Ginger
   b. Garlic
   c. Tea tree oil
   d. Saw palmetto

3. Which of the following herbs can be used in the management of an aphthous ulcer? (p. 297)
   a. Aloe vera
   b. Garlic
   c. Kava kava
   d. St. John's wort

4. Which of the following nutraceuticals may have to be discontinued prior to periodontal surgery? (p. 296)
   a. Aloe vera
   b. Echinacea
   c. Green tea
   d. Kava kava

5. Which of the following nutraceuticals can be used in the treatment of periodontal disease? (p. 297)
   a. Coenzyme Q10
   b. Green tea
   c. Tea tree oil
   d. Aloe vera

Selected References

Abebe W. 2002. Herbal supplements: Any relevancy to dental practice? *NY State Dent J.* 68:26–30.

ADA Guide to Dental Therapeutics, 3rd ed. 2003. Chicago: American Dental Association.

Cheema P, El-Mefty O, Jazieh AR. 2001. Intraoperative haemorrhage associated with the use of extract of Saw Palmetto herb: A case report and review of literature. *J Intern Med* 250:167–169.

Cohan RP, Jacobsen PL. 2000. Herbal supplements: Considerations in dental practice. *J Calif Dent Assoc* 28:600–610.

Cupp MJ. 1999. Herbal remedies: Adverse effects and drug interactions. *Am Fam Physician* 59:1239–1245.

Fugh-Berman A. 1997. Clinical trials of herbs. *Primary Care* 24:889–903.

Lambrecht JE, Hamilton W, Rabinovich A. 2000. A review of herb–drug interactions: Documented and theoretical. *U.S. Pharmacist* 25:42–53.

Philip RB. 2004. *Herbal–drug interactions and adverse effects (an evidence-based quick reference guide).* New York: McGraw-Hill.

Web Sites

http://www.nlm.nih.gov/medlineplus/druginformation.html
http://www.herbal-supplements-guide.com/
www.ars-grin.gov/duke/

Use this address to access the Companion Website created for this textbook. Simply select "Dental Hygiene" from the choice of disciplines. Find this book and log in using your username and password to access video clips of selected tests.

Glossary

Absorption Movement of a drug from its site of administration (e.g., mouth), across body membranes and into the bloodstream (circulation).

Acethylcholine (ACh) Neurotransmitter of the parasympathetic nervous system; also present at the sympathetic preganglionic neurons.

Acquired resistance When a microorganism is no longer affected by an anti-infective drug.

Action potential Electrical changes in the membrane of a nerve cell due to changes in membrane permeability.

Acute Disease that has a sudden onset, severe symptoms, and a short course.

Addiction *See* Dependence.

Adherence Also referred to as compliance. Obeying, following orders as it pertains to taking medications. The opposite is nonadherence.

Adrenal crisis (acute adrenocortical insufficiency) Severe phase or attack characterized by insufficient amounts of the adrenocortical hormones and resulting in nausea, vomiting, low blood pressure, and life-threatening imbalances in electrolytes.

Adrenal glands Two small, triangular-shaped glands located on top of each kidney; consists of the adrenal cortex, which synthesizes and secretes corticosteroids, and the adrenal medulla, which synthesizes, secretes, and stores dopamine, epinephrine, and norepinephrine.

Adrenergic Referring to nerves that release norepinephrine (NE) or epinephrine (EPI).

Adrenergic agonist A drug that acts on or mimics the sympathetic nervous system. *See* Sympathomimetic drug.

Adrenergic blocker (antagonist) A drug that blocks the actions of the sympathetic nervous system.

Adverse drug event An undesirable and unexpected effect of a drug that occurs at a dose used in humans for prophylaxis, diagnosis, or therapy.

Adverse drug reaction An effect that is noxious and unintended, and that occurs at normal doses, during normal use.

Affinity Reversible binding of a drug with a receptor forming a drug–receptor complex. The higher the affinity of the drug to the receptor, the more binding occurs to that receptor versus another receptor.

Agonist Binding of a drug to a receptor that results in a maximal pharmacological response.

Agonist, full An agonist drug that produces the greatest maximal response of any agonist acting on the same receptors on the same tissue.

Agonist, partial An agonist drug that produces a response that is less than the maximal response produced by a full agonist acting at the same receptors on the same tissue.

Akathisia Inability to remain still; constantly moving.

Aldosterone A steroid hormone secreted by the adrenal cortex that regulates the salt and water balance in the body.

Allergen A substance, such as pollen or aspirin, that causes an allergy or allergic reaction.

Allergic response A hyperresponse of body defenses. Signs of allergic reactions include skin rash, itching, edema (swelling), and redness.

Alternative medicine (also referred to as complementary medicine) Use of products that are not considered to be part of conventional healthcare.

Amide Type of chemical linkage found in some local anesthetics involving carbon, nitrogen, and oxygen (–N4–CO–).

Analgesia Loss of pain sensation without loss of consciousness.

Analgesic A drug that relieves pain without the loss of consciousness (patient is awake).

Anaphylaxis A severe type of allergic reaction that causes tachycardia (increased heart rate) and bronchospasm (spasm in lung tissue).

Androgens Steroid sex hormones that promote the appearance of masculine characteristics.

Anesthesia State of total or partial loss of sensation (inability to sense pain) with or without the loss of consciousness, induced by an anesthetic.

Anesthetic A drug that causes loss of sensation. Example: Local anesthetic causes a loss of pain sensation but not a loss of consciousness; general anesthetics cause a loss of pain sensation and a loss of consciousness.

Angina pectoris Heart condition where acute chest pain occurs upon physical or emotional exertion due to inadequate oxygen supply to the heart.

Angiotensin converting enzyme (ACE) Enzyme responsible for converting angiotensin I to angiotensin II.

Angiotensin II Chemical released in response to falling blood pressure that causes vasoconstriction and the release of aldosterone. Angiotensin II receptor antagonists are drugs used in the treatment of hypertension.

Antacid Drug that neutralizes acids in the stomach; used for heartburn (GERD).

Antagonist The effect of two or more drugs is less than the effects produced by each individual drug. The antagonist diminishes the effects of an agonist.

Antibiotic Substance produced by microorganisms that inhibits or kills other microorganisms. Some antibiotics are semisynthetic.

Anticholinergic See *Cholinergic blocker.*

Anticoagulant Drug that inhibits the formation of blood clots.

Anticonvulsant See *Anti-epileptic.*

Antidepressant Drug used in the treatment of depression.

Anti-epileptic Drug used in the management of seizures.

Antifibrinolytic Drug used to prevent and treat excessive bleeding from surgical sites.

Antifungal Drug used to treat fungal infections.

Antihistamine Drug that blocks histamine (H1) receptors, eliminating symptoms of rhinitis.

Anti-inflammatory Medication that reduces inflammation.

Antimicrobial (drug) resistance Bacteria can develop resistance to antibiotics, where the bacteria become insensitive to the antibiotic.

Antioxidant compounds (e.g., vitamins A, C, and E) They inhibit chemical reactions with oxygen and protect cells in the body against damage by free radicals, which are reactive by-products of normal cell activity. Claims are that antioxidants can lower the risk of heart disease and some forms of cancer.

Antipsychotics A group of drugs such as the phenothiazines or butyrophenones that are used to treat psychosis (mental disorder characterized by derangement of personality and loss of contact with reality).

Antipyretic Pertaining to an agent that works against fever.

Antiretroviral Drug used in the treatment of HIV/AIDS.

Antitussive Drug used to suppress a cough.

Antiviral Drug used to treat viral infections (e.g., acyclovir).

Anxiety State of apprehension, tension, or uneasiness from anticipation of danger. Treatment with anti-anxiety (anxiolytics) drugs, including benzodiazepines.

Anxiolysis Anti-anxiety.

Anxiolytics Drugs that have an anti-anxiety effect. The most commonly used anti-anxiety drugs are the benzodiazepines.

Apothecary System of Measurement Older system of measurement using drams; rarely used.

Arrythmias Irregular heart beat.

Asthma Chronic inflammatory disease of the lungs characterized by airway obstruction.

Atherosclerosis Condition characterized by a buildup of fatty plaque and loss of elasticity of the walls of the arteries.

Attention-deficit/hyperactivity disorder (ADHD) Disorder in children and adolescence characterized by hyperactivity, short attention span, poor concentration and behavior control problems.

Autonomic nervous system (ANS) Portion of the nervous system that regulates involuntary body functions including the heart and intestines.

Autoreceptor Binding of a drug to an autoreceptor results in a negative feedback response, whereby norepinephrine is inhibited from being released. Alpha$_2$-autoreceptors are located on postsympathetic nerve endings.

Bactericidal Antibiotic that kills bacteria.

Bacteriostatic Antibiotic that inhibits bacterial multiplication.

Balanced anesthesia Use of multiple medications to rapidly induce unconsciousness, cause muscle relaxation, and maintain deep anesthesia.

Benzodiazepines A category of drugs used to treat anxiety and insomnia.

Beta-blockers Drugs used to decrease high blood pressure.

Beta-lactam ring Chemical structure found in most penicillins.

Beta-receptors Type of receptor found in the sympathetic nervous system.

Bile A greenish-yellow fluid produced in and secreted by the liver, stored in the gallbladder, and released into the intestine.

Bioavailability The amount of drug dose (in percentage) entering the systemic circulation after administration. It is the amount of drug absorbed into the blood. For example, a drug given via IV has 100% bioavailability because the entire amount of drug directly enters the blood.

Bioequivalent (bioequivalence) A drug that acts on the body with the same strength and similar absorption (bioavailability) as the same dosage of a sample of a given substance.

Biotransformation Chemical alteration of a fat-soluble drug into a more water-soluble drug so it can be easily eliminated from the body. Term is used interchangeably with metabolism.

Bipolar disorder (formerly known as manic-depressive disorder) A psychiatric disorder characterized by alternating episodes of mania (excessive enthusiasm, interest, or desire) and depression.

Bisphosphonates Drugs used in the treatment of osteoporosis, metastatic cancer, Paget's disease, multiple myeloma. Concerns in dentistry because there is an association with the development of osteonecrosis of the jaw (ONJ).

Blood–brain barrier Anatomical structure that prevents or allows certain substances from gaining access to the brain.

Bradycardia Decreased heart rate.

Bradykinin Chemical released by cells during inflammation that produces pain and side effects similar to histamine.

Brand name Also called trade name; a name used to identify a drug that may or may not be registered as a trademark.

Broad-spectrum antibiotic Antimicrobial that is effective against many different gram-negative and gram-positive organisms.

Bronchioles Part of the lungs.

Bronchoconstriction Constriction or reduction in the size of a bronchus or bronchial tube of the lung.

Bronchodilation Dilation or widening of the air passages of the lungs, which eases breathing by relaxing bronchial smooth muscle.

Bronchospasm Rapid constriction of the airways.

Bruxism Characterized by grinding of the teeth.

Buccal route Tablet is placed in the oral cavity between the gingiva and the cheek.

Calcium channel blocker Drug that blocks the flow of calcium ions into the heart. Used for hypertension, angina, arrhythmias. They are vasodilators.

Candidiasis Fungal (Candida; *C. albicans*) infection.

Cardiac output Amount of blood pumped by a ventricle in one minute.

Cardiovascular Relating to the heart and blood vessels.

Carotene Class of yellow-red pigments that are precursors to vitamin A.

Catecholamines A group of amines derived from catechol that are important as neurotransmitters, which act in the autonomic nervous system (e.g., epinephrine, norepinephrine, and dopamine).

Ceiling effect The maximum pharmacological effect that can be induced from a drug regardless of how large a dose is administered; increasing the dose will not enhance the pharmacological response. Example: Once the maximum response is achieved with aspirin, increasing the dose does not increase the response.

Central nervous system (CNS) Division of the nervous system consisting of the brain and spinal cord.

Certainly lethal dose (CLD) Five to 10 g of sodium fluoride is considered a certainly lethal dose for a 70-kg adult. One quarter of the certainly lethal dose can be ingested without producing serious acute toxicity and is known as the safely tolerated dose.

Chemical name Name (chemical formula) used for drugs that is established by the International Union of Pure and Applied Chemistry.

Cholecalciferol Vitamin D_3, formed in the skin by exposure to ultraviolet light.

Cholesterol Essential component of cell membranes and precursor to steroids that are synthesized in the body.

Cholinergic Also referred to as parasympathetic; a term relating to nerves that release acetylcholine (ACh).

Cholinergic agonist Drug that acts on or mimics the cholinergic nervous system.

Cholinergic blocker (anticholinergic) Drug that blocks the actions of the parasympathetic nervous system.

Chronic Disease that continues over a long time, showing little change in symptoms or course.

Chronic obstructive pulmonary disease Progressive lung disease process characterized by difficulty breathing, wheezing, and a chronic cough. Complications include bronchitis, pneumonia, and lung cancer.

Chronotropic effect Change in the heart rate.

Clearance The volume of body fluid removed by biotransfomation or excretion.

Coagulation Process of blood clotting.

Coenzyme A substance that enhances or is necessary for the action of enzymes. They are usually smaller than enzymes themselves.

Cold sore (also referred to as herpes labialis) Herpes infection of the vermillion boarder of the lip.

Comorbidity Presence of more than one disease or disorder.

Controlled drug substances Certain drugs (e.g., narcotics) whose use is restricted by the Controlled Substance Act of 1970. Prescribers of drugs must register with the Drug Enforcement Administration (DEA) in order to prescribe narcotics.

Convulsions Uncontrolled muscle contractions or spasms.

Corticosteroids Steroid hormones released by the adrenal cortex; include mineralocorticoids and glucocorticoids.

Cortisone A glucocorticosteroid (corticosteroid) hormone that is isolated from the adrenal cortex; used as an anti-inflammatory agent.

Cyclooxygenase Enzymes found in the body. COX-1 functions to maintain and protect the lining of the stomach from damaging acid; COX-2 is produced during inflammation.

Cytochrome P450 enzymes Enzymes in the liver that metabolize drugs.

Cytokines Proteins such as interleukins that are released by cells of the immune system and regulate the actions of other cells in the generation of an immune response.

Dental infection Pathological state resulting from the invasion of the dental structures by pathogenic microorganisms.

Dependence (dependency) Replaces the obsolete term *addiction*. A physiological or psychological need for a drug or substance.

Depot Long-acting formulation of an injectable drug that is designed to have only weekly or monthly dosing.

Depression Disorder characterized by a depressed mood with feelings of sadness, despair, and discouragement. Treatment is with antidepressants.

Diabetes mellitus Group of hormonal diseases that are characterized by alterations in carbohydrates, protein, and lipid metabolism, the primary manifestation being abnormally high blood glucose levels (hyperglycemia).

Disintegrate Break open. Example: capsules disintegrate or break open before the drug can be dissolved.

Distribution The movement of a drug after it is absorbed in the bloodstream to the tissues/organs that the drug is intended to act on.

Dopamine A neurotransmitter formed in the brain and essential to the normal functioning of the central nervous system. An intermediate substance in the synthesis of norepinephrine. A deficiency in its concentration within the brain is associated with Parkinson's disease. Also, different levels are associated with schizophrenia.

Dosage form The state in which a drug is dispensed to be used; for example, the most common dosage form of aspirin is a tablet.

Dose The amount or quantity of a drug administered. For example, 500 mg (milligrams) of penicillin is given to a patient with an oral infection. 500 mg is the dose of the drug.

Drug Also referred to as a ligand. A chemical that is used in the diagnosis, treatment, or prevention of diseases in the body.

Drug effects Drug has a specific action on different parts of the body; can include intended action and side effects.

Drug laws To protect the public from deceitful and unsafe drug acts.

Drug-protein complex Drugs will bind reversibly to plasma (blood) proteins and circulate in the plasma until they are released or displaced from the drug-protein complex. While bound to the protein, drugs are not available for distribution to the body tissues. Drugs not bound to this complex are called "free drugs."

Duodenal ulcer Ulcer in the duodenum (part of the small intestine).

Duodenum Small intestine.

Dystonia Severe muscle spasms, particularly of the back, neck, tongue, and face; characterized by abnormal tension starting in one area of the body and progressing to other areas.

Edema "Fluid filled"; swelling. Sign of inflammation.

Effective dose (ED_{50}) The dose of a drug that produces a desired effect.

Efficacy The effectiveness of a drug in producing a more intense response as its concentration increases.

Elimination Drug is removed from the body.

Endogenous Produced or growing within the body.

Enteral Drugs administered orally or through a nasogastric tube into the digestive (gastrointestinal) tract. Most common route of drug administration.

Enteric-coated Tablets that have a hard, wax coating so they dissolve in the basic environment of the small intestine rather than the acidic contents of the stomach, which can be irritating to the stomach.

Enterohepatic circulation Some large drug compounds are excreted in the bile rather than in the urine. After the bile empties into the intestines, part of the drug may be reabsorbed into the blood and eventually return to the liver. An example of a drug that undergoes enterohepatic circulation is oral contraceptives.

Enzyme A protein that accelerates the rate of chemical reactions.

Epilepsy Disorder of the CNS (central nervous system) characterized by seizures and/or convulsions.

Epinephrine A catecholamine released by the adrenal medulla upon activation of preganglionic sympathetic nerves. Causes increased heart rate (β_1-receptor stimulation), vasoconstriction in arteries and veins (α_1 and α_2-receptor stimulation), and vasodilation (β_2 stimulation), which decreases blood pressure.

Excretion The removal of drugs from the body. The primary site of excretion is through the kidney via urine. Other routes of drug elimination are lungs, sweat, milk, bile, and feces.

Exogenous Produced or growing outside the body.

Expectorant Drug used to increase bronchial secretions.

Extrapyramidal side effects Symptoms of acute dystonia, akathisia, Parkinsonism, and tardive dyskinesia, often caused by antipsychotic drugs.

Fight-or-flight response Characteristic set of signs and symptoms produced when the sympathetic nervous system is activated.

First-order kinetics Refers to the rate (time) of drug elimination from the body. The rate of elimination depends on the concentration of drug in the blood. As the blood concentration of a drug falls, the amount of drug eliminated or excreted also falls. First-order elimination accounts for elimination of most drugs.

First-pass effect Also referred to as first-pass metabolism. After a drug is swallowed, it is absorbed by the digestive (gastrointestinal) system. It then enters the liver via the portal vein. In the liver the drug is metabolized (broken down) before entering systemic circulation (bloodstream). Some drugs are so extensively metabolized by the liver that only a small amount of unchanged drug enters the systemic circulation (bloodstream) to become available to the whole body. Drugs administered via the sublingual or rectal route undergo less first-pass metabolism than if given by the oral route. Examples of drugs that undergo first-pass metabolism are methyldopa/levodopa for the management of Parkinson's disease, aspirin, estrogens, and analapril (Vasotec; for hypertension).

Fluoride A binary compound of fluorine with another element; helps prevent dental caries.

Folic acid A B vitamin that is a coenzyme in protein and nucleic acid metabolism.

Food and Drug Administration (FDA) An agency of the U.S. Department of Health and Human Services. Responsible for the evaluation and approval of new drugs.

GABA (gamma-aminobutyric acid) Substance found in the central nervous system that is associated with the transmission of nerve impulses.

Ganglion (plural, ganglia) A collection of cell bodies of neurons located outside the central nervous system (CNS).

Gastric ulcer Ulcer in the stomach.

Gastroesophageal reflux disease (GERD) Condition of the upper gastrointestinal tract where there is a reflux or "backing up" of gastric contents from the stomach into the esophagus. Common complaint is heartburn.

Gastrointestinal Refers to the gastrointestinal (GI) tract, which is part of the digestive system that includes the mouth, esophagus, stomach, and intestines.

General anesthesia A controlled state of unconsciousness, accompanied by a partial or complete loss of protective reflexes, including loss of ability to independently maintain airway and respond purposefully to physical stimulation or verbal command, produced by a pharmacologic or nonpharmacological method or combination.

Generic name A drug name assigned by the U.S. Adopted Name Council. Example: acetaminophen is the generic name of the drug Tylenol.

Glomerular filtration Passive filtration (straining) of the blood as blood flows through the kidney. The extent to which a drug is filtered depends on size, protein binding, ionization, polarity, and kidney function.

Glucocorticosteroids Synthetic steroids used as anti-inflammatories in certain medical conditions.

Glucogenolysis Epinephrine is responsible for converting stored glycogen (carbohydrates) into glucose (in the liver).

Half-life (T_2^1) The time required for the concentration of a drug in the blood to be reduced by 50% (or $\frac{1}{2}$). For example, penicillin G has a half-life of 20 minutes. This means that 50% of the drug remains in the blood 20 minutes after its intravenous administration.

Hemorrhage Profuse bleeding.

Hepatic Refers to the liver.

Hepatic cytochrome enzyme system Enzymes found in the liver that are responsible for most biotransformation (or metabolism) of drugs. The primary action of these enzymes is to inactive drugs, which makes them more water-soluble, to be excreted in the urine. Many drug–drug interactions can be explained by changes in the activity of these enzymes. Examples of some enzymes in the liver include CYP3A4 (CYP refers to cytochrome) and CYP2C9. Erythromycin and clarithromycin inhibit the CYP3A4 enzyme in the liver, which decreases the metabolism and elimination of alprazolam (Xanax; anti-anxiety drug) and ketoconazole (Nizoral; antifungal drug), resulting in increased toxic blood levels of these drugs.

Hepatotoxicity (hepatotoxic) Liver damage that is caused by many factors, including certain drugs.

Herbal (as in herbal supplements) Use of medicinal herbs (plants) to prevent and treat diseases and ailments or to promote health and healing.

Herpes simplex virus Virus that causes oropharygeal disease (eyes, lips, mouth, face) (HSV-1) and sexually transmitted disease (HSV-2).

High-density lipoprotein (HDL) Lipid-carrying particle in the blood that contains high amounts of protein and lower amounts of cholesterol; considered to be "good" cholesterol.

Highly active antiretroviral therapy (HAART) Drug therapy for HIV infection that includes high doses of three-drug combination regimens that are given concurrently.

Hormone Chemical secreted by endocrine glands that act as a chemical messenger to effect homeostasis.

Host The recipient (one that receives).

Host flora Normal microorganisms found in or on an individual.

Hydrophilic "Water-loving"; refers to drugs that are water-soluble and do not dissolve easily in the lipid layer of the cell membrane. These drugs must go through pores or channels in the membrane.

Hydroxyapatite Mineral component of bones and teeth.

Hypercholesterolemia High levels of cholesterol in the blood.

Hyperglycemia High glucose level in the blood.

Hyperkalemia High potassium levels in the blood.

Hyperlipidemia Excess amount of lipids in the blood.

Hypertension High blood pressure.

Hypervitaminosis Excessive intake of vitamins.

Hypnotic Drug that induces sleep.

Hypoglycemia Low glucose level in the blood.

Hypokalemia Low potassium levels in the blood.

Immunocompetent Normal immune systems.

Immunocompromised Immune systems are not functioning properly; seen in medically ill patients such as HIV/AIDS.

Inotropic effect Change on the strength of contractility of the heart.

Insulin Hormone secreted by the beta cells of the pancreas. Keeps glucose levels within a normal range within the blood.

Insulin resistance Decreased insulin effectiveness with a reduced sensitivity of the beta cells to respond to the insulin.

Interferons A group of naturally occurring proteins that act as chemical messengers between cells. Three interferons—alpha, beta and gamma—have immune-modulating effects. Used in the treatment of cancer, hepatitis, and autoimmune diseases.

Interleukins A type of cytokine that regulates or stimulates immune cells.

Intradermal (ID) route Drug is administered with a needle into the top layer (dermis) of skin.

Intramuscular (IM) route Drug is administered with a needle into specific muscles.

Intravenous (IV) route Drug is administered with a needle directly into the bloodstream. There is 100% bioavailability.

Ionized Ionized form of a drug has a high water solubility, which means that the drug will diffuse (cross) lipid (fat) membranes with more difficulty than unionized/fat-soluble drugs. Ionized drugs are more water-soluble and are more rapidly excreted in the urine than nonionized drugs.

Ischemia Decreased blood supply to an organ or tissue.

Isoenzymes Any of the chemically distinct forms of an enzyme that perform the same function.

Ligand Refers to a molecule or drug that binds to another chemical entity to form a larger complex (e.g., a drug binding to a receptor resulting in a pharmacological action).

Lipid Refers to "fat."

Lipophylic "Fat-loving"; refers to drugs that are lipid soluble and will dissolve easily in the lipid layer of the cell membrane.

Lipoproteins Transport cholesterol, triglycerides, proteins, and phospholipids in the blood (because lipids are insoluble in plasma). Different types: HDL, LDL, VLDL.

Loading dose A high amount of drug is administered, usually as a first dose, which is intended to supply the blood with a sufficient level to quickly induce a therapeutic response. A maintenance dose is administered afterward.

Local anesthetic Loss of sensation to a limited part of the body without loss of consciousness (e.g., dental local anesthetics).

Low-density lipoproteins (LDL) Lipid-carrying particle that contains relatively low amounts of protein and high amounts of cholesterol; considered to be "bad" cholesterol.

Maintenance dose After a loading dose is administered and before plasma levels drop to zero, a maintenance dose is administered to keep the plasma drug concentration in the therapeutic range.

Manic Disorder characterized by impulsive, excitable, and overreactive actions.

Mechanism of action How a drug exerts its effects.

Median effective dose (ED$_{50}$) Dose required to produce a specific therapeutic response in 50% of a group of patients.

Median lethal dose (LD$_{50}$) Often determined in preclinical trials, the dose of drug that will be lethal (kill) in 50% of a group of patients.

Median toxicity dose (TD$_{50}$) Dose that will produce a given toxicity in 50% of a group of patients.

Megadoses Usually referring to vitamins; doses of a nutrient that are more than the recommended amount.

Metabolism (metabolize) Breakdown of fat-soluble drugs into water-soluble form. Primary site of metabolism is the liver. See also *Biotransformation*.

Migraine Common type of vascular headache involving abnormal sensitivity of arteries in the brain to various triggers.

Minerals Natural compounds formed through geological processes; used as supplements in some medical conditions. Examples: calcium, magnesium.

Minimum effective concentration The amount of a drug required to produce a therapeutic effect or response.

Miosis Constriction of the pupil.

Moderate sedation Formerly referred to as conscious sedation. Administration of drugs for the purpose of sleepiness (sedation), unaware of surroundings, amnesia, or analgesia without loss of consciousness.

Monoamine oxidase inhibitors (MAOIs) Drugs used to treat depression. Inhibit the enzyme monoamine oxidase, which terminates the actions of neurotransmitters such as norepinephrine, epinephrine, dopamine, and serotonin. By inhibiting the enzyme action, the levels of these neurotransmitters are elevated.

Monotherapy Use of one drug to treat a condition because it reduces the incidence of adverse effect (e.g., monotherapy is the prefered treatment option in epilepsy).

Mood disorder Change in behavior such as clinical depression, emotional swings, or manic depression.

Morbidity (rate) The proportion of patients with a particular disease during a given year per given unit of population; the incidence or prevalence rate of a disease.

Mortality Death rate.

Muscarinic receptor Type of cholinergic receptor found in smooth muscle, cardiac muscle, and glands. *See* Receptors.

Mydriasis Dilation of the pupil of the eye.

Myocardial infarction Heart attack.

Narcotic (also refered to as opioids) Natural or synthetic drug related to morphine; may be used as a broader legal term referring to hallucinogens, CNS stimulants, marijuana, and other illegal drugs.

Narrow-spectrum antibiotic Anti-infective (antimicrobial) drug that has an effect against only one or a small number of microorganisms.

Narrow therapeutic index Dose of the desired or therapeutic effect is close to the toxic dose. Examples of drugs with a narrow therapeutic index are lithium and digoxin.

Negative symptoms In schizophrenia, symptoms that subtract from normal behavior including a lack of interest, motivation, responsiveness, or pleasure in daily activities.

Nephrotoxicity (nephrotoxic) Pertaining to kidney failure.

Nerve membrane Nerve sheath that surrounds a nerve cell. Local anesthetic must penetrate the membrane to be effective.

Nervous system

Autonomic nervous system (ANS) Portion of the nervous system that regulates involuntary body functions including the heart and intestines.

Central nervous system (CNS) Portion of the nervous system that consists of the brain and spinal cord.

Peripheal nervous system (PNS) Portion of the nervous system that is outside the brain and spinal cord. The nerves in the PNS connect the CNS to sensory organs (e.g., eyes), other body organs, muscle, blood vessels, and glands.

Neuralgia Sharp, severe pain extending along a nerve or group of nerves.

Neuromuscular blocker Drug used to cause total muscle relaxation.

Neuron Cell that is the functional unit of the nervous system.

Neuropathic pain Pain sustained by abnormal processing of sensory input by the peripheral or central nervous system. It is often described as burning, tingling, or shooting. Examples include cancer-related pain, diabetic neuropathy, HIV-associated pain, postherpetic neuralgia, and trigeminal neuralgia.

Neurotransmitter A chemical released by nerves at synapses and neuromuscular junctions.

Nicotonic receptor Type of cholinergic receptor found in ganglia of both the sympathetic and parasympathetic nervous system. *See* Receptors.

Nitrous oxide A colorless, sweet-tasting gas, N_2O, used as a mild anesthetic in dentistry and surgery.

Nociceptive pain Pain arising from a stimulus (e.g., injury to tissues) that is outside of the central nervous system. Pain comes from skin, bone, joint, muscle, or connective tissue. Pain is often described as throbbing and is well localized. Examples include pulpitis, post-periodontal surgery, post-extraction, and dentinal hypersensitivity.

Nonionized Nonionized form of drugs have a high lipid (fat) solubility that easily crosses cell membranes, made of lipids. During excretion from the body, most nonionized drugs must be reabsorbed into the blood before being excreted in the urine because they need to be in a water-soluble form to be excreted.

Norepineprine (NE) A neurotransmitter released from sympathetic nerves. Causes increased heart rate (β_1-receptor stimulation) and vasoconstriction in arteries and veins (β_1- and β_2-receptor stimulation).

Odontogenic Pertaining to teeth.

Opiate Any preparation or derivative of opium.

Opioid A narcotic substance, either natural or synthetic.

Oral Route of delivery in which drugs are swallowed, chewed, or dissolved in the mouth.

Oral lesion An area of altered tissue in the mouth.

Orofacial Pertaining to the mouth (oro) and face (facial), as in orofacial pain (pain in and around the mouth and the face).

Orthostatic hypotension Fall in blood pressure that occurs when changing position from recumbent to upright.

Osteonecrosis of the jaw (bisphosphonate-associated osteonecrosis of the jaw) Severe condition associated with the use of IV and oral bisphosphonates. Characterized by necrosis of the jawbone.

Over-the-counter drugs (OTC) Medications that can be obtained without a prescription.

Parasympathetic nervous system Part of the autonomic nervous system that is active during resting and digestion periods; produces a relaxation response (e.g., increases gastrointestinal movement and slows heart rate).

Parasympathomimetics Drugs that mimic the actions of the parasympathetic nervous system.

Parenteral route Delivery of a drug by all routes except oral and topical. Drug is administered with a needle into the skin, subcutaneous tissue, muscles, or veins.

Parkinson's disease Degenerative condition of the nervous system caused by a deficiency of the brain neurotransmitter dopamine that results in disturbances of muscle movement.

Parkinsonism Having tremors, muscle rigidity, stooped posture, and a shuffling walk.

Pellagra Deficiency of niacin (vitamin B_3).

Peptic ulcer Erosion of the mucosa of the lining of the esophagus, stomach, or duodenum. Usually caused by the bacterium *Helicobacter pylori* (*H. pylori*). An ulcer in the stomach is called a gastric ulcer, an ulcer in the duodenum is called a duodenal ulcer.

Periocoronitis Infection of the tissue (operculum) overlying a partially erupted tooth.

Peripheral nervous system Division of the nervous system that includes all nerves outside the central nervous system, including the autonomic nervous system.

Permeability (permeable) The flow of a substance through a porous material.

pH A measure of the acidity or alkalinity of a solution. Involved in the absorption and solubility of drugs.

Pharmacodynamics What the drug does to the body: drug action on the body, mechanism of action of the drug.

Pharmacogenetics Convergence of pharmacology and genetics, which deals with genetic factors that influence an organism's response to a drug.

Pharmacokinetics What the body does to the drug: absorption (movement of the drug through the body), distribution, metabolism, and elimination.

Pharmacology Comes from the Greek words *pharmakos*, which means drug or medicine, and *logos*, which means study.

Photosensitivity Condition that occurs when the skin is highly sensitive to sunlight. Some drugs are photosensitive, including doxycycline and ciprofloxacin.

Placebo A pill or injection that has no pharmacological action. It exerts no therapeutic effect and produces no side effects. Used in clinical studies. Patients often report a decrease in symptoms and side effects. This is the power of suggestion.

Plasma The fluid portion of blood. Whole blood does not clot. The red blood cells are centrifuged down.

Plasma half-life *See* Half-life.

Polar Soluble in water.

Polypharmacy (also referred to as polytherapy) Use of multiple medications.

Polytherapy See *Polypharmacy*.

Positive symptoms In schizophrenia, symptoms that add on to normal behavior, including hallucinations, delusions, and a disorganized thought or speech pattern.

Posology Study of the dosages of medicines and drugs.

Postsynaptic neuron Neuron in the synapse that has receptors for the neurostransmitter.

Potency The strength of a drug at a specific concentration or dose.

Pregnancy category Classifying drugs based on how safe they are for the unborn fetus. Category A, B, C, D, or X.

Prescription A prescriber's order (written or oral) to dispense a specific drug.

Prescription drugs Drugs obtained with a prescription (oral or written).

Presynaptic neuron Neuron that releases the neurotransmitter into the synaptic cleft.

Prodrug Drugs that are administered into the body as inactive compounds and must be biotransformed or metabolized in the liver to an active form that will result in a pharmacological effect or response in the body.

Prophylaxis (prophylactically; prophylactic) Prevention of disease with treatment (e.g., antibiotic prophylaxis to prevent infective endocarditis).

Prostaglandins Class of hormones that promotes local inflammation and pain when released by cells in the body.

Protein A large complex molecule made up of one or more chains of amino acids. Proteins perform activities inside the cell.

Protein bound After being absorbed into the blood, a drug may become bound (bind) to proteins (albumin) in the blood. These protein-bound drugs are inactive.

Proton pump inhibitors Drugs that inhibit the enzyme H^+, K^+-ATPase. Used in the treatment of ulcers.

Reabsorption Elimination process whereby after being filtered out of the blood and through the kidneys nonionized, lipid-soluble drugs cross back through the kidney membrane and return to the blood (circulation), and are not eliminated, in order to be further metabolized into a more water-soluble form to be excreted. Ionized and water-soluble drugs generally do not get reabsorbed back into the circulation, but remain in the filtrate for excretion because these drugs are water-soluble and are easily excreted in the urine.

Receptors Component (protein) of a cell to which a drug binds in a dose-related manner to produce a response:

Adrenergic Receptors on sympathetic nerves.

Cholinergic Receptors on nerves that release acetylcholine.

Alpha (α) Type of subreceptor found in the sympathetic nervous system.

Beta (β) Type of subreceptor found in the sympathetic nervous system.

Muscarinic Type of cholinergic receptor found in/on smooth muscle, cardiac muscle, and glands.

Nicotinic Type of cholinergic receptor found in ganglia of both sympathetic and parasympathetic nervous systems.

Recommended daily allowance (RDA) Amount of vitamin or mineral needed each day to avoid a deficiency in a healthy adult.

Recurrent Minor aphthous ulcer (also referred to as canker sore).

Reflex tachycardia If blood pressure decreases, the heart beats faster in an attempt to raise it.

Refractory Resistant to treatment.

Renal Refers to the kidneys.

Renin-angiotensin system Series of enzymatic steps by which the body elevates blood pressure.

Retinoid Compound resembling vitamin A. Indicated in the treatment of severe acne and psoriasis.

Reye's syndrome Potentially fatal complication of infection associated with aspirin use in children.

Rhinitis Inflammation of the nasal mucous membranes.

Risk factor An environmental, behavioral, or biological factor that definitely increases the probability that something will occur.

Scheduled drug Drugs (narcotics) that have a significant potential for abuse. There are five categories based on the abuse potential: Schedule I (high potential for abuse), Schedule II, Schedule III, Schedule IV, and Schedule V (lowest abuse potential).

Schizophrenia Psychosis characterized by abnormal thoughts, withdrawal from people and the outside environment, and preoccupation with one's own mental state.

Secretion (secrete) The passage of material from the inside of a cell to the outside.

Sedative Drug that quiets, calms, or allays excitement.

Sedative/hypnotic Drug that produces a calming, sedative effect in low doses and sleep in higher doses.

Seizures Symptom of epilepsy characterized by abnormal electrical charges within the brain.

Generalized seizures Seizures that go through the entire brain on both sides.

Partial seizures Seizures that start on one side of the brain and go a short distance before stopping.

Selective serotonin reuptake inhibitor (SSRI) Drug that selectively inhibits the reuptake of serotonin into the nerve terminal; used for the treatment of depression.

Selectivity Responses involving any given type of receptor, only elicited by a narrow range of drugs with similar structural properties.

Sensitivity Referring to receptors. Drugs producing marked effects at low doses.

Serotonin A compound formed from tryptophan and found in the brain, blood, and gastric mucous membranes. A neurotransmitter.

Serotonin syndrome A condition that is caused by taking selective serotonin reuptake inhibitors (SSRIs) with MAOIs. This results in increased serotonin levels in the brain. Characterized by agitation, confusion, severe hypertension, and GI symptoms.

Serum Whole blood is allowed to clot. The red blood cells and fibrinogen are centrifuged down. The supernatant fluid is serum.

Sex hormones Any of various hormones, such as estrogen and androgen, affecting the growth or function of the reproductive organs and the development of secondary sex characteristics.

Soluble Dissolves in a solution.

Steroid Type of lipid that makes up certain hormones and drugs.

Subcutaneous (SC, SQ) route Drug is injected with a needle into the deepest layers of the skin. Insulin is given this route.

Sublingual route (SL) Drug is placed under the tongue and allowed to dissolve slowly. Rapid onset of drug action because this area is very vascular (a lot of blood vessels).

Substance P Protein substance that stimulates nerve endings at an injury site and within the spinal cord, increasing pain messages.

Superinfection An infection, usually a fungus such as *Candida albicans*, caused by an organism different from the one causing the initial infection. It is usually an adverse side effect of broad-spectrum antibiotics.

Sympathetic The part of the autonomic nervous system (ANS) that deals with stress or fight or flight. When stimulated, heart rate increases.

Sympatholytic A drug that blocks the actions of the sympathetic nervous system.

Sympathomimetic A drug that stimulates or mimics the sympathetic nervous system.

Synapse Junction between two neurons consisting of a presynaptic (preganglionic) neuron, a synaptic cleft, and a postsynaptic (postganglionic) neuron.

Synaptic cleft Space between two neurons that must be crossed by the neurotransmitter.

Syncope Fainting.

Tachycardia Increased heart rate.

Tachyphylaxis Rapidly decreasing response to a drug following initial doses; a type of tolerance.

Tardive dyskinesia Unusual tongue and face movements such as lip-smacking and wormlike motions of the tongue that occur during treatment with antipsychotic drugs.

Teratogen A chemical substance that harms a developing fetus or embryo.

Teratogenic Causing malformations of an embryo or fetus.

Testosterone Hormone produced by the testes; male sex hormone important in the development of secondary sex characteristics and masculinization.

Therapeutic Index The ratio of a drug's LD_{50} to its ED_{50}.

Therapeutic range The plasma (blood) drug concentration between the minimum effect concentration and the toxic concentration.

Thrombocytopenia Low platelet count.

Thrombosis Enhanced formation of fibrin.

Thyroid gland Gland produces and releases thyroid hormones that are involved in the regulation of basal metabolic rate or the speed by which cells perform their functions. By increasing cellular metabolism, thyroid hormone increases body temperature. The gland also helps to maintain blood pressure and regulate growth and development.

Thyroxine (T_4) Major hormone secreted by the thyroid gland.

Tolerance Need for increased amount of a substance to achieve the same desired effect or intoxication.

Topical The route by which drugs are placed directly onto the skin or mucous membranes. Example: topical dental anesthetic.

Toxic concentration The plasma level of a drug that will result in serious adverse effects.

Trade name Drug name assigned by the company marketing the drug. Example: Tylenol is the trade name of the drug acetaminophen.

Transdermal drug delivery Drug from a patch penetrates the top layer of skin.

Tricyclic antidepressant Class of drugs used in the management of depression.

Triglycerides Type of lipid in the body and the main storage form of energy to support the generation of high-energy compounds.

Triiodothyronine (T_3) At the target tissue, thyroxine is converted to T_3, which enters the target cells and binds to receptors inside the cell; it is the active form of the thyroid hormone.

Tuberculosis Bacterial infection affecting primarily the lungs, more common in urban areas, treatable with antibiotics.

Tyroxine Hormone produced by the thyroid gland; important in growth and development and regulation of the body's metabolic rate and metabolism of carbohydrates, fats, and proteins.

Vascular Referring to blood vessels.

Vasoconstriction The narrowing of blood vessels; causes blood pressure to rise.

Vasoconstrictor A drug added to local anesthetics to counteract the vasodilating effects of the anesthetic agent. Example is epinephrine.

Vasodilation (vasodiliation) Relaxation of the smooth muscles of the blood vessels producing dilated vessels; causes blood pressure to lower.

Very low-density lipoprotein (VLDL) Lipid-carrying particle that is converted to LDL in the liver.

Vitamins Organic compounds required by the body in small amounts.

Withdrawal Physical signs of discomfort associated with drug abuse.

Xerostomia Dry mouth.

Appendix **A**

Pregnancy and Breast Feeding

The Food and Drug Administration requires that all prescription drugs absorbed systemically or that are known to be potentially harmful to the fetus be given a pregnancy category of A, B, C, D or X. The following table lists all categories.

CATEGORY	DESCRIPTION	DURING BREAST FEEDING
A	Controlled studies in women fail to show a risk to the fetus.	Yes
B	Animal or human studies have not shown a significant risk to the fetus. No controlled studies in pregnant women. Drugs that have been found to have adverse effects in animals but no well controlled studies of humans.	Yes
C	Drugs for which there are no adequate studies, either animal or humans, or drugs shown to have adverse fetal effects in animals but for which no human data are available.	Yes
D	Fetal risk in humans is evident.	No
X	Studies in animals or humans have shown definitive fetal risk. These drugs are contraindicated in women who are or may become pregnant.	No

List of Common Dental Drugs: During Pregnancy and Nursing

DRUG	FDA CATEGORY	CAN USE DURING PREGNANCY?	CAN USE DURING NURSING?
Antibiotics			
Penicillin	B	Yes	Yes
Amoxicillin	B	Yes	Yes
Erythromycin	B	Yes (except for esolate form)	Yes
Clarithyromycin	C	No	No
Azithromycin	B	Yes; no human studies	Not enough information
Clindamycin	B	Yes	Yes
Metronidazole	B	Not in first trimester	Discontinue breast feeding for 12–24 hours
Tetracyclines	D	No	No
Analgesics			
Acetaminophen	B	Yes	Yes
Aspirin	C (in low dose)	No	No
Ibuprofen (all NSAIDs)	B (first two trimesters)	Yes (first two trimesters)	Yes
	D (if used in third trimester)	No (not in third trimester)	
Codeine (e.g., acetaminophen with codeine)	C	Can use in second or third trimester	Yes
Hydrodone (e.g., Vicodin)	C	Not in first trimester	Yes
Antifungal Agents			
Nystatin	B	Yes	Yes
Clotrimazole (topical)	B	Yes	Yes
Local Anesthetics			
Lidocaine	B	Yes	Yes
Mepivacaine	C	No	Caution
Bupivacaine	C	No	No
Etidocaine	B	Yes	Yes
Articaine	C	No	Caution
Marcaine	C	No	Caution
Anti-anxiety Drugs			
Benzodiazepines (e.g., diazepam, alprazolam)	D	No	No
	X (Triazolam and Temazepam)		

Drug Interactions in Dentistry

Types of drug interactions (Table 1) and ratings of drug interactions (Table 2) describe the mechanism of a drug interaction and how severe it can be. Metabolism-type drug interactions occur primarily due to metabolism of drugs. Few drugs are eliminated from the body unchanged in the urine. Most drugs are metabolized or chemically altered to a less lipid-soluble compound that is more easily eliminated from the body. One way of metabolizing drugs involves alteration of groups on the drug molecule via the **cytochrome P450 enzymes** (Table 3). These enzymes are found mostly in the liver, but can also be found in the intestines, lungs, and other organs. Each enzyme is termed an isoenzyme because each derives from a different gene. There are more than 30 cytochrome P450 enzymes present in human tissue.

A *substrate* is a drug that is metabolized by a specific CYP450 isoenzyme. An *inhibitor* is a drug that inhibits or reduces the activity of a specific CYP450 isoenzyme. An *inducer* is a drug that increases the amount and activity of that specific CYP450 isoenzyme.

Drug interactions can occur when a drug that is metabolized and/or inhibited by these cytochrome enzymes is taken concurrently with a drug that decreases the activity of the same enzyme system (e.g., an inhibitor). The result is often increased concentrations of the substrate. Another scenario is when a substrate that is metabolized by a specific cytochrome enzyme is taken with a drug that increases the activity of that enzyme (e.g., an inducer). The result is often decreased concentrations of the substrate.

Some substrates are also inhibitors for the same enzyme, probably due to competitive inhibition of enzyme activity. Some inhibitors affect more than one isoenzyme and some substrates are metabolized by more than one isoenzyme.

Tables 4–6 describe clinically significant drug–drug, drug–food, and drug–disease interactions in dentistry and possible ways to avoid or manage an interaction.

TABLE 1 Types of Drug Interactions

There are five main types of interactions:

INTERACTION	DEFINITION
Pharmacokinetic	A change in the pharmacokinetics of one drug caused by the interacting drug
Pharmacodynamic	A change in the pharmacodynamics of one drug caused by the interacting drug
Addition	The effect of two or more drugs when administered together is the same as if the drugs were given separately.
Synergism	The effect of two or more drugs when administered together is greater than if the drugs were given separately; may produce responses equivalent to over dosage.
Antagonism	The effect of two or more drugs when administered together is less than when the drugs are given separately.

TABLE 2 Rating of Drug Interactions

SEVERITY RATING	DOCUMENTATION RATING
Major: Potentially life-threatening or causing permanent body damage	Established: Proven with clinical studies to cause an interaction
Moderate: Could change the patient's clinical status and require hospitalization	Probable: Very likely to cause an interaction
Minor: Only mild effects are evident or no changes seen	Suspected: Supposed to cause an interaction, but more clinical studies are required Possible: Limited data proven Unlikely: Not certain to cause an interaction

TABLE 3	Common Cytochrome P450 Drug Interactions in Dentistry			
ENZYME	SUBSTRATE DRUG*	INHIBITOR DRUG§	INDUCER DRUG¶	MANAGEMENT
CYP1A2	Caffeine **Anti-asthmatic:** theophylline (Aerolate) **Alzhemier's disease:** tacrine (Cognex) **Tricyclic antidepressants:** amitriptyline (Elavil), imipramine (Tofranil) **Antidepressants: SSRIs** [e.g., fluvoxamine (Luvox)] **Antipsychotics:** clozapine (Clozaril), haloperidol (Haldol)	**SSRIs:** fluvoxamine (Luvox) **Fluroquinolones:** ciprofloxacin (Cipro)	Tobacco (smoking) **Anti-ulcer:** omeprazole (Prilosec) **Antiseizure:** phenytoin (Dilantin)	If possible, do not give a substrate with an inducer or inhibitor if they will interact; if necessary to give, then observe the therapeutic and adverse effects.
CYP3A4	**Local anesthetic:** Lidocaine **Antibiotics:** erythromycin, clarithromycin (Biaxin) **Calcium channel blockers:** amlodipine (Norvasc), diltiazem (Cardizem), felodipine (Plendil), nifedipine (Adalat, Procardia), verapamil (Calan, Isoptin)	**Grapefruit juice** (lasts about 24 hours) **Antibiotics:** erythromycin, clarithromycin **Antifunguals:** ketoconazole (Nizoral), fluconazole (Diflucan), itraconazole (Sporanox) **Antidepressants:** fluvoxamine (Luvox), nefazodone (Serzone)	**Trigeminal neuralgia:** carbamazepine (Tegretol) **Antiseizure:** phenytoin (Dilantin) **Barbiturates:** phenobarbital **Antituberculosis:** rifampin (Rifadin, Rimactane)	If possible, do not give a substrate with an inducer or inhibitor if they will interact; if necessary to give, then observe the therapeutic and adverse effects.
	Antidepressants: sertraline (Zoloft), trazodone (Desyrel), nefazodone (Serone) **Benzodiazepines:** diazepam (Valium), midazolam (Versed), triazolam (Halcion) **Cholesterol-lowering drugs (statins):** atorvastatin (Lipitor), lovastatin (Mevacor), simvastatin (Zocor) **Anticoagulant:** warfarin (Coumadin) **Antihistamine:** fexofenadine (Allegra) **Corticosteroid:** hydrocortisone **Antidiabetics:** glyburide (Glynase, Micronase) **Antirejection drugs:** cyclosporine **Hormones:** estradiol, progesterone **HIV protease inhibitors:** ritonavir (Norvir), saquinavir (Invirase), indinavir (Crixivan), nelfinavir (Viracept) **Antigout:** colchicine	**H₂ receptor blocker:** cimetadine (Tagamet)		
CYP2C9	**Nonsteroidal anti-inflammatory drugs:** ibuprofen (Motrin, Advil), naproxen sodium (Aleve), celecoxib (Celebrex) **Antiseizure:** phenytoin (Dilantin) **Anticoagulant:** warfarin (Coumadin)	**Antibiotics:** metronidazole (Flagyl) **Antifungals:** fluconazole (Diflucan), ketoconazole (Nizoril)	**Antituberculosis:** rifampin (Rifadin, Ricmactane)	If possible, do not give a substrate with an inducer or inhibitor if they will interact; if necessary to give, then observe the therapeutic and adverse effects.

*Substrate: A drug that is metabolized by an enzyme system.

§Inhibitor: A drug that decreases the activity of the enzyme which may decrease the metabolism of the substrate and generally lead to increased drug effect.

¶Inducer: A drug that will stimulate the synthesis of more enzymes enhancing the enzyme's metabolizing actions. Inducers increase metabolism of substrates, generally leading to decreased drug effect.

TABLE 4 Clinically Significant Drug–Drug Interactions in Dentistry

ANTIBIOTICS

DRUG	INTERACTING DRUG	EFFECT	WHAT TO DO?
Doxycycline (including doxycycline 20 mg, Atridox)	Antacids (magnesium hydroxide/ aluminum hydroxide), iron (ferrous sulfate)	Decrease doxycycline absorption into the blood	Take doxycycline 1 hour before or 2 hours after antacid.
	Penicillins	Interfere with bactericidal effect of penicillins	Do not take at same time; take penicillin a few hours before doxycycline.
	Oral contraceptives	May interfere with contraceptive effect	May not be clinically significant; some sources say to use alternative methods of birth control
	Phenytoin (Dilantin)	Decrease serum doxycycline levels	Either switch to another antibiotic or monitor.
Minocycline (including Arestin)	Warfarin	Increase anticoagulant effect	Minimal risk; monitor patients for enhanced anticoagulant effects; warfarin dosage may need adjustments
	Oral contraceptives	May interfere with contraceptive effect	May not be clinically significant; some sources say to use alternative methods of birth control
	Antacids (magnesium hydroxide/ aluminum hydroxide), calcium-containing products, iron (ferrous sulfate)	Decrease amount of tetracycline absorption into the blood	Do not take concurrently. Take minocycline 1 hour before or 2 hours after antacid.
	Phenytoin (Dilantin)	Decrease serum doxycycline levels	Either switch to another antibiotic or monitor.
Tetracycline	Antacids (magnesium hydroxide/ aluminum hydroxide), calcium-containing products, iron (ferrous sulfate)	Decrease amount of tetracycline absorption into the blood	Do not take concurrently. Take tetracycline 1 hour before or 2 hours after antacid.
	Warfarin	Increase anticoagulant effect	Minimal risk; monitor patients for enhanced anticoagulant effects.
	Penicillins	Interfere with bactericidal effect of penicillins	Do not take at same time; take penicillin a few hours before tetracycline.
	Digoxin	Digoxin is partially metabolized by bacteria in intestine; increase digoxin blood levels	Either switch antibiotic or monitor for increased serum digoxin levels.
	Oral contraceptives	May interfere with contraceptive effects	May not be of clinical significance; some sources recommend to use alternative birth control.
Penicillins	Erythromycin, tetracyclines	Decrease effectiveness of penicillin	Do not take at same time; give the penicillin a few hours before the tetracycline.
	Probenicid (Benemid): drug for gout	Inhibit penicillin excretion	Can take together; make sure penicillin levels are not excessive.
	Oral contraceptives (including ampicillin)	May interfere with contraceptive effects	May not be clinically significant; some say to use alternative birth control methods.
Erythromycins Clarithromycin	Theophylline	Increase theophylline levels	Avoid together; contact physician; reduce theophylline dosage to avoid toxicity.
	Carbamazepine (Tegretol)	Increase carbamazepine levels	Avoid concurrent use.

(continued)

TABLE 4   *(continued)*

ANTIBIOTICS

DRUG	INTERACTING DRUG	EFFECT	WHAT TO DO?
	Statins: atorvastatin (Lipitor), simvastatin (Zocor)	Increase statin levels (increased myopathy, including muscle pain)	Either switch to azithromycin or to another statin drug like lovastatin (Mevacor) or pravastatin (Pravachol).
	Oral contraceptives	Interfere with contraceptive effects	Some sources recommend alternative birth control.
	Digoxin	Increase digoxin levels (see increase salivation and visual disturbances)	Switch antibiotic to penicillin. Monitor for signs of digoxin toxicity or switch antibiotic.
	Cyclosporine	Cyclosporine toxicity	Cyclosporine doses may need reduction.
	Ergot alkaloids [e.g., ergotamine (Bellergal-S, Cafergot)] (for migraine headache)	Toxic ergot levels (ergotism; pain, tenderness, and low skin temperature of extremities)	Use azithromycin or another antibiotic.
	Midazolam (Versed)	Increase sedation	Avoid combination; use alternative drugs.
	Disopyramide (Norpace)	Prolongation of QTc interval	Switch to another antibiotic or monitor for development of arrhythmias.
	Warfarin	Increase anticoagulant effect	Switch to azithromycin (Zithromax) or monitor for anticoagulant effects; contact physician.
Fluroquinolones [ciprofloxacin (Cipro)]	Antacids, iron (decrease absorption of the drug)	Decrease fluroquinolone effect	Do not take concurrently. Take fluroquinolone 1 hour before or 2 hours after antacid.
	Caffeine	Increase caffeine effects	Do not take together.
Clindamycin (Cleocin)	Neuromuscular blockers (succinylcholine)	Increase neuromuscular blocking effect	Since most dental patients are not taking these drugs, there are no special precautions.
Metronidazole (Flagyl)	Alcohol	Severe disulfiram-like reaction with headache, flushing, and nausea	Avoid alcohol.
	Warfarin	Inhibit warfarin metabolism; increase anticoagulant effect	Contact physician; adjustment of warfarin dosage or select different antibiotic.
	Lithium	Lithium excretion inhibited resulting in toxic levels	Contact physician.

ANALGESICS

DRUG	INTERACTING DRUG	EFFECT	WHAT TO DO?
Aspirin and nonsteroidal anti-inflammatory drugs (NSAIDs) (ibuprofen, naproxen)	warfarin	Synergistic anticoagulant effects (increase bleeding)	Avoid concurrent use/contact patient's physician.
	Angiotensin-converting enzyme (ACE) inhibitors (e.g., enal-april, captopril); beta-blockers, angiotensin II receptor blockers (ARBs)	Decrease antihypertensive response (lowers blood pressure). Short-term course (5 days) may not significantly increase blood pressure.	Interaction causes lowering of blood pressure. Monitor blood pressure. Use alternative analgesic such as acetaminophen or narcotic after 5 days or more of use of NSAIDs.
	Lithium oral antidiabetic drugs (occurs with aspirin)	Inhibit renal clearance of lithium Increase hypoglycemic effects	Decrease lithium dosage. Limited importance.
	Furosemide (Lasix)	Decrease diuretic effect	Monitor patient.

ANALGESICS

DRUG	INTERACTING DRUG	EFFECT	WHAT TO DO?
	Venlafaxine (Effexor)	Possible serotonin syndrome	Avoid concurrent use.
	Phenytoin (Dilantin)	Decrease hepatic phenytoin metabolism (increase serum levels)	No special precautions.
Acetaminophen	Alcohol	Increase incidence of hepatotoxicity (liver disease)	Contraindicated in alcoholics; avoid taking together.
	Warfarin	Increase anticoagulant effect	Avoid concurrent use of adjustment of warfarin dosage.

SYMPATHOMIMETICS (CONTAINED IN LOCAL ANESTHETICS)

DRUG	INTERACTING DRUG	EFFECT	WHAT TO DO?
Epinephrine	Beta-blockers Nonselective ($\beta_1\beta_2$) such as propranolol (Inderal), nadolol (Corgard), timolol (Blocadren), and sotalol (Betapace)	Elevate blood pressure	Epinephrine should be used cautiously. Limit the amount used to 0.04 mg (two cartridges of 1:100,000).
	Selective beta-blockers (β_1) such as atenolol (Tenormin), metoprolol (Lopressor), acebutolol (Sectral), and betaxolol (Kerlone)	No elevation in blood pressure	No concerns.
	Tricyclic antidepressants	Hypertension (enhances sympathomimetic effects)	Treat similar to the cardiac patient; maximum amount is two cartridges of EPI 1:100,000.
	Cocaine	Increase heart contraction leading to death	Do not use epinephrine if the patient used cocaine within 24 hours.
Levonordefrin (contained in mepivicaine)	Nonselective beta-blockers (e.g., propranolol, nadolol)	Stimulate alpha-receptors on heart tissue, causing an increase in blood pressure; limit use of vasoconstrictor	Minimize the amount of levonordefrin.
	Tricyclic antidepressants (e.g., imipramine, amitriptyline)	Enhance sympathomimetic effects	Avoid use of levonordefrin.

ANTI-ANXIETY DRUGS (BENZODIAZEPINES)

DRUG	INTERACTING DRUG	EFFECT	WHAT TO DO?
Diazepam (Valium), alprazolam (Xanax)	Grapefruit juice + midazolam (Versed) or triazolam (Halcion)	Inhibit CYP3A4 enzyme, decreasing metabolism of these drugs and increasing blood levels	The duration of effect of grapefruit juice—do not take juice while on these drugs.
	Cimetidine (Tagamet)	Inhibit diazepam elimination Increase CNS depression	Little clinical importance.
	Opioids (narcotics; codeine, hydrocodone)	Increase CNS depression	Avoid taking together.
	Clarithromycin with midazolam (Versed)	Increase sedation	Avoid combination; use alternative drugs.

Note: Most drug–drug or drug–food interactions occur when two or more drugs are taken at the same time. To avoid these interactions most drug dosing is spaced so as not to administer them concurrently. If in doubt, the patient's physician should be contacted.

TABLE 5 Clinically Significant Drug–Food Interactions in Dentistry

DENTAL DRUG	FOOD	WHAT TO DO?
Tetracycline	Dairy products (e.g., milk, yogurt) (forms a calcium/tetracycline complex that inhibits tetracycline absorption)	Space 1 hour before or 2 hours after meal.
Doxycycline (Vibramycin), minocycline (Minocin)	Dairy products (only 30% decrease in bioavailability)	No special management, can take with dairy.
Ciprofloxacin (Cipro)	Caffeine (decreases absorption of the drug) Food (e.g., orange juice fortified with calcium) and dairy (decreases absorption of the drug)	Space 1 hour before or 2 hours after the calcium-containing supplement or food.
Erythromycins	Food (decreases absorption of the drug)	Take drug 1 hour before or 2 hours after meals.
Azithromycin (Zithromax)	Food (decreases absorption of the drug)	Take 1 hour before or 2 hours after meals.

TABLE 6 Clinically Significant Drug–Disease Interactions in Dentistry

DENTAL DRUG	CONDITION	WHAT TO DO?
Clindamycin (Cleocin)	Ulcerative colitis, Crohn's disease, pseudomembranous enterocolitis	Do not give clindamycin; remember, this antibiotic is given for infective endocarditis prophylaxis if patient is allergic to penicillins.
Tetracyclines (doxycycline, minocycline)	Pregnant and lactating women Children under 8 years	Do not give to these patients.
Clarithromycin (Biaxen)	Prolonged QT interval Ventricular arrhythmias	Do not give to these patients.
Erythromycins	Cardiac arrhythmias Liver disease Prolonged QT interval	Do not give to these patients.
Penicillins	Infectious mononucleosis	Do not give to these patients.
	Pseudomembranous enterocolitis	Do not give to these patients.
	Renal disease	Reduce dosage or don't give depending on severity.
Metronidazole (Flagyl)	Central nervous system disorder, epilepsy, lactating women	Do not give; substitute another antibiotic.
Ciprofloxacin (Cipro)	Achilles tendonitis, pseudo-membranous enterocolitis	Do not give; substitute another antibiotic.
NSAIDs (e.g., Aleve, Motrin); aspirin	Gastrointestinal bleeding (ulcers), nasal polyps with asthma, blood coagulation disorder, pregnancy	Do not give; give acetaminophen.
Epinephrine	Narrow-angle glaucoma, dilated cardiomyopathy	Do not give to these patients.
	Hypertension, diabetes, hyperthyroidism	Use with caution; limited quantities.

Selected References

Anastasio GD, Cornell KO, Menscer D. 1997. Drug interactions: Keeping it straight. *Am Fam Physician* 56:883–894.

Brown CH. 2000. Overview of drug interactions. *U.S. Pharmacist* 25(5):HS-3–HS-30.

Cupp MJ, Tracy TS. 1998. Cytochrome P450: New nomenclature and clinical implications. *Am Fam Physician* 57:107–114.

Haas DA. 1999. Adverse drug interactions in dental practice: Interactions associated with analgesics—Part III in a series. *JADA* 130:397–406.

Hansten PD, Horn JR. 2005. *The top 100 drug interactions: A guide to patient management.* Edmonds, WA: H&H Publications.

Hersh EV. 1999. Adverse drug interactions in dental practice: Interactions involving antibiotics—Part II in a series. *JADA* 130:236–251.

Hersh EV, Moore PA. 2004. Drug interactions in dentistry: The importance of knowing your CYPs. *JADA* 135:298–311.

Hulisz D. 2007. Food–drug interactions: Which ones really matter? *US Pharmacist* 32(3):93–98.

Marek C. 1966. Avoiding prescribing errors: A systematic approach. *JADA* 127:617–623.

Moore PA. 1999. Adverse drug interactions in dental practice: Interactions. *JADA* 130:541–554.

Web Sites

www.PDR.net
www.medwatch.com
www.rxlist.com

Appendix C

Adverse Effects of Common Medications Dental Patients Are Taking

Many drugs can cause oral adverse effects, including fungal infections, xerostomia, hairy tongue, gingival overgrowth, increased salivation, changes in taste, and bleeding. Table 1 lists drug reactions evident in the oral cavity. Table 2 lists commonly used drugs that cause xerostomia.

If the medication cannot be changed or the dose altered, then increase water intake or have the patient suck on sugarless candy or chew sugarless gum. Oral products (e.g., oral rinses, toothpaste, gel) such as Oasis and Biotène may be helpful.

TABLE 1 Adverse Effects of Medications and Dental Management

CONDITION	MEDICATION	DENTAL MANAGEMENT
Candidiasis (fungal/yeast infection)	Inhalation steroids (in asthma)	Patient should rinse mouth and brush after use of asthmatic corticosteroid drugs.
Tardive dyskinesia (abnormal mouth and tongue movements, including lip-puckering and tongue protrusion)	Antipsychotics	There is no definitive treatment; patient management is important and may be difficult.
Orthostatic hypotension (a sudden drop in blood pressure when standing up). The decrease is typically greater than 20/10 mm Hg and may be most pronounced after resting or lying down in dental chair	Diuretics and other heart medications	After moving dental chair from a supine position have the patient sit in an upright position for a few minutes before dismissing.
Esophageal burning/ulcers and dizziness	Tetracyclines	For esopheageal irritation: Take with full glass of water in an upright position. For dizziness: Warn patient about dizziness.
Gingival enlargement	Phenytoin (Dilantin), Nifedipine (Procardia, Adalat), and other calcium channel blockers; cyclosporine	Keep meticulous oral hygiene; sometimes surgical removal of gingival is necessary, but usually the enlargement will return.
Gingival hemorrhages	Coumadin (Warfarin) Clopidogrel (Plavix)	Note petechiae on chart; consult with patient's physician.
Hairy tongue	Mouthrinses (e.g., chlorhexidine) Antibiotics (especially broad spectrum) Steroids	Brush tongue.
Taste changes	Lithium Metrondiazole (Flagyl)	Taste changes are transient for metronidazole, but chronic for lithium because the patient will be on lithium for a long time.
Exaggerated gag reflex	Digitalis/cardiac glycosides	Patient management with impression and radiographs.
Xerostomia	Many; see Table 2	Many OTC products: Orajel gel, spray, toothpaste, Biotène products, Oasis moisturizing mouthrinse, and saliva substitutes (e.g., Xero-Lube, Salivart). Prescription sialagogue may be beneficial; pilocarpine HCl (Salagen) and cevimeline (Evoxac).

TABLE 2   Classification of Commonly Used Drugs Causing Xerostomia

CLASSIFICATION	DRUG
Anti-acne	Isotretinoin (Accutane)
Anti-anxiety	Alprazolam (Xanax)
	Chlorazepate (Tranxene)
	Diazepam (Valium)
	Hydroxyzine (Atarax, Vistaril)
	Lorazepam (Ativan)
	Oxazepam (Serax)
Anticonvulsants	Carbamazepine (Tegretol)
	Gabapentin (Neurontin)
	Lamotrigine (Lamictal)
Antidepressants	Amitriptyline (Elavil)
	Bupropion (Wellbutrin)
	Chlomipramine (Anafranil)
	Desipramine (Norpramin)
	Doxepin (Sinequan)
	Fluoxetine (Prozac)
	Fluvoxamine (Luvox)
	Imipramine (Tofranil)
Antipsychotics	Clozapine (Clozaril), olanzapine (Zyprexa), lithium (Eskalith), haloperidol (Haldol)
Antihistamines	Diphenydramine (Benadryl)
	Triprolidine/pseudoephedrine (Actifed)
	Loratadine (Claritin)
	Brompheniramine (Dimetane)
	Brompheniramine/phenylpropanolamine (Dimetapp)
	Promethazine (Phenergan)
Anticholinergic (antispasmodic/antimotionsickness)	Belladonna alkaloids (Bellergal)
	Dicyclomine (Bentyl)
	Hyoscyamine with atropine
	Phenobarbital (Solfotan)
	Scopolamine (Donnatal, Transderm Scop)
Antidiarrheal	Ioperamide (Imodium AD)
	Diphenoxylate with atropine (Lomotil)
Bronchodilator	Ipratropium (Atrovent)
	Isoproterenol (Isuprel)
	Albuterol (Proventil, Ventolin)
Diuretics	Chlorothiazide (Diuril)
	Furosemide (Lasix)
	Hydrochlorothiazide (Hydrodiuril)
	Triamterene/hydrochlorothiazide (Dyazide)
Sedative/hypnotics	Temazepam (Restoril), triazolam (Halcion)

Case Studies, Answers, and Explanations

CASE I

A 62-year-old male presents to the dental office with a chief complaint of bleeding gums. The patient is very anxious about going to the dentist. The dentist administers midazolam (Versed) for the patient about 30 minutes before the procedure.

Height: 5′ 10″   Weight: 185 lbs
BP: 140/90

Allergies: None
Social History: The patient is a smoker (30-year smoking history).

Medical History
1. Allergic to penicillin and tetracycline (gets a rash).
2. Diabetes mellitus
3. Hypertension
4. Depression
5. Facial pain

Medication History
1. Glyburide (Micronase)
2. Atenolol (Tenormin)
3. Paroxetine (Paxil)
4. Gabapentin (Neurontin)
5. Hydrochlorothiazide (Hydrodiuril)

Self-Quiz

1. Which of the following substances should the patient not take for at least 24 hours before taking midazolam?
   a. Peanut butter
   b. Sugar-free soda
   c. Grapefruit juice
   d. Ice cream

2. The patient has an endodontic abscess with facial swelling and lymphadenopathy. Which of the following antibiotics is recommended?
   a. Penicillin VK
   b. Erythromycin
   c. Clarithromycin
   d. Clindamycin
   e. Trimox

3. The patient had a maxillary first molar extracted and is in pain. Which of the following analgesics is best for this patient?
   a. Aspirin
   b. Acetaminophen
   c. Ibuprofen
   d. Naproxen sodium

4. Which of the following statements is correct concerning the administration of a local anesthetic to this patient?
   a. 2% lidocaine 1:100,000 epinephrine can be administered safely
   b. Benzocaine 20% can be used for profound anesthesia
   c. Lidocaine topical can be used for profound anesthesia
   d. 2% lidocaine 1:50,000 epinephrine can be administered but use only five cartridges,

5. After the dental procedure is finished, the patient should remain sitting in the dental chair and then arise slowly because he is taking which of the following drugs?
   a. Atenolol
   b. Gabapentin
   c. Glyburide
   d. Paroxetine

6. The patient is taking gabapentin. Which of the following dental management techniques is necessary?
   a. Antibiotic prophylaxis is required.
   b. Do not administer epinephrine.
   c. No special precautions.
   d. An antimicrobial mouthrinse is recommended.

7. In which of the following classifications does the antidepressant the patient is taking belong?
   a. Tricyclic antidepressant
   b. Monoamine oxidase inhibitor (MAO)
   c. Anticonvulsant
   d. Selective serotonin reuptake inhibitor (SSRI)

8. The dentist prescribed bupropion (Zyban) to this patient. What is the indication for this drug?
   a. Smoking cessation
   b. Analgesic
   c. Anti-anxiety
   d. Heartburn

9. Which of the following periodontal adjunctive therapies can be used in this patient?
   a. Periostat
   b. Arestin
   c. Atridox
   d. PerioChip

10. Which of the following drugs the patient is taking is a diuretic?
    a. Glyburide (Micronase)
    b. Atenolol (Tenormin)
    c. Paroxetine (Paxil)
    d. Hydrochlorothiazide (Hydrodiuril)

Answers and Explanations to Self-Quiz

Disease	Medications with Potential Dental–Drug Interactions	Dental Management
Diabetes	Glyburide + aspirin	Do not recommend any form of aspirin.
		Acetaminophen is recommended as long as the patient does not take alcohol, which together increase liver toxicity.
Hypertension	Atenolol + epinephrine in local anesthetic	Atenolol is a selective β-blocker. There is minor concern (with increasing blood pressure) about using epinephrine (vasoconstrictor) with selective β-blockers. There is more concern using EPI with a nonselective β-blocker such as propranolol (Inderal) because epinephrine acts on both β_1 and β_2 receptors.
	Hydrochlorothiazide NSAIDs	
Depression	Paroxetine + epinephrine in local anesthetic	Paxil is a selective serotonin reuptake inhibitor (SSRI), not a tricyclic antidepressant. Only two cartridges of 1:100,000 epinephrine should be given to a patient taking a tricyclic antidepressant because epinephrine utilizes the NE reuptake pump, as tricyclic antidepressants do. Thus, EPI will accumulate, resulting in hypertension and cardiac arrythmias. Selective serotonin reuptake inhibitors (SSRIs) have a different mechanism of action, so epinephrine can be given without any precautions.
	Grapefruit juice	
Facial pain	Gabapentin	No special dental precautions
Anxiety	Midazolam grapefruit juice	Do not take these two drugs together. Grapefruit juice has effects up to 24 hours. Excessive sedation occurs.

1. c: Grapefruit juice inhibits the CYP3A4 enzyme in the liver, which breaks down (biotransforms) midazolam. Increased midazolam levels will result in excessive sedation.

2. d: The patient is allergic to penicillin, so penicillin and amoxicillin are contraindicated. Midazolam interacts with erythromycins and clarithromycin, resulting in prolonged sedation. Thus, clindamycin is the only antibiotic that can be used.

3. b: Aspirin with glyburide may increase the risk of hypoglycemia. Five days or more taking nonsteroidal anti-inflammatory drugs (NSAIDs; ibuprofen, naproxen sodium) can reduce the antihypertensive effects of beta-blockers (Atenolol). Acetaminophen is acceptable as long as the patient does not drink alcohol before or during treatment.

4. a: 1:100,000 epinephrine given to a patient taking a cardio-selective β-blocker such as atenolol is of minor concern because epinephrine has a greater affinity to β_2 receptors. This patient is taking an antidepressant called paroxetine. It is not a tricyclic antidepressant but a selective serotonin

reuptake inhibitor (SSRI), which does not have any effect on epinephrine because EPI uses the NE (norepinephrine) reuptake pump, which is how tricyclic antidepressants work.

5. a: Atenolol, a beta-blocker, as well as other antihypertensive drugs cause orthostatic hypotension. If the patient gets up quickly from the dental chair he can faint (syncope).

6. c: Gabapentin is prescribed for facial pain.

7. d: Paroxetine (Paxil) is an selective serotonin reuptake inhibitor (SSRI).

8. a: Bupropion is used for smoking cessation as well as an antidepressant.

9. d: The patient is allergic to tetracyclines. Periostat is doxycycline 20 mg, Arestin contains minocycline, and Atridox containes doxycycline. PerioChip contains chlorhexidine.

10. d: Hydrochlorothiazide is the diuretic. Atenolol is a beta-blocker, glyburide is an antidiabetic drug, and paroxetine is an antidepressant.

CASE II

A 54-year-old male patient presents to the dental office with a chief complaint of "My front teeth are moving."

Height: Weight: 165 lbs.
BP: 130/80
Allergies: None
Social History: Drinks occasionally

Medical History
1. Asthma
2. Hypertension
3. Hyperlipidemia

Medications
1. 81 mg aspirin/day (without physician's approval)
2. Albuterol (Proventil) (oral inhalation)
3. Beclomethasone dipropionate (Beclovent) (oral inhalation)
4. Nifedipine (Procardia)
5. Simvastatin (Zocor)

Self-Quiz

1. Which of the following advice should be given to this patient concerning his asthma medication and dental care?
   a. Drink orange juice after each inhalation dose.
   b. Rinse mouth with water after each inhalation dose.
   c. Eat grapefruit before each inhalation dose.
   d. Gargle with sodium bicarbonate before each inhalation dose.

2. The patient complains of his gingiva being overgrown and bulbous. Which of the following drugs that the patient is taking is the cause of this?
   a. Aspirin
   b. Albuterol
   c. Beclomethasone dipropionate
   d. Nifedipine
   e. Simvastatin

3. The patient requires an antibiotic for a dental infection. Which of the following antibiotics should not be given to this patient?
   a. Clarithromycin (Biaxin)
   b. Penicillin VK
   c. Metronidazole (Flagyl)
   d. Clindamycin (Cleocin)

4. The patient is taking 81 mg of aspirin per day. The patient is taking this drug and dosage to
   a. increase the effectiveness of nifedipine.
   b. keep himself pain free.
   c. prevent strokes.
   d. keep his urine acidic.

5. What advice should the dental hygienist give this patient concerning the aspirin he is taking?
   a. He should contact his physician and only take medications under the supervision of his physician.
   b. Tell him not to take it.
   c. Take it with water.
   d. Take it in the morning.

6. Which of the following analgesics is best for this patient after a tooth extraction?
   a. Aspirin
   b. Advil
   c. Motrin
   d. Acetaminophen with codeine (No. 3)

7. Which of the following foods should be avoided in this patient?
   a. Orange juice
   b. Grapefruit juice
   c. Calcium supplements
   d. Antacids

8. Regarding the use of lidocaine in this patient with 1:100,000 epinephrine, which of the following statements is true?
   a. Epinephrine is contraindicated in this patient because he has hypertension and is taking a calcium channel blocker.
   b. Epinephrine is contraindicated in this patient because he has asthma.
   c. Epinephrine can be used in this patient, but limit the number of cartridges to two because he has hypertension.
   d. Epinephrine can be used in this patient with no special precautions taken.

9. Which of the following precautions should the dental hygienist take regarding the patient's asthmatic medications?
   a. Tell the patient to keep the inhaler within easy reach.
   b. There is no need to bring the medicine if he has not had an attack in the last 3 months.
   c. Keep the medicine in the patient's pocket because it is not under OSHA regulations to keep it on the dental cart.
   d. The dental hygienist should hold the medicine in her or his pocket until the patient requires it.

10. Which of the following should the dental hygienist do before any dental procedures are started on this patient?
    a. Tell the patient to rinse his mouth with chlorhexidine before the dental procedure.
    b. Take vital signs because he is hypertensive.
    c. Limit the appointment time.
    d. Avoid shining the dental light on the patient because nifedipine is a photosensitive drug.

Answers and Explanations to Self-Quiz

Medications with Potential Disease	Dental–Drug Interactions	Dental Management
Asthma	Albuterol (Proventil) aspirin NSAIDs	There is a high percentage of aspirin sensitivity in asthma. Aspirin as well as nonsteroidal anti-inflammatory drugs (NSAIDs) such as ibuprofen (Advil, Motrin, Nuprin) can cause bronchospasm and induce an asthma attack.
		Patients with asthma or nasal polyps should not take aspirin or other NSAIDs. Aspirin-sensitive asthma (ASA) and NSAID sensitivity occurs in up to 10–15% of asthmatics and up to 30–40% of asthmatics with nasal polyps. Thus, asthmatics are much more sensitive to aspirin and NSAIDs.
Hypertension	Nifedipine (Procardia) No significant dental drug interactions	There are no precautions regarding antibiotics or other dental drugs.
		Gingival overgrowth is the only significant side effect of this drug.
Hyperlipidemia	Simvastatin (Zocor) grapefruit juice, erythromycin, and clarithromycin	Avoid grapefruit juice.
		Grapefruit juice inhibits the metabolism of simvastatin.
		Erythromycin and clarithromycin inhibit the metabolism of simvastatin, increasing blood levels. Avoid using these antibiotics.

1. b: Beclomethasone dipropionate (Beclovent) is administered through oral inhalation. It is a corticosteroid and can cause oral candidiasis (fungal infection). The dental hygienist should instruct the patient to rinse the mouth with water after each dose.

2. d: Nifedipine is a calcium channel blocker used for the treatment of hypertension. It causes gingival enlargement. Teach the patient the importance of good oral hygiene and frequent maintenance appointments. Surgical removal of the enlarged gingival may be necessary.

3. a: Erythromycin and clarithromycin inhibit the metabolism of simvastain, increasing blood levels. Avoid using these antibiotics.

4. c: 81 mg (low-dose) aspirin is taken for the prevention of strokes and heart attacks. This patient is also an asthmatic. The hygienist should tell the patient to inform his physician.

5. a: Tell the patient to inform his physician that he is taking aspirin. He is also an asthmatic and if he is sensitive to aspirin, an asthmatic attack may be precipitated.

6. d: Since there is a chance of this patient being sensitive to aspirin and NSAIDs, acetaminophen, or acetaminophen with codeine, are acceptable analgesics.

7. b: Grapefruit juice inhibits the breakdown of simvastatin.

8. c: The patient has hypertension. Epinephrine can be used, but limit the dose to 0.04 mg, which is two cartridges of 1:100,000.

9. a: Ask the patient when his last asthmatic attack was. The patient should always keep the inhaler on hand.

10. b: The hygienist should take vital signs on all patients before treatment is started.

Answers to Board Review Questions

Chapter 1
1. a
2. d
3. a
4. a
5. a
6. a
7. c
8. a
9. c
10. b

Chapter 2
1. c
2. b
3. a
4. b
5. b
6. b
7. b
8. c
9. b
10. a
11. a
12. d
13. d
14. a
15. a

Chapter 3
1. d
2. c
3. d
4. c
5. a
6. d
7. b
8. c
9. c
10. c
11. d
12. a
13. a
14. d
15. b

Chapter 4
1. d
2. b
3. b
4. e
5. b
6. a
7. a
8. d
9. b
10. a

Chapter 5
1. a
2. a
3. b
4. a
5. c
6. c
7. b
8. b
9. c
10. c

Chapter 6
1. a
2. a
3. c
4. c
5. b
6. d
7. d
8. d
9. c
10. d
11. a
12. c
13. a
14. a
15. c

Chapter 7
1. c
2. d
3. b
4. a
5. c
6. b
7. c
8. c
9. a
10. d
11. c
12. d
13. a
14. a
15. c
16. c
17. d
18. c
19. a
20. c
21. a
22. b
23. a
24. b
25. c

Chapter 8
1. d

2. a
3. a
4. b
5. c
6. b
7. a
8. a
9. c
10. b
11. b
12. c
13. d
14. a
15. b

Chapter 9
1. c
2. c
3. a
4. d
5. c

Chapter 10
1. a
2. e
3. d
4. d
5. d

Chapter 11
1. c
2. a
3. c
4. a
5. b
6. c
7. d
8. a
9. b
10. b

Chapter 12
1. c
2. c
3. a
4. a
5. a

Chapter 13
1. c
2. a
3. a
4. a
5. c
6. c
7. c
8. a
9. b
10. c

Chapter 14
1. a
2. d
3. b
4. a
5. b

Chapter 15
1. c
2. d
3. a
4. d
5. d

Chapter 16
1. c
2. a

3. b
4. a
5. d
6. b
7. c
8. a
9. a
10. c
11. b
12. b
13. c
14. b
15. a
16. a
17. b
18. a
19. a

20. a
21. c
22. e
23. e
24. d

Chapter 17
1. a
2. c
3. a
4. d
5. a

Index

Note: Page numbers with *f* indicate figures; those with *t* indicate tables.

A

Absorption, drug, 21–28
  cell membranes/barriers and, 22–24, 22*f*, 23*f*
  pH and, effect on weak acids and basis, 24–25, 24*f*, 24*t*
  rate of, factors altering, 25
  routes of drug administration and, 25–28, 26*f*
ACE inhibitors. *See* Angiotensin-converting enzyme (ACE) inhibitors
Acetaminophen, 96–97
  adverse effects of, 97
  drug interactions, 97
  for orofacial pain, 88, 89, 96–97
  overdose, 6*f*, 97
  pharmacokinetics, 97
Acetylcholine (ACh), 48, 237
Acquired antibiotic resistance, 112
Acquired immune deficiency syndrome (AIDS). *See* HIV/AIDS
Active efflux system, 112
Active transport, 24
Active tubular secretion, 30
Acute migraines (abortive), 240–41, 240*t*
  analgesics for, 240*t*, 241
  ergot derivatives for, 240*t*, 241
  triptans for, 240–41, 240*t*
Acute pseudomembranous candidiasis (thrush), 149, 151
Acute rescue asthma medications, 219
Acute toxicity, 171
Adaptation, 38, 112
Adrenal crisis, 280
Adrenal disease, local anesthetics and, 70
Adrenal glands, 277
Adrenal (steroid) hormones, 277–81
  adrenal glands and, 277–78
  dental hygiene applications, 280–81
  systemic adrenocortical steroids, 278–80, 279*t*
  topical corticosteroids, 280, 281*t*
Adrenal medulla, 44
Adrenergic agonists, 48–51, 49*t*, 183
  adverse effects of, 51
  alpha$_1$-adrenoceptor agonists, 226–27
  direct-acting, 49*t*, 50–51, 60
  drug interactions, 51
  for hypertension, 183
  indirect-acting, 51, 53, 60
  mixed-acting, 51, 60
  sympathetic, 51

Adrenergic antagonists, 49*t*, 51–53, 60
  adverse effects of, 53
  alpha, 52*t*, 60, 248
  antipsychotic drugs binding to, 248
  beta, 52*t*, 53, 60
  drug interactions, 53
  for hypertension, 183
  indirect acting, 53, 60
Adrenergic bronchodilation, 50–51
Adrenergic neurons, 44
Adult Treatment Panel III, 193
Adverse drug event (ADE), 35–36
Adverse drug reaction (ADR), 36, 37*t*
Adverse Event Reporting System (AERS), 36
Agonists, 34. *See also* Adrenergic agonists
Alcohol-free mouthrinses, 130–31
Alcoholics, signs and symptoms of, 102*t*
Aldosterone, 183
Alkylating agents (DNA alkylating drugs), 157*t*, 163
Allergic reactions, 37
  antibacterial agents, 112
  local anesthetics, 68–69
  penicillin, 115
Allergic rhinitis, development of, 225*f*
Alpha$_1$-adrenergic receptors, antipsychotic drugs binding to, 248
Alpha$_1$-adrenoceptor agonists, 226–27
Alpha-adrenergic antagonists, 49*t*, 52
Alpha-glucosidase inhibitors, 272
Alternative drug therapy, 2
Alzheimer's disease, 239, 244
American Dental Association Council on Scientific Affairs (CSA), 169
American Society of Anesthesiologists (ASA), 64, 77
Amides, 63*f*, 64, 65*t*, 74
Aminoglycosides, 124, 138
Aminopenicillins (broad spectrum), 111*t*, 114, 137
Amoxicillin, 114–16
  for endocarditis prophylaxis, 125
  penicillin taken with, 114
Amphetamine, 51
  users, signs and symptoms of, 102*t*
Anabolic steroids, 285
Analgesics
  aspirin, 91
  for migraines, 240*t*, 241
  narcotic, 97–102
  nonnarcotic, 88–94
  NSAIDs, 95

opioid, 97–101, 98*t*
Quick Drug Guide, 245
Androgens steroids, 285
Anesthesia
  general, 76, 81–84
  local, 62–74
  sedation, 76–81
Anesthetic base, 63
Angina pectoris, 53, 185–88, 193*t*
  defined, 185
  dental hygiene applications, 188
  nonselective beta-blockers for, 53
  pathogenesis, 185–86
  pharmacotherapy/treatment, 186–88
Angiotensin-converting enzyme (ACE) inhibitors, 183–84,
    189*t*, 191, 201
Angiotensin-II receptor blockers (ARBs), 184, 201
Angular cheilosis, 152
Antacids, 207–10
Antagonist, 34. *See also* Adrenergic antagonists
Anti-anginal drugs, 186–88, 186*t*, 187*f*, 202
Anti-anxiety agents. *See* Benzodiazepines
Anti-arrhythmic drugs, 192, 192*t*, 202–3
Antibacterial agents, 110–38
  adverse effects of, 111–13
  allergic reactions to, 112
  aminoglycosides, 124
  antimicrobial activity, 111
  antimicrobial resistance, 111–12
  bactericidal antibiotics, 113–18
  bacteriostatic antibiotics, 118–21
  controlled (sustained)-release drug delivery, 131–32
  drug interactions, 113
  in endodontic therapy, 113
  gastronintestinal problems, 112
  in implant dentistry, 113
  infective endocarditis and, prevention of, 124–26
  in periodontal therapy, 113
  photosensitivity and, 113
  Quick Drug Guide, 137–38
  selection of, 113
  sulfonamides, 121, 124
  superinfections, 112
  topical, 127–31
  tuberculosis and, 132–34
  vancomycin, 124
Antibiotic-associated diarrhea, 212, 212*t*
Antibiotic prophylaxis
  conditions recommended for, 124*t*, 125
  for infective endocarditis, 124–27, 126–27*t*
Anticholinergics
  for asthma, 222, 227
  cholinergic transmission, drugs affecting, 54–56, 61
  for Parkinson's disease, 238
  for regulation of airway smooth muscle tone, 222
  for rhinitis, 227
Anticoagulants, 197, 197*f*, 203

Anticonvulsants, 240*t*, 241
Antidepressants, 247, 250–54, 265
  atypical antidepressants, 254
  classification of, 250*t*, 251
  herbal remedies, 254
  mechanism of action, 250
  monoamine oxidase inhibitors, 254
  selective serotonin reuptake inhibitors, 252–54
  serotonin-norepinephrine reuptake inhibitors, 254
  tricyclic antidepressants, 251–52
Antidiabetic drugs, 290
Anti-emetic drugs, 211*t*
Anti-epileptic drugs, 233–36. *See also* individual headings
  benzodiazepines, 235
  carbamazepine, 234–35
  defined, 233
  ethosuximide, 235
  first-generation/traditional drugs, 233–35, 235*t*
  mechanism of action of, 237*f*
  in orofacial pain control, 102, 108
  other indications for, 236
  oxcarbazepine, 235
  phenobarbital, 233–34
  phenytoin, 234
  Quick Drug Guide, 244
  second-generation drugs, 235–36
  valproic acid, 235
Anti-estrogens, 282
Antifungal agents, 148–53
  dental hygiene applications, 152–53
  drug interactions, 152
  mucocutaneous mycoses, 148, 149*t*
  mycosis, 148–52
  for oral candidiasis, 148–49, 151–52
  prescriptions for, samples of, 150–51*f*
  Quick Drug Guide, 155
  subcutaneous, 148, 150*t*, 152
  systemic, 148, 150*t*, 152
Antihistamines, 209, 226
Antihyperlipidemia/hypertriglyceridemia drugs, 203
Antihypertensive drugs
  classification of, 177–80*t*
  Quick Drug Guide, 201
  sites of action, 181*f*
Anti-inflammatories
  aspirin, 91
  glucocorticosteroids, 278
  NSAIDs, 95
Antimetabolites, 157*t*, 163
Antimicrobial activity, 111
Antimicrobial resistance, 111–12
Antimycobacterial drugs, 138. *See also* Tuberculosis
Antineoplastic drugs, 157–60. *See also* Cancer
  adverse effects of, 158–60, 159*t*
  categories of, 157
  common, 157*t*
  Quick Drug Guide, 163–64

Antiplaque/antigingivitis agents, 127
Antiplatelets
  in aspirin, 92
  in NSAIDs, 95
  Quick Drug Guide, 203
Antipseudomonal penicillins (extended spectrum), 111*t*, 114, 137
Antipsychotic drugs, 247–50, 265
  adverse effects of, 248
  alpha₁-adrenergic receptors, binding to, 248
  defined, 247
  dopamine receptors, 247–48
  drug interactions, 249–50
  histamine receptors, 248
  local anesthetics and, 70
  mechanism of action of, 247*f*
  medications and, 248
  muscarinic receptors, 248
  types of, 249, 249*t*
Antipyretic effects of aspirin, 91
Antiretrovial drugs, 145–46, 146*t*
  for oral opportunistic infections, 145–46, 147*t*
  for systemic opportunistic infections, 145
Antiretrovial therapy, 145
Antithyroid drugs, 275–76, 277*t*
Antitumor antibiotics, 157*t*, 158, 163
Antitussives, 227, 231
Antivirals for herpes simplex virus, 140–42, 155
Anxiolytics (anti-anxiety agents), 247, 258–60, 259*t*, 266
Apothecary system of measurement, 9–10, 10*t*, 11*f*
Applied fluorides, 169*t*, 170
Approved Drug Products with Therapeutic Equivalence Evaluations (FDA), 14
Arachidonic acid, 89, 89*f*
Arrhythmias, 191–92, 193*t*
  anti-arrhythmic drugs, 192*t*
  classifications of, 191–92
  defined, 191
  dental hygiene applications, 192
Articaine, 65*t*, 67
Aspirin, 91–94
  adverse effects of, 92–93
  as analgesic, 91
  for angina pectoris, 188
  anti-inflammatory effects of, 91
  antiplatelet effects of, 92
  antipyretic effects of, 91
  ceiling effect, 91, 102
  drug–drug interactions, 93–94
  herbal and natural remedies taken with, 296
  indications for, 91–92
  low-dose, 94
  NSAIDs taken with, 96
  opioid analgesics taken with, 101, 101*t*
  overdose, toxicity and treatment for, 93
  pharmacokinetics, 92
  precautions/contraindications, 93
  profile, 94
  uricosuric effects of, 91
Asthma, 219–24
  anticholinergic agents, 222
  beta adrenergic agonists for, 50–51
  bronchodilators, 221–22, 223
  defined, 217, 220
  drug therapy, basis of, 219–24, 219*f*
  immunomodulators, 224
  inhaled corticosteroids, 222–23
  leukotriene modifiers, 224
  local anesthetics, 70
  long-term medications, 222–24, 223*t*
  mast cell stabilizers, 224
  medications, classification of, 219
  methylxanthines, 223–24
  other agents, 224
  pathogenesis/diagnosis, 217–19
  Quick Drug Guide, 230
  rescue medications, 221, 221*t*
  routes of administration, 220–21, 221*f*
  severity classifications of, 219–20
  step-by-step treatment, age twelve or greater, 220, 220*t*
  systemic corticosteroids, 222
Atherosclerosis, 175, 186*f*
Atrial flutter, 191
Atropine, 55
Attention-deficit/hyperactivity disorder (ADHD) drugs, 260–61, 266
Atypical antidepressants, 254
Atypical antipsychotics, 249, 249*t*
Autonomic drugs, 48
Autonomic nervous system (ANS), 44–48
  effects of, 45*t*
  nerve cell anatomy, 42–44
  neurotransmitters and receptors, 44–48, 46*t*, 47*t*
  parasympathetic nervous system, 42–48
  structure, 42–44, 43*f*
  sympathetic nervous system, 42–43
Autonomic nervous system (ANS) drugs
  adrenergic agonists, 48–51
  adrenergic receptor antagonists, 51–53, 60
  autonomic drugs, 48
  cholinergic transmission, drugs affecting, 53–56
  dental hygiene applications, 56–57
  sympathomimetic, 48
Avoirdupois system of measurement, 10
Axon, 43
Azathioprine, 161
Azithromycine, 119

B

Bacteremia, 125
Bacterial infections, cancer treatment and, 159–60
Bactericidal antibiotics, 113–18
  cephalosporins, 116–17
  nitroimadazole, 117

penicillins, 113–16
Quick Drug Guide, 137
quinolones (fluoroquinolones), 117–18
Bacteriostatic antibiotics, 118–21
lincomycins, 119–20
macrolides, 118–19, 118*t*
Quick Drug Guide, 137–38
tetracyclines, 120–21, 120*t*
Barbiturates (sedative/hypnotics)
injectable anesthetics, 83
intravenous sedation, 78
psychiatric drugs, 260
Quick Drug Guide, 266
Basal insulin, 273
Basal metabolic rate, 275
Benzodiazepines, 258–62, 262*t*
adverse effects of, 259
anti-epileptic drugs, 235
defined, 258
drug-drug interactions, 260
GAD treating, 260
indications, 258–59
mechanism of action, 258
overdose, 78, 259, 260
Quick Drug Guide, 266
as sedative, 78
Benzonatate, 227
Beta-adrenergic antagonists, 49*t*, 53, 60
Beta-blockers
for angina, 53, 186*t*, 187
for glaucoma, 53
for heart failure, 191
for hypertension, 53
for migraines, 240*t*, 241
nonselective, 53, 60
Quick Drug Guide, 201, 202, 245
selective, 52*t*, 60
Beta-lactamases, 111*t*, 114–15, 137
Biguanides, 272
Bile acid sequestrants, 194, 203
Biliary excretion, 30, 30*f*
Bioavailability, 31
Biological variation, 37
drug interactions, 37–38
Biologic drug approval. *See* Drug approval
Biologics, 2
Biotransformation in drug elimination, 29–30, 29*t*
Bipolar disorder (BPD), 255–58
carbamazepine and, 257
defined, 255
depressive episode treatment, 257, 258*t*
divalproex sodium for, 256–57
DSM-IV classifications of, 255
episodes needed for, 255–58
lithium for, 256
maintenance phase, 257–58
manic/mixed (acute) episode treatment, 255–56

olanzapine for, 257
pharmacological treatment, 255, 255*t*
quetiapine for, 257
Bisbiguanides, 129
Bismuth subsalicylate (BSS), 207
Bisphosphonates, 285–87, 285*t*
classification of, 285, 285*t*
clinical presentation, 286, 286*f*
dental hygiene applications, 286–87
indications, 285
management, 286
osteoporosis and, 285–86
osteoporosis and to treat osteolytic tumors, 160
Quick Drug Guide, 164
risk factors, 286
Black box warning, 13
Bleeding, cancer treatment and, 160
Blocking drug, 34
Blood, cancer treatment and, 158
Blood–brain barrier, 22
Blood disorders
local anesthetics and, 69–70
methemoglobinemia, 69–70
Blood dyscrasias
local anesthetics and, 70
Blood pressure for adults
JNC-VII classification of, 175, 175*t*
three factors of, 176*f*
Blood–tissue barrier, 22
Botox, 240*t*, 241, 245
Botulinum toxin type A, 240*t*, 241, 245
Bradykinesia, 236
Bronchioles, changes in, 218*f*
Bronchitis, local anesthetics and, 70
Bronchodilators, 221–22, 221*t*
Bronchospasm, 218
rescue inhalers for, 221*t*
Brush-on gels, 169*t*, 170
Bruxism, 261–62
Buccal drug administration, 19
Bupivacaine, 65*t*, 67
Buprenorphine, 99

C

Calcium channel blockers (CCBs)
for angina, 184, 186*t*, 187–88
for heart failure, 189*t*
for migraines, 240*t*, 241
Quick Drug Guide, 201, 202, 244
Cancer. *See also* Antineoplastic drugs
bacterial infections, 159–60
bleeding, 160
blood, 158
caries, 158
dental hygiene applications, 161
esophagitis, 159
impaired healing, 160

Cancer (*continued*)
  limitations to dental treatment, 160
  oral candidiasis, 159
  oral care, 161*t*
  oral mucositis, 158
  taste, 160
  toxicities, 158
  treatment, 158
  xerostomia, 158
Candida, 148
Candidia albicans, 149, 151
Candidiasis. *See* Oral candidiasis
Carbamazepine
  bipolar disorder, 257
  epilepsy, 234–35
Cardiac glycosides, heart failure treatment and, 188–89
Cardiovascular drugs, 174–203
  for angina pectoris, 185–88
  arrhythmias, 191–92
  bile acid sequestrants, 194
  dental drug-drug interactions, 198–99
  dental hygiene applications, 199
  epinephrine in cardiac patients, 192
  fibric acid drugs, 194
  for heart failure, 188–91
  hematopoeitic drugs, 199
  HMG-CoA reductase inhibitors (statin drugs), 193–94
  for hypertension, 175–85
  introduction to, 175
  lipid-lowering drugs, 193
  low-dose heparins, 199
  natural products, 194–96
  other drugs, 196–97
  Quick Drug Guide, 201–3
  thrombolytic drugs, 197–99
Cardiovascular problems from general anesthesia, 84
Cardiovascular system, 175
Caries
  cancer treatment, 158
  in children, 167
  flouride, 167, 170
Catecholamines, 44
Ceiling effect, 35, 91, 102
Cell body, 43
Cell cycle-nonspecific (CCNS), 157
Cell cycle-specific (CCS) antineoplastic agents, 157
Cell membranes/barriers, drug absorption in, 22–24, 22*f*, 23*f*
Center for Drug Evaluation and Research (CDER), 36
Central alpha$_2$-agonists, 49*t*, 50, 60
Central nervous system (CNS), 42
  local anesthetics, 69
  problems from general anesthesia, 83
Cephalosporins, 116–17, 137
Certainly lethal dose (CLD), 171
Cetuximab, 157
Chemical names of drugs, 8
Chemistry of inhalational anesthetics, 82

Chemotherapy. *See* Antineoplastic drugs
Children
  asthma in, 218, 220*t*
  certainly lethal dose and, 171
  dental caries in, 167
  doses for, 33
  fluoride and, 168–71, 168*t*
  local anesthetics for, 68
  mouthrinses for, 170
  prescriptions for, 15
  sedation for, 77
Chloral hydrate, 79, 260
Chlorhexidine, 129
Chlorhexidine gluconate chip, 131
Cholinergic fibers, 44
Cholinergic receptors, 55, 56*t*, 61
Cholinergics, 53–54, 61
Cholinergic transmission, drugs affecting, 53–56
  anticholinergic drugs, 54–56, 61
  parasympathomimetic drugs, 53–54, 61
Cholinesterase inhibitors, 54–55
Chronic atrophic candidiasis (denture sore mouth), 151–52
Chronic obstructive pulmonary disease (COPD), 224, 224*t*
Clindamycin, 119–20
Clozapine, 249
Cocaine, 51, 63
Cocaine user
  local anesthetics and, 70
  signs and symptoms of, 102*t*
Codeine
  adverse effects of, 100
  for coughs, 227
  drug–drug interactions, 100
  guidelines for taking, 100*t*
  indications, 100
Coenzyme Q10 (CoQ10), 196
Colds, drugs for, 225–27, 230
Cold sores, 140–42, 140*f*
Colon, 205
Combination drugs
  antibiotic, 215
  antidiabetic agent, 272
  gastrointestinal, 215
  for LDL reduction, 197, 203
  opioid analgesics with nonnarcotic
    analgesics, 101, 101*t*
Combined moderate sedation, 76
Community water fluoridation, 167
Competitive antagonist, 34
COMT (catechol-O-methyltransferase) inhibitors, 238, 244
Congestive heart failure. *See* Heart failure
Conscious sedation, 76
Constant percent of elimination, 31–32*f*
Constipation, 211
Continuation treatment, 257
Controlled dangerous substances (CDS), 12. *See also* Sched-
    uled drugs

Controlled (sustained)-release drug delivery, 131–32, 131*t*
  chlorhexidine gluconate chip, 131
  dental hygiene applications, 132
  doxycycline hyclate gel, 131
  minocycline hydrochloride microsphere, 131–32
  resorbable, 131–32
Controlled substances. *See* Scheduled drugs
Controlled Substances Act, 12
Corpus striatum, 237
Corticosteroids
  adrenal glands, 277–78
  dental hygiene applications, 280–81
  drug interactions, 280
  inhaled, 222–23, 223*t*
  Quick Drug Guide, 231
  withdrawal of, 279
Cough, drugs for, 227, 230
Cromolyn, 227
Cyclooxygenase, 90
Cylcooxygenase pathway, 89–90
CYP enzymes, 29
Cytochrome P450 enzymes, 29

D

Deep sedation, 76
Dendrites, 43
Dental
  drug–drug interactions, 198–99
Dental drug–drug interactions
  cardiovascular drugs, 198–99
Dental hygiene applications, 213
  adrenal (steroid) hormones, 280–81
  angina pectoris, 188
  antifungal agents, 152–53
  arrhythmias, 192
  autonomic nervous system drugs, 56–57
  bisphosphonates, 286–87
  cancer treatment, 161
  cardiovascular drugs, 199
  cephalosporins, 116–17
  controlled (sustained)-release drug delivery, 132
  corticosteroids, 280–81
  diabetes mellitus, 275
  drug action, 38
  endocrine and hormonal drugs, 287
  epilepsy, 236
  fluoride, 171
  gastrointestinal drugs, 213
  for headache, 242
  heart failure, 191
  herbal and natural remedies, 297–98
  HIV/AIDS, 146, 148
  hypertension, 185
  infective endocarditis, 127
  lincomycins, 120
  local anesthetics, 71–72
  macrolides, 119

mycosis, 152–53
nitroimadazoles, 117
nitrous oxide, 80
oral candidiasis, 152–53
oral rinses, 132
pain control, 102
Parkinson's disease, 239
penicillins, 115–16
in pharmacology, 8–9
prescriptions, 16
psychiatric drugs, 262–63
respiratory drugs, 227–28
tetracyclines, 121
thyroid drugs, 277
tuberculosis, 134
Dental hygiene process of care in pharmacology, 2
DentiPatch, 65*t*
Denture sore mouth (chronic atrophic candidiasis), 151–52
Depressant users, signs and symptoms of, 102*t*
Depression, 250–54. *See also* Antidepressants
Depressive episodes, 255
Dermatological symptoms, 37
Desflurane, 83
Dextromethorphan, 100, 227
Diabetes mellitus, 267–73. *See also* Insulin; Insulin formulations
  complications, 270, 270*f*
  control and management, 270, 270*t*
  defined, 267
  dental hygiene applications, 275
  diagnosing, 269–70
  local anesthetics and, 70
  signs and symptoms of, 269
  treatment agents for, 271–72, 271*t*
  type 1, 268
  type 2, 268
Diarrhea, 211–12
  acute, treatment of, 212
  antibiotic-associated, 212
  defined, 211
  nonspecific, therapy for, 212*t*
Dietary Supplement and Health Education Act (DSHEA), 295
Diflunisal, 94
Diphenoxylate, 100
Direct-acting adrenergic agonists, 49*t*, 50–51, 60, 61
Direct-acting cholinergic agonists, 54*t*, 61
Dissociatives, 83
Distribution of drugs, 28–29
  distribution phase in, 28
  factors affecting, 28–29, 28*f*
  volume of distribution in, 28
Distribution phase, 28
Diuretics
  defined, 181
  heart failure and, 188, 189*t*, 202
  loop, 182, 201
  potassium-sparing, 183, 201

Diuretics (*continued*)
   site of action, 182f
   thiazide, 181–82, 201
Divalproex sodium, 256–57
DNA (deoxyribonucleic acid), 37
   alkylating drugs (alkylating agents), 157t, 163
   synthesis inhibitors, 157t, 163
Dopamine, 48, 236
   agonists, 238, 244
   antagonists, 248
   level of, decreasing, 237–38
   receptors, 247, 247f, 248
   replacement, 244
Dopaminergic drugs, 237–38
Dose-response curve, 34
Doses
   certainly lethal dose, 171
   for children, 33
   effect dose, 35
   lethal dose, 35
   loading dose, 32, 32f
   of local anesthetics, 66t, 68, 69t
   maintenance dose, 32
   multiple-dose kinetics, 31–33
   for older adults, 33
   safely tolerated dose, 171
   single-dose kinetics, 31
Doxycycline hyclate gel, 131
Drug accumulation, 31–32
Drug action, 18–40
   dental hygiene applications, 38
   drug administration, 31–33
   drug effects of, 35–38
   pharmacodynamics, 33–35
   pharmacokinetics, 21–33, 21f
   routes of administration, 19–21
   site of, 22
Drug administration, 31–33
   absorption via routes of, 25–28, 26f
   in asthma, 220–21, 221f
   multiple-dose kinetics, 31–33
   single-dose kinetics, 31
Drug administration routes, 19–21
   absorption and, 25–28, 26f
   advantages and disadvantages of, 20t
   enteral, 19, 25–26, 76
   parenteral, 19–21, 26, 76
   summary of, 27t
   topical, 21, 26, 28
Drug approval, 6–8
   clinical human studies in, 7
   clinical investigations in, 7
   drug recalls, 8
   postmarketing surveillance in, 7
   preclinical investigations in, 6–7
   review of new drug applications (NDA), 7
   time line, 7t

Drug clearance, 30
Drug container, 12–13, 13t
Drug dependency, 101–2, 102t
Drug development, 4–5
Drug dosing in multiple-dose kinetics, 32
Drug–drug interactions
   aspirin, 93–94
   benzodiazepines, 260
   codeine, 100
   dental, 198–99
   gastrointestinal drugs, 209
Drug effects, 35–38
   adverse drug events, 35–36
   adverse drug reactions, 36, 37t
   classifications of, 36t
   drug idiosyncrasies, 37, 38
   drug interactions, 37–38
   toxicity or toxic reactions, 36–37
Drug Enforcement Administration (DEA), 11, 12
Drug idiosyncrasies, 37, 38
Drug-induced Parkinsonism, 237
Drug information sources. *See* Pharmacology references
Drug interactions, 37–38
   acetaminophen, 97
   adrenergic agonists, 51
   adrenergic antagonists, 53
   antibacterial agents, 113
   antifungal agents, 152
   biological variation, 37–38
   corticosteroids, 280
   drug effects, 37–38
   morphine, 99
   NSAIDs, 96
   penicillins, 115
   placebo response, 38
   sex hormones, 285
   tetracyclines, 121
   thrombolytic drugs, 198–99
   tricyclic antidepressants, 252, 252f
   warfarin, 198–99
Drug laws, 4–5. *See also* Drug regulation and classification
Drug names and properties, 8
Drug-receptor complex, 33f, 34
Drug-receptor interaction, 33–34, 33f
Drug regulation and classification, 4–6
   drug development and drug safety, 4–5
   drug laws, 4–5
   Food and Drug Administration, 4–5
   labeling requirements for over-the-counter drugs, 5–6
Drug-response relationships, 34–35, 34f
Drug safety, 4–5
Drug types, 11–14
   over-the-counter (OTC) drugs, 11
   prescription drugs, 11–14
   scheduled drugs, 11–12, 13t
Duodenal ulcer (DU), 205, 206
Duodenum, 205

E

Effect dose (LD_{50}), 35
Efficacy, 35–36*f*
Elderly. *See* Older adults
Electronic prescriptions, 15
Elimination, drug, 29–31
  biotransformation, 27*f,* 29–30, 29*t*
  constant percent of (first-order kinetics), 31–32*f*
  excretion, 30
  half-life (t½) of, 31
Emesis (vomiting), 211
Endocrine and hormonal drugs, 267–92
  adrenal (steroid) hormones, 277–81
  bisphosphonates/osteoporosis, 285–87
  dental hygiene applications, 287
  for diabetes mellitus, 267–73
  formulations, 273–74
  Quick Drug Guide, 290–92
  sex hormones and contraceptives, 281–85
  thyroid drugs, 275–77
Endodontic therapy, antibacterial agents in, 113
Endogenous insulin, 273
Enteral drug administration, 25–26, 76
Enteric-coated tablets, 25
Enterohepatic recirculation, 30
Enzymes, 29
Ephedrine, 51
Epilepsy, 233–36
  anti-epileptic drug therapy, 233–36, 235*t*
  defined, 233
  dental hygiene applications, 236
  drugs for, 244
  pathophysiology, 233
Epinephrine, 50, 56, 68, 192
Ergot derivatives, 240*t,* 241, 245
Erythromycins, 118–19, 118*t,* 137–38
Esophageal ulcer, 205
Esophagitis, cancer treatment and, 159
Esters, 63*f,* 64, 65*t,* 74
Estrogen/hormonal replacement therapy, 284
Estrogen + progesterone products, 292
Estrogen + progestin products, 292
Estrogens, 282, 291
Ethosuximide, 235
Etidocaine, 65*t,* 67
Excretion, drug
  biliary, 30, 30*f*
  drug clearance and, 30
  local anesthetics and, 64
  renal, 30
Expectorants, 227, 231
Extrapyramidal, 236
Extrapyramidal side effects (EPS), 248
Ezetimibe, 196

F

Facilitated diffusion, 24

Fax prescriptions, 15
FDA MedWatch and Patient Safety, 36
FDA Modernization Act (FDAMA), 12
Fentanyl, 100
Fever, NSAIDs and, 95
Fibric acid drugs, 194, 203
"Fight-or-flight response," 44
First-generation antihistamines, 226, 226*t,* 230
First-generation/traditional anti-epileptic drugs, 233–35, 235*t*
  benzodiazepines, 235
  carbamazepine, 234–35
  ethosuximide, 235
  oxcarbazepine, 235
  phenobarbital, 233–34
  phenytoin, 234
  valproic acid, 235
First-order kinetics in elimination, 31–32*f*
First-pass effect, 25–26
Fluoride, 165–71
  chemical composition of, 166
  defined, 166
  deliveries of, 167
  dental hygiene applications, 171
  in oral rinses, 130
  pharmacokinetics, 166
  products, 169*t*
  Quick Drug Guide, 173
  sources, 166
  systemics, 167–68
  topicals, 168–70
  toxicology of, 171
  treatment methods, choosing, 170–71
  uses, 166–67
Fluoroquinolones (quinolones), 117–18, 137
Fluorosis, 168
Food and Drug Administration (FDA), 4–5
  adverse drug event categorized by, 35–36
  adverse drug reaction categorized by, 36
  Adverse Event Reporting System, 36
  black box warning, 13
  bottled water labeling and, 166
  Center for Drug Evaluation and Research, 36
  drug regulation and, 4–5, 11
  herbal remedies approved by, 254
  hypertensive drugs approved by, 176
  intravenous Acredia and Zometa precautions, 160
  Modernization Act (FDAMA), 12
  orange book, 14
  package insert requirements, 12–13
  pregnancy categories, 16*t*
  prescription abbreviations, 15
Fungal infections. *See* Mycosis
Fusion (entry) inhibitors, 145

G

GABA (gamma-aminobutyeric acid), 258
Ganglionic-blocking drugs, 61

Gastric ulcer (GU), 205
Gastroesophageal reflux disease. *See* GERD
Gastrointestinal drugs, 204–15
    for constipation, 211
    dental hygiene applications, 213
    for diarrhea, 211–12
    drug–drug interactions, 209
    introduction to, 205
    for irritable bowel syndrome, 210–11
    for nausea and vomiting, 211
    for peptic ulcer disorders, 205–10
    Quick Drug Guide, 215
    for ulcerative colitis, 212–13
Gastrointestinal problems
    antibacterial agents for, 112
    aspirin and, 92
    in cancer treatment, 158
    from general anesthesia, 84
    NSAIDs and, 94, 95, 95*t*
    penicillins for, 115
    ulcers, 95, 95*t*
Gastrointestinal (GI) tract, defined, 205
General anesthesia, 76–77, 81–84
    classification and chemistry of, 82
    history of, 81
    indications, 81
    inhalational, 82–83
    injectable, 83
    monitoring, 79
    patient physical status classification, 77*t*
    postoperative problems, 83–84
    stages (Guedel's signs), 81–82, 81*t*
    therapeutic uses of, 76
Generic names of drugs, 8
GERD, 206–10
    defined, 206
    pharmacotherapy, 206–10, 208*t*
    risk factors for, 206
    treatment guidelines, summary of, 210
Gingival crevicular fluid (GCF), 120
Gingival enlargement, 185*f*
Ginkgo biloba, 296
Glaucoma, 53
Glomerular filtrate, 30
Glucocorticoids, 278
    adverse effects of, 278–79
    systemic products, 278, 279*t*
Glucose, 268, 268*f*, 269*f*
Glycopeptide antibiotic, 124, 138
Glycosated hemoglobin levels, 270, 270*t*
GOAL (Gaining Optimal Asthma controL) study, 223
Gonadocorticoids, 278
Guedel's signs, 81–82, 81*t*

H

Habit-forming drugs. *See* Scheduled drugs
Hahnemann, Samuel, 294

Half-life (t½), 31
Halogenated drugs, 82–83
Halothane, 83
Halsted, William, 63
Harrison Narcotics Act of 1914, 11
Headache, 239–42
    alternative treatments for, 241–42
    classifications of, 239
    dental hygiene applications, 242
    drug therapy for, 240–41
    medication-overuse, 240
    migraines, 239
Healthy People 2010, 167
Heart, normal conduction pathway of, 191*f*
Heart failure, 188–91, 193*t*
    defined, 188
    dental hygiene applications, 191
    drugs in treatment of, 189*t*, 190*f*, 202
    local anesthetics and, 70
    pharmacotherapy, 188–91
Helicobacter pylori (H. pylori), 206, 208*t*, 210
Hematopoeitic drugs, 199
Hemolytic anemia, aspirin and, 93
Herbal and natural remedies, 293–97
    active ingredients in, 294–96, 295–96*t*
    adverse effects of, 296
    aspirin taken with, 296
    dental hygiene applications, 297–98
    dental implications, 296, 297*t*
    dietary supplements, 294
    homeopathy and, 294
    for major depression, 254
    NSAIDs taken with, 296–97
    safety concerns, 294
    standardizations, 296
Herbal dietary supplements, 294
Herpes labialis, 140–42, 140*f*
Herpes simplex virus, antivirals for, 140–42
    antiherpetic drugs, 141–42, 141*t,* 155
    over-the-counter drugs, 142*t*
    prescriptions for, samples of, 143–44*f*
    primary herpes infection, 140
    Quick Drug Guide, 155
    recurrent herpes infection, 140–42
Highly active antiretroviral therapy (HAART), 145
Histamine receptors, 226, 248
HIV/AIDS, 142, 144–48
    antiretroviral drugs for, 145, 146*t*
    antiretroviral therapy for, 145
    dental hygiene applications, 146, 148
    diagnosis of, 144*f*
    introduction to, 142, 144
    oral opportunistic infections in, 145–46, 147*t*
    Quick Drug Guide, 155
    replication of HIV, 144*f*
    structure of HIV, 144*f*
    systemic opportunistic infections in, 145

HMG-CoA reductase inhibitors (statin drugs), 193–94, 203
Homeopathic Pharmacopoeia of the United States/Revision
    Service (HPRS), 294
Homeopathy, 294. *See also* Herbal and natural remedies
Hormonal drugs. *See* Endocrine and hormonal drugs
Hormone replacement therapies (HRTs), 160, 292
Hormones, 157*t*, 163
Household system of measurement, 10
Human immunodeficiency virus (HIV). *See* HIV/AIDS
Human insulin preparations, recombinant, 273–74
Hydrocodone, 100
Hydroxyapatite, 166
Hypercalcemia of malignancy (HCM), 160
Hypercholestolemia, 193
Hyperglycemia, 268
Hyperinsulinemia, 269
Hyperlipidemia, 193, 195*t*
Hyperresponsive individuals, 38
Hypertension, 175–85, 193*t*
    algorithm for, 180*f*
    antihypertensive agents, classification of, 177–80*t*
    defined, 175
    dental hygiene applications, 185
    nonselective beta-blockers for, 53
    pathogenesis, 175
    pharmacotherapy, 181–85
    risk factors for, 176*t*
    treatment, 175–76
Hypoglycemia, aspirin and, 93
Hypomanic episodes, 255
Hypothyroidism, 276–77, 277*t*

I

Ibuprofen and ibuprofen-like drugs, 94–96. *See also* Nonster-
    oidal anti-inflammatory drugs (NSAIDs)
Idiosyncratic response, 37, 38
Immunomodulators, 157*t*, 163, 223*t*, 224
Immunosuppressant drugs, 160–61, 164
Impaired glucose tolerance, 269
Impaired healing, cancer treatment and, 160
Implant dentistry, antibacterial agents in, 113
Indirect-acting adrenergic antagonists, 53, 60
Indirect-acting agonists, 51, 60, 61
Indirect-acting cholinergic agonists, 54*t*, 61
Indirect drug reaction, 34
Induction in general anesthesia, 82
Infective endocarditis, 124–26
    antibiotic prescriptions, 128–29*f*
    antibiotic prophylaxis, 124–27, 126–27*t*
    dental hygiene applications, 127
Inflammatory bowel disease. *See* Ulcerative colitis
Inhalation administration of drugs, 21
Inhalational anesthetics, 82–83
    adverse effects of, 82
    chemistry and pharmacokinetics, 82
    classification of, 82*t*
    for general anesthesia, 82–83

    halothane, 83
    isoflurane, 83
    nitrous oxide, 79–80
    routes of administration, 76
    sevoflurane/desflurane, 83
    volatile liquids and halogenated drugs, 82–83, 82*t*
Inhalation moderate sedation, 76
Inhaled corticosteroids (ICSs), 222–23
Inhaled insulin, 274
Injectable anesthetics for general anesthesia, 83
Injectable general anesthesia, 83
Insulin, 268, 269*f*
    adverse effects of, 274
    delivery services, 274
    mixing, 274
    pharmacology history, 272–73
    regimen, 273
    secretion and absorption, 273
    therapy, goal of, 273
Insulin formulations
    insulin analogs, 273
    intermediate-acting insulin, 273
    long-acting insulin analog, 274
    mixing, 274
    rapid-acting insulin analogs, 273
    short or rapid-acting insulin, 273
Insulin preparations and premixed insulin preparations, mix-
    ing, 274
Insulin resistance, 268–69, 268*f*
International Classification of Headache Disorders, The, 239
International normalized ratio (INR) values, 197–98, 198*t*,
    199
Intestinal mucosa–blood barrier, 22
Intolerant individuals, 38
Intradermal injection of drug administration, 20–21
Intramuscular (IM) injection of drug administration, 19, 20
Intranasal drugs
    administration of, 21
    antihistamines, 226
    corticosteroids, 227, 231
Intrathecal injection of drug administration, 21
Intravenous (IV) injection of drug administration, 19
Intravenous moderate sedation, 76
Intravenous sedation, 77–78
    barbiturates, 78, 83
    benzodiazepines, 78
    classification of, 78*t*
    narcotics, 78–79, 83
    nonbarbiturates, 78–79
    propofol, 78, 83
    routes of administration, 77
    sequence of events for, 83
Involuntary nervous system. *See* Autonomic nervous system
    (ANS)
Iodine, 276
Ionized drug form, 24, 24*f*
Ipratropium bromide (Atrovent), 222, 227

Irritable bowel syndrome (IBS), 210–11
Isoflurane, 83

K
Kava kava, 296
Ketamine, 83
Koller, Carl, 63

L
Labeled and off-labeled uses of drugs, 13–14
Labeling
  black box warning, 13
  drug container and package insert, 12–13, 13*t*
  labeled and off-labeled uses of drugs, 13–14
  over-the-counter drugs, 5–6
Latin abbreviations in prescriptions, 10, 12*t*
Laughing gas. *See* Nitrous oxide
Laxatives, types of, 211
Lethal dose (LD$_{50}$), 35
Leukotriene modifiers, 223*t*, 224, 230
Levo-alpha-acetyl-methadol (LAAM), 99
Levonordefrin, 50, 57, 68
Lidocaine, 56, 57, 64–65, 65*t*, 67, 74
Lidocaine and prilocaine gel, 67, 74
Ligand, 34
Lincomycins, 119–20
Lipid-lowering drugs, 193
Lipid solubility, 22
Lipid-soluble (lipophilic) drugs, 22
Lipoproteins, composition of, 194*f*
Lithium, 256
Liver
  biotransformation and, 29
  impairment in multiple-dose kinetics, 33
  local anesthetics and liver disease, 70
Loading dose, 32, 32*f*
Local anesthetic agents, 64–67, 65*t*. *See also* Local anesthetics
  amides, 63*f*, 64, 65*t*, 74
  articaine, 67
  benzoncaine, 63, 65*t*, 67
  bupivacaine, 67
  doses of, recommended, 66*t*, 68, 69*t*
  epinephrine, 68
  esters, 63*f*, 64, 74
  etidocaine, 67
  levonordefrin, 68
  lidocaine, 64–65, 67, 74
  lidocaine and prilocaine gel, 67, 74
  mepivacaine, 65–66
  prilocaine, 66
  Quick Drug Guide, 74
  topical anesthetics used before, 65*t*, 67
  vasoconstrictors, 66*t*, 67–68
Local anesthetics, 62–74. *See also* Local anesthetic agents
  allergic reactions to, 68–69
  blood disorders and, 69–70
  central nervous system and, 69
  chemical properties of, 63
  for children, 68
  defined, 63
  dental hygiene applications, 71–72
  excretion and, 64
  history of, 63
  liver disease and, 70
  mechanism of action of, 63, 64*f*
  medically compromised patients and, 70–71
  metabolism of, 64
  for older adults, 68
  patient physical status classification and, 64*t*
  pH and, 63–64
  pK$_a$ and, 63–64
  pregnancy and, 68
  selection of, 70
  tissue inflammation and, 64
  toxicity/overdose of, 67, 68, 69, 70
Log dose, 34, 34*f*
Long-term control asthma medications, 219, 222–23, 223*t*, 230
Look alike–sound alike drugs, 8, 8*t*
Loop diuretics, 182
Loop of Henle, 182
Loperamide, 100
Low-dose aspirin, 94
Low-dose heparins, 199
Low-molecular-weight heparins, 199
LSD users, signs and symptoms of, 102*t*
Lung anatomy, 217, 217*f*, 218*f*

M
Macrolides, 118–19, 118*t*, 137–38
Maintenance doses, 32
Maintenance in general anesthesia, 82
Major depression, 250. *See also* Antidepressants
Manic episodes, 255
Margin of safety, 33
Marijuana users, signs and symptoms of, 102*t*
Mast cell stabilizers, 20, 223*t*, 224
Maximal response, 34
Measurement in prescriptions, units of, 9–10, 10*t*, 11*f*
  apothecary system, 9–10, 10*t*, 11*f*
  avoirdupois or household system, 10
  metric system, 9, 10*t*
Median effective dose (ED$_{50}$), 35
Medical history, 2
Medication errors, prescriptions and, 15
Medication-overuse headache (MOH), 240
Meglitinides, 272
Membrane affinity, 28
Meperidine, 99–100
Mepivacaine, 65–66, 65*t*
Metabolism
  in drug elimination, 27*f*, 29–30, 29*t*
  of local anesthetics, 64
Metabolite, 29
Methadone, 99

Methemoglobinemia, 69–70
Methohexital, 83
Methylxanthines, 223–24, 223*t*, 230
Metric system of measurement, 9, 10*t*
Metronidazole, 117
Migraine
    drugs for, 244
    phases of attack, 239
    prophylaxis, treatment of, 240*t*, 241
    with/without aura, 239
Mineralocorticoid, 277–78
Minimal alveolar concentration (MAC), 82
Minimal sedation, 76
Minimum effective concentration (MEC), 32
Minocycline hydrochloride microsphere, 131–32
Misuse resistance, 112
Mitotic inhibitors, 157*t*, 163
Mixed-acting adrenergic agonists, 51, 60
Mixed episodes, 255
Moderate sedation, 76
Monoamine oxidase B (MAO-B) inhibitors, 238, 244
Monoamine oxidase inhibitors (MAOIs), 70, 254
Mood disorders
    bipolar disorder, 255–58
    depression, 250–54
    drugs for, 250–58
Morphine, 98–99
    actions and adverse effects of, 99
    characteristics of, 99
    drug interactions, 99
    indications, 99
    profile, 98
Morton, William, 81
Mouthrinses, 169*t*, 170
Multiple-dose kinetics, 31–33
    adjustment of dosage, 33
    drug accumulation and steady-state principle, 31–32
    drug dosing, 32
    therapeutic drug responses, 33
Muscarine, 54, 248
Muscarinic blocking agents, 55*t*
Muscarinic cholinergic receptors, 48
Muscarinic-receptor antagonists, 61, 248
Muscle relaxants, 83
Muscular rigidity, 236
Mutagenic effects, 37
Mycobacterium tuberculosis (MTB), 132
Mycosis, 148–52
    dental hygiene applications, 152–53
    mucocutaneous mycoses, 148, 149*t*
    oral candidiasis and, 148–49, 151–52
    subcutaneous, 148, 152
    systemic, 148, 150*t*, 152

N

Naloxone, 34, 100–101
Narcotic analgesics, 97–102
    abusers, signs and symptoms of, 102*t*
    drug dependency and, 101–2, 102*t*
    nonnarcotic analgesics taken with, 101, 101*t*, 108–9
    opioid analgesics and, 97–101
    overdose, 34, 51, 98, 100–101
    prescription, sample of, 104*f*
    Quick Drug Guide, 107, 108–9, 245
    selecting, criteria for, 101
Narcotics, intravenous, 78–79, 83
Nasal decongestants, 50, 60, 226–27
National Diabetes Data Group (NDDG), 269
Naturally fluoridated water, 168
Natural penicillins (narrow spectrum), 111*t*, 114, 137
Natural plant alkaloids, 54
Natural products, 194–96
    coenzyme Q10, 196
    nicotinic acid, 194–95
    vitamin E, 195–96
Nausea and vomiting, 211
Nedocromil, 227
Negative symptoms, 247
Nerve cell anatomy, 42–44
    neurons, 42–43, 43*f*
    neurotransmitters, 43, 44*f*
    receptors, 43
Nerve membrane, 63
Nervous system, 42–44. *See also* Autonomic nervous system (ANS)
    cell anatomy, 42–44
    divisions of, 42, 42*f*
Neuroleptics. *See* Antipsychotic drugs
Neurological drugs, 232–45
    for Alzheimer's disease, 239
    for epilepsy, 233–36
    for headache, 239–42
    for Parkinson's disease, 236–38
    Quick Drug Guide, 244–45
Neurological problems from general anesthesia, 83
Neuromuscular blocking agents, 61, 83
Neuropathic dental pain, 88, 88*t*. *See also* Pain
Neurotransmitters, 44–48, 46*t*
    adrenergic neurotransmitters, 44
    affinity of, for receptors, 47*t*
    dopamine, 48
    parasympathetic, 46*t*, 48
    serotonin, 48
    sympathetic nervous system and, 44–48, 46*t*
New drug applications (NDA), 7
Nicotine, 54
Nicotinic acid, 194–95, 203
Nicotinic cholinergic receptors, 48
Niemann, Albert, 63
Nitrates, 186–87, 186*t*
Nitroimadazole, 117, 137
Nitrous oxide, 79–80
    abuse of, 80
    adverse effects of, 80

Nitrous oxide (*continued*)
  contraindications, 80
  dental hygiene applications, 80
  indications, 79
  method of administration, 80
  occupational exposure, 80
  pharmacokinetics, 79–80
  pregnancy and, 80
  properties, 79, 80*t*
Nociceptive acute dental pain, 88, 88*t. See also* Pain
Nonbarbiturates (sedative/hypnotics), 78–79
Nongenetic transformation, 112
Nonionized drug form, 24, 24*f*
Nonnarcotic analgesics, 88–94
  in drug therapy for dental pain, 88–90, 88*t*
  narcotic analgesics taken with, 101, 101*t*, 108–9
  NSAIDs, 94–97
  Quick Drug Guide, 107
  salicylates (aspirin), 91–94
Nonnitrates, 188
Nonprescription drugs. *See* Over-the-counter (OTC) drugs
Nonsedating antihistamines, 226, 226*t*
Nonselective alpha-blockers, 60
Nonselective beta-blockers, 53, 60
Nonspecific drug reaction, 34
Nonsteroidal anti-inflammatory drugs (NSAIDs), 94–97
  acetaminophen, 96–97
  adverse effects of, 36, 37*t*, 95
  analgesic effect, 95
  anti-inflammatory effect, 95
  antiplatelet effect, 95
  ceiling effect, 102
  drug interactions, 96
  fever and, 95
  gastrointestinal ulcers and, 95, 95*t*
  herbal and natural remedies taken with, 296–97
  ibuprofen and ibuprofen-like drugs, 94–96
  mechanism of action, 94–95
  for pain control, 94–97
  precautions/contraindications, 95
  prescriptions, samples of, 103–4*f*
  Quick Drug Guide, 107
  selective COX-2 inhibitors, 96
Nonsteroidal estrogens, 282
NSAIDs. *See* Nonsteroidal anti-inflammatory drugs (NSAIDs)
Nucleoside reverse transcriptase inhibitors (NRTIs), 145
Nutritional dietary supplements, 294

O

Ocular decongestants, 50
Olanzapine, 257
Older adults
  adjustment of dosage in multiple-dose kinetics, 33
  local anesthetics for, 68
Omeprazole, 210
Ophthalmic administration of drugs, 21
Opiates, 97

Opioid agonists, 98–100
  buprenorphine, 99
  codeine, 100
  dextromethorphan, 100
  diphenoxylate, 100
  fentanyl, 100
  hydrocodone, 100
  loperamide, 100
  meperidine, 99–100
  methadone, 99
  mixed agonist/antagonists, 100
  moderate potency, 100
  morphine, 98–99
  oxycodone, 100
  propoxyphene, 100
  strong potency, 98–100
  tramadol, 100
Opioid analgesics, 97–101, 98*t. See also* Opioid agonists;
    Opioid antagonists
  classification of, 98
  combination with nonnarcotic analgesics, 101, 101*t*
  introduction to, 97
  mechanism of action, 97–98
  opioid receptors, 97–98, 98*f*
  opioid responses, 98*t*
  pharmacokinetics, 98
  Quick Drug Guide, 107
Opioid antagonists, 100–101
Oral antidiabetic agents, 271–72
Oral candidiasis, 148–49, 151–52
  acute pseudomembranous candidiasis (thrush), 149, 151
  angular cheilosis, 152
  cancer treatment, 159
  chronic atrophic candidiasis (denture sore mouth), 151–52
  dental hygiene applications, 152–53
  treatments, 148–49
Oral contraceptives, 115, 284–85, 292
Oral Health in America, 167
Oral hypoglycemics, 271, 271*t*
Oral moderate sedation, 76
Oral mucosa-blood barrier, 22
Oral mucositis (OM), 158
Oral rinses, 127–31
  alcohol-free, 130–31
  antiplaque/antigingivitis agents, 127
  bisbiguanides, 129
  classifications of, 127, 127*t*, 129
  fluorides, 130
  indications for, 127
  oxygenating agents, 130
  phenolic compounds in, 129–30
  povidone-iodine, 130
  prebrushing, 130
  quaternary ammonium compounds in, 130
Oral route (PO) of drug administration, 19, 25–26
Oraqix, 65*t*, 67
Orofacial pain, 88, 88*t*, 108. *See also* Pain

Osteonecrosis of the jaw (ONJ), 160, 285, 286*t. See also*
 Bisphosphonates
Osteoporosis
 bisphosphonates and, 285–86
 fluoride absorption and, 167
Otic administration of drugs, 21
Overdose
 acetaminophen, 6*f,* 97
 aspirin, 93
 benzodiazepines, 78, 259, 260
 chloral hydrate, 79
 diphenoxylate, 100
 halothane, 83
 local anesthetics, 67, 68, 69, 70
 naloxone for narcotic overdose, 34, 100–101
 narcotics, 34, 51, 98, 100–101
 tricyclic antidepressants, 252
Over-the-counter (OTC) drugs, 11
 for herpes simplex virus, 142*t*
 labeling requirements for, 5–6
 regulation of, 11
Oxcarbazepine, 235
Oxycodone, 100
Oxygenating agents, 130

P

Package insert (PI), 12–13
Pain
 arachidonic acid and, 89, 89*f*
 components, 88
 cyclooxygenase pathway and, 89–90
 drug therapy for, 88–90. *See also* Pain control, drugs for
 introduction to, 88
 neurophysiology and, 88
 nociceptive and neuropathic, 88, 88*t*
 prostaglandin synthesis pathway and, 89–90, 89*f*
Pain control, drugs for, 87–109
 anti-epileptics, 102, 108
 dental hygiene applications, 102
 drug dependency, 101–2, 102*t*
 nonnarcotic analgesics, 88–94
 nonsteroidal anti-inflammatory drugs, 94–97
 opioid analgesics, 97–101
 Quick Drug Guide, 107–9
 tricyclic antidepressants, 102, 108
Parasympathetic nervous system, 42–48, 46*f*
Parasympathetic neurotransmitters and receptors, 48
Parasympatholytics (anticholinergics), 54–56, 61
Parasympathomimetics (cholinergics), 53–54, 61
Parenteral drug administration, 19–21, 26, 76
Parkinson, James, 236
Parkinsonism, 237
Parkinson's disease, 236–39
 clinical presentation, 236
 defined, 236
 dental hygiene applications, 239
 drug-induced Parkinsonism, 237

drugs used in, 237*t*, 244
pathophysiology and, 236–37
pharmacological treatment, 237–38
Partial agonists, 34
Passive diffusion, 24
Passive reabsorption, 30
Pathological anxiety, 258
Penicillinase-resistant penicillins, 114, 137
Penicillins, 111*t*, 113–16
 actions, 113
 adverse effects of, 115
 aminopenicillins (broad spectrum), 111*t*, 114, 137
 amoxicillin taken with, 114
 antipseudomonal penicillins (extended spectrum), 111*t*,
  114, 137
 beta-lactamase inhibitors, 111*t*, 114, 137
 dental hygiene applications, 115–16
 drug interactions, 115
 how supplied, 115
 indications, 115
 mechanism of action, 113, 114*f*
 microbial activity, 113, 114*f*
 natural (narrow spectrum), 111*t*, 114, 137
 penicillinase-resistant penicillins, 114, 137
 pharmacokinetics, 115
 pregnancy and, 115
 resistance to, 114–15
 spectrum of activity, 114
Peptic ulcer disease (PUD), 205–6
 defined, 205
 mechanism of formation, 205*f*
 pharmacotherapy, 206–10, 207*f*, 208*t*
 treatment guidelines, summary of, 210
Peptic ulcer disorders, 205–10
 gastroesophageal reflux disease, 206–10
 peptic ulcer disease, 205–6
Periodontal therapy, antibacterial agents in, 113
Peripheral nervous system (PNS), 42
P450 enzymes, 29
PH
 drug absorption and, 24–25, 24*f*, 24*t*
 local anesthetics and, 63–64
Pharmacodynamics, 2, 33–35
 ceiling effect, 35
 drug–receptor complex, drug classifications in, 33*f,* 34
 drug–receptor interaction, 33–34, 33*f*
 drug–response relationships, 34–35, 34*f*
 efficacy, 35–36*f*
 potency, 35
 toxicity, 35
Pharmacogenetics, 2
Pharmacognosy, 294
Pharmacokinetics, 2, 21–33, 21*f*
 of absorption, 21–28
 of acetaminophen, 97
 of aspirin, 92
 of distribution, 28–29

Pharmacokinetics (*continued*)
  of drug action, 21–33, 21*f*
  of elimination, 29–31
  of fluoride, 166
  of inhalational anesthetics, 79–80, 82
  of metabolism (biotransformation), 27*f*, 29–30, 29*t*
  of nitrous oxide, 79–80
  of opioid analgesics, 98
  of penicillins, 115
  two-compartment model of, 21, 22*f*
Pharmacology, 1–17
  defined, 2
  dental hygiene applications and, 8–9
  in dental hygiene process of care, 2
  drug approval, therapeutic and biologic, 6–8
  drug names and properties, 8
  drug regulation and classification, 4–6
  drug types, 11–14
  introduction to, 2
  medical history and, 2
  prescriptions, 9–10, 15–16
  references, 2–4
  terminology used in, 2
Pharmacology references, 2–4
  computer resources, 4
  online resources, 4
  printed resources, 2–4, 3*t*
Pharmacotherapeutics, 2
Pharmacotherapy
  for angina pectoris, 186–88
  for constipation, 211
  for GERD, 206–10, 208*t*
  for heart failure, 188–91
  for *Helicobacter pylori*, 208*t*, 210
  for hypertension, 181–85
  for irritable bowel syndrome, 211
  for peptic ulcer disease, 206–10, 207*f*, 208*t*
Phenobarbital, 233–34
Phenolic compounds, 129–30
Phenytoin, 234
Photosensitivity, antibacterial agents and, 113
Pilocarpine, 54
Pinocytosis, 24
PK$_a$, local anesthetics and, 63–64
Placebo response, 38
Placenta barrier, 22
Plant alkaloids or extracts, 157*t*, 163
Plasma drug concentration curve, 31, 32*f*
Plasma protein binding, 28, 28*f*
Positive inotropic effect, 188
Positive symptoms, 247
Posology, 2
Postprandial hyperglycemia, 269
Postural instability, 236
Potassium-sparing diuretics, 183
Potency, 35
Povidone-iodine, 130

Prandial insulin, 273
Prebrushing rinses, 130
Prediabetes, 269
Pregnancy
  cephalosporins and, 116
  FDA categories and, 16*t*
  local anesthetics and, 68
  macrolides and, 119
  nitrous oxide and, 80
  penicillins and, 115
  prescriptions and, 15–16, 16*t*
  tetracyclines and, 121
Premedication in general anesthesia, 81
Prescription drugs, 11–14. *See also* Prescriptions
  bioavailability of, 14
  bioequivalence of, 14
  black box warning and, 13
  drug container and package insert, 12–13, 13*t*
  labeled and off-labeled uses of, 13–14
  regulation of, 11
Prescription pads, 15
Prescriptions, 9–10, 15–16. *See also* Prescription drugs; Prescription samples
  for children, 15
  defined, 9
  for dental hygiene applications, 16
  electronic and fax, 15
  Latin abbreviations in, 10, 12*t*
  medication errors in, 15
  parts of, 9, 10*f*
  patient adherence to, 15
  pregnancy and, 15–16, 16*t*
  prescription pads used in, 15
  units of measurement used in, 9–10, 10*t*, 11*f*
  writing, goals of, 9
Prescription samples
  of antifungal agents, 150–51*f*
  of antivirals for herpes simplex virus, 143–44*f*
  of narcotic analgesics, 104*f*
  of NSAIDs, 103–4*f*
Priestley, Joseph, 79
Prilocaine, 65*t*, 66
Primary herpes simplex virus, 140
Procaine, 63
Progestin inhibitors, 284
Progestins, 282, 284, 291
Prokinetic drugs, 210
Propofol, 78, 83
Propoxyphene, 100
Prostacyclin (PGI$_2$), 90
Prostaglandins (PG$_s$), 89–90
  supplementation, 210
  synthesis pathway, 89–90
Protease inhibitors (PIs), 145
Protective barrier drugs, 210
Proton pump inhibitors (PPI), 209–10
Pseudoephedrine, 51

Pseudomembranous colitis, 115
Psychiatric drugs, 246–66
  anti-anxiety drugs, 261–62
  antipsychotic drugs, 247–50
  anxiolytics, 258–60
  for attention-deficit/hyperactivity disorder, 260–61
  dental hygiene applications, 262–63
  introduction to, 247
  for mood disorders, 250–58
  pharmacology, 247
  Quick Drug Guide, 265–66
  sedative/hypnotic drugs, 260
Psychopharmacology, 247
Psychosis, defined, 247

Q

Quaternary ammonium compounds, 130
Quetiapine, 257
Quinolones (fluoroquinolones), 117–18, 137

R

Radioactive iodine (RAI), 276, 290
Ranitidine, 210
Receptors, 44–48, 47t
  adrenergic, 44–45, 48
  affinity of neurotransmitters for, 47t
  classification of, 47t
  dopamine, 48
  parasympathetic, 47t, 48
  serotonin, 48
  sympathetic nervous system, 44–48, 47t
Recombinant human insulin, 273–74
Recovery in general anesthesia, 82
Rectal route (PR) of drug administration, 19
Recurrent herpes simplex virus infection, 140–42, 140f
Referred pain, 88
Reflux esophagitis, 206
Reliever asthma medications, 219
Renal dysfunction, aspirin and, 93
Renal excretion, 30
Renal impairment in multiple-dose kinetics, 33
Renin-angiotensin system, 184f
Repolarization, 191
Rescue inhalers, 221t
Rescue medications, asthma, 221
Resorbable controlled (sustained)-release
    devices, 131–32
Respiratory drugs, 216–31
  for asthma, 217–24, 219f
  for colds, 225–27
  delivery methods for, 220–21, 221f
Respiratory problems from general anesthesia, 83
Respiratory system, 217f
"Resting and digestive response," 44
Resting tremor, 236
Rhinitis, 225–26, 225f
  drugs for, 225–27, 230

  symptoms associated with, 226
  treatment of, 226

S

Safely tolerated dose (STD), 171
St. John's wort, 254, 296
Salicylate-like drugs, 94
Salicylates. *See* Aspirin
Scheduled drugs, 11–12
  categories of, 12, 13t
  regulation of, 11–12
Schizophrenia, 247, 247f
School water fluoridation, 167
Scopolamine, 55
Second-generation anti-epileptic drugs, 235–36, 235t
Second-generation antihistamines, 226t, 230
Sedating (first-generation) antihistamines, 226, 226t
Sedation, 76–81. *See also* General anesthesia
  barbiturates, 78, 83, 260
  of children, 77
  deep, 76
  in dental office, 77
  intravenous, 77–78
  introduction to, 76
  minimal, 76
  moderate, 76
  monitoring, 79
  nitrous oxide, 79–80
  oral, 78–79
  patient physical status classification, 77t
  routes of administration, 76
  terminology used in, 76
  types of, 76
Sedative/hypnotic drugs, 247, 260, 261t. *See also* Sedation
Seizures
  classifications of, 233t
  defined, 233
  penicillins and, 115
  types of, 233
Selective alpha-blockers, 52t, 60
Selective beta-blockers, 52t, 60
Selective COX-2 inhibitors, 96
Selective long-acting beta$_2$-agonists (LABA), 223, 223t, 230
Selective serotonin reuptake inhibitors (SSRIs),
    252–54, 253f
  adverse effects of, 253–54
  drug–drug–food interactions, 254
  local anesthetics and, 70
Self-applied dentifrices, 169–70, 169t, 173
Serotonin, 48
Serotonin-norepinephrine reuptake inhibitors (SNRIs), 254
Severity classifications for asthma, 219–20
Sevoflurane, 83
Sex hormones, 281–85
  androgens and anabolic steroids, 285
  anti-estrogens, 282
  drug interactions, 285

Sex hormones (*continued*)
    estrogen/hormonal replacement therapy, 284
    estrogens, 282
    nonsteroidal estrogens, 282
    oral contraceptives, 284–85
    products, 283–84*t*
    progestin inhibitors, 284
    progestins, 282, 284
Short-acting beta$_2$-agonists (SABAs), 221–22, 221*t*
Single-dose kinetics, 31
Sinus bradycardia, 191
Sinus tachycardia, 191
Site of drug action, 22
Snow capping, 168
Somatic nervous system, 42, 47*t*
Spectrum of activity, 111, 114
SSRIs. *See* Selective serotonin reuptake inhibitors (SSRIs)
Stable angina, 186–87
Statin drugs. *See* HMG-CoA reductase inhibitors (statin drugs)
Steady-state principle, 31–32
Step-by-step treatment, asthma, 220, 220*t*
Subcutaneous (SC or SQ) injection of drug administration, 20
Subgingival drug administration, 21, 26, 28
Sublingual drug administration, 19
Substance abuse and dependency, 101–2, 102*t*
Substance Abuse and Mental Health Services Administration (SAMHSA), 99
Substantia nigra, 236
Sulfonamides, 121, 124, 138
Sulfonylureas, 271
Superinfections, 112, 115
Sweat glands, 44
Sympathetic agonists, 51
Sympathetic nervous system, 42–43
Sympatholytics, 51
Sympathomimetics, 48, 60, 191, 201, 231
Synapse, 43, 44*f*
Systemic adrenocortical steroids, 278–80, 279*t*
Systemic corticosteroids, 222, 291
Systemic fluorides, 167–68, 169*t*, 173
    community water fluoridation, 167
    fluorosis, 168
    naturally fluoridated water, 168
    prescriptions and supplements, 168, 168*t*
    school fluoridation, 167

T

Tachyphlaxis, 38
Taste, cancer treatment and, 160
Teratogenic defect, 37
Teratogenic drug, 37
Terminology used in pharmacology, 2
Tetracyclines, 120–21, 120*t*
    actions, 120
    adverse effects of, 120
    anticollagenase feature, 120
    dental hygiene applications, 121

    drug interactions, 121
    gingival crevicular fluid, 120
    how supplied, 121
    indications, 120
    pregnancy and, 121
    Quick Drug Guide, 137
Therapeutic drug approval. *See* Drug approval
Therapeutic drug responses, 33
Therapeutic index (TI), 35
Therapeutic range, 33
Therapeutics, 2
Thiazide diuretics, 181–82
Thiazolidinediones (TZDs), 272
Thioamide drugs, 276
Thrombocytopenia, 148, 160
Thrombolytic drugs, 197–99
    adverse effects of, 198
    defined, 197
    drug interactions, 198–99
    indications, 197
    warfarin as, 197–98
Thromboxane A$_2$, 90
Thrush (acute pseudomembranous candidiasis), 149, 151
Thyroid disease, local anesthetics and, 70
Thyroid drugs, 275–77, 290
    antithyroid drugs, 275–76
    dental hygiene applications, 277
    for hypothyroidism, 276–77, 277*t*
    thyroid gland hormones, 275
Thyroid gland, 275, 275*f*, 276*f*
Thyroxine, 275
Tissue inflammation, 64. *See also* Anti-inflammatories
Tolerance, 38
Tonic-clonic seizures, 233
Topical antibacterial agents, 127–31. *See also* Oral rinses
Topical corticosteroids, 227, 280, 291
Topical fluorides, 168–70, 169*t*, 173
    brush-on gels, 169*t*, 170
    mouthrinses, 169*t*, 170
    professionally applied, 169*t*, 170
    self-applied dentifrices, 169–70, 169*t*
Topiramate, 240*t*, 241
Toxic concentration, 32*f*, 33
Toxicity or toxic reactions, 35, 36–37. *See also* Overdose
    of aspirin, 93
    of cancer treatment, 158
    of fluorides, 171
    of local anesthetics, 69, 70
Toxicology, 2
Trade (or brand) names of drugs, 8
Tramadol, 100
Transdermal administration of drugs, 21, 76
Tricyclic antidepressants (TCAs)
    adverse effects of, 251–52, 251*f*, 252*t*
    drug interactions, 51, 252, 252*f*
    local anesthetics and, 70
    for migraines, 240, 241*t*

in orofacial pain control, 102, 108
overdose, 252
Quick Drug Guide, 245, 265
Triiodothyronine, 275
Triptans, 240–41, 240*t*, 244
Tuberculosis, 132–34
active, treatment of, 134
dental hygiene applications, 134
latent tuberculosis infection (prophylaxis), 133–34, 133*t*
pharmacology treatment, 133, 133*t*
Quick Drug Guide, 138
special situations, 134
testing for, 132
Tylenol. *See* Acetaminophen
Type 1 diabetes mellitus, 268–69
Type 2 diabetes mellitus, 268–69, 268*f*
Typical antipsychotics, 249, 249*t*, 265

U

Ulcerative colitis, 212–13, 213*t*
U.S. Pharmacopoeia (USP), 4
Unstable angina, 186
Uricosuric effects of aspirin, 91

V

Valproic acid, 235, 240*t*, 241
Vancomycin, 124, 138
Variant angina, 186
Vasoconstrictors, 66*t*, 67–68
alpha-adrenergic agonists, 50
doses of, 66*t*
effects of, 67–68
epinephrine, 68
levonordefrin, 68
Vasodilators, direct-acting, 184–85, 189*t*, 191, 201–2
Ventricular tachycardia, 191
Viral rhinitis, 225
Vitamin E, 195–96, 203
Volatile liquid anesthetics, 82–83, 82*t*
Volume of distribution (V$_d$), 28
Voluntary nervous system. *See* Somatic nervous system
Vomiting, 211*t*

W

Warfarin, 197–99
dental management of patients on, 197–98
drug interactions with, 198–99
Water fluoridation, 167
Water-soluble (hydrophilic) drugs, 22
Weak acids and basis, 24–25, 24*f*, 24*t*
World Health Organization (WHO), 36, 269
pain treatment, stepladder for, 102
tuberculosis, 132

X

Xerostomia, 158

Z

Zaleplon, 260
Zero-order kinetics, 31
Zolpidem, 260